D1495649

2004
YEAR BOOK OF
MEDICINE®

The 2004 Year Book Series

Year Book of Allergy, Asthma, and Clinical Immunology™: Drs Rosenwasser, Boguniewicz, Milgrom, Routes, and Spahn

Year Book of Anesthesiology and Pain Management™: Drs Chestnut, Abram, Black, Lang, Roizen, Trankina, and Wood

Year Book of Cardiology®: Drs Gersh, Cheitlin, Graham, Kaplan, Sundt, and Waldo

Year Book of Critical Care Medicine®: Drs Dellinger, Parrillo, Balk, Bekes, Dries, and Roberts

Year Book of Dentistry®: Drs Zakariasen, Boghosian, Burgess, Hatcher, Horswell, McIntyre, and Zakariasen

Year Book of Dermatology and Dermatologic Surgery™: Drs Thiers and Lang

Year Book of Diagnostic Radiology®: Drs Osborn, Birdwell, Dalinka, Gardiner, Groskin, Levy, Maynard, and Oestreich

Year Book of Emergency Medicine®: Drs Burdick, Cone, Cydulka, Hamilton, Handly, and Quintana

Year Book of Endocrinology®: Drs Mazzaferri, Becker, Kannan, Kennedy, Kreisberg, Meikle, Molitch, Osei, Poehlman, and Rogol

Year Book of Family Practice®: Drs Bowman, Apgar, Dexter, Miser, Neill, and Scherger

Year Book of Gastroenterology™: Drs Lichtenstein, Dempsey, Ginsberg, Katzka, Kochman, Morris, Nunes, Reddy, Rosato, and Stein

Year Book of Hand Surgery®: Drs Berger and Ladd

Year Book of Medicine®: Drs Barkin, Frishman, Klahr, Loehrer, Mazzaferri, Phillips, Pillinger, and Snydman

Year Book of Neonatal and Perinatal Medicine®: Drs Fanaroff, Maisels, and Stevenson

Year Book of Neurology and Neurosurgery®: Drs Gibbs and Verma

Year Book of Nuclear Medicine®: Drs Coleman, Blaufox, Royal, Strauss, and Zubal

Year Book of Obstetrics, Gynecology, and Women's Health®: Drs Mishell, Kirschbaum, and Miller

Year Book of Oncology®: Drs Loehrer, Arceci, Glatstein, Gordon, Morrow, Schiller, and Thigpen

Year Book of Ophthalmology®: Drs Rapuano, Cohen, Eagle, Grossman, Myers, Nelson, Penne, Regillo, Sergott, Shields, and Tipperman

Year Book of Orthopedics®: Drs Morrey, Beauchamp, Peterson, Swiontkowski, Trigg, and Yaszemski

Year Book of Otolaryngology-Head and Neck Surgery®: Drs Paparella, Keefe, and Otto

2004

The Year Book of MEDICINE®

Editors

Jamie S. Barkin, MD
William H. Frishman, MD
Saulo Klahr, MD
Patrick J. Loehrer, Sr, MD
Ernest L. Mazzaferri, MD
Barbara A. Phillips, MD, MSPH
Michael H. Pillinger, MD
David R. Snydman, MD

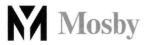

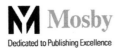

Dedicated to Publishing Excellence

Vice President, Continuity Publishing: Timothy M. Griswold
Managing Editor: David Orzechowski
Developmental Editor: Nell McShane Wulfhart
Senior Manager, Continuity Production: Idelle L. Winer
Senior Issue Manager: Pat Costigan
Composition Specialist: Betty Dockins
Senior Illustrations and Permissions Coordinator: Chidi M. Nwaseki

2004 EDITION

Printed in the United States of America
Composition by Thomas Technology Solutions, Inc.
Printing/binding by Sheridan Books, Inc.

Editorial Office:
Elsevier
300 East
170 South Independence Mall West
Philadelphia, PA 19106-3399

International Standard Serial Number: 0084-3873
International Standard Book Number: 0-323-01578-6

Eric T. Poehlman, PhD
Professor of Medicine and Nutrition, University of Montreal, Montreal, Quebec, Canada

Alan D. Rogol, MD, PhD
Professor of Clinical Pediatrics, University of Virginia Hospital; Clinical Professor of Internal Medicine, Medical College of Virginia, Charlottesville, Virginia

Joan H. Schiller, MD
Melanie Heald Professor of Medical Oncology, University of Wisconsin Hospital, Madison, Wisconsin

James Tate Thigpen, MD
Professor of Medicine; Director, Division of Oncology, University of Mississippi Medical Center, Jackson, Mississippi

Table of Contents

Journals Represented

Mosby and its editors survey approximately 500 journals for its abstract and commentary publications. From these journals, the Editors select the articles to be abstracted. Journals represented in this YEAR BOOK are listed below.

Acta Radiologica
American Journal of Cardiology
American Journal of Gastroenterology
American Journal of Human Genetics
American Journal of Kidney Diseases
American Journal of Medicine
American Journal of Obstetrics and Gynecology
American Journal of Respiratory and Critical Care Medicine
Annals of Internal Medicine
Annals of Rheumatic Diseases
Annals of Thoracic Surgery
Archives of Internal Medicine
Archives of Surgery
Arthritis and Rheumatism
British Journal of Clinical Pharmacology
British Medical Journal
Cancer Epidemiology, Biomarkers and Prevention
Chest
Circulation
Clinical Endocrinology (Oxford)
Clinical Infectious Diseases
Critical Care Medicine
Diabetes Care
Diabetic Medicine
Digestive Diseases and Sciences
European Journal of Vascular and Endovascular Surgery
European Respiratory Journal
Gastroenterology
Gastrointestinal Endoscopy
Gut
Heart
Hepatology
Hypertension
Intensive Care Medicine
International Journal of Cancer
Journal of Allergy and Clinical Immunology
Journal of Bone and Mineral Research
Journal of Clinical Endocrinology and Metabolism
Journal of Clinical Investigation
Journal of Clinical Oncology
Journal of Computer Assisted Tomography
Journal of Diabetes and Its Complications
Journal of General Internal Medicine
Journal of Hypertension
Journal of Immunology
Journal of Infectious Diseases
Journal of Internal Medicine

Journal of Nuclear Medicine
Journal of Pediatric Hematology/Oncology
Journal of Rheumatology
Journal of Urology
Journal of the American Geriatrics Society
Journal of the American Medical Association
Journal of the American Society of Nephrology
Journal of the National Cancer Institute
Kidney International
Lancet
Medicine
Nature
Nephrology, Dialysis, Transplantation
New England Journal of Medicine
Obstetrics and Gynecology
Pain
Pediatrics
Pituitary
Proceedings of the National Academy of Sciences
Public Health Reports
Radiology
Scandinavian Journal of Rheumatology
Sleep
Thorax
Transplantation
World Journal of Surgery

STANDARD ABBREVIATIONS

The following terms are abbreviated in this edition: acquired immunodeficiency syndrome (AIDS), cardiopulmonary resuscitation (CPR), central nervous system (CNS), cerebrospinal fluid (CSF), computed tomography (CT), deoxyribonucleic acid (DNA), electrocardiography (ECG), health maintenance organization (HMO), human immunodeficiency virus (HIV), intensive care unit (ICU), intramuscular (IM), intravenous (IV), magnetic resonance (MR) imaging (MRI), ribonucleic acid (RNA), and ultrasound (US).

NOTE

The YEAR BOOK OF MEDICINE is a literature survey service providing abstracts of articles published in the professional literature. Every effort is made to assure the accuracy of the information presented in these pages. Neither the editors nor the publisher of the YEAR BOOK OF MEDICINE can be responsible for errors in the original materials. The editors' comments are their own opinions. Mention of specific products within this publication does not constitute endorsement.

To facilitate the use of the YEAR BOOK OF MEDICINE as a reference tool, all illustrations and tables included in this publication are now identified as they appear in the original article. This change is meant to help the reader recognize that any illustration or table appearing in the YEAR BOOK OF MEDICINE may be only one of many in the original article. For this reason, figure and table numbers will often appear to be out of sequence within the YEAR BOOK OF MEDICINE.

RHEUMATOLOGY

MICHAEL H. PILLINGER, MD

Introduction

This year continued the astonishing advances that we have seen in rheumatology over the past half-decade or so, particularly in regard to inflammatory arthritis and the use of biologic therapies. In this year's Rheumatology section, we learn that targeting costimulatory pathways for T cells is a potentially useful strategy for treatment of rheumatoid arthritis; that patients with lupus get more atherosclerosis than the rest of us (but not necessarily the lupus patients you'd suspect); and that uric acid crystals may actually play a critical role in the immune system. We scan the fields of osteoarthritis, osteoporosis, pain, vasculitis, and others; in each field there are either new treatments, new knowledge, or new ideas, or sometimes an old idea comes around again. And always, progress.

As in past years, my criteria for selection have been simple. I aim to select the important large-scale clinical trials of the past year; these trials provide convincing insights into important diseases. I also strive to include small-scale trials, where the question is pressing and the results appear solid. I also include large-scale retrospective outcomes studies, where the question is of interest. Finally, I select a small number of basic science studies, specifically studies that either make or break a paradigm, and so shed light on the way that rheumatic diseases operate. In the past few years, I have had no difficulty in finding interesting studies; with all that is happening in rheumatology, the hard part has been narrowing down the choices to just a few.

Michael H. Pillinger, MD

1 Rheumatoid Arthritis

Introduction

Research into the pathogenesis and treatment of rheumatoid arthritis (RA) continues to advance more rapidly than perhaps any other rheumatic disease. The newest treatment options, including anti-TNF-antibodies, have become almost commonplace (see also Chapter 12, "Pharmacology of Anti-Rheumatic Agents"), and our understanding of synovitis has advanced beyond the critical role of the T cell to embrace a variety of other players, including the macrophage, the synovial fibroblast, the osteoclast, the mast cell, and even—to bring back a couple of somewhat neglected players—the B cell and the neutrophil.

The articles selected here touch on 3 aspects of RA: natural history of the disease, diagnosis, and finally, treatment. From Solomon et al (Abstract 1–1) comes a study that firmly establishes what some smaller studies had already suggested: that patients with RA have an increased risk of cardiovascular morbidity. Zeng et al (Abstract 1–3) establish the diagnostic utility of antibodies to cyclic citrullinated peptides in RA. These antibodies are about as sensitive, but much more specific than rheumatoid factor, and may allow more accurate diagnosis in early or ambiguous cases; whether they also play a role in disease pathogenesis remains to be determined. Finally, Kremer et al (Abstract 1–4) report on the results of the first phase III study with a new biologic agent, one that targets a completely different aspect of the immune process than previous biologics. Articles by Navarro-Cano et al (Abstract 1–2), Nakamachi et al (Abstract 1–5), and Krishnan and Fries (Abstract 1–6), respectively, touch on overall mortality in RA, the mechanisms of inflammation in the RA joint, and a reduction in RA disability over the past decade. Taken together, these 3 represent meaningful advances in our ongoing efforts to understand and manage this defining rheumatologic condition.

Michael H. Pillinger, MD

Cardiovascular Morbidity and Mortality in Women Diagnosed With Rheumatoid Arthritis

Solomon DH, Karlson EW, Rimm EB, et al (Harvard Med School, Boston; Harvard School of Public Health, Boston; Merck Research Labs, West Point, Pa)
Circulation 107:1303-1307, 2003   1–1

Background.—Rheumatoid arthritis affects approximately 2.1 million Americans, making it the most common systemic autoimmune disease. Of these patients, 1.5 million are women. Several studies have documented increased morbidity and mortality among persons with rheumatoid arthritis. Recently, the relationship between rheumatoid arthritis and cardiovascular disease has become a focus of attention, in part because of increased recognition of the inflammatory basis of atherosclerosis. The incidence rates of myocardial infarction and stroke were compared in persons with and without rheumatoid arthritis.

Methods.—This prospective cohort study used the 114,342 women participating in the Nurses' Health Study who were free of cardiovascular disease and rheumatoid arthritis at baseline in 1976. Self-reported cases of rheumatoid arthritis were confirmed by medical record review, as were cases of fatal and nonfatal myocardial infarctions and strokes. Multivariate pooled logistic regression was used to adjust for potential cardiovascular risk factors.

Results.—A total of 527 incident cases of rheumatoid arthritis and 3622 cases of myocardial infarctions and strokes were confirmed during 2.4 million person-years of follow-up. The adjusted relative risk of myocardial infarction in women with rheumatoid arthritis, in comparison with women without rheumatoid arthritis, was 2.0 (95% confidence interval [CI], 1.23-

TABLE 2.—Age-Adjusted and Multivariate Relative Risks for Cardiovascular End Points According to Presence of Rheumatoid Arthritis in Nurses' Health Study, 1977 to 1996

Cardiovascular End Point	Rheumatoid Arthritis	No Rheumatoid Arthritis	P
Person-years of follow-up	6259	2 381 418	...
Myocardial infarction			
Incidence/100 000 person-years	272	96	...
No. of cases	17	2279	...
Age-adjusted relative risk* (95% CI)	2.07 (1.28 to 3.34)	1.0	0.002
Multivariable relative risk† (95% CI)	2.00 (1.23 to 3.29)	1.0	0.005
Stroke			
Incidence/100 000 person-years	112	55	...
No. of cases	7	1319	...
Age-adjusted relative risk (95% CI)	1.47 (0.70 to 3.08)	1.0	0.31
Multivariable relative risk (95% CI)	1.48 (0.70 to 3.12)	1.0	0.31

*Relative risk compared with participants without rheumatoid arthritis. Adjusted for age in 5-year categories.
†Relative risk compared with participants without rheumatoid arthritis. Adjusted for age in 5-year categories, hypertension, diabetes, high cholesterol level, parental history of myocardial infarction before age 60 years, body mass index, cigarette use, physical activity, alcohol use, aspirin use, menopausal status, hormone replacement therapy use, oral glucocorticoid use, nonsteroidal anti-inflammatory drug use, folate intake, omega-3 fatty acid intake, and vitamin E supplement intake.
Abbreviation: CI, Confidence interval.
(Courtesy of Solomon DH, Karlson EW, Rimm EB, et al: Cardiovascular morbidity and mortality in women diagnosed with rheumatoid arthritis. *Circulation* 107:1303-1307, 2003.)

3.29) (Table 2). The adjusted relative risk for stroke was 1.48 (95% CI, 0.70-3.12). For women with rheumatoid arthritis for at least 10 years, the risk of myocardial infarction was 3.10 (95% CI, 1.64-5.87).

Conclusions.—Patients with rheumatoid arthritis had a significantly increased risk of myocardial infarction, but not stroke, in comparison with women who did not have rheumatoid arthritis. Confirmation of these findings would point to a need for testing of aggressive coronary heart disease prevention strategies for patients with rheumatoid arthritis.

▶ The past decade has brought us a new-found appreciation of the morbidity and mortality of rheumatoid arthritis (RA), with studies by Pincus[1] and others showing that RA may significantly alter not only quality of life, but life expectancy in our RA patients. An increased frequency of cardiovascular morbidity and mortality in RA has been an area of particular interest in recent years, and accumulating evidence supports the notion that this is a particular problem. Less clear is the magnitude of the problem, and whether cardiovascular disease in RA stems from the RA itself, or the agents (such as steroids) that we use to treat it.

To address these questions, Solomon et al enlisted the formidable resources of the Nurses' Health Study. Using the Nurses' Health Study database, they identified 114,342 participating women who were free of RA and cardiovascular disease at study inception in 1976. From among this group they identified 527 incident cases of RA, and used the remainder of the study participants as their controls to identify the risk of myocardial infarction (MI) and stroke in a prospective cohort analysis ending in 1996. They observed that women with RA had a greater than 2-fold relative risk of MI compared with women without RA. Indeed, for women with more than 10 years of RA, the relative risk rose to greater than 3-fold. Although the women with RA had some life- and treatment-related potential cardiovascular risk factors (eg, somewhat increased parental history of MI, greater smoking history, steroid use), the relative risk for MI in RA patients did not change when corrected for these other risk factors. The only good news? The relative risk for stroke was not similarly elevated.

This is a sobering study, as its large numbers suggest that it is likely to be the largest prospective study we will ever have on this subject. How can we lower the risk of MI in this population? That remains unclear. It is, of course, reasonable to try to control the disease, and as our therapies have improved, it is possible that we have already lowered the MI risk in our RA patients simply through more effective arthritis treatment. Time will tell, but we would be irresponsible if we did not pay more attention to our patients' hearts, even as we see their synovitis improve. So while we administer our disease-modifying antirheumatic drugs and cytokine blockers, let's not forget to control serum cholesterol and glucose, reduce steroid use wherever possible, give aspirin where appropriate, and generally provide the best medical care we possibly can to these high-risk patients.

Also noted: a very large database study by Watson et al,[2] confirming increased all-cause mortality as well as major vascular events in patients with RA.

M. H. Pillinger, MD

References

1. Pincus T: Long-term outcomes in rheumatoid arthritis. *Br J Rheumatol* 34:59-73, 1995.
2. Watson DJ, Rhodes T, Guess HA: All-cause mortality and vascular events among patients with rheumatoid arthritis, osteoarthritis, or no arthritis in the UK general practice research database. *J Rheumatol* 30:1196-1202, 2003.

Association of Mortality With Disease Severity in Rheumatoid Arthritis, Independent of Comorbidity

Navarro-Cano G, del Rincón I, Pogosian S, et al (Univ of Texas, San Antonio)
Arthritis Rheum 48:2425-2433, 2003　　　　　　　　　　　　　　　　1–2

Background.—Patients with rheumatoid arthritis (RA) are at increased risk of dying compared to healthy controls. Whether this is due to their higher burden of comorbidity or to the disease itself is not well understood. To assess the contribution of RA to mortality, disease severity and comorbidity were assessed in a large cohort of patients with RA.

Study Design.—The study group consisted of 779 patients with RA who were recruited from January 1996 to April 2000. Severity of disease was assessed with the Duke Severity of Illness Checklist. This was separated into the RA component and the comorbid component. A physician-rated global RA evaluation was also used, as well as the Charlson Comorbidity Index. Patients were followed up for up to 6 years for mortality data. The impact of both disease severity and comorbidity on mortality was estimated by Kaplan-Meier survival curves, Cox proportional hazard models and logistic regression analyses.

Findings.—The total follow-up period was 2315 patient-years. During this time, 75 patients died, for a total mortality rate of 3.2/100 patient-years. Both disease severity (Fig 3) and comorbidity were significantly and independently associated with mortality.

Conclusion.—RA disease severity is significantly and independently associated with mortality, in addition to mortality due to comorbid disease. Further studies are needed to understand the contribution of RA severity to mortality in these patients.

► Ever since Pincus' ground-breaking study,[1] rheumatologists have appreciated that patients with RA (particularly severe RA) have diminished life expectancy relative to similar individuals without RA. But why? Clearly, one reason, as outlined elsewhere in this chapter,[2] is the fact that patients with RA have more coronary artery disease than matched controls. But it is obvious that other reasons may also supervene. Patients with RA may have other associ-

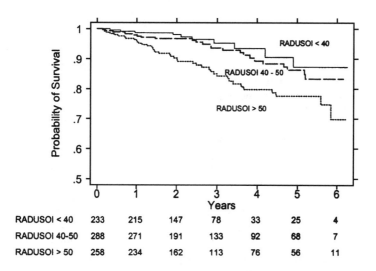

RADUSOI < 40	233	215	147	78	33	25	4
RADUSOI 40-50	288	271	191	133	92	68	7
RADUSOI > 50	258	234	162	113	76	56	11

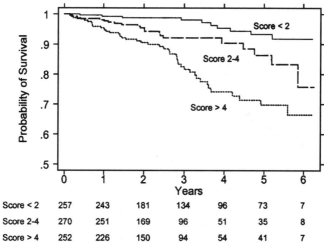

Score < 2	257	243	181	134	96	73	7
Score 2-4	270	251	169	96	51	35	8
Score > 4	252	226	150	94	54	41	7

FIGURE 3.—Estimated survival curves for each rheumatoid arthritis severity scale, using the Kaplan-Meier technique. **Top,** Survival according to the RADUSOI categories. The difference in survival probability among the 3 categories was significant (log-rank χ^2 [with 2 degrees of freedom] = 15.03, P = .0001). **Bottom,** Survival according to the rheumatoid arthritis global severity scale (log-rank χ^2 [with 2 degrees of freedom] = 33.5, P = .0001). Values next to the categories are number of patients in each category in each year of follow-up. *Abbreviation: RADUSOI,* Rheumatoid arthritis component of the Duke Severity of Illness Checklist. (Courtesy of Navarro-Cano G, del Rincón I, Pogosian S, et al: Association of mortality with disease severity in rheumatoid arthritis, independent of comorbidity. *Arthritis Rheum* 48:2425-2433, 2003. Copyright American College of Rheumatology.)

ated (or unrelated) comorbidities, including such classic risk factors as hypertension, diabetes, osteoporosis, renal disease, etc. Such comorbidities may be "side-effects" of RA in some cases, or side-effects of RA therapy in others; in still other cases, they may occur at random. But are comorbidities the entire explanation for mortality in RA?

Navarro-Cano et al think not. They performed a prospective study of 779 RA patients from 1996 to 2002. RA patients in 6 outpatient clinics were carefully assessed for severity of RA, as well as for severity of comorbidities, using 2 different scales for each. They then followed patient survival. The resulting data permitted 2 observations, 1 expected, the other a bit surprising. First, the authors observed that a higher rate of comorbidity resulted in an increase in mortality among the patients surveyed. So much for the expected result.

The unexpected result was that, even when the comorbidities were expurgated from the analysis, RA patients continued to have a rate of mortality that was directly related to the degree of severity of the patient's RA. Because at least 1 of the scales they used to rate comorbidity was an open-ended metric that permitted inclusion of any observed problems in addition to RA, the authors conclude that RA is associated with increased mortality, even beyond any recognizable secondary consequences of RA. This means that there are mechanisms for RA mortality that we have not yet begun to recognize.

The authors hazard a guess that such factors may include treatment toxicities, chronic metabolic or endocrinologic stress, or other factors that could lead to unexpected death in the absence of well-defined causes. Whether better treatments of synovitis will reduce this component (or the comorbidity component) of RA mortality will require further study. For the present, these data would seem to argue for a more aggressive approach to RA therapy, with the caveat that our treatments may, of course, have consequences of their own.

M. H. Pillinger, MD

References

1. Pincus T, Callahan LF, Sale WG, et al: Severe functional declines, work disability, and increased mortality in seventy-five rheumatoid arthritis patients studied over nine years. *Arthritis Rheum* 27:864-872, 1984.
2. Solomon DH, Karlson EW, Rimm EB, et al: Cardiovascular morbidity and mortality in women with rheumatoid arthritis. *Circulation* 107:1303-1307, 2003.

Diagnostic Value of Anti-Cyclic Citrullinated Peptide Antibody in Patients With Rheumatoid Arthritis
Zeng X, Ai M, Tian X, et al (Peking Union Med College, China; Capital Univ of Medical Science, Beijing, China)
J Rheumatol 30:1451-1455, 2003   1–3

Background.—Rheumatoid arthritis can result in irreversible damage to joints, even in the first 2 years of the disease. The most effective management approach to patients with rheumatoid arthritis is early diagnosis and treatment with disease-modifying antirheumatic drugs (DMARDs), which prevent the exacerbation of disease, reduce the probability of joint destruction, and improve the outcome. At present the immunoglobulin M rheumatoid factor (RF) is the only serologic indicator used routinely in the diagnosis of rheumatoid arthritis. RF has a low specificity because it can be found in patients with other autoimmune diseases and in healthy people (though at a lower frequency). This study explored the diagnostic value of a new serologic indicator, anticyclic citrullinated peptide antibody (anti-CCP) detected by enzyme-linked immunosorbent assay (ELISA) in patients with rheumatoid arthritis.

Methods.—The synthetic cyclic citrullinated peptide was used as substrate for ELISA. Anti-CCP antibody was evaluated by ELISA in 191 patients with rheumatoid arthritis, 132 patients with rheumatic diseases other than rheumatoid arthritis, and 98 patients with nonrheumatic diseases. These patients were also tested for the antiperinuclear factor (APF), the antikeratin antibody (AKA), rheumatoid factor (RF), and HLA-DR4 gene complex. Results of these tests were compared with anti-CCP antibody to examine the correlation between them.

Results.—ELISA indicated that 90 patients with rheumatoid arthritis (47.1%), 4 patients with other rheumatic diseases (3%), and 2 patients with nonrheumatic diseases (2%) were anti-CCP antibody positive. The sensitivity of anti-CCP antibody was 47.1%, with a high specificity (97.4%) in rheumatoid arthritis. Anti-CCP antibody correlated with APF, AKA, RF, and HLA-DR4 gene complex.

Conclusion.—Testing for anticyclic citrullinated peptide antibody was evaluated in this study and found to have a moderate sensitivity of 47.1% but a high specificity of 97.5% in patients with rheumatoid arthritis. Anti-CCP was found to be a valuable supplement to the diagnosis of rheumatoid arthritis. Anti-CCP correlated with APF, AKA, RF, and HLA-DR4 gene complex but did not completely overlap with these factors. Anti-CCP may be considered a new diagnostic marker for rheumatoid arthritis.

▶ Although anti-CCP antibody assays for rheumatoid arthritis have been under study for a number of years, I've selected this article because these serologic tests appear to be achieving increased acceptance among the academic rheumatologic community. Indeed, the interest in these tests is sufficiently great that the American College of Rheumatology elected to issue a "hotline" e-mail bulletin on the subject, even as I was preparing this selection.[1]

Citrulline is a nonstandard amino acid that is created by enzymatic deimination of arginine residues, including on connective tissue proteins. Patients with rheumatoid arthrisis (RA) appear to have immune systems that are prone to the generation of these antibodies. The benefit of these antibodies resides in their sensitivity. When compared with immunoglobulin M RF, the type of RF most laboratories test for, anti-CCP has a roughly similar sensitivity but an exceptional specificity in "gold-standard" RA patients. In this study by Zeng et al, anti-CCP antibodies were found in 47% of RA patients but in less than 3% of patients with other rheumatic diseases, and in only 1 of 90 healthy controls. The sensitivity of the test was 47%, but its specificity was more than 97%.

Of course, the authors already knew their test patients had RA, so who really needs the test? Rheumatologists know well that many patients with RA present initially with a nondescript disease that is hard to specifically diagnose. Since RF is present in a large number of other diseases—including diseases like hepatitis and endocarditis that can cause arthritis and/or arthralgia—its utility in the early setting is limited. If the anti-CCP antibodies can identify such patients as having RA, it would make possible not only early diagnosis but also early treatment; and increasing evidence suggests that in RA, early treatment may be more efficacious.

At least 1 preliminary study suggests that anti-CCP positivity in early arthritis is a good predictor of progression to RA.[2] Another issue is prognosis. The early studies suggest that anti-CCP positivity is predictive of erosion.[3] When utilized in conjunction with RF studies, the results may be both more specific and more predictive of erosion than either agent alone.

Are anti-CCP antibodies ready for prime time? Maybe not prime time exactly. Although we increasingly appreciate the value of early RA diagnosis, for example, we have not quite figured out how to modulate our treatments in a way that makes such early diagnosis truly useful. Still, I think the potential value of anti-CCP antibodies is such that it may be time for those of us not rigorously studying them to begin at least to get a feel for their usage. For example, my own personal strategy is to begin to order these tests for patients for whom the picture is not clear—patients with early disease, rheumatoid factor–negative patients, and patients for whom I'm not sure how aggressive to be in my approach. In so doing and by following this literature as it evolves, I hope to learn for myself how best to apply this potentially useful test.

M. H. Pillinger, MD

References

1. Wiik AS, van Venrooij WK: The use of anti-cyclic citrullinated peptide (anti-CCP) antibodies in RA. American College of Rheumatology Hotline 2003:http://www.rheumatology.org/research/hotline/1003anticcp.asp
2. van Gaalen FA, Linn-Rasker SP, van Venrooij WJ, et al: In undifferentiated arthritis autoantibodies to cyclic citrullinated peptides (CCP) predict progression to rheumatoid arthritis: A prospective cohort study. *Arthritis Rheum* 48(9)(suppl):168, 2003.
3. Kroot EJ, de Jong BA, van Leeuwen MA, et al: The prognostic value of anti-cyclic citrullinated peptide antibody in patients with recent-onset rheumatoid arthritis. *Arthritis Rheum* 43:1831-1835, 2000.

Treatment of Rheumatoid Arthritis by Selective Inhibition of T-Cell Activation With Fusion Protein CTLA4Ig

Kremer JM, Westhovens R, Leon M, et al (Ctr for Rheumatology, Albany, NY; Universitaire Ziekenhuizen Leuven, Belgium; Free Univ of Brussels, Belgium; et al)
N Engl J Med 349:1907-1915, 2003   1–4

Introduction.—Cytokines such as tumor necrosis factor alpha (TNF-α) and interleukin-1 (IL-1) are therapeutic targets in rheumatoid arthritis, but drugs that block TNF-α fail to bring substantial improvement to approximately 60% of patients. Because T cells play an important role in the disease, a fusion protein (cytotoxic T-lymphocyte-associated antigen 4-IgG1 [CTLA4Ig]) was evaluated for the treatment of rheumatoid arthritis. The efficacy of CTLA4Ig was assessed in a randomized double-blind study.

Methods.—The study included those patients who had active rheumatoid arthritis that failed to respond adequately to methotrexate therapy. Participants in the study were divided into 3 groups. Group 1 (n = 105) received 2 mg of CTLA4Ig per kilogram of body weight, group 2 (n = 115) received 10 mg of CTLA4Ig per kilogram of body weight, and group 3 (n = 119, control group) received placebo. Methotrexate therapy continued during the study. The extent of response to treatment was assessed at 6 months with the use of American College of Rheumatology (ACR) criteria: 20% (ACR 20), 50% (ACR 50), or 70% (ACR 70). Patients completed a survey designed to assess health-related quality of life and were asked to report adverse events (Fig 3).

Results.—Patients treated with the higher dose of CTLA4Ig were more likely to have an ACR 20 response (60%) than were patients who received placebo (35%). Both CTLA4Ig groups had significantly higher rates of ACR 50 and ACR 70 responses than did the placebo group. Group 2 (10 mg of CTLA4Ig per kilogram of bodyweight) had clinically important and statistically significant improvements in all 8 subscales of the Medical Outcomes 36-Item Short-Form General Health Survey. The active treatment was well tolerated, with rates of adverse events similar or lower than in the placebo group. No antibody responses to the fusion protein were detected.

Conclusion.—Treatment with CTLA4Ig, the first in a new class of drugs known as costimulation blockers, significantly improved the signs and symptoms of disease and health-related quality of life in patients who had rheumatoid arthritis despite ongoing methotrexate therapy. Response to the drug was dose-dependent.

▶ For all that they have revolutionized the treatment of rheumatoid and seronegative inflammatory arthritides, the first generation of biologic therapies is far from perfect. While most people have a dramatic response to TNF or interleukin1 (IL-1) blockade, not everyone has complete remission. Moreover, agents must be continued or relapse will almost certainly occur. And the potential toxicities of TNF blockade (tuberculosis reactivation, autoimmunity, congestive heart failure), while not common, make these agents inadvisable for a meaningful number of patients. Accordingly, new strategies continue to

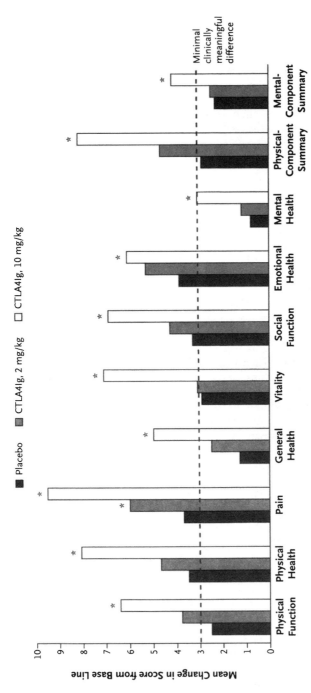

FIGURE 3.—Effect of CTLA4Ig on the health-related quality of life. Health-related quality of life was assessed with the use of the Medical Outcomes Study 36-Item Short-Form General Health Survey (SF-36). Scores on the 8 subscales of the SF-36 were aggregated to derive the physical-component summary score and the mental-component summary score. The 8 subscales, physical-component summary, and mental-component summary were scored with the use of norm-based methods that standardize the scores to a mean (±SD) of 50 ± 10 on the basis of an assessment of the general US population of persons without chronic conditions. Scores on each subscale range from 0 to 10, and the summary scores range from 0 to 100, with higher scores indicating better health. Asterisks indicate a significant difference (P < .05) for the comparison with the placebo group with the use of an analysis of covariance model with the baseline value as covariate. Values were carried forward from the last efficacy observation. Changes from baseline were also significant for each subscale score and for the summary scores in the 10-mg CTLA4Ig group. (Reprinted by permission of *The New England Journal of Medicine* from Kremer JM, Westhovens R, Leon M, et al: Treatment of rheumatoid arthritis by selective inhibition of T-cell activation with fusion protein CTLA4Ig. *N Engl J Med* 349:1907-1915, 2003. Copyright 2003, Massachusetts Medical Society. All rights reserved.)

be needed. IL-1 and TNF antagonists are directed at cytokines—soluble extracellular molecules that present a ready target for the large, antibody-based agents that technology currently permits. But extracellular targets need not be cytokines, and in this article, Kremer et al test an agent that targets a cell-surface protein critical to immune responses.

One of the more important insights of recent years has been the idea of "costimulation"—the notion that antigen presentation to a T cell is not enough to drive an immune response, and that 1 of several satellite interactions between the antigen-presenting cell and the T cell is required to complete the presentation. One such interaction is between CD28 on T cells and CD80 or CD86 on antigen-presenting cells. In the absence of such an interaction, antigen presentation either fails to stimulate a response, or more profoundly, may induce T-cell anergy or apoptosis. To take advantage of that knowledge, Kremer et al tested CTLA4Ig. This molecule consists of an immunoglobulin fused to CTLA4, a natural receptor that binds CD80 and CD86 far more avidly than CD28 does. Thus, in theory at least, CTLA4Ig should bind, and block CD80 and CD86, preventing T-cell activation.

Does it work? In this 6-month, double-blind, placebo-controlled trial, the tentative answer would appear to be "yes." All patients received methotrexate, but the CTLA4Ig group (actually, the 10 mg dose—the 2 mg dose was much less effective) had dramatically improved responses as measured by ACR 20, 50, and 70 indices (these indices provide a global assessment of joint swelling, tenderness, patient and physician assessment). Side effects, in this brief study, were essentially the same as placebo, including infection.

Many questions remain, of course, including the question of whether CTLA4Ig will inhibit joint erosion (not measured in this study), and the question of whether long-term use will lead to side effects. Another issue concerns when we might wish to use this agent. At first glance, it would seem that CTLA4Ig is about as effective as TNF blockade, but not necessarily more effective. Should it be considered a substitute for TNF blockade? An adjunct? An alternative? Will other new agents render it redundant by proving even better? Even if CTLA4Ig is only as good as what we have available now, it is clearly a harbinger of more to come. The next train of biologics is readying to leave the station.

M. H. Pillinger, MD

Specific Increase in Enzymatic Activity of Adenosine Deaminase 1 in Rheumatoid Synovial Fibroblasts

Nakamachi Y, Koshiba M, Nakazawa T, et al (Kobe Univ, Japan; Kyowa Hakko Kogyo Co Ltd, Shizuoka, Japan)
Arthritis Rheum 48:668-674, 2003   1–5

Background.—Elevated levels of serum adenosine deaminase (ADA) have been reported in patients with diseases that involve stimulation of cellular immunity. ADA1 activity is elevated in patients with acute lymphoblastic leukemia or acute hepatitis, while ADA2 activity is elevated in patients with

HIV infection. Most ADA activity in human tissues and cells is derived from ADA1, but the prevalent form in serum is ADA2. The tissue source of ADA2 in human cells is not clear, although the monocyte/macrophage cell system is thought to be a major source.

It is also known that total ADA activity is significantly more elevated in the synovial fluid of patients with rheumatoid arthritis than in the synovial fluid of patients with osteoarthritis. Methotrexate is one of the most effective antirheumatic drugs and has been reported to be associated with increased levels of extracellular adenosine. The role of ADA1 and ADA2 in the pathogenesis of rheumatoid arthritis was investigated.

Methods.—ADA1 and ADA2 activity was measured in the synovial fluid obtained from patients with rheumatoid arthritis and those with osteoarthritis, in sera from patients with rheumatoid arthritis, in lysates prepared from mononuclear and polymorphonuclear cells from the synovial fluid of patients with rheumatoid arthritis, peripheral blood from patients with rheumatoid arthritis, and fibroblast-like synoviocytes (FLS) from patients with rheumatoid arthritis and osteoarthritis. The effects of proinflammatory cytokines on ADA1 activity and ADA mRNA expression in rheumatoid arthritis FLS were determined by real-time polymerase chain reaction. Radioimmunoassay was used to measure the adenosine concentration in rheumatoid arthritis synovial fluid.

Results.—In synovial fluid from patients with rheumatoid arthritis, the adenosine concentration ranged from 0.027 μM to 0.508 μM. ADA1 would be expected to be functionally dominant at these concentrations because of its greater affinity for adenosine. ADA1 activity was significantly greater in the synovial fluid from patients with rheumatoid arthritis than in synovial fluid from patients with osteoarthritis or sera from patients with rheumatoid arthritis. In addition, ADA1 activity in FLS lysate from patients with rheumatoid arthritis was the highest among the cell lysates tested. ADA1 activity and ADA mRNA expression in rheumatoid arthritis FLS were not affected by proinflammatory cytokines.

Conclusion.—Elevated ADA1 activity is an intrinsic characteristic of FLS in rheumatoid arthritis, which is a likely contributing factor in the pathogenesis of rheumatoid arthritis through neutralization of the antirheumatic properties of endogenous adenosine.

▶ One of the more interesting observations to come out of disease-modifying anti-rheumatic drug research in recent years has been the fact that methotrexate, and probably sulfasalazine, act on rheumatoid arthritis via mechanisms distinct from their previously appreciated effects.[1] In particular, these agents appear to work, in part if not in whole, via a capacity to increase extracellular adenosine levels. Because adenosine has potent anti-inflammatory effects, the net result may be to increase the production of natural anti-inflammation.

Now Nakamachi et al have shown that adenosine metabolism may play an important role in rheumatoid arthritis, even in the absence of methotrexate or sulfasalazine therapy. They observed that adenosine levels were quite low in rheumatoid synovial fluid (though they failed to compare these levels with those of normal or osteoarthritic joints) and that ADA—the enzyme that inactivates adenosine—was present in high concentrations in rheumatoid synovial fluid compared to osteoarthritis. ADA levels in rheumatoid synovial fluid were also much lower than ADA levels in serum from patients with rheumatoid arthritis, indicating that ADA production was a local phenomenon in the joint.

Interestingly, the cell that appeared to be most responsible for the production of ADA in the joint was the synovial fibroblast, a cell whose importance to the rheumatoid process is becoming increasingly apparent. Thus, increased ADA production by the rheumatoid fibroblast may serve to lower extracellular adenosine levels, contributing to an inflammatory state. Interestingly, ADA expression in vitro was not affected by the addition of cytokines such as tumor necrosis factor–α (TNFα). It is well known that TNF antagonists work better when used in conjunction with methotrexate. One might speculate that the reason for this is that TNF antagonists and methotrexate operate on distinct processes (cytokine and adenosine levels, respectively) which are independently important in the pathogenesis of rheumatoid arthritis.

M. H. Pillinger, MD

Reference

1. Cronstein BN: The antirheumatic agents sulphasalazine and methotrexate share an anti-inflammatory mechanism. *Br J Rheumatol* 34(suppl 2):30-32, 1995.

Reduction in Long-term Functional Disability in Rheumatoid Arthritis From 1977 to 1998: A Longitudinal Study of 3035 Patients
Krishnan E, Fries JF (Stanford Univ, Calif; Clinical Research Ctr of Reading, West Reading, Pa)
Am J Med 115:371-376, 2003   1–6

Background.—Disease-modifying antirheumatic drugs should reduce disability in patients with rheumatoid arthritis. To determine whether more recent, aggressive therapy with newer agents was reducing patient disability, trends in disability were prospectively tracked over time.

Study Design.—The study group consisted of 3035 patients with rheumatoid arthritis tracked from 1977 to 1998 in the Arthritis, Rheumatism and Aging Medical Information System. Patients were followed up with semiannual questionnaires that included the Health Assessment Questionnaire disability index. The calendar year of symptom onset was used as a surrogate for treatment strategy. Disability was evaluated as disability score measured over time. The relationship between successive annual cohorts was assessed, with control for sex, race, education, clinical center, disease duration, follow-up, and attrition.

Findings.—Average patient disability declined by approximately 2% to 3% per calendar year of disease onset in univariate models and 2% in multivariate models, after controlling for possible confounding variables (Figure).

Conclusion.—The findings provide evidence that more aggressive treatment of rheumatoid arthritis results in decreased patient disability. After ac-

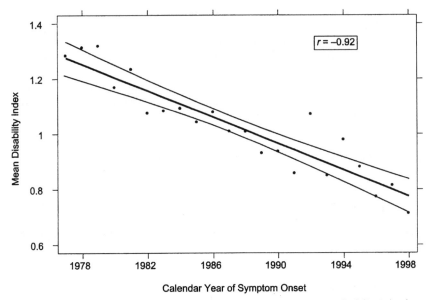

Calendar Year of Symptom Onset

FIGURE.—Time trends in mean cumulative Health Assessment Questionnaire disability index from 1977 through 1998. The *regression line* has a correlation coefficient of −0.92. The *curved lines* represent the 95% confidence limits. (Reprinted from the *American Journal of Medicine* courtesy of Krishnan E, Fries JF: Reduction in long-term functional disability in rheumatoid arthritis from 1977 to 1998: A longitudinal study of 3035 patients. *Am J Med* 115:371-376. Copyright 2003, with permission from Excerpta Medica Inc.)

counting for potential confounding variables, disability levels have declined approximately 40% since 1977.

▶ Having reported elsewhere in this chapter that rheumatoid arthritis is associated with both increased cardiovascular mortality in particular and increased mortality in general, I felt honor bound to also include some good news. And here it is: Despite all the problems, appreciated and unappreciated, that our rheumatoid patients are plagued with, they've been doing better than ever, even before the advent of the new biologics and other mechanism-based therapies.

In this study, Krishnan and Fries prospectively studied (by combining 8 prospective data banks) more than 3000 patients with rheumatoid arthritis entered into the study between 1977 and 1998. On average, patients entered the study with a little more disability in the earlier years than in the later years. (Disability was calculated from the Health Assessment Questionnaire, an index common to all the databases included in the study). However, the average overall disability of each patient—essentially indicating the level of disability over time—declined steadily from 1978 to 1998 at a rate of about 2% per year. Thus, over the 20-odd years of the study, the mean disability score of enrolled patients fell by about 30%.

The authors attribute this improvement in disability to increased use of aggressive treatment, noting that during the period in question the standard treatment of rheumatoid arthritis moved from the "pyramid" to the "inverted pyramid" (ie, moved from saving the most effective treatments for last to using them at the beginning of care) and that methotrexate use in the study group went from 0.5% at the beginning of the study to 49% at the end. If advances in care resulted in reduced functional disability between 1977 and 1998, that is very good news indeed, especially since it seems pretty clear that our newer agents are doing as well as, or even better than, the tried-and-true disease-modifying anti-rheumatic drugs tracked in this report.

M. H. Pillinger, MD

2 Osteoarthritis

Introduction

This year, we report on 2 studies in osteoarthritis—one that follows up on a very new question, one that follows up on a very old one. First, the new. Readers of the 2002 YEAR BOOK OF MEDICINE may recall that we included a study by Felson et al detailing the fact that bone marrow "edema"—which looks like edema on MRI but is actually something more like bone "scar tissue" on pathologic examination—is associated with pain in osteoarthritis. This year, we report on a follow-up by Felson (Abstract 2–2) indicating that bone marrow "edema" has prognostic value—it is a marker for disease progression in osteoarthritis. And the old? Raynauld et al (Abstract 2–1) investigate an age-old question—whether steroid injections into the knees of osteoarthritis patients are safe and effective. The conclusion? See below.

Michael H. Pillinger, MD

Safety and Efficacy of Long-term Intraarticular Steroid Injections in Osteoarthritis of the Knee: A Randomized, Double-blind, Placebo-controlled Trial

Raynauld J-P, Buckland-Wright C, Ward R, et al (Centre Hospitalier de l'Université de Montréal; King's College, London; American Univ of Beirut, Lebanon; et al)
Arthritis Rheum 48:370-377, 2003   2–1

Background.—With osteoarthritis (OA) of the knee, pain, stiffness, and loss of joint motion develop gradually. Pain relief is one of the primary goals of therapy, although tempered by the understanding that pain prevents the patient from engaging in activities that may further injure the knee joint and cartilage. Intra-articular injections of corticosteroids are used to relieve pain in patients with OA, but studies have not evaluated more long-term use of corticosteroid injections and their possible effects on the cartilage structure of the knee.

Methods.—At 3-month intervals over a period of 2 years, 68 participants with OA received injections into the knee of either triamcinolone acetonide 40 mg (34 patients) or saline solution (34 patients). The degree of joint space narrowing present after 2 years was determined radiographically, and clinical efficacy was determined with the pain subscale from the Western Ontario

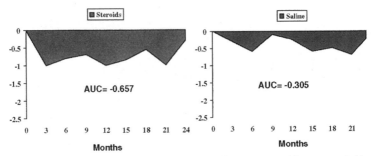

FIGURE 2.—Changes over time in levels of knee pain at night in patients with knee osteoarthritis treated for 2 years with intra-articular steroids or saline, as assessed by visual analog scales. Area under curve (AUC) of normalized values for night pain is shown for each group. Difference between 2 treatment groups was significant (P = .0047). (Courtesy Raynauld J-P, Buckland-Wright C, Ward R, et al: Safety and efficacy of long-term intraarticular steroid injections in osteoarthritis of the knee: A randomized, double-blind, placebo-controlled trial. *Arthritis Rheum* 48:370-377, 2003. Copyright 2003, American College of Rheumatology. Reprinted by permission of John Wiley & Sons, Inc.)

and McMaster Universities Osteoarthritis Index (WOMAC). The patients' clinical symptoms were evaluated before each injection. In addition, assessments were carried out for patient's and physician's global assessment, subjective assessment of pain, range of motion (ROM) of the knee, and time required to walk 50 feet.

Results.—Sixty-six patients completed the study. No differences in mean joint space width developed between the 2 groups, and disease progression did not occur. Those receiving steroid had a significantly greater change in ROM than those receiving placebo after 1 year. The WOMAC pain subscale and night pain scores for the steroid group tended toward greater improvement than was seen in the placebo group at the 1-year evaluation (Fig 2). However, neither primary nor secondary efficacy variables showed significantly different values after 2 years between the 2 groups. Both groups had significantly improved knee pain and stiffness as evaluated on the WOMAC questionnaire after both 1 and 2 years.

Conclusions.—ROM increased significantly, and pain showed a slight improvement with the use of corticosteroid injections of the knee after 1 year, with somewhat improved values at 2 years. There was no difference in the radiographic joint space measurements between the 2 groups.

▶ Intra-articular steroid injections are a mainstay of office-based treatment of OA, but relatively little data supports their use. Some animal studies suggest that steroid injections may slow the rate of OA progression, presumably by reducing the production of inflammatory mediators, metalloproteinases, and other enzymes that contribute to joint inflammation and damage. On the other hand, many physicians—as well as their patients—worry that repeated injections of steroids into an OA joint may lead to softening and/or damage to both the cartilage and other soft tissue structures of the joint. The current injunction followed by most rheumatologists—to limit injection frequency to no more than every 3 months—has relatively little hard data to support it. What is needed, then, are better studies to address these questions.

Raynauld et al have performed just such a study. They recruited 68 patients for a 2-year controlled study comparing triamcinolone injection (40 mg) every 3 months with saline injections over a 2-year period. This is the longest such study yet on record, and it provides some useful practical insights.

Both the control and treatment regimens were well tolerated, with no infections and no injection-induced flairs of OA pain over more than 500 injections. More importantly, perhaps, within the limits of their study, the authors observed no increased progression of osteoarthritic changes or other bony deformities in the triamcinolone relative to the control group. Although the study was only of moderate size, these data are convincing that regular injection of steroids do not advance the process of joint destruction in OA. Thus, when we repeatedly inject our patients with steroids in their painful, arthritic knees, we can probably rest easy that we are doing them no harm.

But are we doing them any good? The answer from this study would seem to be "a bit." At the end of the first year, patients who received steroid injections had statistically significant improvement in range of motion. Night pain showed a strong but not quite significant trend toward improvement ($P = .08$), and other indexes, including the WOMAC score, showed a weaker trend. By the end of 2 years most of these parameters had evened out, and even range of motion differences ceased to be significant. Moreover, if triamcinolone did not speed joint destruction, it also did not prevent it, since no differences were seen between the saline control group and the steroid group.

However, most physicians and patients suspect that the effects of steroids are transient; if that is the case, then it is not the end point that is important, but rather how the patients feel along the way. Seen from that perspective, the steroid arm did in fact win out. The area under the curve for both night pain and knee stiffness favored the triamcinolone arm over the 2-year course of the study. And while other parameters did not reach significance, all showed a trend toward improvement with steroid injection. Moreover, the design of the study actually disfavored the steroid group. For one thing, all patients were allowed to continue taking nonsteroidal anti-inflammatory drugs, probably mitigating differences between treatment arms. For another, it is possible that saline injection may not be the ideal control, as some studies have suggested that saline washout of OA joints may be beneficial—again suggesting that the study design may actually make it harder to see differences between the control and treatment arms.

So what can we say about steroid injection in OA knees? They are probably safe, and symptomatically effective to a greater or lesser extent. On the other hand, they probably don't slow the progression of OA, though the "right" study remains to be done. Since they don't seem to improve long-term end points, I for one will not be putting my patients on a rigid regimen of 4-times-yearly injections, but I will also not hesitate to utilize steroid injections for flares, exacerbations, and whenever the patient feels the need for symptomatic improvement.

M. H. Pillinger, MD

Bone Marrow Edema and Its Relation to Progression of Knee Osteoarthritis

Felson DT, McLaughlin S, Goggins J, et al (Boston Univ; Veterans Affairs Boston Health Care System; Univ of Rochester, NY)
Ann Intern Med 139:330-336, 2003   2–2

Background.—Osteoarthritis is the most common form of arthritis and is the leading cause of mobility-related disability in elderly persons. The prevalence of osteoarthritis is increasing with the increasing age of the population in the United States. Factors that affect the course of osteoarthritis in the knee are largely unknown, but it has been shown that lesions on bone scan and mechanical malalignment increase the risk for radiographically evident deterioration. Bone marrow edema lesions on MRI scans have been shown to correspond to bone scan lesions. Whether edema lesions in the subarticular bone in patients with knee osteoarthritis identify knees at high risk for radiographic progression was investigated. Also investigated was whether these lesions are associated with limb malalignment.

Methods.—This natural history study was conducted in a Veterans Administration hospital and enrolled patients 45 years of age and older with symptomatic knee osteoarthritis. A total of 256 patients were assessed at baseline with MRI imaging of the knee and fluoroscopically positioned radiography. During follow-up at 15 and 30 months, patients underwent repeated radiography. Long-limb films were obtained at 15 months to assess mechanical alignment. Progression was defined as an increase at follow-up in medial or lateral joint space narrowing on the basis of a semiquantitative grading scale. Generalized estimating equations were used for evaluation of the relationship of medial bone marrow edema lesions to medial progression and the relationship of lateral lesions to lateral progression, before and after adjustment for limb alignment.

Results.—A total of 223 of 256 patients (87.1%) participated in at least 1 follow-up examination. Medial bone marrow lesions predominated in patients with varus limbs, and lateral lesions were seen mainly in patients with valgus limbs. Of the 75 knees with medial lesions, 27 (36%) showed medial progression compared with 12 of 148 knees without lesions (8.1%). About 69% of knees with medial progression had medial lesions, and lateral lesions were a significant risk factor for lateral progression. These increased risks were attenuated by 37% to 53% after adjustment for limb alignment.

Conclusion.—Bone marrow edema is a significant risk factor for structural deterioration in patients with knee osteoarthritis. The relationship of bone marrow edema to progression can be attributed at least in part to its association with limb alignment.

▶ In the 2002 YEAR BOOK, I included an article by Felson et al indicating that bone marrow edema seen on MRI correlated with knee pain in osteoarthritis (OA).[1] This was interesting work, in part because cartilage has no nerves, and the cause of pain in OA remains to some extent a mystery. What the MR radiologist calls marrow edema, by the way, probably isn't edema at all. Histopathologic correlation suggests that such "edema" is really abnormal bone with fibrosis, osteonecrosis, and remodeling, suggesting a response similar to that occurring after fatigue fractures.

Now Felson et al have extended their studies by looking at what such "edema" means with regard to OA progression. Two hundred fifty-six patients met criteria for knee OA and the presence of marrow edema in the subchondral tibia and were studied both initially and longitudinally. The authors found a strong association between the presence of edema and knee malalignment. Varus limbs had medial marrow edema, whereas valgus limbs had primarily lateral edema. The authors also found a strong association between edema in a particular compartment and progression of OA in that compartment. Knees with lateral edema lesions showed much more lateral progression of OA, and knees with medial lesions showed medial OA progression.

Interestingly, medial lesions were associated with an apparent protective effect on lateral OA progression and vice-versa. Much of the edema effect on progression could be accounted for by its relation to joint malalignment, but the association between edema and OA progression persisted even after statistical correction for the malalignment effect was carried out.

These studies shed interesting light on the mechanisms of OA progression, emphasizing that subchondral bone plays an integral part in the osteoarthritis process. Less clear is whether marrow edema is a cause or consequence of OA progression. One can easily imagine that the development of compartmental marrow edema might arise as a response, as malalignment and cartilage destruction put ever more pressure on the underlying bone. Equally plausible, though, is that the development of mechanically abnormal bone skews the arthritic response—either mechanically or biochemically—toward further progression and damage. Perhaps both occur.

The strong predictive value of the marrow lesions raises the question of whether routine MRI of OA joints should be recommended. For now, the authors demur, suggesting that (a) there is no treatment for marrow lesions anyway and (b) it has not yet been determined how much information MRI adds to other less expensive studies, such as long-limb radiographs to assess knee alignment. The use of MRI to identify edema may be a worthwhile adjunct to clinical studies, however, where stratification of risk of OA progression is likely to be particularly valuable.

Also noted: a study by McQueen et al, indicating that the presence of bone edema of the dominant carpus in patients with rheumatoid arthritis was predictive of radiographic joint damage six years later.[2]

M. H. Pillinger, MD

References

1. Felson DT, Chaisson CE, Hill CL, et al: The association of bone marrow lesions with pain in knee osteoarthritis. *Ann Intern Med* 134:541-549, 2001. (2002 YEAR BOOK OF MEDICINE, pp 39-41.)
2. McQueen FM, Benton N, Perry D, et al: Bone edema scored on magnetic resonance imaging scans of the dominant carpus at presentation predicts radiographic joint damage of the hands and feet six years later in patients with rheumatoid arthritis. *Arthritis Rheum* 48:1814-1827, 2003.

3 Lupus and Lupus-like Illnesses

Introduction

Systemic lupus erythematosus (SLE) is one of the most fascinating and complex of the rheumatic diseases. Much is known, and much is not known, about the natural history and pathogenesis of SLE. In this YEAR BOOK OF MEDICINE, we select just a few of the many interesting SLE studies that have transpired this year. From Arbuckle et al (Abstract 3–1) comes a very interesting study that traces the development autoantibodies in patients with lupus—long before their lupus was ever diagnosed. Cervera et al (Abstract 3–2) also report on the natural history of lupus—in this case after diagnosis—to give insight into the differences between the first, and second decade of the disease. Roman et al (Abstract 3–3) examine the risk of atherosclerosis in lupus. Crowther et al (Abstract 3–4) provide insight into the treatment of an important aspect of SLE that also can exist as an independent entity, the anti-phospholipid antibody syndrome. Finally, I have included a case report from Stengaard-Pedersen et al (Abstract 3–5) of an illness that is not strictly lupus but undoubtedly involves some of the same mechanisms. As our readers may know, various hereditary complement deficiencies may predispose to SLE. However, no deficiencies in the oldest part of the complement system—the mannose-binding lectin pathway—have previously been reported in autoimmune diseases. Stengaard-Pedersen define just such an entity, suggesting that this pathway may also play a role in lupus and lupus-like illnesses.

Michael H. Pillinger, MD

Development of Autoantibodies Before the Clinical Onset of Systemic Lupus Erythematosus

Arbuckle MR, McClain MT, Rubertone MV, et al (Oklahoma Med Research Found, Oklahoma City; Univ of Oklahoma, Oklahoma City; Dept of Veterans Affairs, Oklahoma City, Okla; et al)
N Engl J Med 349:1526-1533, 2003   3–1

Background.—Systemic lupus erythematosus (SLE) is almost always accompanied by the production of autoantibodies, and it has been shown that autoantibodies contribute directly to the pathologic changes of SLE. Autoantibodies are central to the pathogenesis of the disorder, so their development must coincide with or precede clinical disease. The prevalence of SLE autoantibodies among patients with confirmed SLE has been established; however, little is known of the autoimmune history of patients before the diagnosis of SLE. The onset and progression of autoantibody development before clinical diagnosis of SLE were investigated.

Methods.—This study utilized the Department of Defense Serum Repository, which contains about 30 million specimens prospectively collected from over 5 million armed forces personnel. Serum samples obtained from 130 persons before they received a diagnosis of SLE were evaluated along with samples from matched controls.

Results.—At least 1 SLE autoantibody tested was present before the diagnosis (up to 9.4 years earlier; mean, 3.3 years) in 115 of the 130 patients (88%). Antinuclear antibodies were present in 78% of patients (at a dilution of 1:120 or more); anti–double-stranded DNA antibodies in 55%; anti-Ro antibodies in 47%; anti-La antibodies in 34%; anti-Sm antibodies in 32%; antinuclear ribonucleoprotein antibodies in 26%; and antiphospholipid antibodies in 18%. Antinuclear, antiphospholipid antibodies, anti-Ro, and anti-La autoantibodies were present earlier than anti-Sm and antinuclear ribonucleoprotein antibodies (a mean of 3.4 years before the diagnosis vs 1.2 years).

Anti–double-stranded DNA antibodies, with a mean onset of 2.2 years after the diagnosis, were found later than antinuclear antibodies and earlier than antinuclear ribonucleoprotein antibodies. The earliest available serum sample was positive in many patients; thus, these measures of the average time from the first positive antibody test to the diagnosis are underestimates of the time from the development of the antibodies to the diagnosis. Among the 130 initial matched control subjects, 3.8% were positive for 1 or more autoantibodies.

Conclusion.—Autoantibodies are usually present many years before the diagnosis of SLE. The appearance of autoantibodies in patients with SLE often follows a predictable course, with a progressive accumulation of specific autoantibodies before the onset of SLE.

▶ What is the natural history of lupus before the illness becomes clinically apparent? Most of us would probably assume that serologic autoimmunity precedes clinical symptoms of autoimmunity, but until now, it's been an almost impossible question to answer. You would need to be able to identify and follow lupus patients before their disease has become apparent. That, in essence, is what Arbuckle et al have managed to accomplish in this study. They took advantage of the fact that the United States military keeps both accurate medical records and serum samples on every one of its recruits. They were able to screen more than 5 million medical records for a diagnosis of lupus and identified 130 individuals with a diagnosis of SLE. They then removed at least 1 serum sample from each patient that preceded the onset of clinically appreciated SLE and tested it for standard lupus autoantibodies.

Several interesting facts were revealed. First, the development of serologic autoimmunity preceded clinical autoimmunity in almost 90% of the cases. Moreover, serologic autoimmunity preceded clinical disease by a significant period—on average, 3.3 years but frequently much longer. In terms of the specific antibodies that were present prior to illness, the authors observed a sequence of autoimmunity in which, in most cases, autoantibody formation evolved in a clearly defined pattern.

Antiphospholipid, anti-Ro, and anti-La antibodies were seen earliest. In keeping with their general nature, antinuclear antibody tests were also positive at this early stage. Later, anti–double-stranded DNA antibodies developed. Last came the occurrence of anti-Sm and antiribonucleoprotein antibodies. It is not clear from these studies whether formation of an earlier autoantibody in some way influences the formation of the next autoantibody (for example, by epitope spreading, in which related antigens become progressively more susceptible to response as the immune system undergoes stimulation). What is clear is that lupus is a more rational disease than we have come to expect and that its evolution into a particular immunologic picture plays by a set of rules that we can now try to understand.

For the clinician, it is possible that these data suggest increased vigilance when evaluating a patient with a positive antinuclear antibody but no symptoms, since we now know a bit more about how early markers develop into late ones. On the other hand, this study specifically examined patients with a known outcome of clinical lupus, so it actually tells us very little about patients with 1 or 2 autoantibodies but no signs or symptoms of disease. For those individuals, prudence must remain the watchword.

M. H. Pillinger, MD

Morbidity and Mortality in Systemic Lupus Erythematosus During a 10-Year Period: A Comparison of Early and Late Manifestations in a Cohort of 1,000 Patients
Cervera R, Khamashta MA, Font J, et al (Univ of Barcelona; St Thomas' Hosp, London; Ospedale San Camillo de Lellis, Rome; et al)
Medicine 82:299-308, 2003   3–2

Background.—Some authorities have proposed that the spectrum of clinical manifestations of systemic lupus erythematosus (SLE) and the causes of death depend on the time of SLE evolution. Some researchers have suggested that SLE tends to remit in many patients after a long evolution. Others have reported that patients with a long duration of SLE still have active disease. To clarify the long-term evolution of SLE, a multicenter observational study was begun in 1990 in Europe.

Methods.—The study included 1000 patients from 7 European countries with documented medical histories. All underwent interviews and a general physical examination on study entry. One team of physicians followed up the patients from 1990 until 2000.

Findings.—Forty-eight percent of the patients had 1 or more episodes of arthritis at some time during follow-up. Thirty-one percent had malar rash; 27.9%, active nephropathy; 19.4%, neurologic involvement; 16.6%, fever; 16.3%, Raynaud's phenomenon; 16%, serositis; 13.4%, thrombocytopenia; and 9.2%, thrombosis. Most manifestations were more frequent in the initial 5 years. Thirty-six percent of the patients had infections; 16.9%, hypertension; 12.1%, osteoporosis; and 8.1%, cytopenia from immunosuppressive agents. Malignancies developed in 2.3% of the patients. The most common sites of such malignancies were the uterus and breast (Table 3). The mortality rate was 6.8%. The most common causes of death were equally divided between active SLE, thromboses, and infections. The 10-year survival probability was 92%. Survival rate was less for patients who initially had nephropathy. Active SLE and infections appeared to be the most common causes of death in the first 5 years, whereas thromboses were the most common cause of death in the next 5 years.

Conclusions.—Most inflammatory manifestations of SLE appear to be less common after long-term evolution of SLE. This probably reflects the effects of treatment and progressive remission in many patients. Thrombotic events play a more prominent role later in the disease, influencing morbidity and mortality.

TABLE 3.—Associated Medical Problems That Appeared in the Total Cohort During the 10-Year Prospective Study (1990-2000)

Associated Medical Problem	1990-2000 (n = 1,000) No. (%)	1990-1995 (n = 1,000) No. (%)	1995-2000 (n = 840)* No. (%)	P Value†
Infection	360 (36)	270 (27)	161 (19.2)	<0.001
Urinary	169 (16.9)	113 (11.3)	84 (10)	
Cutaneous	102 (10.2)	76 (7.6)	39 (4.6)	0.01
Respiratory	117 (11.7)	74 (7.4)	60 (7.1)	
Abdominal	43 (4.3)	34 (3.4)	17 (2)	
Central nervous system	7 (0.7)	5 (0.5)	3 (0.4)	
Sepsis	26 (2.6)	25 (2.5)	5 (0.6)	0.002
Other		62 (6.2)	31 (3.7)	0.019
Hypertension	169 (16.9)	113 (11.3)	108 (12.9)	
Osteoporosis	121 (12.1)	75 (7.5)	83 (9.9)	
Drug-induced cytopenia	81 (8.1)	59 (5.9)	40 (4.8)	
Gastrointestinal bleeding	49 (4.9)	31 (3.1)	28 (3.3)	
Cataracts	47 (4.7)	29 (2.9)	26 (3.1)	
Diabetes	30 (3)	27 (2.7)	10 (1.2)	
Avascular necrosis of bone	29 (2.9)	23 (2.3)	14 (1.7)	
Retinopathy	22 (2.2)	17 (1.7)	10 (1.2)	
Malignancy	23 (2.3)	16 (1.6)	7 (0.8)	
Uterus	8 (0.8)	7 (0.7)	1 (0.1)	
Breast	4 (0.4)	3 (0.3)	1 (0.1)	
Non-Hodgkin lymphoma	2 (0.2)	2 (0.2)	0 (0)	
Colon	1 (0.1)	1 (0.1)	0 (0)	
Lung	3 (0.3)	1 (0.1)	2 (0.2)	
Other	5 (0.5)	2 (0.2)	3 (0.4)	

*Number of patients that continued in the study in 1995.
†All P values are a comparison between the frequencies in the 1990-1995 and in the 1995-2000 periods.
(Courtesy of Cervera R, Khamashta MA, Font J, et al: Morbidity and mortality in systemic lupus erythematosus during a 10-year period: A comparison of early and late manifestations in a cohort of 1,000 patients. *Medicine* 82:299-308, 2003.)

▶ Okay, we're probably getting better at handling crises in lupus—getting patients through an attack of nephritis, a CNS change, or an antiphospholipid catastrophe. But how are our lupus patients doing in the long run—not over a week or month, but over the many years of their disease? Relatively few studies have addressed the long-term outcome in patients with lupus. This one, by Cervera et al, is both the latest (thereby reflecting as nearly as possible the outcomes of lupus in the present era) as well as one of the biggest ever performed. The European Working Party on Systemic Lupus Erythematosus began this prospective cohort study in 1990, enrolling 1000 patients. They now report on 10 years of patient follow-up and compare the first and second 5 years of the study. Some interesting data emerge. First, it would seem that rheumatologists really are not doing that badly in managing this potentially unstable disease. Overall, the 10-year mortality rate was a relatively modest 8%. Since the mean age of the patients at the time of study entry was 37 years, and since the mean age at death was 44 years, it is clear that most deaths (nearly all, in fact) were related to lupus. Still, the 92% survival rate this study found would probably be at the optimistic end of most rheumatologists' estimates. The major causes of death are pretty much what would be expected—the most common overall were active lupus, infection, and thrombosis—all at about 25 %, with malignancy a distant fourth at 5.9%. These data are slightly different than a previous study by Abu-Shakra et al, which found that infection caused most lupus deaths (32%), followed by lupus activity and thrombosis (each about 16%).[1] One of the strongest predictors of mortality was the presence of nephropathy at the time of diagnosis; patients whose initial presentation included nephropathy had a survival rate of about 87%, compared with that of 94% for patients without initial nephropathy. Again, this isn't particularly surprising, since nephropathy is no doubt a marker not only for lupus activity, but also for more aggressive immunosuppression and increased hypercoagulability, owing to nephrotic syndrome.

On an interesting note, Cervera et al also compare the outcomes of lupus in the first 5 years of the study with those in the second 5 years. Their observations tend to confirm an impression shared by many rheumatologists: that patients later in their disease tend to have less disease activity than patients earlier on. Compared with the first 5 years, patients in the second 5 years of the study experienced fewer major infections (19.2% vs 27%), less nephropathy (6.8% vs 22.2%), less arthritis (28.6% vs 41.3%) and overall less lupus activity. Patients also died less frequently, and died less frequently from lupus activity (21.7% of all deaths vs 28.9%) and infection (17.4% of all deaths vs 28.9%) in the second 5 years. Of course, these data may be at least partly skewed by the early mortality of the sickest of all lupus patients. Of important note, the rate of thrombosis, and death from the same, did not decrease over 10 years, and so in the late period, thrombosis advanced to become the leading cause of death.

Following a very large cohort of sick patients is an extremely difficult accomplishment. Like all such studies, this one is necessarily flawed and cannot answer all the questions we might like to ask of it. One major limitation is the fact that the study was done in Europe, and almost all the enrollees were white. Those of us in the United States and other parts of the world are acutely aware of the fact that lupus patients of African and Asian descent tend to be sicker than white patients, and so, at the very least, we clinicians outside of Europe will need to apply a mental correction factor to these data, anticipating that studies in our own countries would show a somewhat poorer outcome (as indeed they have[2-4]). Still, as we begin (one hopes!) to enter an era of better, highly targeted approaches to lupus therapy, this impressive study shows us an important window on how we are doing right now—both how far we have come and how much farther we have to go.

M. H. Pillinger, MD

References

1. Abu-Shakra M, Urowitz MB, Gladman DD, et al: Mortality studies in systemic lupus erythematosus. Results from a single center: I. Causes of death. *J Rheumatol* 1995;22:1259-1264.
2. Alarcon GS, McGwin G Jr, Petri M, et al: Baseline characteristics of a multiethnic lupus cohort: PROFILE. *Lupus* 2002;11:95-101.
3. Petri M: The effect of race on the presentation and course of SLE in the United States. *Arthritis Rheum* 1997:40:S162.
4. Wang F, Wang CL, Tan CT, et al: Systemic lupus erythematosus in Malaysia: A study of 539 patients and comparison of prevalence and disease expression in different racial and gender groups. *Lupus* 1997:6:248-253.

Prevalence and Correlates of Acclerated Atherosclerosis in Systemic Lupus Erthyematosus
Roman MJ, Shanker B-A, Davis A, et al (Cornell Univ, New York; State Univ of New York at Stony Brook)
N Engl J Med 349:2399-2406, 2003   3–3

Background.—The focus of the diagnostic criteria for systemic lupus erythematosus is on its major clinical manifestations, particularly renal, neurologic, and hematologic disease. There have been cardiovascular manifestations of this disease reported, but these outcomes are based on relatively few events, and the prevalence of atherosclerosis among patients with lupus and its relationship to the prevalence in a control population are unknown. The hypothesis that atherosclerosis would be more prevalent among patients with lupus and would not be attributable to traditional risk factors was investigated.

Methods.—A total of 197 patients with lupus and 197 matched control subjects underwent carotid US, echocardiography, and assessment for risk factors for cardiovascular disease. Patients were also evaluated with respect to their clinical and serologic features, inflammatory mediators, and disease treatment.

Results.—Patients and control subjects had similar risk factors for cardiovascular disease. Atherosclerosis was more prevalent among the patients than among the control subjects (37.1% vs 15.2%). Multivariate analysis indicated that the only factors independently related to the presence of plaque were older age, the presence of systemic lupus erythematosus, and higher serum cholesterol levels. Patients with plaque were older, had a longer duration of disease, and had more disease-related damage. Patients were also less likely to have multiple autoantibodies or to have undergone treatment with prednisone, cyclophosphamide, or hydroxychloroquine. Multivariate analysis showed that independent predictors of plaque were a longer duration of disease, a higher damage-index score, a lower incidence of cyclophosphamide use, and the absence of anti-Smith antibodies.

Conclusion.—Atherosclerosis is a premature occurrence in patients with systemic lupus erythematosus and is independent of the traditional risk factors for cardiovascular disease. The clinical profile of patients with lupus and atherosclerosis suggests a role for disease-related factors in atherogenesis.

▶ By now, it's pretty well accepted that patients with lupus have an increased risk of myocardial infarction compared with the general population. But why? Is it because they have more atherosclerosis than the rest of us? And if so, is the atherosclerosis driven by routine factors, by their disease itself, or by the drugs we use to treat lupus? Based on this article (as well as a complementary study by Asanuma et al published in the same issue of the *New England Journal of Medicine*[1]), we may conclude that it is lupus itself that in some way predisposes to accelerated atherosclerosis.

Roman et al studied 197 patients with lupus and 197 matched controls. Instead of trying to look for cardiovascular outcomes (which would probably have shown a low incidence, based on a sample this size), they used carotid US to search for the presence of arterial plaque—the sine qua non of atherosclerosis. With the exception of blood pressure (the control group actually had more hypertension than the lupus group), the authors observed no significant differences in traditional risk factors between patients and controls. Nonetheless, the lupus patients had double the incidence of plaque compared with the controls. Thus, the authors conclude that the increased incidence of atherosclerosis in lupus must have had something to do with the disease itself.

To understand this effect more fully, they next compared lupus patients with and without plaque to see if there were differences in these groups. The results were interesting. On balance, lupus patients with accelerated atherosclerosis tended to be less sick by our standard notions of lupus activity. That is, they had fewer autoantibodies (including lower rates of antiphospholipid antibodies), lower disease activity, and less treatment than the patients without plaque. Indeed, although steroid use is postulated as a cause of cardiovascular disease in lupus, it was the patients without plaque who had a higher level of steroid use.

On the other hand, the patients with plaque had a longer history of disease, a higher damage-index score, and more diabetes and hypertension. While it is possible that the increased rates of diabetes and hypertension were independent correlates of disease activity (ie, that a chance increase in diabetes and hypertension in the high-plaque group was actually responsible for the increase in atherosclerosis), the authors instead suggest that they were able to segregate their lupus patients into 2 groups. The first, with more active disease and more treatment, had less plaque. The second, with more of a "smouldering" lupus picture, got less treatment and had more atherosclerosis. Whether this represents a different sort of lupus disease (Could other, unrecognized autoantibodies target the vascular lining?) or a consequence of not treating (since the patients weren't sick by routine standards) was not evaluated.

The other study, by Asanuma et al, took a similar approach but used electron beam CT to look for calcium in coronary arteries as a marker of atherosclerosis. This group also found an increase in atherosclerosis in lupus patients, and then compared lupus patients with and without coronary artery calcification. This group's data were somewhat different than those of Roman et al in that they failed to show an inverse association with autoantibodies and disease activity. Why these studies should differ remains unclear. But like Roman et al, the Asanuma group found that traditional risk factors could not account for the increase in cardiovascular disease among lupus patients. Thus, we are left with the inevitable conclusion that lupus itself is associated with atherosclerosis. Now comes the fun and hard part: figuring out why.

M. H. Pillinger, MD

Reference

1. Asanuma Y, Oeser A, Shintani AK, et al: Premature coronary-artery atherosclerosis in systemic lupus erythematosus. *N Engl J Med* 349:2407-2415, 2003.

A Comparison of Two Intensities of Warfarin for the Prevention of Recurrent Thrombosis in Patients With the Antiphospholipid Antibody Syndrome

Crowther MA, Ginsberg JS, Julian J, et al (McMaster Univ, Hamilton, Ont, Canada; Univ of Toronto; Dalhousie Univ, Halifax, NS, Canada; et al)
N Engl J Med 349:1133-1138, 2003   3–4

Background.—Antiphospholipid antibodies, including anticardiolipin antibodies and lupus anticoagulant, are associated with both venous and arterial thrombosis. After the initial episode of thrombosis, patients with antiphospholipid antibodies are at a higher risk of recurrent thrombosis than patients without these antibodies. Many patients with antiphospholipid antibody syndrome and recurrent thrombosis receive warfarin at doses that are adjusted to achieve an international normalized ratio (INR) of more than 3.0. However, there are no prospective data to support this approach to thromboprophylaxis. Whether high-intensity warfarin therapy is required in these patients was investigated, and the hypothesis that high-intensity warfarin would be more effective than moderate-intensity therapy was tested.

Methods.—This randomized double-blind trial enrolled 114 patients with antiphospholipid antibodies and previous thrombosis. The patients were random to receive enough warfarin to achieve an INR of 2.0 to 3.0 (moderate intensity) or 3.1 to 4.0 (high intensity).

Results.—Recurrent thrombosis occurred in 6 of 56 patients (10.7%) assigned to receive high-intensity warfarin and in 2 of 58 patients (3.4%) assigned to moderate-intensity warfarin. Major bleeding occurred in 3 patients in the high-intensity warfarin group and in 4 patients in the moderate-intensity warfarin group.

Conclusion.—High-intensity warfarin does not perform better than moderate-intensity warfarin for thromboprophylaxis in patients with antiphospholipid antibodies and previous thrombosis. The low rate of recurrence in patients in the moderate-intensity group (target INR, 2.0 to 3.0) suggests that moderate-intensity warfarin is appropriate for patients with antiphospholipid antibody syndrome.

▶ The proper treatment of the antiphospholipid antibody syndrome remains a muddle. For most patients with prior proven thrombotic events, physicians "in the know" would almost certainly recommend warfarin therapy. But how much? And for how long? The trend of late has been to advance the dose of warfarin into the high therapeutic range, specifically, to an INR greater than 3.0. Surprisingly, not a single solid prospective study has existed to support this strategy, which is, naturally, associated with an increased risk of bleeding.

The study by Crowther et al set out to support the use of high therapeutic doses of warfarin, but the authors ended up concluding exactly the opposite. One hundred fourteen patients with documented thrombosis and either lupus anticoagulant or antiphospholipid antibodies were enrolled to receive either moderate (INR, 2.1-3.0) or high (INR, 3.1-4.0) dose warfarin anticoagulation and were monitored for a mean of 2.7 years. In the end, the group receiving moderate-dose warfarin had fewer thromboses than the high-dose group. Although the numbers of bleeding events were nearly identical in the 2 groups, all 3 bleeding events that required study withdrawal occurred in the high-dose group. The authors conclude that there is no basis for using high-dose warfarin in most patients being anticoagulated for antiphospholipid syndrome.

This study is not without its flaws, it should be noted. Chief among them, in my opinion, is the fact that many of the patients on the so-called high-intensity regimen actually failed to achieve their target INR for at least some of the study (patients in this group actually had an INR in the 2.1-3.0 range for fully 43% of the study time). This failure to achieve the target means that many of the people in the high-intensity group actually spent a significant amount of time on what, practically speaking, was a moderate-intensity regimen.

On the other hand, the failure to achieve the high-intensity response, even in a group of study patients, also testifies to the difficulty in maintaining too high an INR. Am I convinced by this data? Not entirely. I suspect I will still struggle to reach an INR greater than 3 in patients with life-threatening thromboses, as well as patients who have thromboses develop on moderate-dose regimens. But for all other patients, this work by Crowther et al warns us that we should carefully consider the potential risks and benefits before pushing the warfarin dose up beyond a standard level.

M. H. Pillinger, MD

Inherited Deficiency of Mannan-Binding Lectin–Associated Serine Protease 2

Stengaard-Pedersen K, Thiel S, Gadjeva M, et al (Aarhus Univ, Denmark; John Radcliffe Hosp, Oxford, England; Univ of Lund, Sweden)
N Engl J Med 349:554-560, 2003   3–5

Background.—The complement system contributes to innate immunity. The mannan-binding lectin pathway of the complement system is activated when mannan-binding lectin binds to mannan in the membranes of microorganisms through autoactivation of the mannan-binding lectin–associated serine protease 2 (MASP-2). This case report described a patient with an inherited deficiency of MASP-2.

Case Report.—A male patient was healthy from birth in 1967 until diagnosed with ulcerative colitis in 1980. He was successfully treated with prednisolone. He had erythema multiforme bullosum develop and was again successfully treated with prednisolone. Between 1995 and 1997, the patient had 3 episodes of severe pneumococcal pneumonia. In 1997, progressive lung fibrosis was detected. Hypocomplementemia was diagnosed, but results of the Coomb's test and tests for autoantibodies were negative.

Severe deficiency of the MASP complexes was detected. These complexes did not contain either MASP-2 or MASP-19. Sequencing of the MASP-2 gene revealed that it contained a mutation in the CUB1 domain, causing glycine to be substituted for a conserved aspartic acid, preventing formation of functional MASP-2 complex.

Conclusion.—A patient with chronic inflammatory disease and susceptibility to infection was found to have a genetic deficiency in MASP-2, which led to nonfunctional mannan-binding complexes. The prevalence of this mutation and its influence on disease should be examined in a larger population.

▶ I've chosen this case report because it is fascinating, but also because it reminds us that complement deficiencies commonly result in both immune deficiencies and, paradoxically, autoimmunity. Some of the best-appreciated complement deficiencies—C1q and C4 deficiencies, for instance—are associated with lupus or lupus-like syndromes and represent deficiencies of the classical complement pathway.

In this article, Stengaard-Pedersen describe a deficiency of the most recently described of the complement pathways: the mannose-binding lectin pathway. Under normal circumstances, this pathway uses a protein known as mannose-binding lectin to recognize bacteria by virtue of the fact that bacterial, but not mammalian, membrane glycoproteins incorporate mannose. Binding of mannose-binding lectin to bacterial mannose leads to formation of a complex including several mannose-binding lectin–associated serine proteases—MASPs—that can, in turn, activate a complement cascade similar to that of the classical pathway.

The patient that Stengaard-Pedersen et al describe had an autosomal recessive deficiency in MASP-2 expression and, in consequence, developed inflammatory bowel disease, erythema multiforme bullosa, joint symptoms, myalgia, lung fibrosis, and a weakly positive anti–nuclear antibody test. In the case of classical pathway complement deficiencies, the mechanism(s) of autoimmune disease is often presumed to relate to impaired clearance of immune complexes, but the mechanism is even less clear in this case. Given the fact that, at least in the Swedish population studied, the frequency of heterozygotes for the disease was approximately 1 in 10, it is likely that MASP-2 deficiency is present but undiagnosed in as much as 1% of the population. Add this to the other complement deficiencies and we can see that these deficiencies should not be overlooked.

M. H. Pillinger, MD

4 Psoriatic Arthritis

Introduction

When it comes to pathogenesis and treatment, psoriatic arthritis is like the younger sibling of rheumatoid arthritis—it usually has to settle for the hand-me-downs. Methotrexate, sulfasalazine, and more recently anti-TNF antibodies all came to be used in psoriatic arthritis only after they were developed for use in rheumatoid arthritis. If we are going to have truly disease-specific therapies for psoriatic arthritis, we must first develop a specific understanding of the mechanisms of this disease.

In this section, we have included 2 studies that specifically address the pathogenesis of psoriatic arthritis. Reporting from the laboratory bench, Ritchlin et al (Abstract 4–2) suggest an important role for osteoclast maturation and activity in psoriatic joint damage. Reporting from the clinic, Rahman et al (Abstract 4–1) perform a genome wide scan of 187 patients with psoriatic arthritis and report on the first non-HLA gene—CARD15—to be associated with psoriatic arthritis. Perhaps rheumatoid arthritis' "younger sibling" is beginning to grow up.

Michael H. Pillinger, MD

***CARD15*: A Pleiotropic Autoimmune Gene That Confers Susceptibility to Psoriatic Arthritis**
Rahman P, Bartlett S, Siannis F, et al (Mem Univ of Newfoundland, Canada; Inst of Public Health, Cambridge, England; Univ of Toronto)
Am J Hum Genet 73:677-681, 2003   4–1

Background.—Recently, a genome-wide scan of psoriatic arthritis (PsA) demonstrated a susceptibility locus at 16q, a region that overlaps *CARD15*, a susceptibility gene in Crohn's disease. Epidemiologic studies also support the possibility of a common susceptibility gene between PsA and Crohn's disease, as patients with Crohn's disease have an increased incidence of psoriasis. A new screening study was discussed.

Methods.—The study included 187 patients with PsA and 136 healthy persons. All were from Newfoundland. Screening for 3 common, independent sequence variants of *CARD15* (R702W, leu1007fsinsC, G908R) was performed using polymerase chain reaction with allele-specific primers and visualization through gel electrophoresis.

Findings.—At least 1 *CARD15* gene variant was documented in 28.3% of probands with PsA and in 11.8% of the control group. In the patient group, allele frequencies of R702W were 10.4%; of leu1007fsinsC, 3.2%; and of G908R, 1.6%. In the control group, these frequencies were 3.3%, 2.6%, and 0.4%, respectively.

Conclusions.—These data suggest that *CARD15* represents a pleiotropic autoimmune gene. This is the first non-major histocompatibility complex (non-MHC) gene to be correlated with PsA.

▶ Both the mechanism and the genetic origins of PsA remain relatively obscure. Several human leukocyte antigen (HLA) types have been associated with psoriasis, but only 1 of these, HLA-Cw*0602, is associated with PsA. Still, the familial clustering of PsA is well established. Are there other genes that regulate the onset of this disease?

Rahman et al. took a classic genetic approach to evaluating a candidate gene. From the extensive, ongoing studies of the population of Iceland, it was recognized that a region of chromosome 16q was highly associated with PsA. Within that region, the gene *CARD15* was a good candidate, as it had already been associated with both Crohn's disease (ie, an overlapping condition) as well as with cellular responses to inflammatory stimuli in vitro. With these facts in mind, the authors used 3 single nucleotide polymorphisms (SNPs) to study the prevalence of different versions of *CARD15* in 187 patients with PsA versus unaffected control subjects. (SNPs, which represent nucleotides that commonly vary in a particular gene, can be used to recognize different variants of that gene in a population. They are, therefore, labels of variance, but in and of themselves, they do not necessarily represent the important mutations that lead to phenotypic differences.) By this method, the authors found a strong relationship between less common variants of *CARD15* and the presence of PsA. Indeed, the odds ratio for *CARD15* (2.97) was pretty similar to that for HLA-Cw*0602 (3.72), suggesting the potential importance of this gene for PsA. As the authors point out, *CARD15* is the first candidate susceptibility gene for PsA outside of the MHC locus.

Of course, these genetic studies can only begin to raise questions that need to be answered by a variety of disciplines. For instance, what, if any, is the mechanism(s) through which *CARD15* acts? Is it a gene that is truly specific to PsA (and Crohn's), and if so, does it regulate the onset, or severity of the disease? Alternatively, does *CARD15* regulate an inflammatory response that is important for other diseases as well? Is *CARD15* a general susceptibility gene for PsA, or does it apply specifically to the population studied—the generally homogeneous residents of Newfoundland, almost exclusively white and of Northern European descent? And finally, are there other genes that are equally, or even more important in PsA? The answer to that question is almost certainly, yes.

Also noted: in a similar vein, Brown et al.[1] searched for genetic loci associated with disease activity in ankylosing spondylitis. They observed that regions on chromosome 18p, 2q, and, perhaps, 11p were associated with disease activity. Although they did not identify the putative genes involved, none of these regions encodes the MHC, again indicating that non-MHC genes clearly regulate the members of the seronegative spondyloarthropathy group.

M. H. Pillinger, MD

Reference

1. Brown MA, Brophy S, Bradbury L, et al: Identification of major loci controlling clinical manifestations of ankylosing spondylitis. *Arthritis Rheum* 48:2234-2239, 2003.

Mechanisms of TNF-α- and RANKL-Mediated Osteoclastogenesis and Bone Resorption in Psoriatic Arthritis
Ritchlin CT, Haas-Smith SA, Li P, et al (Univ of Rochester, NY; Cleveland Clinic, Ohio)
J Clin Invest 111:821-831, 2003   4–2

Background.—Extensive bone resorption occurs in psoriatic arthritis (PsA), an inflammatory joint disease. However, the mechanisms underlying bone loss in this setting have not been defined. To determine these mechanisms, a study was done.

Methods and Findings.—During joint replacement surgery, synovium, cartilage, and bone specimens were obtained from 5 patients with PsA, 4 with rheumatoid arthritis (RA), and 4 with osteoarthritis (OA). Blood samples from patients with PsA, especially those with bone erosions on plain radiographs, showed a marked increase in osteoclast precursors (OCPs) compared with samples from healthy persons. In addition, peripheral blood mononuclear cells (PBMCs) from patients with PsA readily formed osteoclasts in vitro, with no exogenous receptor activator of NF-κB ligand (RANKL) or macrophage colony-stimulating factor (MCSF). Osteoclast formation was inhibited by osteoprotegerin (OPG) as well as anti-TNF-α antibodies. Compared with the control group, cultured PBMCs in the PsA group spontaneously secreted greater concentrations of TNF-α. After anti-TNF treatment, OCP frequency markedly decreased in vivo in patients with PsA. In PsA specimens, immunohistochemical analysis of subchondral bone and synovium demonstrated RANK-positive perivascular mononuclear cells and osteoclasts. The expression of RANKL was upregulated substantially in the synovial lining layer, whereas OPG immunostaining was limited to the endothelium.

Conclusions.—A model is proposed for understanding the pathogenesis of aggressive bone erosion in patients with PsA (Fig 12). Osteoclast precursors may arise from TNF-α-activated PBMCs, which migrate to the inflamed synovium and subchondral bone. Here they are exposed to unopposed RANKL and TNF-α. This results in osteoclastogenesis at the erosion front and in subchondral bone, effects that lead to a bidirectional assault on psoriatic bone.

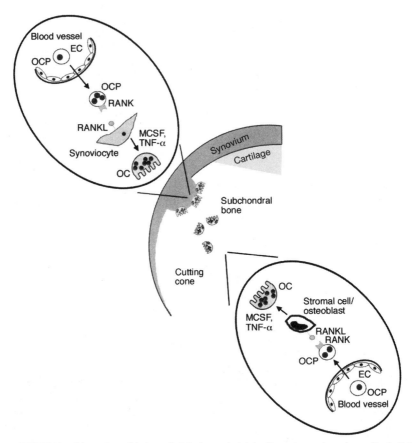

FIGURE 12.—Schematic model of osteolysis in the psoriatic joint. Extensive erosions observed in the PsA joint are mediated by a bidirectional attack on bone. We propose that circulating OCPs enter the synovium and are induced to become osteoclasts by RANKL expressed by synoviocytes (outside-in). In parallel, OCPs traverse endothelial cells in the subchondral bone and undergo osteoclastogenesis following RANKL stimulation from osteoblasts and stromal cells (inside-out). (Republished with permission of the *Journal of Clinical Investigation* from Ritchlin CT, Haas-Smith SA, Li P, et al: Mechanisms of TNF-α- and RANKL-mediated osteoclastogenesis and bone resorption in psoriatic arthritis. *J Clin Invest* 111:821-831, 2003. Reproduced by permission of the publisher via Copyright Clearance Center, Inc.)

▶ Relatively few studies have specifically addressed the mechanisms through which PsA damages joints. In this report, Ritchlin et al describe an elegant series of studies that examine the role of osteoclasts in PsA. The authors observe that the bony lesion of PsA is characterized by an infiltrate of osteoclasts at the bone-synovial junction. Interestingly, osteoclasts were seen not only at the bone-synovial junction, but also within subchondral bone itself, suggesting a 2-faced attack on bone by these cells. Moreover, osteoclastogenesis appeared to be a systemic process: osteoclast precursors were found in dramatically increased numbers in the peripheral blood of patients with PsA compared with those of controls, suggesting that they influx into bone from the bloodstream. Additionally, the bloodstream of PsA patients contained a factor—almost certainly TNF-α—that stimulated osteoclastogenesis, as transfer of serum from PsA patients to monocytes of normal controls in vitro resulted in osteoclast formation. Both in vitro and in vivo, anti-TNF therapy resulted in reduced transformation of osteoclast precursors to osteoclasts, the reduced presence of osteoclasts in bone, and the reduced destruction of bone by osteoclasts. These sorts of studies are going to be critical to understanding the precise mechanisms of PsA and developing specific treatments for this potentially crippling disease.

M. H. Pillinger, MD

5 Osteoporosis

Introduction

The past few years have seen tremendous advances in the treatment of osteoporosis. The advent of bisphosphonates, the more recent introduction of parathyroid hormone, and even the appreciation of cardiovascular risk in the use of estrogen have all represented opportunities for us to improve the treatment of our patients with this "silent" disease. It would only be natural to expect that, with each new year, we would be able to report additional advances in osteoporosis therapy. This year, however, was marked by 2 significant disappointments. As discussed below, Black et al (Abstract 5–1) show that the next logical step in osteoporosis treatment—combination therapy using simultaneous administration of a bisphosphonate and parathyroid hormone—appears to be a bust. And LaCroix et al (Abstract 5–2) show that statins—which have recently been touted for their possible utility in a variety of diseases—are probably not useful for treating osteoporosis. These are important studies, albeit disappointing ones. The work, of course, goes on.

Michael H. Pillinger, MD

The Effects of Parathyroid Hormone and Alendronate Alone or in Combination in Postmenopausal Osteoporosis

Black DM, for the PaTH Study Investigators (Univ of California, San Francisco; et al)
N Engl J Med 349:1207-1215, 2003   5–1

Background.—The use of antiresorptive drugs is established practice for the prevention of osteoporotic fractures in patients with osteoporosis. Studies have shown that nitrogen-containing bisphosphonates, such as alendronate and risedronate, reduce the risk of fracture and increase bone mineral density by suppressing bone resorption. Unlike bisphosphonates, parathyroid hormone is anabolic when administered intermittently for osteoporosis. Tested was the hypothesis that concurrent administration of alendronate and parathyroid hormone would increase bone density more than the use of either agent alone.

Methods.—A total of 238 postmenopausal women not using bisphosphonates were enrolled in this study. All of the women had low bone mineral density at the hip or spine as determined by a T score of less than -2.5 or a T score of less than -2.0 with an additional risk factor for osteoporosis. The women were randomly assigned to daily treatment with parathyroid hormone (100 μg, 119 women), alendronate (10 mg, 60 women) or both (59 women) and were followed up for 12 months. Dual-energy x-ray absorptiometry and quantitative CT were used to assess bone mineral density at the spine and hip. Markers of bone marrow turnover were measured in fasting blood samples.

Results.—An increase in the bone mineral density at the spine was manifest in all treatment groups, and there was no significant difference in the increase between the parathyroid hormone group and the combination therapy group. The volumetric density of the trabecular bone at the spine was significantly increased in all groups; however, the increase in the parathyroid hormone group was nearly twice that in the other groups. Bone formation was significantly increased in the parathyroid hormone group but not in the combination-therapy group. Bone resorption decreased in the combination-therapy group and the alendronate group.

Conclusion.—No evidence of synergy between parathyroid hormone and alendronate was found in this study. However, changes in the volumetric density of trabecular bone, the cortical volume at the hip, and levels of markers of bone turnover provide evidence that the concurrent use of alendronate may reduce the anabolic effects of parathyroid hormone. There is a need for longer-term studies of fractures to determine whether and how antiresorptive drugs can be optimally used in conjunction with parathyroid hormone therapy.

▶ The treatment of osteoporosis has undergone tremendous advances in recent years, and physicians now have an effective, if not yet ideal, panel of drugs for this condition. Bisphosphonates, calcitonin, selective estrogen receptor modulators, estrogen in some instances (less so now that the adverse effects of estrogen on coronary artery disease and malignancy are appreciated),[1] and, most recently, parathyroid hormone (PTH). Each has established a place in the treatment of osteoporosis. But how do we choose among them? And, can we use any of these agents together to achieve synergistic effects?

A combination of a bisphosphonate and PTH would seem to be a particularly intriguing combination. Since bisphosphonates block bone resorption and PTH stimulates bone formation, the 2 agents might complement each other to optimal effect. Alas, Black et al show that this is likely not the case. In an exceptionally well-done, fully blinded study, they compared the effects of alendronate, PTH, or both over the course of a year. Their end points were bone density—measured by both dual energy x-ray absorptiometry and quantitative CT, and analyzed as total, trabecular, and cortical density—and serum markers of bone turnover. At the very least, they observed no synergy between alendronate and PTH.

Indeed, in a number of outcomes where PTH led to more bone density increase than alendronate, treatment with the 2 together most resembled the alendronate group. Thus, alendronate may actually impair the effects of PTH. This actually makes some logical sense, as PTH is most active on actively remodeling bone, and bisphosphonates actually reduce overall bone remodeling. Still, many questions remain. Is this effect generalizable to other bisphosphonates and to the PTH peptide also currently in use? Would sequential use of PTH and bisphosphonate (in either order) result in synergy where concurrent use does not? Or does prior use of a bisphosphonate render subsequent PTH use ineffective? These are fascinating and important questions and testify not to our failure to understand osteoporosis, but rather to our ongoing success in this area.

Also noted: a smaller study by Finkelstein et al[2] looking at combination therapy with PTH and alendronate in men and reaching the same conclusions as the Black study.

M. H. Pillinger, MD

References

1. Rossouw JE, for the Women's Health Initiative Investigators: Risks and benefits of estrogen plus progestin in healthy postmenopausal women: Principal results from the Women's Health Initiative randomized controlled trial. *JAMA* 288:321-333, 2002. (2003 YEAR BOOK OF MEDICINE, pp 49-51.)
2. Finkelstein JS, Hayes A, Hunzelman JL, et al: The effects of parathyroid hormone, alendronate, or both in men with osteoporosis. *N Engl J Med* 349:1216-1226, 2003.

Statin Use, Clinical Fracture, and Bone Density in Postmenopausal Women: Results From the Women's Health Initiative Observational Study

LaCroix AZ, Cauley JA, Pettinger M, et al (Fred Hutchinson Cancer Research Ctr, Seattle; Univ of Pittsburgh, Pa; George Washington Univ, Washington, DC; et al)

Ann Intern Med 139:97-104, 2003   5–2

Background.—Several large multicenter trials have established the long-term efficacy and safety of 3-hydroxy-3-methylglutaryl coenzyme A (HMG-CoA) reductase inhibitors, or statins, for the prevention of coronary events in both men and women. Recent studies have also shown that statins stimulate bone formation in vitro and in vivo. In early epidemiologic studies, findings showed a lower risk for hip fracture among statin users than among nonusers. However, subsequent studies have produced mixed results. The association of statin use with the incidence of hip, lower arm or wrist, and other clinical fractures and with baseline levels of bone density was evaluated.

Methods.—The Women's Health Initiative Observational Study was a prospective study conducted in 40 clinical centers in the United States. A total of 93,716 postmenopausal women aged 50 to 79 years were enrolled in the study, which compared rates of hip, lower arm or wrist, and other clinical fractures among 7846 statin users and 85,870 nonusers over a median follow-up of 3.9 years. In 6442 women enrolled at 3 clinical centers, baseline levels of total hip, posterior-anterior spine, and total-body bone density measured by dual-energy x-ray absorptiometry were compared on the basis of statin use.

Results.—Statin users and nonusers were found to have similar age-adjusted rates of hip, lower arm or wrist, and other clinical fractures, regardless of the duration of statin use. There was no statistically significant difference in bone density levels between statin users and nonusers at any skeletal site after adjustment for age, ethnicity, body mass index, and other factors.

Conclusion.—The Women's Health Initiative Observational Study found that statin use did not improve fracture risk or bone density. The use of statins for the prevention or treatment of osteoporosis is not supported by the cumulative evidence.

▶ Statins are fascinating drugs. Because they inhibit HMG-CoA–mediated biosynthesis of prenyl groups, they reduce cholesterol biosynthesis but also have the capacity to block the synthesis of prenyl groups that modify and modulate the actions of a number of families of intracellular signaling molecules. One of the most interesting possible effects of statins has seemed to be on bone metabolism. Both in vitro and in animal models, statins stimulate bone formation, and initial epidemiologic human studies seemed to confirm a similar effect in people. These human studies were small, however, and some follow-up studies have failed to support a beneficial effect.

More data were needed, and LaCroix et al have now supplied an important study, to disappointing effect. They took advantage of the Women's Health Initiative Observational Study to look at fracture rates among 93,716 postmenopausal women aged 50 to 79 years. The results showed no decrease in fracture rate at any site, nor any improvement in bone density in statin users versus nonusers.

Alas, what works in rodents does not always work in humans. So although statins remain among our best drugs for lowering serum lipids (and although this study doesn't rule out the possibility that a specific group of patients might still respond to statins for osteoporosis), we are forced to conclude that clinicians cannot kill the two birds of hypercholesterolemia and osteoporosis with the single stone of HMG-CoA reductase inhibition. Newer and better drugs will continue to be required.

Also noted: a study by Leung et al indicating that, in a murine model at least, simvastatin markedly inhibits not only developing but also clinically-evident collagen-induced arthritis.[1]

M. H. Pillinger, MD

Reference

1. Leung BP, Sattar N, Crilly A, et al: A novel anti-inflammatory role for simvastatin in inflammatory arthritis. *J Immunol* 170:1524-1530, 2003.

6 Pain and Pain Syndromes

Introduction

Rheumatologists are trained to manage and/or treat the inflammatory autoimmune processes that lead to tissue damage. We probably spend less time thinking about pain management, despite the fact that almost all of our patients suffer from pain of one form or another. In this chapter, we report a few of the more interesting and/or important articles of the year concerning rheumatologic pain. In the first report, Zelman et al (Abstract 6–1) describe a very interesting study that defines the meaning of numerical pain scales in osteoarthritis and low back pain (one hopes that they will go on to do the same for pain scales in inflammatory arthritis). The second report by Dobkin et al (Abstract 6–2) documents an interesting phenomenon: that patients think their rheumatologists do a better job with fibromyalgia than the rheumatologists themselves do. In the last article, Assendelft et al (Abstract 6–3) perform a meta-analysis of spinal manipulation for low back pain. They conclude that the data do not support spinal manipulation as a valid treatment in most patients with this sometimes incapacitating and always frustrating condition.

Michael H. Pillinger, MD

Development of a Metric for a Day of Manageable Pain Control: Derivation of Pain Severity Cut-Points for Low Back Pain and Osteoarthritis
Zelman DC, Hoffman DL, Seifeldin R, et al (California School of Professional Psychology-Alliant Internatl Univ, Alameda; Purdue Pharma LP, Stanford, Conn)
Pain 106:35-42, 2003
6–1

Background.—Methods to quantify pain are needed both for research and for clinical practice. One approach derives from the "episode-free day" concept that emerged in the asthma literature and is now used for other conditions. This study attempted to quantify a day of manageable pain control or a "manageable day." The term "manageable day" emerged from focus group findings that for patients with persistent moderate to severe pain, a "pain-free day" was unrealistic, but a day with enough pain control to be manageable was a realistic daily goal. The primary research objective was to derive a single cut-point on a 0 to 10 numeric scale of average pain that would support the concept of the manageable day metric. A secondary objective was to derive double cut-points.

Study Design.—The study group consisted of 96 patients with chronic low back pain (LBP) and 98 patients with osteoarthritis (OA). Participants were required to be at least 18 years of age, have pain that they rated as an average of "4" of at least 1-year duration, and to use analgesic medication daily. All participants completed the Brief Pain Inventory (BPI) and the Medical Outcomes Study (OAS). Participants with LBP completed the Oswestry Questionnaire and the Roland Morris Questionnaire. Those with OA completed the Western Ontario McMaster Universities Osteoarthritis Index.

One week before the structured interview, participants completed pain and functional interference assessments at home. One week later, they were interviewed with the use of the same assessments. The 2 scores were averaged. Analyses were conducted separately for the 2 patient groups. The first analyses were used to derive a single cut-point on the 0 to 10 BPI Average Pain scale. The second analyses were used to derive a double cut-point to be used for classifying pain as "low, medium, high" or "mild, moderate, severe." A third set of analyses derived a single cut-point from measures of functional disability.

Findings.—For each patient group, "5" was the cut-point on the BPI 0 to 10 numeric scale of average daily pain that optimally distinguished a manageable day of pain relief. For patients with LBP, "5" and "7" were the double cut-points and for patients with OA, "5" and "8" were the double cut-points. These cut-points were confirmed with assessments of functional disability.

Conclusion.—This research establishes "5" as the optimal BPI Average Pain cut-point that distinguishes manageable pain for patients with persistent moderate to severe OA or LBP. This result was stable across both groups, who have different pain severity and functional disability. This supports the use of "5 or less" on the numeric 0 to 10 BPI Average Pain scale as a possible criterion for a "manageable day" metric for patients with chronic pain.

▶ As rheumatologists, most of us ask our patients the question many times a day: "On a scale of 1 to 10, how badly does your arthritis hurt?" But when our patients answer us with a number, what exactly do they mean? In this interesting study, Zelman et al examine this question from a rigorous, psychometric perspective. They studied 96 patients with LBP and 98 patients with OA and obtained these patients' responses to a 0 to 10 scale of an average daily pain. They also obtained the patients' responses to a number of questions about function and then used statistical techniques to compare the pain and functional reports.

The result was the derivation of a so-called "cut-point"—a pain number that best separates dysfunction from the ability to function. The results for both the OA patients and the LBP patients were the same: the cut-point between function and dysfunction depended upon whether the patient's pain report was above or below 5.

The authors also used a similar technique to identify a double cut-point (for high, intermediate, and low function, useful in some studies). In the case of the double cut-point, the OA and LBP scales gave slightly different results. In particular, the double cut-points for OA and LBP were 5 to 7 and 5 to 8, respectively, suggesting that pain may mean something slightly different for the 2 distinct problems.

One interesting result that came out of this and a related study was the psychological meaning of the scores above and below 5. With some other medical diagnoses, the goal of treatment in studies is a "symptom-free" or "attack-free" day; in the case of some cancers, a "pain-free" day is a target of treatment. In these musculoskeletal diseases, however, the authors used focus group methodology to confirm what rheumatologists knew already: that for many of our patients with chronic pain, a symptom-free day is not yet achievable. However, the authors also identified a theme among OA and LBP patients, specifically, their recognition that they would not be pain free but that they could achieve manageable levels of pain that would permit them to function in their routine activities. Such a "manageable day" correlated well with the cut-point report of a pain score less than 5.

In treating our OA and LBP patients then, we should recognize that getting a patient's pain score from above to below 5 is a significant step along the way to restoring the patient to a manageable, if not yet normal, life. Whether 5 is the right cut-point for pain in other rheumatologic diseases remains to be determined, but the same principles applies and it should be possible to rigorously ascertain the right cut-point for these conditions as well.

M. H. Pillinger, MD

Patient-Physician Discordance in Fibromyalgia
Dobkin PL, De Civita M, Abrahamowicz M, et al (McGill Univ, Montreal)
J Rheumatol 30:1326-1334, 2003   6–2

Background.—The prevalence of fibromyalgia is estimated at 3.4% for women and 0.5% for men. Fibromyalgia is the second most common diagnosis in rheumatology clinics, and data from Europe, South America, the United States, and Canada collectively indicate that fibromyalgia is a major cause of morbidity. Fibromyalgia may coexist with other rheumatic diseases, such as lupus, and in many patients it presents in conjunction with a number of conditions, such as irritable bowel syndrome and chronic fatigue syndrome. Heath care providers tend to avoid contact with fibromyalgia patients, and these patients may, in turn, believe themselves to be misunderstood and rejected by health care providers. The discordance between patients' and physicians' health perceptions and satisfaction with the office visit in fibromyalgia was examined.

Methods.—A group of 182 women with fibromyalgia were examined by a rheumatologist to confirm the diagnosis. The patients and physicians inde-

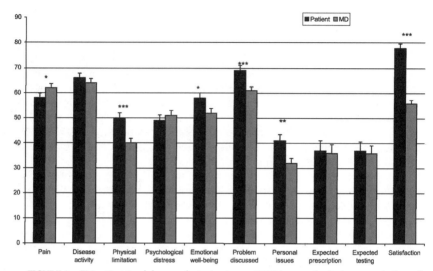

FIGURE 1.—FM patients' and rheumatologists' ratings on PPDS items and paired t test results for each item. *$P < .01$, **$P < .001$, ***$P < .0001$. *Abbreviations: FM*, Fibromyalgia; *PPDS*, Patient-Physician Discordance Scale. (Courtesy of Dobkin PL, De Civita M, Abrahamowicz M, et al: Patient-physician discordance in fibromyalgia. *J Rheumatol* 30:1326-1334, 2003.)

pendently completed the Patient-Physician Discordance Scale regarding their perceptions of health and satisfaction with the office visit. The patients also completed questionnaires concerning sociodemographics, social support, disability, perceived stress, and psychological distress after the office visit. Separate generalized estimating equations with forward selection were modeled for each measure of discordance, with control for the possible dependence of outcomes among patients of the same physician.

Results.—The highest discordance score occurred in the rating of satisfaction with the office visit, as physicians systematically underestimated the patients' level of satisfaction (Fig 1). Higher levels of satisfaction with social support and increased psychological distress were marginally associated with greater discordance in rating of physical functioning. Higher levels of satisfaction with social support, younger age, and lower disability were associated with greater discordance on well-being. A history of sexual abuse was significantly associated with greater discordance on ratings of satisfaction with the office visit.

Conclusions.—A gap exists between what patients with fibromyalgia and rheumatologists examining them experience during the office visit.

▶ If some of us inwardly groan each time a fibromyalgia patient comes into the office, it's not from any innate lack of sympathy. On the contrary, I would argue exactly the opposite: it is actually our desire to help, coupled with our expectations of futility in treating this condition, that leads us to sometimes regret that fibromyalgia is a rheumatic condition. But is our sense of futility a proper one? Or is it our expectations that may be awry?

In this study, Dobkin et al examine the perceptions of patients and physicians after a fibromyalgia visit. Patients and physicians independently completed the Patient-Physician Discordance Scale, and patients also filled in details about their demographics, social support, disability, and psychological distress, among others. Patients and physicians were in accord on most features of the visit, including the patient's level of pain, disease activity, limitation, distress, and the appropriate level of testing and treatment. But a striking discrepancy was observed regarding the question of patient satisfaction with the visit. In fact, patients had significantly more positive opinions about their visit than their physicians predicted they would have. Patients with stonger social supports and better functioning were even more satisfied than the rest (and even more discordant with their physician's assessment of patient satisfaction), but the bottom line remained that in general, fibromyalgia patients seemed to like what their doctors were doing for them better than their doctors thought they should. Is the difference really one of expectations, and is it possible that physicians think they should be doing more for their patients than their patients think possible? If so, perhaps we physicians need to be a bit easier on ourselves and support our patients through their problems. We may not be curing our patients with fibromyalgia, and we may not be doing as well as we'd like, but just by being there, we may be doing well enough for now.

M. H. Pillinger, MD

Spinal Manipulative Therapy for Low Back Pain: A Meta-analysis of Effectiveness Relative to Other Therapies
Assendelft WJJ, Morton SC, Yu EI, et al (Cochrane Back Review Group, Toronto; Cochrane Back Review Group, Amsterdam; Dutch College of Gen Practitioners, Utrecht, The Netherlands; et al)
Ann Intern Med 138:871-881, 2003   6–3

Background.—Low back pain is burdensome, both to the individual patient and to western societies as a whole, because of lost work time and increased medical expenditures. Spinal manipulative therapy has been widely used for the treatment of low back pain, but the previous systematic reviews and practice guidelines have reached conflicting conclusions on the effectiveness of spinal manipulative therapy for the treatment of low back pain. The discrepancies related to use of spinal manipulative therapy were examined. Previous estimates of the effectiveness of spinal manipulative therapy were updated by comparing it with other therapies and then incorporating data from recent high-quality randomized controlled trials (RCTs) into the analysis.

Methods.—Data from MEDLINE, EMBASE, CINAHL, the Cochrane Controlled Trials Register, and previous systematic reviews were used. RCTs that evaluated spinal manipulative therapy in patients with low back pain with at least 1 day of follow-up and at least one clinically relevant outcome measure were reviewed.

Results.—A total of 39 RCTs were identified. Meta-regression models were developed for acute or chronic pain and for short-term and long-term pain and function. For patients with acute low back pain, spinal manipulative therapy was superior only to sham therapy or to therapies determined to be ineffective or even harmful. Spinal manipulative therapy provided no statistically significant advantage over care provided by a general practitioner, use of analgesics, physical therapy, exercises, or back school. Similar results were obtained in patients with chronic low back pain. Radiation of pain, study quality, profession of manipulator, and use of manipulation alone or in combination with other therapeutic approaches did not affect these results.

Conclusions.—This meta-analysis found no evidence to support the contention that spinal manipulative therapy is more beneficial than other standard treatments for patients with acute or chronic low back pain.

▶ Low back pain remains one of the most common problems that rheumatologists, and general practitioners, face in their day-to-day practice. Moreover, low back pain is a problem of both medical and economic importance, since it is a major cause of disability and missed work. The therapies for low back pain are legion, and each—analgesia, anti-inflammatory drugs, physical therapy, back school, surgery, and the like—has its adherents. The data, alas, remain poor, and true believers in one treatment or another generally have no reason to convert to another spinal cult.

One of the most highly utilized and highly regarded treatments has been spinal manipulation. The notion that manipulation of tender, inflamed, or malaligned spinal structures may improve pain and function seems reasonable enough, and it even has studies to support it. But how good those studies are, and whether they trump studies advocating other therapies, has remained a mystery. In this report, the Cochrane Group has turned its focus to low back pain to try and determine whether the evidence supports the superiority, or even use, of spinal manipulative therapy. Assendelft and colleagues have performed a meta-analysis of 53 articles detailing the use of spinal manipulation. Their study differs from previous meta-analyses and reviews in a number of significant ways. First, they benefit from the availability of a number of newer, more rigorously performed studies of the subject (much of the older literature is of limited statistical value). Second, they benefit from the latest meta-analytic techniques and the experience of the Cochrane group in evidence-based medicine. Finally, they structure their evaluations to compare spinal manipulation not merely with all comers, but with specific, individual treatments or groups of treatments.

The results provide some ammunition for both detractors and supporters of spinal manipulation. For the detractors, spinal manipulation was no better than just about any other reasonable treatment for low back pain, including physical therapy, exercise, general practitioner's care, and analgesia, as well as back school. In fact, the only treatments that spinal manipulation appeared to be superior to were either sham treatments or treatments considered to lack evidence of benefit or to show evidence of harm, including traction, corset, bed rest, diathermy, and topical agents. If you are a supporter of spinal manipulation, you will now note that, in fact, these latter observations indicate that spinal manipulation is really better than no useful treatment at all. Fair enough; but the benefits of manipulation—as well as for other "effective" therapies— are modest at best, and back pain remains a pain in the back for patients and clinicians alike.

Also noted: a review by Cherkin et al,[1] in the same issue of the *Annals of Internal Medicine*, comparing acupuncture, massage therapy, and spinal manipulation for back pain. The authors concluded that the quality of the acupuncture studies was too poor to permit interpretation, that manipulation had a small clinical benefit, and that massage was probably better, and cheaper than the other 2 alternatives.

M. H. Pillinger, MD

Reference

1. Cherkin DC, Sherman KJ, Deyo RA, et al: A review of the evidence for the effectiveness, safety, and cost of acupuncture, massage therapy, and spinal manipulation for back pain. *Ann Intern Med* 138:898-906, 2003.

7 Periodic Fever Syndromes

Introduction

Periodic fever syndromes—familial Mediterranean fever (FMF), TRAPS (tumor necrosis factor receptor-associated periodic syndrome, formerly called familial Hibernian fever), and the hyper-IgD syndrome—are characterized by intermittent paroxysms of organ-based inflammation, accompanied by fever and, in many cases, by secondary amyloidosis. Beyond that, it is fair to say that, until several years ago, we knew virtually nothing about these diseases. However, in the last decade, pioneering studies have led to the identification of genes responsible for each of these diseases and, to a limited extent at least, the beginning of an understanding of how they occur. While these diseases are rare events for many physicians, they are common in their traditional geographic areas. Moreover, their biology provides insight into the mechanisms of other rheumatologic diseases.

The studies abstracted here perform a useful task: they redefine the scope of our ignorance. In the case of FMF, Cazeneuve et al (Abstract 7–1) use sophisticated population genetics to conclude that, at least in a small percentage of cases, the gene for what we call FMF must in fact be different from the one that we have so recently come to take for granted. Aganna et al (Abstract 7–2) use more traditional genetic analyses to show that a percentage of patients with TRAPS have no mutation at all in the gene recently identified as responsible for that disease. Again, in these patients the offending gene must lie elsewhere. These studies in no way diminish the accomplishments of the past few years. Rather, they remind us that there are many roads to Rome, and that multiple genotypes can lead to a single phenotype. They also remind us what an exciting, unending endeavor investigative medicine can and must be.

Michael H. Pillinger, MD

Familial Mediterranean Fever Among Patients From Karabakh and the Diagnostic Value of *MEFV* Gene Analysis in All Classically Affected Populations
Cazeneuve C, Hovannesyan Z, Geneviève D, et al (Hôpital Henri-Mondor, Crèteil, France; Natl Academy of Sciences, Yerevan, Armenia; Stepanakert Clinic, Karabakh)
Arthritis Rheum 48:2324-2331, 2003   7–1

Background.—Familial Mediterranean fever (FMF) is characterized by recurrent episodes of fever and serosal inflammation associated with increased erythrocyte sedimentation rate and increased serum levels of acute-phase proteins. It is most common among Armenian, Sephardic Jewish, Turkish, and Arabic populations. The diagnosis of FMF is one of exclusion. Recently, mutations in the gene *MEFV* have been associated with this condition in many, but not all, cases. A cohort of FMF patients was analyzed in Karabakh to further clarify the value of *MEFV* analysis for diagnosis.

Study Design.—The study group consisted of 50 consecutive FMF patients from 39 unrelated families living in Karabakh. All patients had *MEFV* mutation analysis. The expected distribution of alleles was compared to that expected by the Hardy-Weinberg equilibrium.

Findings.—There were 6 different *MEFV* mutations present in the Karabakh FMF population. The distribution of genotypes among the Karabakhian patients was significantly different from the Hardy-Weinberg equilibrium. Literature review confirmed that this was true of all populations analyzed. This suggests the existence of an FMF-like syndrome that is not related to mutations in the *MEFV* gene.

Conclusion.—Results of a molecular analysis of the *MEFV* gene performed in a cohort of patients from Karabakh with familial Mediterranean fever suggest that there is an FMF-like syndrome that is not related to mutations in the *MEFV* gene. The identification of this gene(s) will be essential for defining the nature of FMF in these populations.

▶ One of the most exciting stories in rheumatology in recent years has been the identification of the gene that causes FMF. That gene, known as *MEFV1*, encodes a protein called pyrin that is found almost exclusively in neutrophils and, to a lesser extent, in microphages. While the exact role of this gene is not known, it appears to play a role in the regulation of inflammation, and any one of several identified mutations in *MEFV1* has been associated with the phenotype of FMF.

Indeed, testing for the better-known mutations is now commercially available and is extremely helpful in making the diagnosis of FMF, especially when the presentation is atypical or—as is the case in the United States—the penetration of the disease is low. With the identification of *MEFV1*, the hard nut of FMF appeared to be cracked.

On the other hand, a small percentage of patients with seemingly classic FMF routinely test negative for known *MEFV1* mutations. What are we to make of this? Does it imply the existence of *MEFV1* mutations that have not yet been identified? Or do some patients with typical (or atypical) FMF actually have a different disease?

Cazeneuve et al have employed population genetics to address these questions. The population they examined included patients with clinical FMF from Karabakh, a country with a high penetrance of the disease. They also compared their data to previously obtained data from Armenians, Sephardic Jews, Turks, and Arabs. They observed that the groups varied in the prevalence of known *MEFV1* mutations, implying a likely founder effect for each population. What each group had in common, however, was the fact that at least 10% of FMF patients had no recognizable *MEFV1* mutations.

By analyzing the distribution of mutation according to Hardy-Weinberg principles, the authors were able to show that the number of FMF patients with no identifiable *MEFV1* mutation far exceeded what would be expected from a binomial distribution of previously unidentified alleles. That is, there were too many patients without identifiable *MEFV1* mutations to be accounted for by a simple failure to identify some unknown mutations in the gene. Rather, the authors conclude that their data point to the presence of at least 1 additional, non-*MEFV1* gene capable of causing an FMF-like picture. In fact, among patients with FMF symptoms but no identifiable *MEFV1* mutations, the likelihood that a new gene was involved was extremely high, ranging from 85% to 99% in the different populations.

In essence, therefore, the authors appear to have defined a new disease very like the traditional *MEFV1* disease but driven by a different engine. Whether they are correct remains to be seen, and the newly implicated gene (s) remains unidentified. Meanwhile, these observations provide some insight into FMF patients who lack an identifiable *MEFV1* mutation.

We are wondrously mysterious creatures, and our questions are like swords, cutting one by one through the mysteries of human biology. But like Hercules battling the multiheaded Hydra, each time we smote a question, 2 new ones spring up to take its place. How wonderful to be living in this heroic age of science!

M. H. Pillinger, MD

Heterogeneity Among Patients With Tumor Necrosis Factor Receptor-Associated Periodic Syndrome Phenotypes

Aganna E, Hammond L, Hawkins PN, et al (MRCPI, London; Royal Free Hosp, London; IDIBAPS, Barcelona; et al)
Arthritis Rheum 48:2632-2644, 2003   7–2

Background.—Tumor necrosis factor receptor-associated periodic syndrome (TRAPS) is a relapsing, remitting multisystem chronic inflammatory disorder that is dominantly inherited. The phenotype and clinical severity of this disorder vary. Characteristic features are recurrent fever, abdominal pain, and cutaneous and synovial inflammation lasting for several days to weeks or more. The prevalence of TRAPS among outpatients seeking care for recurrent fevers and clinical features consistent with the disorder was investigated.

Methods.—The affected members of 18 families including multiple members with TRAPS-like symptoms underwent mutational screening. One hundred seventy-six consecutive patients with nonfamilial TRAPS-like symptoms were also studied. Plasma levels of soluble tumor necrosis factor receptor superfamily 1A (sTNFRSF1A) were measured. Fluorescence-activated cell sorter analysis was also done to determine TNFRSF1A shedding from monocytes.

Findings.—Analysis identified 8 novel and 3 previously reported TNFRSF1A missense mutations. These included an amino acid deletion in a Northern Irish family and a C70S mutation in a Japanese family, both reported for the first time. Patients with nonfamilial TRAPS had only 3 TNFRSF1A variants. Three members of a "prototype familial Hibernian fever" family did not have C33Y, which was present in 9 other affected members, suggesting a nonalleleic heterogeneity in TRAPS-like disorders. Plasma sTNFRSF1A concentrations were low in patients with no renal amyloidosis, in mutation-negative symptomatic persons in 4 families, and in 8% of patients with nonfamilial TRAPS. Patients with the T50M and T50K variants, but not patients with other variants, had reduced shedding of TNFRSF1A from monocytes.

Conclusions.—The genetic basis of TRAPS-like features is heterogeneous. Not uncommonly, TNFRSF1A mutations correlate with nonfamilial recurrent fevers of unknown origin.

▶ The familial Hibernian fever syndrome (FHF) has recently been renamed TRAPS, based on an increased understanding of its pathogenesis. This syndrome, found most frequently among Europeans (particularly of Scottish and Irish descent), presents with fever, abdominal pain, rash and inflammatory arthritis, along with other symptoms. Amyloidosis may also occur. In contrast to familial Mediterranean fever (FMF; autosomal recessive) TRAPS is autosomal dominant; as in the case of FMF, a gene has recently been identified in its etiologic pathogenesis. In TRAPS, the gene is question encodes the TNF receptor superfamily 1A (TNFRSF1A). Missense mutations in a limited number of TNFRSF1A codons results in impaired cleavage of TNF receptors on the cell surface, and hence, a paucity of soluble TNF receptor (sTNFR) to sop up extracellular TNF. TRAPS, thus, becomes a disease of TNF overactivity, due to failed regulation. Case closed.

Well, maybe not always. In this rigorous study, Aganna et al examined the *TNFRSF1A* gene in 18 families with TRAPS, as well as 176 nonfamilial (sporadic) cases of TRAPS-like illness. What they observed did not always fit the prevailing paradigm. First, not all patients with TRAPS had the gene mutations previously described. In fact, more than twice as many patients with *TNFRSF1A* mutations had novel, as opposed to previously established mutations in the gene. In 1 family with TRAPS, 3 affected family members failed to show any mutation in the gene (the rest of the family had a common mutation), suggesting that other factors must be in play. The role of *TNRFSF1A* was even more questionable in the sporadic cases of TRAPS: only 4 of 176 had any mutation in the receptor superfamily gene. The failure of affected individuals to shed TNFR was usually associated with *TNFRSF1A* mutations, but some patients with *TNFRS1A* mutations failed to show reduced levels of sTNFR. On the other hand, 4 families and 14 patients with sporadic TRAPS had decreased sTNFR despite no mutation in *TNFRSF1A*, suggesting that other genes or proteins or both must also regulate TNFR shedding.

These data are humbling, but in a good way. They indicate that while we have learned a lot about TRAPS in the last few years, there is ample opportunity to learn more, and to consider new ways to help our patients. And while TRAPS itself is not a common condition, the importance of TNF to so many rheumatologic illnesses suggests that a better understanding of TRAPS and TNF regulation may ultimately reap benefits for a much larger group of patients.

M. H. Pillinger, MD

8 Progressive Systemic Sclerosis

Introduction

Systemic sclerosis and its variants continue to arouse both intrigue and frustration among rheumatologists. We have gotten much better at managing the adverse consequences of these conditions—particularly scleroderma renal crisis and, more recently, scleroderma lung disease and pulmonary hypertension—but control of the basic process continues to elude us. Indeed, because systemic sclerosis is such a slowly progressive disease, even assessing the disease activity and determining short- or long-term prognosis are as much guesswork as anything else. Serologies have been no help; certain antibodies are helpful in diagnosing scleroderma, but they have not been thought to vary with disease severity or activity.

For this chapter, we include 2 selections. The first from Hill et al (Abstract 8–1) provides strong evidence of a relatively unappreciated problem in systemic sclerosis. The authors show that malignancies—both before and after the initial recognition of the disease—are significantly more common among patients with scleroderma than in the general population. Hu et al (Abstract 8–2) address the topic of serologies in systemic sclerosis. This group, from the University of Pittsburgh, is one of the foremost systemic sclerosis research groups in the world. In this case, they have developed a highly reproducible assay for a typical systemic sclerosis antibody, directed at DNA topoisomerase I. Using this assay—which should readily lend itself to future commercialization—they demonstrate that anti-topoisomerase I antibodies do, in fact, vary with disease activity. Not only that, they may also predict systemic sclerosis flares. Like the disease itself, our understanding of systemic sclerosis proceeds slowly, sometimes almost unnoticeably. But our progress is also inexorable, and someday, the disease itself will not be.

Michael H. Pillinger, MD

Risk of Cancer in Patients With Scleroderma: A Population Based Cohort Study

Hill CL, Nguyen A-M, Roder D, et al (Queen Elizabeth Hosp, Woodville, Australia; Dept of Human Services, Adelaide, Australia; Anti-Cancer Found, Eastwood, Australia; et al)
Ann Rheum Dis 62:728-731, 2003   8–1

Background.—It has been suggested that scleroderma is associated with an increased risk of cancer. This population-based, retrospective cohort study examined the association between scleroderma and cancer.

Study Design.—Patients with scleroderma (78 men and 363 women) were identified from the South Australian Scleroderma Registry. They were further subdivided by scleroderma type: limited, diffuse, and overlap or other. Patients with scleroderma were followed up until January 1, 2001, or their death. Cancer diagnoses were obtained from the South Australian Cancer Registry. The number of cancers expected for this cohort were calculated. Standardized incidence ratios (SIRs) were obtained indirectly by dividing cancers observed by cancers expected and deriving 95% confidence intervals. Analyses were performed for all cancers and for specific types of cancer when numbers were sufficient. Analyses were also performed for total scleroderma and for each subtype. Cancers occurring before scleroderma diagnosis were also analyzed.

Findings.—Of the 441 patients with scleroderma, there were 90 cases of cancer. Of these cancers, 47 developed after diagnosis of scleroderma. The SIRs for all cancers among all scleroderma patients were significantly increased (Table 2) compared with cancer incidence rates of the general population. The SIRs for cancer were most increased among those with diffuse scleroderma. The SIRs for lung cancer were specifically significantly increased. The SIRs for breast cancer were also increased, but they tended to occur before the diagnosis of scleroderma. Bladder and prostate cancer were also more common among scleroderma patients.

TABLE 2.—Standardized Incidence Ratios and 95% Confidence Intervals of Cancer

Type (ICD-9 Code)	Obs	Men SIR (95% CI)	Obs	Women SIR (95% CI)	Obs	Total SIR (95% CI)
All cancer sites (140-208)	16	2.79 (1.59 to 4.53)	31	1.73 (1.18 to 2.46)	47	1.99 (1.46 to 2.65)
Lung (162)	8	9.32 (4.02 to 18.37)	4	3.41 (0.93 to 8.72)	12	5.9 (3.05 to 10.31)
Breast (174)			8	1.62 (0.7 to 3.19)		
Prostate (185)	3	2.41 (0.5 to 7.03)				
Bladder (188)	1	2.71 (0.08 to 15.07)	2	3.93 (0.47 to 14.19)	3	3.42 (0.71 to 9.99)
Haematological (200-208)	0	0.00 (0.00 to 7.98)	2	1.56 (0.19 to 5.64)	2	1.15 (0.14 to 4.14)
Gastrointestinal (150-154)	0	0.00 (0.00 to 3.49)	4	1.22 (0.33 to 3.13)	4	0.92 (0.25 to 2.36)
Remainder	4	2.29 (0.63 to 5.87)	11	1.86 (0.93 to 3.33)	15	1.96 (1.10 to 3.23)

Abbreviations: SIRs, Standardized incidence ratios; *CI,* confidence interval.

Conclusion.—All types of scleroderma are associated with increased malignancy risk. The greatest risk is associated with lung cancer.

▶ Rheumatologists are generally aware that dermatomyositis is accompanied by an increased risk of solid tumors and that Sjögren's syndrome brings an increased risk of lymphoma. But do any of our other diseases bring with them an increased risk of malignancy? In this study, Hill et al have taken advantage of the fact that South Australia maintains mandated registries on both scleroderma and malignancy, in order to ask about the relationship between scleroderma and cancer risk. They observe that nearly 20% of all scleroderma patients had cancer develop at some point or another, translating into a 2-fold increased risk of malignancy for these patients.

Patients with diffuse, as opposed to limited and other forms of scleroderma, had an even greater malignancy risk—up to almost 3-fold over the general population. The most common malignancy seen was lung cancer, which appeared 5 times more frequently in scleroderma patients than in the general population (9 times more frequently in men!). The authors speculate that the increased risk of lung malignancies may relate to the lung inflammation and/or damage seen in diffuse scleroderma, although the possibility also exists, for lung or other cancers, that the disease process itself (eg, a genetic background common to both scleroderma and cancer) or the treatments used may all have contributed to cancer risk.

Interestingly, the second most common malignancy seen—breast cancer—appeared to occur most commonly before rather than after the onset of scleroderma, prompting the authors to speculate that in these cases, scleroderma may actually have been a paraneoplastic consequence of breast malignancy. Other tumors that appeared more commonly included bladder (3- to 4-fold increased risk overall, and higher among women) and prostate (2- to 3-fold increased risk). These data indicate a need to be on the lookout for malignancy in our scleroderma patients, with proper regular screening, especially for lung, prostate, and perhaps bladder cancer.

M. H. Pillinger, MD

Correlation of Serum Anti-DNA Topoisomerase I Antibody Levels With Disease Severity and Activity in Sytemic Sclerosis
Hu PQ, Fertig N, Medsger TA Jr, et al (Univ of Pittsburgh, Pa)
Arthritis Rheum 48:1363-1373, 2003   8–2

Background.—Systemic sclerosis (SSc) or scleroderma is a connective tissue disease characterized by fibrosis and loss of vascularity. Antinuclear antibodies are detected in almost all patients with SSc. Anti-DNA topoisomerase I (anti-topo I) is found almost exclusively among SSc patients and has been considered a marker of SSc that does not play a role in pathogenesis. This article described the development of a highly sensitive enzyme-linked immunosorbent assay (ELISA) specific for anti-topo I and investigation of the role of anti-topo I in SSc with this assay.

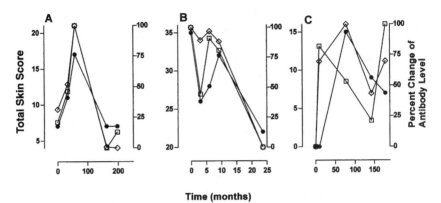

Time (months)

FIGURE 5.—Changes in levels of anti-topoisomerase I immunoglobulin G (IgG) and immunoglobulin A (IgA) with changes in the total skin score (TSS) in systemic sclerosis patients over time. The TSS values (*black circles*) (*left y-axis*) paralleled changes in the IgG (*white squares*) and IgA (*white diamonds*) levels (*right y-axis*) in patient 6 (A) and patient 3 (B) and preceded the change in IgG and IgA levels in patient 2 (C). IgG and IgA levels are presented as the percentage of change in antibody level, which is the percentage of the increase above the lowest recorded level divided by the total increase. For patients 2, 3, and 6, respectively, the increases in total IgG were from 13 to 73 U, 20.3 to 88.1 U, and 4.4 to 66.5 U. The increases in total IgA were from an optical density at 405 nm value of 0.176 to 0.564, 0.025 to 0.119, and 0.0004 to 0.125. The total increases in the TSS were from 0 to 15, 22 to 35, and 7 to 17. (Courtesy of Hu PQ, Fertig N, Medsger TA Jr, et al: Correlation of serum anti-DNA topoisomerase I antibody levels with disease severity and activity in systemic sclerosis *Arthritis Rheum* 48: 1363-1373, 2003. Copyright 2003 American College of Rheumatology. Reprinted by permission of John Wiley & Sons, Inc.)

Study Design.—The study group consisted of 59 patients with anti-topo I–positive SSc. The severity of their skin involvement was measured by the modified Rodnan skin scoring method. The total skin score (TSS), a measure of disease severity, was assessed by grading skin surfaces in 17 different areas. Disease activity was evaluated globally and for 9 organ systems. Levels of anti-topo I antibody, determined by specific ELISA, were compared to TSS.

Findings.—Titers of serum anti-topo I antibody, both immunoglobulin A and immunoglobulin G, were positively correlated with the TSS (Fig 5). In 8 of the 11 patients with serial serum samples, changes in the level of anti-topo I correlated with changes in the TSS. In 3 patients, increases in anti-topo I titers preceded increases in the TSS. Patients with highly active disease had significantly greater average anti-topo I titers than those with inactive disease.

Conclusion.—With the use of a newly developed, highly specific ELISA, a close relationship, both cross-sectional and longitudinal, has been observed between serum anti-topo I antibody titers and scleroderma disease severity . Anti-topo I titers predict or parallel changes in skin involvement and may be useful in clinical trials.

▶ Some autoantibodies (for example, anti–double-stranded DNA antibodies) are thought to reflect autoimmune disease activity; others are generally considered markers for disease that do not fluctuate in any meaningful way. Antibodies to topoisomerase I (anti-topo I, formerly called anti-scl-70 antibodies) have always been considered to be in the latter category. Now Hu et al seriously question that assumption.

They developed their own highly specific, highly reproducible ELISA assay, using recombinant topo I (thus assuring an unlimited supply of completely reproducible antigen for the assay) and used it to look at anti-topo I levels in 59 patients with the diffuse SSc. Their data indicate that anti-topo I antibodies do indeed correlate with severity of SSc. First, they observed an excellent correlation between TSS and anti-topo I titers. Next, they showed that, based on expert physician assessment of disease activity, anti-topo I titers correlated with the activity of patients' SSc in a cross-sectional analysis of all patients in the study.

Finally, in 11 patients from whom multiple serum samples were available, they showed that anti-topo I antibody levels waxed and waned in concert with worsening or improvement in TSS. Interestingly, a few patients who had high titers of anti-topo I but relatively mild disease quickly went on to increased activity and/or worsening TSS, suggesting that rises in anti-topo I may be predictive of an SSc flare. Both IgG and IgA antibodies correlated with disease activity, and although some IgG subtypes were better than others, essentially all IgG subtypes responded in parallel.

These studies raise some important questions. Can we use anti-topo I antibodies to follow SSc, a disease whose activity has been difficult to define? (Of course, we have to recognize that, at present, only Hu et al have access to this better assay.) Moreover, can we use anti-topo I antibodies to predict worsening disease, possibly steering us to try (or, conversely, defer in the case of low antibody titers) therapies that we might otherwise withhold? (One needs a good reason to use disease-modifying drugs in scleroderma, since none of them are well established and the best-tested of the lot—D-penicillamine—can be quite toxic.)

Indeed, can we use anti-topo I titers as surrogates for measuring the effectiveness of current or future therapies? Does the fact that a better assay can detect fluctuations in anti-topo I antibodies suggest that other disease autoantibodies that are not thought to fluctuate (eg, anti-Ro, anti-La, anti-Smith, and others) may actually do so, if only we could get the assay right? And finally, does the fact that anti-topo I antibodies fluctuate with, and even precede, disease activity suggest that these antibodies may actually be pathogenic for the disease, rather than simply markers? A lot of questions, yes, but not one firm answer. Stay tuned.

M. H. Pillinger, MD

9 Lyme Disease

Introduction

Lyme disease continues to be a biologically interesting, therapeutically maddening disease for rheumatologists and infectious disease specialists alike. Of course, the maddening part is that we have good antibiotics that work well for Lyme disease—yet patients continue to complain of symptoms, even after treatment. Is this because the treatment is actually inadequate? Or because the disease is cured, but residual symptoms remain? Or because the patient's continuing symptoms actually have nothing to do with their Lyme disease? No one really knows.

In this chapter, we include 2 articles published this year. The first, by Wormser et al (Abstract 9–1), suggests that for early Lyme disease (ie, patients with erythema migrans), the shortest recommended therapy—10 days of oral doxycycline—is as adequate for treating symptoms and preventing long-term complications, as longer doxycycline treatments or treatments including ceftriaxone. The second article, by Pausa et al (Abstract 9–2), is a fascinating study that suggests that one way that *Borrelia burgdorferi* may elude the immune system is by mimicking our own defenses against complement, and inactivating complement that attaches to the borrelial surface.

Michael H. Pillinger, MD

Duration of Antibiotic Therapy for Early Lyme Disease: A Randomized, Double-blind, Placebo-controlled Trial
Wormser GP, Ramanathan R, Nowakowski J, et al (New York Med College, Valhalla)
Ann Intern Med 138:697-704, 2003   9–1

Introduction.—The optimal duration of antibiotic therapy for patients with early Lyme disease and the need to treat for potential central nervous system involvement remain controversial. These issues were addressed in a placebo-controlled study comparing 10 days of doxycycline with both 10 days of doxycycline plus a single dose of IV ceftriaxone and 20 days of doxycycline only.

Methods.—The double-blind study included 180 patients with erythema migrans. Randomization was stratified by whether patients were asymptomatic or symptomatic so that the 3 treatment groups might have similar

TABLE 3.—Clinical Response Based on an Intention-to-Treat Analysis of Patients for Whom Information Was Available*

Evaluation	Complete Response			Partial Response			Failure			Not Assessable†		
	Doxycycline–Ceftriaxone Group	10-Day Doxycycline Group	20-Day Doxycycline Group	Doxycycline–Ceftriaxone Group	10-Day Doxycycline Group	20-Day Doxycycline Group	Doxycycline–Ceftriaxone Group	10-Day Doxycycline Group	20-Day Doxycycline Group	Doxycycline–Ceftriaxone Group	10-Day Doxycyline Group	20-Day Doxycyline Group
						n (%)						
20 days	36 (65.4)	37 (71.2)	34 (59.6)	19 (34.5)	14 (26.9)	23 (40.4)	0	1 (1.9)	0	5	9	2
3 months	40 (76.9)	41 (74.5)	39 (75.0)	12 (23.1)	13 (23.6)	13 (25.0)	0	1 (1.8)‡	0	8	6	7
12 months	42 (82.4)	44 (86.3)	39 (78.0)	9 (17.6)	6 (11.8)	11 (22.0)	0	1 (2.0)‡	0	9	10	9
30 months	39 (83.0)	35 (85.4)	35 (85.4)	8 (17.0)	5 (12.2)	6 (14.6)	0	1 (2.4)‡	0	13	20	18
Last§	51 (85.0)	50 (83.3)	50 (86.2)	9 (15.0)	9 (15.0)	8 (13.8)	0	1 (1.7)‡	0	0	1||	1||

*Percentages given are percentages of patients for whom information was available at each time point. See the Figure for the flow of patients through the study. For all comparisons of proportions of complete responders, $P > .2$.
†No information at a particular time point.
‡Refers to the patient deemed to have treatment failure at 20 days.
§Refers to last contact with patient regardless of time point.
||Did not return after baseline visit.
(Courtesy of Wormser GP, Ramanathan R, Nowakowski J, et al: Duration of antibiotic therapy for early Lyme disease: A randomized, double-blind, placebo-controlled trial. Ann Intern Med 138:697-704, 2003.)

proportions of patients with dissemination of *Borrelia burgdorferi*. Patients were assessed for treatment efficacy and safety at 20 days, 3 months, 12 months, and 30 months. Evaluations included clinical examination and neurocognitive testing. Outcome was characterized as complete response, partial response, or failure (Table 3).

Results.—The 3 treatment groups were similar in baseline demographic characteristics, clinical findings, and laboratory test results. Systemic illness was present in approximately three fourths of patients. In both on-study and intention-to-treat analyses, the complete response rate was similar for the 3 groups at all time points. Thirty-month complete response rates in the on-study analysis were 83.9% in the 20-day doxycycline group, 90.3% in the 10-day doxycycline group, and 86.5% in the doxycycline plus ceftriaxone group. In the only case of treatment failure at any time point, a patient in the 10-day doxycycline group was diagnosed with meningitis on day 18. A 2-week course of ceftriaxone was successful, and the results of neurocognitive testing were normal. Significantly more patients in the combination therapy group reported diarrhea.

Conclusion.—All 3 treatment groups had generally favorable outcomes. Extending doxycycline treatment from 10 days to 20 days or adding ceftriaxone to a 10-day doxycycline course did not enhance the resolution of erythema migrans or associated systemic symptoms in early, uncomplicated Lyme disease.

▶ Even as the biology of Lyme disease becomes ever more fascinating and complex (see Abstract 9–2), the treatment seems to become simpler and simpler. One somewhat nagging question has been whether the standard short course of doxycycline for early Lyme disease is adequate. In this manuscript, Wormser et al report that it is. They performed a double-blind, placebo-controlled trial on 180 patients with early Lyme disease—either erythema chroniicum migrans alone, or single or multiple erythema chroniicum migrans lesions plus or minus fever, unilateral facial palsy, or or other systemic symptoms. One group got doxycycline for 10 days; another, doxycycline for 20 days; and the final group received doxycycline for 10 days plus a single dose of ceftriaxone (these treatment arms replicate typical regimens in use in the community). The patients were then followed for approximately 2.5 years. At the end of the study, nearly 90% of each group had had a complete remission, and there was no statistical difference between any group, either in initial analysis or in a reanalysis as intention to treat. In fact, there were no significant differences between the groups at any time point along the way. A single individual was deemed a treatment failure (central nervous system Lyme, which responded to 2 weeks of IV ceftriaxone); this patient was in the 10-day doxycycline group, but it is impossible to know whether the appearance of a treatment failure in this group was due to less-aggressive treatment or simply a stochastic event. A small number of patients in each group acquired a second case of Lyme sometime after treatment; there was no significant difference between the 3 treatment arms in this regard, although the largest number of new cases was actually seen in the most aggressive (doxycycline plus ceftriaxone) arm.

In sum, early Lyme disease is an extremely responsive disease.[1] Except in unique situations, it is almost always adequate to treat with a simple 10-day course of doxycyline.

M. H. Pillinger, MD

Reference

1. Smith RP, Schoen RT, Rahn DW, et al: Clinical characteristics and treatment outcome of early lyme disease in patients with microbiologically confirmed erythema migrans. *Ann Intern Med* 136:421-428, 2002. (2003 YEAR BOOK OF MEDICINE, pp 40-41.)

▶ There are few controlled trials of the treatment of the erythema migrans that characterizes early Lyme disease. There seems to be an inordinate fear of CNS infection, and therapy has evolved to encompass longer and longer courses. This set of highly regarded and experienced Lyme investigators demonstrate with a reasonable degree of confidence that 10 days of doxycycline is equivalent to a longer course of therapy or addition of a dose of parenteral ceftriaxone. Failure was extremely rare and should give the clinician confidence in using a shorter course of therapy with less toxicity, especially diarrhea. It is important to note that meningitis symptoms or heart block was an exclusionary criteria.

D. R. Snydman, MD

Serum-Resistant Strains of *Borrelia burgdorferi* Evade Complement-Mediated Killing by Expressing a CD59-like Complement Inhibitory Molecule

Pausa M, Pellis V, Cinco M, et al (Univ of Trieste, Italy; Istituto Ricovero Cura a Carattere Scientifico "Burlo Garofolo," Trieste, Italy)
J Immunol 170:3214-3222, 2003
9–2

Background.—Most pathogenic microorganisms, particularly those that circulate in the bloodstream, have developed an array of strategies to evade the host immune defense, including evasion of complement-activation or complement attack, or both. *Borrelia burgdorferi*, the etiologic agent of Lyme disease, comprises 3 genospecies that exhibit different pathogenicity and differ in their susceptibility to complement-mediated killing. One mechanism that enables some strains of *B burgdorferi* to evade complement attack has been partially elucidated, and these strains have been shown to selectively bind the complement regulatory proteins factor H and factor H–like protein. These proteins interact with several outer membrane proteins including Osp-E, and reduce the numbers of C3 molecules deposited on the bacterial surface. However, it has recently been shown that the amount of C3 and its degradation products deposited on the bacterial surface does not differ in complement-susceptible and complement-resistant strains of *B burgdorferi*. This finding suggests that the ability of surface-bound factor H to control C3 activation is not the only mechanism used by *B burgdorferi* to evade complement-dependent killing. Complement-sensitive and complement-resistant strains of B burgdorferi were examined for deposition of C3 and late complement components.

Methods.—Fluorescence microscopy and flow cytometry were used to evaluate the amount of C3 and late complement components bound to complement-resistant and complement-sensitive strains of B burgdorferi.

Results.—Comparable deposition of C3 was observed on the 2 strains, but the resistant strain exhibited reduced staining for C6 and C7, barely detectable staining for C9, and undetectable staining for poly C9. On the basis of these findings, a search was conducted for a protein that inhibits assembly of complement membrane attack complex and documented an anti-human CD59-reactive molecule on the surface of complement-resistant spirochetes by flow cytometry and electron microscopy. Sodium dodecylsulfate–polyacrylamide gel electrophoresis (SDS-PAGE) and Western blot analysis revealed a molecule of 80 kd recognized by polyclonal and monoclonal anti-CD59 antibodies in the membrane extract of complement-resistant strains. This molecule was released from the bacterial wall by using deoxycholate and trypsin, which suggests its insertion into the bacterial membrane. This CD59-like molecule acts as a complement inhibitor on *Borrelia* because incubation with F(ab')$_2$ anti-CD59 leaves the resistant strain susceptible to complement-mediated killing.

Conclusions.—Some complement-resistant strains of B burgdorferi have the ability to evade complement-dependent killing by expressing a molecule that is structurally and functionally similar to human CD59. However, the structure of this molecule is still to be defined.

▶ How does *B burgdorferi* manage to establish human infections? Last year, we referenced an article by Malawista et al[1] indicating that although neutrophils are excellent killers of *Borrelia* when antibody is present, they are poor at killing the organisms in the absence of humoral immunity. Thus, *Borrelia* may have evolved in such a way as to resist the early, innate immune response. By the time humoral immunity to the spirochete develops, the organism has managed to find an immune privileged niche in the body, and therefore, to persist.

Now, Pausa et al have demonstrated another evolutionary trick by which *Borrelia* may evade the innate immune response. This time the focus is on complement. The investigators observed that some strains of *Borrelia* are resistant to killing by complement, one of the earliest components of innate immunity. Upon further investigation, they observed that the complement-resistant strains showed diminished deposition of late-stage complement components (the ones that punch holes in target membranes). How could this be? The authors were astute to note that the same things happen on our own cells, and that we use cell surface enzymes to degrade deposited complement before it becomes a problem. Could *Borrelia* be using a similar strategy?

Actually, it turned out that *Borrelia* was probably using an almost identical one. By using antibodies to the human complement-decaying enzyme CD59, the authors identified an anti–CD59-reactive antigen on the surface of complement-resistant, but not complement-sensitive strains. Moreover, these anti-CD59 antibodies appear to block the spirochetal enzyme, because exposure to the antibody renders the complement-resistant strains complement sensitive. Indeed, the authors show that bacterial extracts from complement-resistant strains can protect other cells from complement-mediated lysis, an effect that is blocked by the anti-CD59 antibodies. Further work is clearly needed, but these studies suggest that *Borrelia* has either evolved, or stolen, another mechanism to protect itself from innate immunity. Since chronic *Borrelia* infection may be harder to eradicate than the acute phase, studies such as these suggest that we may do well to focus on helping the immune system clear the invader in the early days of infection.

M. H. Pillinger, MD

Reference

1. Montgomery RR, Wang X, Malawista SE: Murine Lyme disease: No evidence for active immune down-regulation in resolving of subclinical infection. *J Infect Dis* 183:1631-1637, 2001.

10 Vasculitis

Introduction

The antineutrophil cytoplasm antibody (ANCA)-positive vasculitides—Wegener's granulomatosis, microscopic polyangiitis, and renal-limited vasculitis—usually respond to therapy, but the therapy (typically prednisone and cyclophosphamide) is potentially toxic and the duration of therapy not much clearer than a guessing game. We need better or at least safer therapies for these potentially life-threatening illnesses. One strategy that has arisen in recent years is based on the notion of maintenance therapy. Specifically, treatment is begun aggressively with accepted therapies, but once remission is achieved, a more benign agent is used for an extended time to prevent relapse. The best-studied agent for such a purpose has been methotrexate, but not everyone can tolerate the marrow and/or liver toxicity associated with this agent. Now, Jayne et al present a study (Abstract 10–1) that uses azathioprine for maintenance therapy—and they conclude that it is an acceptable alternative to methotrexate for this purpose.

In another study, Salvarani et al (Abstract 10–2) test the ability of TNF blockade to treat polymyalgia rheumatica in patients who could not be tapered off of prednisone. They show, in a small number of cases, that treatment with infliximab can be useful as a steroid-sparing agent. More to the point, only a short course of infliximab therapy was required to induce a durable effect, making the use of a biologic potentially justifiable. Since many if not all vasculitides appear to be driven in large part by TNF, this approach may have broad validity in vasculitis therapy.

Michael H. Pillinger, MD

A Randomized Trial of Maintenance Therapy for Vasculitis Associated With Antineutrophil Cytoplasmic Autoantibodies
Jayne D, for the European Vasculitis Study Group (Addenbrooke's Hosp, Cambridge, England; et al)
N Engl J Med 349:36-44, 2003   10–1

Background.—Wegener's granulomatosis and microscopic polyangiitis are 2 of the primary systemic vasculitides typically associated with autoantibodies to neutrophil cytoplasmic antigens. Whether exposure to cyclophosphamide in patients with generalized vasculitis could be decreased by substituting azathioprine at remission was determined.

Methods.—One hundred fifty-five patients newly diagnosed as having generalized vasculitis and with a serum creatinine level of 5.7 mg/dL or less were studied. All had had at least 3 months of treatment with oral cyclophosphamide and prednisolone. After remission, patients were randomly assigned to continued cyclophosphamide treatment, 1.5 mg/kg of body weight/d, or to a substitute regimen of azathioprine, 2 mg/kg/d. All patients continued to take prednisolone. Follow-up was for 18 months from study entry.

Findings.—Ninety-three percent of the patients entered remission and were randomly assigned to azathioprine or cyclophosphamide. Eight patients died, 7 in the first 3 months, for a mortality rate of 5%. Relapse occurred in 15.5% of the azathioprine group and in 13.7% of the cyclophosphamide group. Ten percent of patients had severe adverse events during the induction phase, 11% in the azathioprine group in the remission phase, and 10% in the cyclophosphamide group in the remission phase. Patients with microscopic polyangiitis had a lower relapse rate than those with Wegener's granulomatosis.

Conclusion.—Cyclophosphamide withdrawal and substitution with azathioprine after remission of generalized vasculitis does not appear to increase relapse rates. This substitution allowed cyclophosphamide exposure duration to be safely reduced.

▶ The institution of combination cyclophosphamide and prednisolone therapy for necrotizing vasculitis, by Fauci et al in 1979,[1] was a breakthrough that turned a dreaded class of diseases into a treatable one. As every rheumatologist knows, however, cyclophosphamide is a difficult drug, causing immune suppression, infertility, cystitis, and bladder and other forms of malignancy. Moreover, although the majority of vasculitis patients treated with cyclophosphamide enter into partial or complete remission, the relapse rate is high—as high as 25%.

Longer cyclophosphamide treatment might reduce relapse but would undoubtedly also increase toxicity. To address these problems, rheumatologists have lately been considering a different strategy: induction of remission with cyclophosphamide, followed by substitution of a more benign agent for long-term maintenance therapy. At present, the best-studied substitute agent for such a strategy is probably methotrexate, but methotrexate may be contraindicated in people with hepatitis, alcohol use, or liver disease.

Jayne et al tested the utility of azathioprine for maintenance therapy in vasculitis. The 155 patients in their study had either Wegener's granulomatosis, microscopic polyangiitis, or renal-limited vasculitis; all patients were anti-neutrophil cytoplasmic antibody (ANCA)–positive and/or had biopsy confirmation of vasculitis. Remission was induced with oral cyclophosphamide in 144 patients, and these were then randomized to either receive continued cyclophosphamide (1.5mg/kg) or azathioprine (2mg/kg) daily and were monitored for 18 months. There were no significant differences in the relapse rates between the 2 groups (about 15% each).

Although open-label, this is an extremely rigorous and well-done study, and I for one am convinced of the utility of azathioprine as maintenance therapy for these diseases. Problems with the study include the fact that the authors group 3 different kinds of ANCA-positive vasculitis together. It is at least possible that the 3 different entities might respond differently to different therapies (the authors do report that the relapse rate was lower for microscopic polyangiitis than for Wegener's but don't discuss differences between the treatment arms).

In addition, the study was not powered to detect small differences (ie, less than 20%) between the treatment groups (despite being an extremely large study for these kinds of vasculitis), so it is still possible that small differences exist. Moreover, it must be recognized that azathioprine is not without its own toxicities. Indeed, there were no significant differences in adverse event rates between the 2 groups.

Nonetheless, most rheumatologists would agree that azathioprine is easier to administer and easier to monitor and that its use is associated with fewer problems than cyclophosphamide. For a meaningful percentage of our ANCA-positive vasculitis patients, remission induction with cyclophosphamide followed by maintenance with azathioprine is probably a strategy worth considering.

M. H. Pillinger, MD

Reference

1. Fauci AS, Haynes BF, Katz P, et al: Cyclophosphamide therapy of severe systemic necrotizing vasculitis. *N Engl J Med* 301:235-238, 1979.

Treatment of Refractory Polymyalgia Rheumatica With Infliximab: A Pilot Study
Salvarani C, Cantini F, Niccoli L, et al (Arcispedale S Maria Nuova, Reggio Emilia, Italy; Istituto Rizzoli, Bologna, Italy; Ospedale S Carlo, Potenza, Italy)
J Rheumatol 30:760-763, 2003   10–2

Background.—Corticosteroids are used as the drug of choice for the treatment of polymyalgia rheumatica (PMR). In the absence of giant cell arteritis, an initial dosage of 10 to 20 mg/d of prednisone or its equivalent is usually adequate for most cases of PMR. However, in 30% to 50% of patients, exacerbation of the disease occurs on prednisone withdrawal, and a prolonged course of treatment for several years may be necessary. Corticosteroid-related adverse effects are frequently observed during the course of such prolonged treatment. The purpose of this study was to determine whether infliximab, a chimeric monoclonal anti–tumor necrosis factor (TNF)-α antibody, has a steroid-sparing effect in the treatment of patients with PMR who are resistant to corticosteroid therapy and have experienced corticosteroid-related side effects.

Methods.—Infliximab, 3 mg/kg, was administered at weeks 0, 2, and 6 in 4 patients with relapsing PMR who were unable to reduce their prednisone dosage below 7.5 to 12.5 mg/d and who had experienced multiple vertebral fractures. The patients were monitored for clinical signs and symptoms and erythrocyte sedimentation rate (ESR), C-reactive protein (CRP), and interleukin-6 (IL-6) during the 1-year follow-up period.

Results.—Two patients responded completely to infliximab, with clinical remission occurring 2 weeks after the first infusion. At that time, ESR and IL-6 values were normal, and the patients were able to suspend prednisone therapy. Normal ESR, CRP, and IL-6 levels persisted after the suspension of infliximab and prednisone during the follow-up period, in concert with the clinical remission. The third patient had a complete and persistent clinical remission 2 weeks after the first infusion, although IL-6 levels were elevated during follow-up despite normalization of ESR values. These 3 patients were free of symptoms, with normal ESR and CRP levels at the end of a year-long follow-up period. The fourth patient had continuous clinical activity in association with persistently elevated acute-phase reactants. However, her IL-6 levels during follow-up were lower than baseline values, and she was able to reduce her prednisone dosage to 5 mg/d.

Conclusions.—The results of this study are encouraging and suggest that a controlled study would be appropriate for assessment of the efficacy of infliximab as a corticosteroid-sparing drug for the treatment of PMR.

▶ Most cases of PMR can be easily treated with steroids, but stopping the treatment is another matter altogether. Although some textbooks suggest that steroid treatment in PMR can be withdrawn in a matter of weeks, most rheumatologists know that PMR therapy with steroids typically requires months, and sometimes years before the prednisone can be safely tapered. In the meantime, the patient has probably experienced one or more flares of this painful, incapacitating condition. Moreover, the consequences of long-term steroid use—diabetes, atherosclerosis, obesity, avascular necrosis, osteoporosis, psychiatric alterations, etc—are well known to physicians and patients alike. The alternatives to steroids are slim. Methotrexate has been suggested, but the data as to its efficacy are conflicting. New and effective approaches are clearly needed.

Salvarani et al propose that infliximab might be one such alternative. They identified 4 patients with unequivocal PMR who had responded to steroids but had repeatedly failed steroid taper. In each case, the use of steroids had been required for 2 or more years; in each case, vertebral fractures had ensued. And 3 of the 4 cases had also failed methotrexate. When treated with infliximab, however, each of these patients had a rapid and dramatic response in their symptoms, as well as improvement in some or all of the classic markers of PMR—ESR, CRP, and IL-6 levels. Three patients were able to discontinue prednisone altogether, and the fourth to reduce prednisone consumption to 5 mg/d.

Is treatment with infliximab practical? Maybe. Although infliximab as used in rheumatoid arthritis (ie, indefinitely) is extremely expensive, one of the interesting features of this study was that patients appeared to require only a single cycle of treatment—that is, treatments at 0, 2, and 6 weeks—to have a durable response. Given the cost of steroid monitoring and side effects, the cost of short-term treatment with infliximab might not be prohibitive. Questions, of course, remain. This open-label study involved only 4 patients, so no statistical significance is established. Moreover, it would be interesting to know whether other anti-TNF agents might also be effective. Still, this is a step forward, and for patients with PMR who can't stop and can't tolerate prednisone, infliximab might be an attractive option.

Also noted: a pilot study by the same authors, indicating that infliximab may also be a useful alternative in giant cell arteritis.[1]

M. H. Pillinger, MD

Reference

1. Cantini F, Niccoli L, Salvarani C, et al: Treatment of longstanding active giant cell arteritis with infliximab: Report of 4 cases. *Arthritis Rheum* 44:2933-2935, 2001.

11 Crystal Disease

Introduction

This year, I've chosen to include only a single article about crystal disease, but that article is particularly interesting and may have extremely wide implications. Shi et al (Abstract 11-1) started with a known observation—that cellular lysates can act as adjuvant in immune responses—and carried it to a novel finding: that the active "ingredient" in the adjuvant response is likely to be crystallized uric acid. Why on earth would this be desirable? Consider the scenario in which a cell, infected with a virus, dies. That cell needs to send a "danger signal" to nearby T cells, saying in effect "I'm dying and infected; respond to me for the good of the organism." Uric acid is an excellent candidate for such a danger signal. Normally expressed at low levels, cell apoptosis or necrosis would lead to the breakdown of nucleic acids and a very local increase in uric acid levels. If the observation of Shi and colleagues is true, it will have implications not only for immunity but also for autoimmunity; and the question of whether lowering uric acid levels (easily achieved through drugs such as allopurinol and probenecid) reduces autoimmunity will become a pressing one.

Michael H. Pillinger, MD

Molecular Identification of a Danger Signal That Alerts the Immune System to Dying Cells
Shi Y, Evans JE, Rock KL (Univ of Massachusetts, Worcester)
Nature 425:516-521, 2003   11–1

Objective.—Dying cells or their cytosols can function as adjuvant in animals. This report described the purification of a low molecular weight fraction from the cytosol that has adjuvant activity and its identification as uric acid. These findings provide a molecular link between cell injury and immunity and have implications for vaccines, inflammation, and autoimmunity.

Methods and Results.—Cytosol from ultraviolet-irradiated cells was fractionated by high performance liquid chromatography, and fractions were tested for their adjuvant activity. A pool of low molecular weight fractions had adjuvant activity. These fractions were further purified and uric acid was identified as the active agent. Incubation of the purified fraction with uricase, an enzyme that specifically breaks down uric acid, destroyed both the purified molecule and its activity. Commercially available purified uric acid was also found to have adjuvant activity.

As injured cells degraded their DNA and RNA, uric acid would be created, which would enable dying cells to produce this "danger signal." Uric acid increased in the cytosol of injured cell, as would be expected. When cells were treated with allopurinol, a specific inhibitor of uric acid production, and then injured, both uric acid production and adjuvant activity were reduced.

Uric acid also stimulated primary cultures of dendritic cells to mature. The concentrations that were stimulatory contained uric acid crystals. Preformed monosodium urate crystals were also stimulatory. Uric acid is close to saturation within the body. Thus, a localized increase in uric acid released by dying cells could cause supersaturation and the formation of uric acid crystals. This phase transition could be the signal these cells send to the immune system of cell death and potential danger.

Conclusion.—This research has identified uric acid crystals as an endogenous immunologic signal of cell death and danger. When released from injured and dying cells, it stimulates dendritic cells to mature and primes T-cell responses to antigen. These results further suggest that uric acid crystals are not always pathologic, as in gout, but form part of the normal response of the body to cell death. On the other hand, uric acid may be involved in the development of autoimmune disease in some individuals. As an endogenous adjuvant, uric acid may also be useful in the production of human vaccines.

▶ Why do humans make uric acid anyway? After all, only humans and some other primates have sustained mutations that inactivate uricase, the enzyme that converts uric acid to allantoic acid and renders it soluble for secretion. Is gout just a cosmic joke, a minor goof-up in the great experiment of life? Well, probably not. Last year, we reported on a study by Watanabe et al[1] suggesting that uric acid might convey a survival advantage by inducing hypertension or, in an earlier salt-poor dietary era, by maintaining normotension in the context of hyponatremia. Now comes another fascinating paradigm. According to Shi et al, uric acid may actually serve as an endogenous adjuvant, allowing the immune system to respond to dying, apoptotic cells.

The authors began their studies with the recognition that injured or dying cells, or the cytosol of such cells, can serve as an adjuvant for injected antigen. They therefore proceeded to fractionate the adjuvant activity in cytosol until they came up with a single molecular weight species that possessed adjuvant activity in cytotoxic T-lymphocyte reactions. On chemical analysis, that species turned out to be uric acid. Confirmation that uric acid was "adjuvant X" came from the ability of uricase to abrogate the adjuvant effect and from the ability of "off-the-shelf" uric acid to duplicate the adjuvant activity. (Another purified fraction of cytosol had a similar effect but has not yet been identified by the authors.)

Is it a good thing that uric acid can function as an adjuvant? The authors suggest that it might be. Since intracellular viral infections and/or tumors lead to cell death, and cell death leads to nucleotide breakdown and uric acid production, the authors propose that the death of virally infected cells or tumor cells may lead to the presentation of foreign antigen in the presence of uric acid as an adjuvant (in contrast to extracellular bacterial infection, in which the bacteria provides its own adjuvant in the form of lipopolysaccharides or glycoproteins). Interestingly, the authors suggest that only the crystal form of uric acid possesses adjuvant qualities. Thus, our ability to fend off intracellular infections may be forever and inextricably tied to our ability to suffer gout.

M. H. Pillinger, MD

Reference

1. Watanabe S, Kang D-H, Feng L, et al: Uric acid, hominoid evolution, and the pathogenesis of salt-sensitivity. *Hypertension* 40:355-360, 2002. (2003 YEAR BOOK OF MEDICINE, pp 46-48.)

12 Pharmacology of Antirheumatic Agents

Introduction

For the first time, I have elected to devote a separate chapter to the pharmacology of antirheumatic agents. In past years, these selections would likely have been incorporated into sections on specific conditions. Given the centrality of mediators such as cytokines and prostaglandins in a wide number of rheumatic diseases, however, it seems more apposite to give these agents their own section. Moreover, these selections are not about drug efficacy but about drug mechanisms and toxicity. For instance, we have elected to showcase articles (Abstracts 12–1 and 12–2) about potential important adverse events encountered during TNF blockade—not because these agents should not be used, but because, if we are going to use them, we are obliged to know their disadvantages as well as their advantages. Another selection by Spiegel et al (Abstract 12–3) addresses the cost effectiveness—or lack thereof—of COX-2 inhibitors. Finally, the study by Reid et al (Abstract 12–4) identifies a novel new mechanism for the action of nonsteroidal anti-inflammatory drugs (NSAIDs) and COX-2 inhibitors. Rather than blocking prostaglandin synthesis, some NSAIDs may block prostaglandin secretion out of the cell.

Michael H. Pillinger, MD

Case Reports of Heart Failure After Therapy With a Tumor Necrosis Factor Antagonist
Kwon HJ, Coté TR, Cuffe MS, et al (US Food and Drug Administration, Rockville, Md; Duke Clinical Research Inst, Durham, NC)
Ann Intern Med 138:807-811, 2003   12–1

Background.—Etanercept and infliximab are tumor necrosis factor (TNF) antagonists. Etanercept has been approved for the treatment of rheumatoid, juvenile rheumatoid, and psoriatic arthritis, whereas infliximab is approved for the treatment of Crohn's disease and, in conjunction with methotrexate, rheumatoid arthritis. Congestive heart failure is frequently accompanied by elevated TNF-α levels; however, controlled trials in patients with heart failure have shown no benefits from TNF antagonists and, in the case of infliximab, have suggested worse outcomes. In this study, adverse event reports of heart failure after TNF antagonist therapy for arthritis or Crohn's disease were described.

Methods.—Data were obtained from the US Food and Drug Administration's MedWatch program. The study group included 47 patients who had new or worsening heart failure develop, as determined by clinical and laboratory reports, while receiving TNF antagonist therapy.

Results.—According to the MedWatch program, 38 of 47 patients developed new-onset heart failure and 9 patients experienced exacerbation of heart failure after TNF antagonist therapy. Of the 38 patients with new-onset heart failure, 19 (50%) had no identifiable risk factors. Ten patients younger than 50 years had new-onset heart failure develop after TNF antagonist therapy. After termination of TNF antagonist therapy and initiation of heart failure therapy in these 10 patients, 3 patients had complete resolution of heart failure, 6 patients improved, and 1 patient died.

Conclusions.—The cases presented in this report, along with recent data from clinical trials, suggest that TNF antagonists may induce new-onset heart failure or exacerbate existing heart disease in a subset of patients.

▶ Last year, I included in the YEAR BOOK a report of one potential risk associated with the use of TNF antagonists: the reactivation of latent tuberculosis.[1] This year, I want to take the opportunity to include a report informing readers of another potential risk: the initiation or exacerbation of congestive heart failure (CHF). The link between TNF antagonists and CHF began on a note of promise: cardiologists, noting that severe CHF is often associated with elevated TNF levels, hypothesized that TNF might be contributing to the disease, and initiated large-scale placebo-controlled trials to test the effects of TNF blockade on CHF. Not only did these studies fail to show a benefit to TNF blockers in CHF, but one study, using infliximab, actually suggested increased mortality. The studies were halted, and the hope of a treatment for CHF was discarded.

As a rheumatologist, I use TNF blockers with some regularity for rheumatoid arthritis, because they are extremely effective and, for most people, well tolerated. My gastroenterology colleagues use TNF blockade for inflammatory bowel disease based on a similar rationale. But are we putting at least some of our patients at risk for CHF? And if so, which ones?

Kwon et al report on the accumulating case reports of CHF during TNF antagonist therapy submitted to the US Food and Drug Administration's MedWatch program. Up to the time of publication, 47 such patients had been reported. Thirty-eight developed new-onset heart disease, and 9 experienced CHF exacerbations. Most had rheumatoid arthritis, but of course this is the disease for which these agents are most used. Others had Crohn's disease, psoriatic arthritis, and juvenile rheumatoid arthritis, so at present there is not a clear link between a specific diagnosis and the risk for CHF. Males and females were both reported, so sex does not appear to be a key difference, at least to date. Patients who developed CHF were receiving both infliximab and etanercept, so the effect does not appear to be agent specific. While some of the patients had risk factors for CHF, others had none. Indeed, 10 patients who developed new-onset CHF were younger than 50 years, and only 3 of these had underlying risk factors. These case reports in no way constitute a controlled study, and it is theoretically possible that the onset of CHF had nothing to do with the use of anti-TNF agents. However, of the 10 patients younger than 50 who developed new-onset CHF, all or nearly all experienced resolution with withdrawal of the anti-TNF agent.

How are we as physicians supposed to respond to this report? Well, for the time being, I'd say with prudence and caution. These events appear to be rare, and the usefulness of TNF antagonists in rheumatoid arthritis is so clear-cut that we must be careful not to throw the baby out with the bath water. In my own practice, I screen for a history or for signs and symptoms of CHF, following up with an echocardiogram if need be. I then generally withhold anti-TNF therapy from patients with previously documented or newly diagnosed CHF. When my patients have risk factors for CHF but no actual disease, I try to get those risk factors under control and exercise a judgment as to whether TNF blockade is really necessary for control of their rheumatoid arthritis (which itself is, of course, a cause of increased mortality; see the report by Solomon et al [Abstract 1–1]). If no other options for arthritis treatment are tenable, I go ahead with an anti-TNF agent, but follow-up the patient closely for any signs or symptoms of CHF. This approach seems reasonable, but is unlikely to be helpful for those arthritis patients (no one knows how many) who develop CHF without any prior known risk factors. More knowledge, both clinical and scientific, is clearly needed.

M. H. Pillinger, MD

Reference

1. Mayordomo L, Marenco JL, Gomez-Mateos J, et al: Pulmonary miliary tuberculosis in a patient with anti-TNF-alpha treatment. *Scand J Rheumatol* 31:44-45, 2002. (2003 Year Book of Medicine, pp 59-61.)

Antinuclear Antibodies Following Infliximab Treatment in Patients With Rheumatoid Arthritis or Spondylarthropathy

De Rycke L, Kruithof E, Van Damme N, et al (Ghent Univ Hosp, Belgium)
Arthritis Rheum 48:1015-1023, 2003   12–2

Background.—Rheumatoid arthritis (RA) and spondylarthropathy (SpA) are the 2 most frequent types of autoimmune arthritis, with a prevalence of 1% to 2%. The standard therapy for RA includes a combination of disease-modifying antirheumatic drugs (DMARDs) and nonsteroidal anti-inflammatory drugs (NSAIDs). For SpA, the standard therapy is treatment with NSAIDs, eventually in combination with sulfasalazine for peripheral arthritis or methotrexate for psoriatic arthritis. However, this approach often results in only partial control of the inflammation and structural damage. In recent years, there have been new insights into the cellular and molecular mechanisms of RA and SpA, and new therapies, such as tumor necrosis factor (TNF) antagonists, have been developed on the basis of these insights.

Anecdotal reports suggest that TNF antagonists may occasionally induce the formation of autoantibodies of unknown significance. A study was undertaken to investigate the effects of the TNF antagonist infliximab on the development of antinuclear antibodies (ANAs), anti–double-stranded DNA (anti-dsDNA), antinucleosome, antihistone, and anti–extractable nuclear antigen (anti-ENA) antibodies in patients with RA and SpA (Table 1).

Methods.—Sera were obtained from 62 patients with RA and 35 patients with SpA treated with infliximab and tested at baseline and at week 30 (RA group) or week 34 (SpA group). ANAs were tested by indirect immunofluorescence on HEp-2 cells. Anti-dsDNA antibodies were detected by indirect immunofluorescence on *Crithidia luciliae* and by enzyme-linked immunosorbent assay with further isotyping with γ, μ, and α chain-specific conjugates at various time points. Enzyme-linked immunosorbent assay was used to test antinucleosome antibodies, and anti-ENA antibodies were detected by line immunoassay.

Results.—Initial testing identified 32 of the 62 RA patients and 6 of the 35 SpA patients as positive for ANAs. After infliximab treatment, 51 of the 62 RA patients and 31 of the 35 SpA patients tested positive for ANAs. At baseline, none of the RA or SpA patients had anti-dsDNA antibodies. After infliximab therapy, 7 RA patients and 6 SpA patients became positive for anti-dsDNA antibodies. All 7 anti-dsDNA-positive RA patients had immunoglobulin (Ig) M and IgA anti-dsDNA antibodies. Among the SpA patients, 3 of the 6 anti-dsDNA-positive patients had IgM and IgA anti-dsDNA antibodies, and 2 had IgM anti-dsDNA antibodies only. The IgM anti-dsDNA antibodies appeared before the IgA anti-dsDNA antibodies in both RA and SpA. No IgG anti-dsDNA antibodies or lupus syndromes were noted during the observation period. Some patients had antinucleosome, antihistone, or

TABLE 1.—Autoantibody Profile in RA and SpA Patients After Infliximab Treatment*

Antibody, Detection Method	RA (n = 62)		SpA (n = 35)	
	Week 0	Week 30	Week 0	Week 34
ANA, IIF on HEp-2 cells	32 (51.6)	51 (82.3)†	6 (17.1)	31 (88.6)†
Anti-dsDNA				
IIF on *Crithidia luciliae*	0 (0)	27 (43.5)†	0 (0)	20 (57.1)†
ELISA	2 (3.2)	10 (16.1)‡	6 (17.1)	6 (17.1)
Both IIF on *Crithidia luciliae* and ELISA	0 (0)	7 (11.3)§	0 (0)	6 (17.1)§
Antinucleosome, ELISA	1 (1.6)	5 (8.1)	3 (8.6)	4 (11.4)
Antihistone, LIA	3 (4.8)	6 (9.7)	2 (5.7)	5 (14.3)
Anti-SmD, LIA	1 (1.6)	1 (1.6)	0 (0)	0 (0)
Anti-RNP, LIA	0 (0)	0 (0)	0 (0)	0 (0)
Anti-SSA, LIA	0 (0)	0 (0)	0 (0)	0 (0)
Anti-SSB, LIA	1 (1.6)	2 (3.2)	1 (2.9)	1 (2.9)
Anticentromere, IIF/anti-CENP, LIA	1 (1.6)	1 (1.6)	0 (0)	0 (0)

*Values are the number (%).
Abbreviations: RA, Rheumatoid arthritis; *SpA*, spondylarthropathy; *ANA*, antinuclear antibody; *IIF*, indirect immunofluorescence; *anti-dsDNA*, anti–double-stranded DNA; *ELISA*, enzyme-linked immunosorbent assay; *LIA*, line immunoassay.
†$P \le .001$ versus baseline.
‡$P \le .01$ versus baseline.
§$P \le .05$ versus baseline.
(Courtesy of De Rycke L, Kruithof E, Van Damme N, et al: Antinuclear antibodies following infliximab treatment in patients with rheumatoid arthritis or spondylarthropathy. *Arthritis Rheum* 48:1015-1023, 2003. Copyright 2003, American College of Rheumatology. Reprinted by permission of John Wiley & Sons, Inc.)

anti-ENA antibodies develop after infliximab treatment, but the number was not statistically significant.

Conclusions.—Treatment with infliximab may induce antinuclear antibodies and particularly IgM and IgA anti-dsDNA antibodies in patients with RA and SpA. However, this study found no anti-dsDNA IgG antibodies or lupus symptoms in RA and SpA patients, and the development of antinucleosome, antihistone, or anti-ENA antibodies was not statistically significant. However, further follow-up is necessary because the findings of this study do not exclude potential induction of clinically significant lupus in the long term.

▶ One of the more interesting phenomena associated with the use of anti-TNF agents in RA have been reports of increased prevalence of ANAs. These ANAs have been seen with both infliximab and etanercept but have not been well characterized. De Rycke et al have now studied the serologic responses of both RA patients as well as SpA patients treated with infliximab. They confirm that a significant increase in ANAs occurs in RA and, not previously reported, in SpA as well. Thus, the ANA response to infliximab is not disease specific, despite the common paradigm that RA is a disease of humoral immunity (and not infrequently associated with ANAs as well as anti-Ro and anti-La antibodies, in the case of secondary Sjögren's syndrome) whereas the spondylopathic diseases are seronegative. They extend their ANA observations by testing a wide panel of serologies, and in so doing discover that treatment with infliximab is associated with a statistically significant increase in anti-dsDNA antibodies as well. Interestingly these anti-dsDNA antibodies are predominantly IgM and IgA rather than the IgG anti-dsDNA antibodies typical of lupus nephritis. The generation of other autoantibodies was also looked for, and new accumulations of antinucleosome and anti-Sm antibodies were also observed, though these failed to achieve statistical significance.

Is the production of these antibodies of clinical significance? For the sake of our patients, we would prefer not, and De Rycke et al give us some hope that this may be the case. During the 30- (RA) or 34- (SpA) week follow up, no new clinical features of lupus were documented in any patient, with the possible exception of 1 case each of mild lymphopenia or leukopenia. Still, we should not lose sight of the fact that a study of less than half a year may not be definitive in this regard. I'm not sure whether we should be checking routinely for the appearance of these antibodies in our patients on anti-TNF therapy (would we stop the agent if the antibodies appeared?), but we should certainly remain vigilant for any signs of new-onset lupus or other autoimmune diseases.

M. H. Pillinger, MD

The Cost-Effectiveness of Cyclooxygenase-2 Selective Inhibitors in the Management of Chronic Arthritis

Spiegel BMR, Targownik L, Dulai GS, et al (Univ of California, Los Angeles)
Ann Intern Med 138:795-806, 2003
12–3

Background.—Nonsteroidal anti-inflammatory drugs (NSaids) are widely used for the treatment of chronic arthritis pain and account for 3% of the US prescription market. Despite the association of NSaids with clinically significant peptic ulcer complications, these drugs are a mainstay of treatment. Cyclooxygenase-2 selective inhibitors, including rofecoxib and celecoxib (coxibs), have been developed as safer alternatives to nonselective NSaids. Rofecoxib and celecoxib have been found to effectively treat chronic arthritis pain and to reduce ulcer complications by 50% compared with NSaids. However, the absolute risk reduction of the coxibs is small, and the cost-effectiveness of treatment has not been established. Whether the degree of risk reduction in gastrointestinal complications by coxibs offsets their increased cost compared with a generic nonselective NSAID was determined.

Methods.—This cost-utility analysis used a systematic review of MEDLINE and published abstracts that included patients with osteoarthritis or rheumatoid arthritis who were not taking aspirin and who required long-term NSAID therapy for moderate to severe arthritis pain. Naproxen, 500 mg twice daily, and coxib, once daily, were administered. Patients were also switched to a coxib if they were intolerant of naproxen. The main outcome measure was the incremental cost per quality-adjusted life-year (QALY) gained. Base-case and sensitivity analyses were performed.

Results.—The base-case analysis showed that the use of a coxib instead of a nonselective NSAID in average-risk patients cost an incremental $275,809 per year to gain 1 additional QALY. The sensitivity analysis showed that the incremental cost per QALY gained decreased to $55,803 when the analysis was limited to the subset of patients with a history of bleeding ulcers. The coxib strategy was dominant when the cost of coxibs was reduced by 90% of the current average wholesale price. A probabilistic sensitivity analysis showed that if a third-party payer was willing to pay $150,000 per QALY gained, then 4.3% of average-risk patients would fall within the budget.

Conclusions.—The risk reduction obtained with coxibs does not offset their increased cost compared with nonselective NSaids in the treatment of average-risk patients with chronic arthritis. However, the incremental cost-effectiveness ratio of coxibs may be acceptable when they are used in the subgroup of patients with a history of bleeding ulcers.

▶ By now, most of us probably accept the evidence that coxibs (selective cyclooxygenase-2 [COX-2] inhibitors) have less gastrointestinal toxicity than traditional NSaids. But can we afford them? Depending on the agents compared, coxibs may be more than 20 times more expensive than their nonselective counterparts. From a societal perspective—or is it from a business perspective?—the safety benefits of switching to a coxib obviously need to be substantial to make these agents cost-effective.

To address this issue, Spiegel et al have used a sophisticated mathematical model to compare the cost-effectiveness of coxibs in patients with chronic arthritis. They rigorously input data and assumptions from the literature, and establish parameters that conservatively favor the use of a coxib. (For example, they test their model by using a hypothetical "best" coxib that has an efficacy and safety profile reflecting the best qualities of rofecoxib and celecoxib combined.) The results are instructive, in that they show that the general use of coxibs on a population of people with inflammatory arthritis turns out to be exceptionally expensive. In particular, the authors found that using a coxib on all comers with chronic arthritis would be about twice as expensive, on a cost-benefit basis, as providing dialysis to patients with end-stage renal failure. Moreover, from a cost-effectiveness point of view, the use of coxibs would only be favored over an NSAID for general arthritis use if the cost of the of these agents were to be reduced by about 90%. In one sense, the authors' model isn't fair, since it sets the use of coxibs against NSAIDs without misoprostal or a proton pump inhibitor (PPI), only adding a PPI if gastrointestinal symptoms or signs occur. If the model presumed that NSAIDs were always prescribed with a protective agent (to bring the safety of the NSAID to something like coxib equivalence), the cost-effectiveness of NSAIDs would be reduced, undoubtedly making the difference between coxibs and NSAIDs smaller. On the other hand, it is likely that in clinical practice, most traditional NSAIDs are not automatically prescribed with gastroprotection (I for one almost always prescribe a PPI for anybody with moderate to high risk for whom I do not prescribe a coxib, but perhaps I'm atypical), so maybe the model accurately reflects the general (rather than most conservative) standard of practice. The model also does not factor in other theoretic risks of coxibs, or the possible benefits of coxibs versus NSAIDs in patients on aspirin, both still murky subjects.

Can we rescue the use of coxibs from the clutches of cost-effectiveness? Possibly Spiegel et al show us the way. When they changed their model to assume a high-risk population (in their case, a subset of patients with a history of bleeding ulcers), they observed that the cost-benefit ratio became somewhat reasonable. As physicians, it is our duty when prescribing drugs to weigh risk versus benefit, not cost versus benefit. Still, we also have some obligations to society at large. In practice, it is probably appropriate to reserve coxibs for patients who will really benefit from them—chronic anti-inflammatory users with gastrointestinal risk factors such as older age, diabetes, gastritis or ulcer history, or steroid or (in my opinion) aspirin use—at least until the price of coxibs falls.

Also noted: 2 studies that ask questions similar to that of Spiegel et al, but take a different point of view. Maetzel et al[1] conclude that COX-2 inhibitor use is cost-effective in high-risk and elderly patients. Solomon et al[2] suggest that adverse event–related costs may be excessive when using nonselective NSAIDs.

M. H. Pillinger, MD

References

1. Maetzel A, Krahn M, Naglie G: The cost effectiveness of rofecoxib and celecoxib in patients with osteoarthritis or rheumatoid arthritis. *Arthritis Rheum* 49:283-292, 2003.
2. Solomon DH, Glynn RJ, Bohn R, et al: The hidden cost of nonselective nonsteroidal anti-inflammatory drugs in older patients. *J Rheumatol* 30:792-798, 2003.

The Human Multidrug Resistance Protein MRP4 Functions as a Prostaglandin Efflux Transporter and Is Inhibited by Nonsteroidal Antiinflammatory Drugs

Reid G, Wielinga P, Zelcer N, et al (Netherlands Cancer Inst, Amsterdam)
Proc Natl Acad Sci U S A 100:9244-9249, 2003   12–4

Background.—There is a critical role for prostaglandins in the regulation of many physiologic processes. However, the mechanism by which prostaglandins are released by the cells is not fully understood. Prostaglandins are poorly membrane permeable but are believed to exit cells by passive diffusion. The recently characterized multidrug resistance protein MRP4 has been shown to transport several physiologic substrates, such as cyclic nucleotides, steroid conjugates, and folate. Like MRP1, MRP4 is inhibited by the leukotriene antagonist MK571. There is circumstantial evidence to suggest that MRP4 may also interact with prostaglandins. The interaction between members of the MRP family and prostaglandins was investigated.

Methods.—The interaction between prostaglandins and members of the adenosine triphosphate (ATP)-binding cassette transporter ABCC (MRP) family of membrane export pumps was investigated.

Results.—In inside-out membrane vesicles derived from insect cells or HEK293 cells, MRP4 catalyzed the time-dependent and ATP-dependent uptake of prostaglandin E_1 (PGE_1) and PGE_2. However, MRP1, MRP2, MRP3, and MRP5 did not transport either PGE_1 or PGE_2. Saturation kinetics were demonstrated by the MRP4-mediated transport of PGE_1 and PGE_2, with K_m values of 2.1 and 3.4 µM, respectively. It was further demonstrated that PGF_{1a}, PGF_{2a}, PGA_1, and thromboxane B_2 were high-affinity inhibitors, and presumably substrates, of MRP4.

In addition, several nonsteroidal anti-inflammatory drugs were found to be potent inhibitors of MRP4 at concentrations that did not inhibit MRP1. The steady-state accumulation of PGE_1 and PGE_2 was reduced in proportion to MRP4 expression in cells expressing the prostaglandin transporter PGT. This accumulation deficit was reversed by inhibition of MRP4 by an MRP4-specific RNA interference construct or by indomethacin.

Conclusions.—The suggestion of these findings is that MRP4 can release prostaglandins from cells and that, in addition to inhibiting prostaglandin synthesis, some nonsteroidal antiinflammatory drugs may also act by the inhibition of this release.

▶ Now that we've all become comfortable with the idea of multiple cyclo-oxygenases, selectively inhibited, it's time we recognized that the synthesis and activity of prostaglandins is actually an even more complicated process. For example, investigators are increasingly interested in the fact that PGH_2, the product of both COX-1 and COX-2, is merely the substrate for a variety of different enzymes that variously generate E prostaglandins, thromboxanes, and the like. So, for example, an agent that inhibits PGE synthase, the enzyme that makes PGEs,[1] would be more selective than a COX-2 inhibitor in that it would have no effect on other synthetic branches of the pathway.

In this article, Reid et al address another interesting and potentially relevant question: Once made, how do prostaglandins get out of the cell? Many of our readers may not be aware that cyclooxygenases are actually localized mainly on intracellular membranes. Thus, prostaglandins are synthesized in the cytosol and, being hydrophilic, they are not readily permeable to the plasma membrane. If the PGEs can't get out, they can't exert many of their effects, since they act extracellularly to interact with cellular receptors.

What Reid et al show is that PGEs are actually extruded from the cell through the actions of an energy-dependent transporter designated MRP4, for multidrug resistance protein 4; and yes, this protein is one of a series that are better known for their ability to extrude drugs and induce drug resistance. Inhibition of this transporter's actions resulted in diminished extrusion of PGEs, and accumulation of those PGEs intracellularly.

Whether inhibition of MRP4 actually results in clinically relevant diminishment of extracellular PGE (and whether the accumulation of PGE intracellularly has its own effects!) is not yet known, but certainly these observations suggest a potential target for anti-inflammatory strategies. In fact, such strategies may already be in use, as the authors demonstrate that several nonselective COX inhibitors (indomethacin, ibuprofen, flubiprofen, and ketoprofen, each at clinically relevant or near-relevant concentrations) inhibit the efflux of prostaglandin by MRP4. Interestingly, selective COX-2 inhibitors (rofecoxib, celecoxib) did not share this effect on MRP4.

While the translation of these observations into clinical uses is undoubtedly many years away, they testify to the fascinating and complex world of the cell. We should celebrate that complexity, for it is precisely what we don't yet know about ourselves that holds the greatest promise of new knowledge and new therapies.

M. H. Pillinger, MD

Reference

1. Stichtenoth DO, Thoren S, Bian H, et al: Microsomal prostaglandin E synthase is regulated by proinflammatory cytokines and glucocorticoids in primary rheumatoid synovial cells. *J Immunol* 167:469-474, 2001.

PART TWO

INFECTIOUS DISEASES

DAVID R. SNYDMAN, MD

Introduction

The past year in infectious diseases has been one in which emerging and newly described infections were in the limelight. Chief among them was the reporting and description of the causative agent of the Severe Acute Respiratory Syndrome (SARS). The SARS coronavirus agent discovery was probably the most important disease to emerge in 2003 and serves as a testament to molecular microbiology since the causative agent was discovered within several months of the appearance of this potentially lethal infection. In addition, the emergence of the animal-associated coronavirus, which adapted to humans and spread very rapidly, serves to warn us about the potential of other animal-to-human diseases that may become adapted under specific circumstances. SARS had an enormous economic impact on the world when transmission was noted to be very common, even on airplanes and in hotels. Billions of dollars in economic hardship resulted for countries and airlines alike when travel to the Far East came to a halt. Airlines flirted with bankruptcy and health care workers became ill and died of SARS. Such cases put the spotlight on hand washing and infection control measures. The development of diagnostic tests was rapid and will serve to diagnose and treat patients in the future, should SARS reemerge. Another newly emerging infection, namely West Nile virus infection, also is highlighted since transmission by blood transfusion or organ donation was first reported.

I have also chosen a number of articles that provide information on pneumococcal vaccine and influenza vaccine. These articles should help the internist manage patients who deserve or require such immunizations. New aspects of HIV therapy, such as structured treatment interruption, and prognostic factors for survival have also been recently published and help the internist make decisions about therapy and provide prognostic information to patients. There was the licensure of a new drug, tenofovir, which had important clinical trial data published.

In selecting the articles I have for this volume, I have tried to strike a balance between articles that are useful for managing common problems seen in the clinical practice of internal medicine and those that so significantly advance the science of medicine as to be extremely important.

David R. Snydman, MD

13 Emerging Infectious Diseases

Identification of Severe Acute Respiratory Syndrome in Canada
McGeer AJ, for the National Microbiology Laboratory, Canada, and the Canadian Severe Acute Respiratory Syndrome Study Team (Mount Sinai Hosp, Toronto; et al)
N Engl J Med 348:1995-2005, 2003   13–1

Introduction.—Severe acute respiratory syndrome (SARS) is a condition with an unknown cause that has been identified in patients in Asia, North America, and Europe. The initial epidemiologic findings, clinical description, and diagnostic findings that followed the identification of SARS in Canada were described.

Methods.—The initial cases in Toronto were identified in members of a multigenerational family of Hong Kong descent who live in Toronto and had visited relatives in Hong Kong from February 13 through February 23, 2003 (Fig 2). Epidemiologic, clinical, and diagnostic data were gathered prospectively from the initial 10 cases as they were recognized. Specimens from all patients were sent to local, provincial, national, and international laboratories to identify an etiologic agent.

Results.—The ages of the patients ranged from 24 to 78 years; 60% were male. Transmission occurred only with close contact. The most frequent presenting symptoms were fever (100%) and malaise (70%), followed by nonproductive cough (100%) and dyspnea (80%) associated with infiltrates on chest radiographs (100%). Lymphopenia (89% of those with available data), elevated lactate dehydrogenase levels (80%), elevated aspartate aminotransferase levels (78%), and elevated creatinine kinase levels (56%) were frequently observed (Table 1). Empirical therapy often included antibiotics, oseltamivir, and IV ribavirin. Five patients needed mechanical ventilation. Three patients died. Clinical improvement was seen in 5 patients. Laboratory findings were either negative or not clinically significant, except for the amplification of human metapneumovirus from respiratory specimens from 5 of 9 patients and the isolation and amplification of a novel coronavirus from 5 of 9 patients. Both pathogens were isolated in 4 cases.

Conclusion.—The identification of SARS in Canada only a few weeks after an outbreak on another continent underscores the ease with which infec-

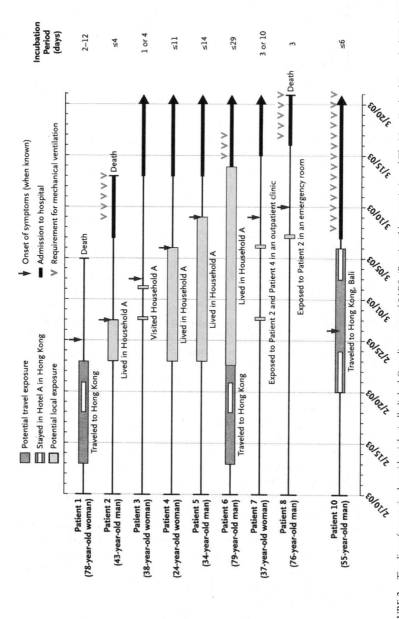

FIGURE 2.—Timeline of events in the epidemiologically linked Canadian cases of SARS. (Reprinted by permission of *The New England Journal of Medicine*, courtesy of Poutanen SM, for the National Microbiology Laboratory, Canada, and the Canadian Severe Acute Respiratory Syndrome Study Team: Identification of severe acute respiratory syndrome in Canada. *N Engl J Med* 348:1995-2005, 2003. Copyright 2003, Massachusetts Medical Society. All rights reserved.)

TABLE 1.—Clinical Features of the Canadian Patients With SARS at Presentation

Variable	Value
	no./
	no. with
	results
	(%)
Symptoms	
Fever	10/10 (100)*
Nonproductive cough	10/10 (100)
Dyspnea	8/10 (80)
Malaise	7/10 (70)
Diarrhea	5/10 (50)
Chest pain	3/10 (30)
Headache	3/10 (30)
Sore throat	3/10 (30)
Myalgias	2/10 (20)
Vomiting	1/10 (10)
Investigations	
Infiltrate on chest radiography	9/9 (100)
Oxygen saturation on room air <95%	7/9 (78)
Leukopenia (cell count <4×10^9/liter)	2/9 (22)
Lymphopenia (cell count <1.5×10^9/liter)	8/9 (89)
Thrombocytopenia (cell count <130×10^9/liter)	3/9 (33)
Lactate dehydrogenase (above upper limit of normal)	4/5 (80)
Aspartate aminotransferase (> 1.5× upper limit of normal)	7/9 (78)
Alanine aminotransferase (>1.5 × upper limit of normal)	5/9 (56)
Creatine kinase (above upper limit of normal)	5/9 (56)

*Although all 10 patients had a history of fever at presentation to the hospital, on examination only 5 of 9 were febrile (temperature, 38.4°C to 40°C; 1 had a low-grade fever (temperature, 37.9°C), and 3 had hypothermia (temperature, 35.5°C to 36.5°C).

(Reprinted by permission of *The New England Journal of Medicine*, courtesy of Poutanen SM, for the National Microbiology Laboratory, Canada, and the Canadian Severe Acute Respiratory Syndrome Study Team: Identification of severe acute respiratory syndrome in Canada. *N Engl J Med* 348:1995-2005, 2003. Copyright 2003, Massachusetts Medical Society. All rights reserved.)

tious agents can be transmitted as a result of international travel. It appears that SARS had a viral origin, with patterns indicative of droplet or contact transmission.

▶ The sudden appearance of SARS in China, Hong Kong, Taiwan, Hanoi, and then Toronto caught the attention of the medical community in March/April 2003. This report details the nature of the transmission within a cluster in Canada. Investigators isolated 2 viruses, a new variant of a coronavirus and a metapneumovirus. In their studies the Canadian investigators suggest that the disease could be caused by either the coronavirus or metapneumovirus, or coinfection with both pathogens. However, as noted below in 2 articles (Abstracts 13–2 and 13–3), one from the Centers for Disease Control and Prevention and the World Health Organization, with collaborations from investigative units in Hanoi, Hong Kong, Bangkok, Singapore, and Thailand, and the other from Germany, France, and The Netherlands, the causative agent appears to be a novel coronavirus. What is remarkable is that it took about 2 months for investigators to isolate the causative agent. This is a testament to molecular biology. When compared with the 4 years it took to isolate HIV, one can see that in 20 years we have come a long way in our ability to use molecular biology to detect pathogens, especially when such a dramatic introduction of the disease captures the world's attention.

The Canadian study underscores the relative ease of nosocomial and horizontal transmission within families. As the Canadian investigators point out, treatment is really supportive. Isolation is critically important to prevent nosocomial spread. Canadian investigators also point out the possible role of smoking as a risk factor. As of this writing, the clinical criteria are still reliant on epidemiologic risk factors for exposure since the disease does not really have features that distinguish it from other forms of multiorgan failure and pneumonia with acute respiratory distress syndrome (ARDS).

D. R. Snydman, MD

▶ This seminal article describes the early cases of SARS in North America. The typical viral illness prodrome and lab data are outlined in Table 1. To date, there is no effective therapy known for this life-threatening disorder. Thus, the most effective therapy at present is preventive (quarantine).

J. A. Barker, MD

A Novel Coronavirus Associated With Severe Acute Respiratory Syndrome
Ksiazek TG, and the SARS Working Group (Ctrs for Disease Control and Prevention, Atlanta, Ga; et al)
N Engl J Med 348:1953-1966, 2003   13–2

Introduction.—A worldwide outbreak of severe acute respiratory syndrome (SARS) has been linked with exposures originating from a single ill health care worker from Guangdong Province, China. The etiologic agent of this outbreak was examined.

Methods.—Clinical specimens were received from patients in 7 countries and underwent testing with virus isolation techniques, electron-microscopic and histologic studies, and molecular and serologic assays to detect a wide range of potential pathogens.

Results.—None of the previously described respiratory pathogens were consistently detected. A novel coronavirus was isolated from patients who fulfilled the case definition of SARS. Cytopathologic characteristics were identified in Vero E6 cells inoculated with a throat swab specimen (Figs 1 and 2). Electron-microscopic examination showed ultrastructural features that were characteristic of coronaviruses. Immunohistochemical and immunofluorescence staining demonstrated reactivity with group I coronavirus polyclonal antibodies. Consensus coronavirus primers designed to amplify a fragment of the polymerase gene by reverse transcription–polymerase chain

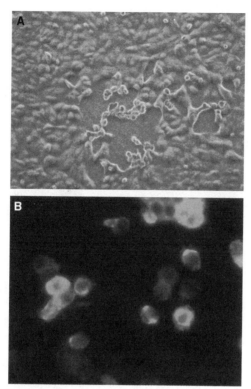

FIGURE 1.—Vero E6 cells inoculated with oropharyngeal specimens from patients with SARS. The typical early cytopathic effects seen with coronavirus isolates from patients with SARS is shown in **Panel A** (×40). Infected Vero cells are shown reacting with the serum of a convalescent patient in an indirect fluorescence antibody assay in **Panel B** (×400). (Reprinted by permission of *The New England Journal of Medicine*, courtesy of Ksiazek TG, and the SARS Working Group: A novel coronavirus associated with severe acute respiratory syndrome. *N Engl J Med* 348:1953-1966, 2003. Copyright 2003, Massachusetts Medical Society. All rights reserved.)

reaction (RT-PCR) were used to determine a sequence that clearly identified the isolate as a unique coronavirus only distantly associated with previously sequenced coronaviruses. With the use of specific diagnostic RT-PCR primers, several identical nucleotide sequences were identified in 12 patients from several locations. This finding was consistent with a point-source outbreak. Indirect fluorescence antibody tests and enzyme-linked immunosorbent assays made with the new isolate have been used to illustrate a virus-specific serologic response. This virus may never have been previously circulated in the US population.

Conclusion.—A novel coronavirus is linked with the worldwide outbreak of SARS, with evidence suggesting that this virus has an etiologic role in SARS.

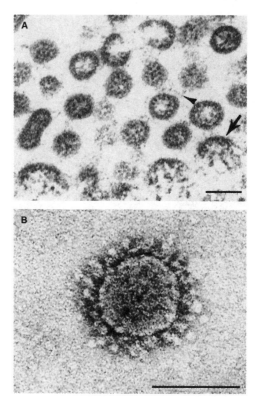

FIGURE 2.—Ultrasound characteristics of SARS-associated coronavirus grown in Vero E6 cells. Panel A shows a thick-section electron-microscopical view of viral nucleocapsides aligned along the membrane of the rough endoplastic reticulum (*arrow*) as particles bud into the cisternae. Enveloped virions have surface projections (*arrowhead*) and an electron-lucent center. Directly under the viral envelope lies a characteristic ring formed by the helical nucleocapsid, often seen in cross section. Negative-stain electron microscopy (Panel B) shows a stain-penetrated coronavirus particle with an internal helical nucleocapsid-like structure and club-shaped surface projections surrounding the periphery of the particle, a finding typical of coronaviruses (methylamine tungstate stain). The *bars* represent 100 nm. (Reprinted by permission of *The New England Journal of Medicine*, courtesy of Ksiazek TG, and the SARS Working Group: A novel coronavirus associated with severe acute respiratory syndrome. *N Engl J Med* 348:1953-1966, 2003. Copyright 2003, Massachusetts Medical Society. All rights reserved.)

Identification of a Novel Coronavirus in Patients With Severe Acute Respiratory Syndrome

Drosten C, Günther S, Preiser W, et al (Natl Reference Ctr for Tropical Infectious Diseases, Hamburg, Germany; Johann Wolfgang Goethe Univ, Frankfurt am Main, Germany; Philipps Univ, Marburg, Germany; et al)
N Engl J Med 348:1967-1976, 2003   13–3

Background.—The severe acute respiratory syndrome (SARS) emerged in spring, 2003 as a new clinical entity. The epidemic began in Asia, and most of the cases occurred in China and the Asia-Pacific region. However, international air travel enabled the SARS epidemic to spread from Asia to other continents. The identification of a novel coronavirus in SARS patients is discussed.

Methods.—The index patient was a 32-year-old male physician in Singapore who, in the first week of March 2003, treated a patient from Hong Kong for atypical pneumonia. On day 1 (March 9), the physician experienced an abrupt onset of fever (39.4 °C) while in New York. A dry cough and sore throat developed on day 4, accompanied by erythema on trunk. On day 7, while on a stopover in Frankfurt, Germany en route to Singapore, the physician was admitted to a hospital isolation unit with suspected SARS. He was treated with levofloxacin, vancomycin, imipenem, doxycycline, and oseltamivir. Two contacts of the index patient, his wife and his mother-in-law, were also isolated. Contact 1 reported a headache on admission on day 1, followed by development of fever and myalgia on day 2. Her temperature then decreased, but fever recurred on day 7 accompanied by crackles over her lungs, dry cough, and hypoxemia. She was treated with erythromycin and ceftriaxone. Contact 2 had similar symptoms and was treated with imipenem, levofloxacin, doxycycline, and oseltamivir. Clinical specimens were obtained from these patients, from 15 patients with probable or suspected SARS, and from 21 healthy contacts of these patients. In addition, stool samples for 54 patients in Germany were used as control agents.

Results.—A novel coronavirus isolate termed *FFM-ic* was identified in the SARS patients (Fig 1C). The virus was isolated in cell culture, and a sequence 300 nucleotides long was obtained by polymerase chain reaction (PCR)-based random-amplification procedure. Genetic analysis showed that this virus is only distantly related to known coronaviruses. Conventional and real-time PCR assays for specific and sensitive detection of the novel virus

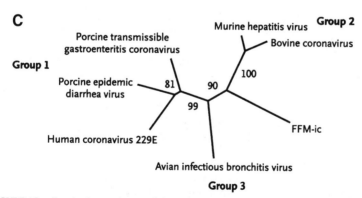

FIGURE 1C.—Genetic characterization of the novel coronavirus. A phylogenetic tree shows relations among coronavirus polymerase gene fragments (corresponding to BNI-1) according to the neighbor-joining method. The maximum likelihood method revealed the same relations (data not shown). Genetic distances are indicated by the lengths of the branches. Analyses were performed on a bootstrapped data set (100 replicates). In addition to the coronavirus isolate FFM-ic, avian infections bronchitis virus (IBR31131), bovine coronavirus (AF220295), human coronavirus 229E (12175745), murine hepatitis virus (9629812), porcine epidemic diarrhea virus (19387576), and porcine transmissible gastroenteritis coronavirus (13399293) were included in the analysis. (Reprinted by permission of *The New England Journal of Medicine* from Drosten C, Günther S, Preiser W, et al: Identification of a novel coronavirus in patients with severe acute respiratory syndrome. *N Engl J Med* 348:1967-1976, 2003. Copyright 2003, Massachusetts Medical Society. All rights reserved.)

TABLE 3.—Proportion of Patients with a Positive RT-PCR Result for Coronavirus*

Group	Mean No. of Samples per Patient	Fraction of Patients Testing Positive	
		IN-6/IN-7 and Nested SAR1S/ SAR1As	BNIoutS2/ BNIoutAs and Nested BNIinS/BNIinAs
Patients with probable SARS†	2.2	5/5	5/5
Patients with suspected SARS‡	1.3	3/13	3/13
Contacts	1.0	0/21	0/21

*RT-PCR denotes reverse-transcriptase polymerase chain reaction.
†Samples were from the lower respiratory tract in five patients and nasopharyngeal swabs in one patient (all positive); samples were obtained 3 to 13 days after the onset of illness.
‡Nasopharyngeal samples from 13 patients were used; they were obtained 3 to 12 days after the onset of illness.
(Reprinted by permission of *The New England Journal of Medicine* from Drosten C, Günther S, Preiser W, et al: Identification of a novel coronavirus in patients with severe acute respiratory syndrome. N *Engl J Med* 348:1967-1976, 2003. Copyright 2003, Massachusetts Medical Society. All rights reserved.)

were established. The virus was detected in a variety of clinical specimens from the patients with SARS but was not detected in the control subjects (Table 3). Sputum samples from the patients contained high concentrations of viral RNA of up to 100 million molecules/mL. Viral RNA was also detected at extremely low concentrations in plasma during the acute phase and in feces in the late convalescence phase. In the SARS-infected patients, seroconversion was observed on the Vero cells in which the virus was isolated.

Conclusion.—Patients with SARS are acutely infected with the novel coronavirus identified in this study.

► These 2 articles (Abstracts 13–2 and 13–3) identify the Urbani strain of coronavirus, putatively the agent associated with SARS. While the YEAR BOOK OF MEDICINE normally would concentrate on clinical descriptions, I chose these articles to underscore the power of a cooperative approach to disease tracking. The investigators relied on a broad multidisciplinary approach, incorporating clinical, epidemiologic, and laboratory investigation. As clinicians, without epidemiologic features to document exposure, we will be lost without the diagnostic tests that are becoming available. And if the virus reappears next year, more broadly disseminated, then every patient with community-acquired ARDS and multiorgan failure will be candidates for testing. Therefore, the testing will be paramount to any diagnostic consideration.

Notable in these articles is the absence of antibody to the coronavirus, and the development of specific antibody during infection. The absence of antibody in all subjects tested also points out that this virus has not spread widely prior to this outbreak. Future studies will be necessary to establish the prevalence of infection in certain populations and to establish the link with Guangdong Province in China, the origin of the index case in Hong Kong.

The second study from European colleagues (Abstract 13–3) points out the high viral RNA in sputum from the index patient, which is consistent with a high degree of infectivity. The detection of viral RNA in serum at day 9 also points out that replication may take place in extrapulmonary sites, even the blood. They also cite the fact that viral RNA can be found in stool even during convalescence. This has important infection control implications for isolation and cleaning of the enviroment. They also point out that nasal and throat swabs seem less suitable for diagnosis since less viral RNA can be detected in these specimens than in sputum.

D. R. Snydman, MD

Clinical Progression and Viral Load in a Community Outbreak of Corona-virus-Associated SARS Pneumonia: A Prospective Study
Yuen KY, and members of the HKU/UCH SARS Study Group (Univ of Hong Kong, China; et al)
Lancet 361:1767-1772, 2003   13–4

Introduction.—Severe acute respiratory syndrome (SARS) investigations have primarily been retrospective or limited to initial clinical, hematologic, radiologic, and microbiological findings. Reported is the temporal progres-

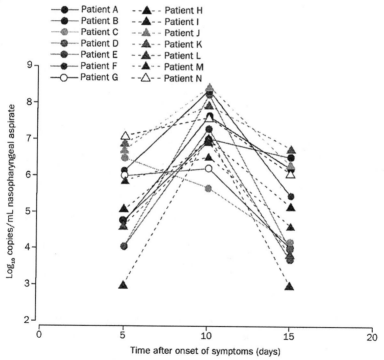

FIGURE 4.—Sequential quantitative RT-PCR for SARS-associated coronavirus in nasopharyngeal aspirates of 14 patients with SARS. *Abbreviations: RT-PCR,* Reverse transcriptase polymerase chain reaction; *SARS,* severe acute respiratory syndrome. (Courtesy of Peiris JS, for members of the HKU/UCH SARS Study Group: Clinical progression and viral load in a community outbreak of coronavirus-associated SARS pneumonia: A prospective study. *Lancet* 361:1767-1772, 2003. Reprinted with permission from Elsevier Science.)

TABLE 4.—Subsequent Analysis of Clinical Samples of 20 Patients With Initial RT-PCR–Positive Nasopharyngeal Aspirates and Antibody Seroconversion to SARS-Associated Coronavirus

	Time After Onset of Symtoms (Days; n=20)				
	10	13	16	19	21
Sample (positivity rate)					
Nasopharyngeal aspirate	19 (95%)	18 (90%)	18 (90%)	15 (75%)	9 (47%)*
Stool	20 (100%)	20 (100%)	19 (95%)	12 (80%)†	10 (67%)†
Urine	10 (50%)	9 (45%)	7 (35%)	6 (30%)	4 (21%)*

*In 19 patients.
†In 15 patients.
Abbreviations: RT-PCR, Reverse transcriptase polymerase chain reaction; SARS, severe acute respiratory syndrome.
(Courtesy of Peiris JS, for the Members of the HKU/UCH SARS Study Group: Clinical progression and viral load in a community outbreak of coronavirus-associated SARS pneumonia: A prospective study. Lancet 361:1767-1772, 2003. Reprinted with permission from Elsevier Science.)

sion of the clinical, radiologic, and virologic changes in residents of a housing estate placed under close surveillance by the Department of Health soon after identification of a SARS outbreak.

Methods.—Between March 24 and 28, 2003, 75 patients were managed for 3 weeks with a standard treatment protocol of ribavirin and corticosteroids. The pattern of clinical disease, viral load, risk factors for poor clinical outcome, and the usefulness of virologic diagnostic methods were examined.

Results.—A fever and pneumonia initially improved; however, 64 patients (85%) had recurrent fevers at a mean of 8.9 days, 55 (73%) had watery diarrhea after 7.5 days, 60 (80%) had radiologic worsening after 7.4 days, and respiratory symptoms worsened in 34 patients (45%) after 8.6 days (all mean values). An improvement in initial pulmonary lesions was linked to the appearance of new radiologic lesions at other sites. Nine patients (12%) experienced spontaneous pneumomediastinum, and 15 (20%) had acute respiratory distress syndrome (ARDS) in week 3. Quantitative reverse transcriptase polymerase chain reaction of nasopharyngeal aspirates in 14 patients (4 with ARDS) revealed a peak viral load at day 10, and at day 15, the load was lower than that at admission (Fig 4 and Table 4). Both age and chronic hepatitis B virus infection treated with lamivudine were independent significant risk factors for progression to ARDS ($P = .001$). On day 14, SARS-related coronavirus in feces was found on reverse transcriptase polymerase chain reaction in 65 of 67 patients (97%). The mean time to seroconversion was 20 days.

Conclusion.—The consistent clinical progression, shifting radiologic infiltrates, and an inverted V viral load profile indicate that worsening in week 2 is unrelated to uncontrolled viral replication and may be associated with immunopathologic damage.

▶ This study is unique in that it was a prospective evaluation of a housing unit placed under surveillance. Thus, the data were prospectively collected from a cohort of patients admitted to the hospital. These authors show that the virus can be detected in fecal and urine samples, as well as in nasopharyngeal secretions. The importance of SARS-associated coronavirus detection in the stool is not entirely clear, although a fecal–oral route of transmission has been suggested and has been related to a faulty sewage system in at least 1 outbreak. Furthermore, watery diarrhea was seen in a number of patients. The infection control aspects of transmission through feces is also unclear. From a diagnostic perspective, serologic seroconversion was detectable in 93% of patients at 1 month after the onset of symptoms.

D. R. Snydman, MD

Critically Ill Patients With Severe Acute Respiratory Syndrome
Fowler RA, for the Toronto SARS Critical Care Group (Univ of Toronto; et al)
JAMA 290:367-373, 2003   13–5

Background.—Severe acute respiratory syndrome (SARS) produces an acute respiratory illness that leads to critical illness in 23% to 32% of patients. The health care system has been strained by the influx of SARS patients and the concerns related to quarantine and SARS infection among health care workers (HCWs). Understanding SARS-related critical illness is required to plan more effectively for the care needed. The epidemiology, clinical characteristics, and outcomes at 28 days for SARS patients who are critically ill were outlined, with an estimate of the impact accompanying SARS transmission from critically ill patients to HCWs.

Methods.—The medical records of 38 adult patients with SARS-related critical illness were reviewed retrospectively. All had been admitted to ICUs in the Toronto area. Daily data collection was undertaken for the first 7 days in the ICU, with 28 days of follow-up.

Results.—One hundred ninety-six patients had probable or suspected SARS, with 38 (19%) developing critical illness. Eighteen percent of the patients were HCWs. Patients ranged in age from 39.0 to 69.6 years (median, 57.4 years), with a predominance of older non-HCWs seen in the critically ill group. In addition, the critically ill patients were more likely to have co-morbid conditions such as diabetes.

Eighty-two percent of the critically ill patients met the diagnostic criteria for acute respiratory distress syndrome, with 29 patients (15% of all SARS patients) requiring mechanical ventilation. Over the first 7 days in the ICU, 34% of the ventilated patients suffered barotrauma, 37% developed cardiovascular dysfunction, 21% hepatic dysfunction, and 11% renal dysfunction.

Eight days was the median time between the onset of symptoms and admission to the ICU; 19 days was the median time from symptom onset to death. At 28 days, mortality was 34% of the total number of patients and 45% of those requiring mechanical ventilation. At 28 days, 6 patients were still requiring mechanical ventilation. At 8 weeks, mortality for those requiring mechanical ventilation was 52%, while the overall mortality rate was 39%, with 3 patients still requiring mechanical ventilation.

Poor outcome occurred in patients of older age, with a history of diabetes mellitus, with tachycardia on admission, or with elevated creatine kinase levels. Patients who required ICU care tended to have bilateral radiographic lung infiltrates at a higher rate than other patients. ICU patients transmitted SARS to HCWs on 2 occasions. As a result, 10-day closures of 35 critical care beds in a tertiary care university medical-surgical ICU (38% of those in Toronto) were required; 38 concurrent bed closures (33% of the Toronto community medical-surgical ICU bed capacity) also occurred because of ICU SARS transmission and quarantine of HCWs.

Conclusion.—A high proportion of the patients who had probable or suspected SARS developed critical illness requiring care in an ICU. While the median time from symptom onset until death was 19 days, many deaths occurred after the follow-up time of 28 days. Older age, preexisting diabetes mellitus, tachycardia on admission, and elevated creatine kinase levels were associated with higher mortality rates. Because HCWs tended to be younger than other SARS patients, they were less likely to die. Half of the SARS patients who required mechanical ventilation died. In addition, the critical care resources of the region were significantly strained by the outbreak.

▶ The authors identify several characteristics of patients with SARS associated with a worse outcome, namely, older age, diabetes mellitus, tachycardia, and elevated creatine kinase. Mortality was much higher among those aged 65 years or older. Among those who did require mechanical ventilation, mortality may have been similar to that seen with influenza outbreaks. The strain on medical resources was enormous, and the authors calculate that one third of the ICU capacity in Toronto was compromised by the SARS outbreak. Clearly, should SARS reappear again to the same or greater extent, we will need greater capacity and improved infection control to avoid the nosocomial spread that also compromised the intensive care capacity in Toronto and elsewhere.

D. R. Snydman, MD

Neurologic Manifestations and Outcome of West Nile Virus Infection
Sejvar JJ, Haddad MB, Tierney BC, et al (Ctrs for Disease Control and Prevention, Atlanta, Ga; Ochsner Clinic, New Orleans, La; Methodist Rehabilitation Ctr, Jackson, Miss)
JAMA 290:511-515, 2003   13–6

Background.—Acute neurologic illness develops in less than 1% of the human cases of West Nile virus (WNV), with most human infections being either subclinical or manifest as mild febrile illness. The neurologic manifestations, laboratory and neurodiagnostic results, and long-term outcomes of WNV infection were investigated.

Methods.—A community-based prospective evaluation was carried out from August 1 to September 2, 2002, in St Tammany Parish, Louisiana.

Thirty-nine suspected cases of WNV were identified and clinical data collected. Follow-up extended for 8 months.

Results.—Of the 39 suspected cases, 16 were confirmed to be WNV infection; the other patients were diagnosed with viral meningitis, headache, viral encephalitis, unspecified viral illness, and encephalopathy. Five patients had West Nile meningitis (WNM), 8 had West Nile encephalitis (WNE), and 3 had acute flaccid paralysis (AFP); 1 patient had AFP plus encephalitis. The median age of patients with WNE was 70 years, while that for patients with WNM was 35 years.

Hospitalization began a median of 2.5 days after symptom onset and lasted a median of 12 days. Five patients spent between 3 and 19 days in intensive care. All patients reported similar symptoms, including frontal/retro-orbital headache, rash, and shakiness or twitching. Patients with WNE complained most about behavioral personality changes. Difficulty with balance and gait as well as weakness (focal in the AFP patients and generalized in other) were reported. Changes in mental status occurred a median of 3 days after symptom onset. AFP patients had areflexia or hyporeflexia, while WNE and WNM patients had abnormal hyperreflexia. Dyskinesias (with tremor that was static or kinetic, asymmetric, and involved the upper extremities), myoclonus, and parkinsonism were also seen. AFP patients reported asymmetric limb weakness plus bladder and bowel dysfunction.

No abnormal CT findings were noted, but MRI showed nonacute abnormalities in 8 patients and bilateral focal lesions of the basal ganglia, thalamus, and pons in 2 severely ill patients. AFP patients had findings consistent with menigitis plus diffuse degenerative changes without spinal cord abnormalities. Electroencephalography showed electrographic seizures, focal sharp waves, and diffuse irregular slow waves. Electromyographic and nerve-conduction studies showed a severe, asymmetric process of the anterior horn cells.

One patient with WNE died 2.5 months after symptom onset, 3 patients with AFP and 2 patients with WNE required long-term rehabilitation care, 11 patients returned home and were functioning normally, 3 were home but dependent, and 1 was in rehabilitation at 8 months. Fatigue, myalgias, and headache persisted. WNE patients reported persistent cognitive deficits. WNM patients had no neurologic deficits, while tremor and parkinsonism were seen in WNE and AFP patients. Most WNE patients recovered to normal or near-normal functioning within 4 months. AFP patients had the lowest overall functioning scores, needing a wheelchair for ambulation and aid with daily activities.

Conclusion.—Acute WNV illness produced disorders of movement (especially tremor, myoclonus, and parkinsonism) more often than previously thought, but the prognosis is generally favorable. Fatigue, headache, and myalgia may persist. Patients with WNE have variable long-term outcomes, but severe encephalopathy is not always indicative of poor prognosis. When meningitis or encephalitis is associated with a syndrome resembling poliomyelitis, the long-term outcome tends to be poor.

▶ The introduction of WNV infection in New York City in 1999, with subsequent dissemination throughout the United States, has heightened our awareness of the diverse clinical manifestations as more cases are reported from regions of the United States where the virus is now endemic. This report from Louisiana underscores the diverse clinical manifestations of WNV infection. Clinical features that differentiate it from other forms of encephalitis include tremor, myoclonus and a Parkinson-like syndrome. In addition, acute flaccid paralysis has become recognized with a polio-like syndrome.

What the authors point out in this very nicely studied population is that the patients without flaccid paralysis do well, and at 8 months' follow-up, all have returned to work and reported normal or near-normal functioning. Interestingly, severe initial encephalopathy did not necessarily portend a poor prognosis; however, persistent fatigue, headache, and myalgia may also be quite common. Not surprisingly, imaging studies show involvement of the pons, thalamus, and basal ganglia. To my knowledge, this is the most comprehensive clinical description of WNV infection to date.

D. R. Snydman, MD

Transmission of West Nile Virus From an Organ Donor to Four Transplant Recipients
Iwamoto M, for the West Nile Virus in Transplant Recipients Investigation Team (Ctrs for Disease Control and Prevention, Atlanta, Ga; et al)
N Engl J Med 348:2196-2203, 2003   13–7

Purpose.—West Nile virus is spread to human beings via infected mosquitoes and birds. Viral transmission by way of blood or organs has not previously been reported. West Nile virus transmission from an organ donor to 4 separate transplant recipients was reported (Table 2).

Patients.—The recipients underwent transplantation of the heart, liver, and kidneys from a single donor who died of trauma. This patient received more than 50 units of blood products before she was declared brain dead. A week or 2 after transplantation, encephalitis developed in 3 of the organ recipients and a febrile illness developed in the fourth. On investigation, 3 of these patients were shown to be seropositive for West Nile virus immunoglobulin M antibody. In the fourth patient—1 of the kidney recipients—isolation and nucleic acid and antigen assays demonstrated brain tissue positivity for West Nile virus. The other 3 organ recipients recovered from their illness.

No West Nile virus was found in serum specimens taken from the donor before or immediately after her blood transfusions. However, serum and plasma samples taken at the time of organ harvest tested positive on viral nucleic acid testing and viral culture. Review and follow-up of blood donors identified 1 donor who had West Nile viremia at the time of donation. Over

TABLE 2.—Selected Laboratory Results for Organ Recipients During Acute West Nile Virus Illness

Variable	Patient 1	Patient 2	Patient 3	Patient 4*
Blood†				
Hemoglobin (g/dl)	10.0	10.9	12.7	9.1
White-cell count (10^{-3}/mm^3)	15.8	4.8	8.0	4.1
Neutrophils (%)	90	73	94	84
Lymphocytes (%)	8	19	4	7
Other (%)	2	8	2	9
Platelet count (10^{-3}/mm^3)	237	121	140	46
Tacrolimus level (ng/ml)	6.7	12.0	17.5	3.4
Cerebrospinal fluid‡				
Protein (mg/dl)	87	71	75	—
White-cell count (per mm^3)	675	10	1	—
Neutrophils (%)	92	43	24	—
Lymphocytes (%)	6	48	16	—
Other (%)	2	9	60	—
Glucose (mg/dl)§	67	56	74	—

*CSF fluid was not obtained from patient 4.
†Blood samples were obtained at the time of the onset of symptoms or re-admission to the hospital.
‡CSF samples were obtained while patients were having symptoms of febrile encephalopathy.
§To convert values for glucose to millimoles per liter, multiply by 0.05551.
(Reprinted by permission of *The New England Journal of Medicine* from Iwamoto M, for the West Nile Virus in Transplant Recipients Investigation Team: Transmission of West Nile virus from an organ donor to four transplant recipients. *N Engl J Med* 348:2196-2203, 2003. Copyright 2003, Massachusetts Medical Society. All rights reserved.)

the subsequent 2 months, this patient became seropositive with West Nile virus immunoglobulin M antibodies.

Conclusion.—This is the first reported case of West Nile virus transmission from a donor to organ recipients. The previously healthy donor probably acquired the virus via transfusion of blood products. Immunosuppressed organ transplant recipients may be at elevated risk for severe disease should they be infected with West Nile virus.

▶ The first recognition of transmission of West Nile virus from blood and organ transplantation has set into motion changes in organ and blood donation screening. This outbreak best illustrates the potential for transmission via such routes, a heretofore postulated but unproven concept. In addition, the severity of illness in the transplant recipients—with a 75% mortality rate—stands in sharp contrast to the cases cited below.

There are a couple of notable features. One, the incubation period of 7 to 17 days was a bit longer in the transplant recipients than has been generally seen (2-14 days). And pleocytosis was not as common in the CSF of the transplant recipients. It may well be that immunosuppression masks some of the traditional findings in West Nile infection.

Diagnostically, molecular studies may be necessary to detect viremia, since the immunoglobulin M antibody assay may be negative in the setting of viremia. New guidelines for tissue and blood transfusion have been issued, and new diagnostic tests will be needed for routine screening. We also know that most patients with West Nile virus infection are asymptomatic, so screening will be essential to eliminate units of blood with viremia.

D. R. Snydman, MD

Transmission of West Nile Virus Through Blood Transfusion in the United States in 2002
Pealer LN, for the West Nile Virus Transmission Investigation Team (Ctrs for Disease Control and Prevention, Atlanta, Ga and Fort Collins, Colo; et al)
N Engl J Med 349:1236-1245, 2003   13–8

Introduction.—During the 2002 West Nile virus epidemic in the United States, some patients had a West Nile virus illness that was temporarily linked with the receipt of transfused blood and blood components. The findings from recipients suspected of acquiring West Nile virus through transfusion of blood components are reported in a study that also investigated the transfusion donors.

Methods.—Patients with laboratory evidence of recent West Nile virus infection within 4 weeks after receipt of a blood component from a donor with viremia were considered to have a confirmed transfusion-associated infection. Donors of the components were interviewed about whether they had symptoms compatible with the presence of a viral illness before or after their donation. Blood specimens retained from the time of donation and collected at follow-up were analyzed for West Nile virus.

Results.—Twenty-three patients were verified to have acquired West Nile virus through transfused leukoreduced and nonleukoreduced red cells, platelets, or fresh-frozen plasma. Of the 23 recipients, 10 (43%) were immunocompromised because of transplantation or cancer. Eight patients (35%) were 70 year or older. Immunocompromised recipients tended to have longer incubation periods than did nonimmunocompromised recipients and infected individuals in mosquito-borne community outbreaks. Sixteen donors with evidence of viremia at donation were linked to the 23 recipients with West Nile virus infection. Of these, 9 donors reported viral symptoms before or after donation, 5 were asymptomatic, and 2 were lost to follow-up. Fevers, new rashes, and painful eyes were independently linked with being a donor with viremia rather than a donor without viremia. All 16 donors had negative test results for West Nile virus-specific IgM antibody at donation (Table 3).

Conclusion.—It is possible for transfused red cells, platelets, and fresh-frozen plasma to transmit West Nile virus. Screening of potential donors with the use of nucleic acid–based assays for West Nile virus may decrease this risk.

▶ In an earlier selection for this volume (see Abstract 13–7), West Nile virus transmission was noted from an organ donor to a series of multiple recipients. This study demonstrates that transmission may occur though blood transfusion, either leukocyte reduced or not. The ideal screening tests have not yet

TABLE 3.—Demographic, Clinical, and Laboratory Data for Donors Implicated in the Transfusion-Related Transmission of West Nile Virus in the United States, 2002

Donor No.	Age (yr)/Sex	Date of Donation	Time of Symptom Onset	Symptoms Reported*												Analysis of Sample Obtained at Donation†	
				Fever	Chills	Headache	Eye Pain	Muscle Pain	Swollen Glands	New Rash	New Difficulty Thinking	Generalized Weakness	Muscle Weakness	Joint Pain	Abdominal Pain	Retention Segment	Plasma
			days before or after donation														pfu/ml
1	44/F	July 22	7 to 14	+	+	+	+	–	+	–	–	+	–	–	+	45.22	5.9§
2	27/F	Aug. 15	Before‡	+	+	+	–	–	–	+	–	+	–	–	–	0.57	3.5
3	56/F	Aug. 30	2 After	–	–	–	–	–	–	–	–	–	–	–	–	Negative	10.5
4	65/M	Sept. 6	1 After	+	+	+	+	–	–	–	–	+	–	+	–	0.78	60.1
5	54/F	Aug. 23	5 Before to 4 after‡	+	+	+	+	+	–	+	–	+	+	+	–	11.21	NA
6	65/F	Aug. 21	1 to 21 After‡	+	+	+	–	–	–	+	–	–	+	+	–	Equivocal	NA
7	44/F	Sept. 9	11 After	+	+	+	–	–	+	+	–	+	+	–	–	Negative	0.8¶
8	46/F	Aug. 19	0	+	+	+	–	–	–	–	+	+	+	+	–	6.34	75.1§
9	47/M	Sept. 20	—	–	–	–	–	–	–	–	–	–	–	–	–	Equivocal	1.4‖
10	27/F	Aug. 31	5 After	+	–	+	–	+	–	–	–	+	–	+	–	Negative	39.8
11	32/M	Sept. 18	—	–	–	–	–	–	–	–	–	–	–	–	–	Equivocal	NA
12	18/M	Oct. 6	—	–	–	–	–	–	–	–	–	–	–	–	–	NA	4.6
13	25/M	July 25	14 to 15	+	–	+	+	–	+	+	+	+	–	–	+	Negative	21.9
14	45/F	Sept. 25	Before‡	–	–	–	–	–	–	+	+	+	–	–	–	Negative	0.8¶
15**	72/F	Aug. 19	—	–	–	–	–	–	–	–	–	–	–	–	–	Negative	11.9§
16**	46/M	Sept. 16	—	–	–	–	–	–	–	–	–	–	–	–	–	Negative	13.2§

*Plus signs indicate that the donor reported the symptom, and minus signs indicate that the donor did not report the symptom.

†*Retention segment* refers to the tubing attached to the original collection bag or the red-cell component. NA denotes sample not available for testing.

‡The donor could not recall the exact time of onset of symptoms, so the date is given as a range.

§West Nile virus was isolated from the unit of plasma.

‖The polymerase chain reaction (PCR) assay was positive only when a more sensitive assay was used.

¶The leukoreduced red-cell unit from this donation tested negative on PCR.

**Virus was isolated from an all initial donation sample; the donor did not return for a follow-up serologic analysis or interview.

(Reprinted by permission of *The New England Journal of Medicine* from Pealer LN, for the West Nile Virus Transmission Investigation Team: Transmission of West Nile virus through blood transfusion in the United States in 2002. *N Engl J Med* 349:1236-1245, 2003. Copyright 2003, Massachusetts Medical Society. All rights reserved.)

been developed. Only 3 of 14 implicated donors who were interviewed, all of whom had passed traditional screening tests, had symptoms of a fever, a headache, or both before the donation, and the viral analysis of retention segments did not always detect the virus. As a result of the findings of these studies, a rapid investigational nucleic acid–based test has been implemented for screening and may have prevented 163 donations that might have been infected.

D. R. Snydman, MD

14 Nosocomial Infections

Introduction

The diagnosis and treatment of ventilator-associated pneumonia continue to be quite problematic for the practicing intensivist, hospitalist, or internist in practice in a small community hospital. We still do not know how to reliably make a diagnosis, nor do we know how long to treat. The next 3 selections discuss and outline some new approaches or confirm the clinical utility of approaches already used.

David R. Snydman, MD

Diagnosing Pneumonia During Mechanical Ventilation: The Clinical Pulmonary Infection Score Revisted
Fartoukh M, Maître B, Honoré S, et al (Hôpital Henri Mondor, Créteil, France)
Am J Respir Crit Care Med 168:173-179, 2003   14-1

Introduction.—The clinical evaluation of ventilator-associated pneumonia (VAP) is typically based on the presence of fever (core temperature, >38.3°C), blood leukocytosis (>10,000/mm³) or leukopenia (<4000/mm²), purulent tracheal secretions, and the presence of a new or persistent radiographic infiltrate. The clinical pulmonary infection score (CPIS) in either the original or the modified form has been proposed for the diagnosis and management of VAP.

Methods.—Seventy-nine episodes of suspected pneumonia in the medical and surgical ICUs were prospectively followed up between May 2000 and September 2001. The diagnostic accuracy of the physicians' clinical evaluation of probability and of the modified CPIS, both measured before (pretest) and after (posttest) incorporating Gram stain results, with bronchoalveolar lavage fluid culture as the reference test, was examined.

Results.—The pretest clinical estimate was not accurate (sensitivity, 50%; specificity, 58%). The mean CPIS score at baseline was 6.5 (range, 3-9) for the 40 confirmed episodes and 5.9 (range, 3-0) for the 39 nonconfirmed episodes (*P* = .07). The CPIS was only slightly more accurate (sensitivity, 60%; specificity, 59%) than the clinical prediction. Incorporation of the Gram stain results of either directed or blind protected sampling enhanced the diagnostic accuracy (sensitivity and specificity of 85% and 49% and 78% and

TABLE 4.—Accuracy of Diagnosis in Suspected Episodes of Ventilator-Associated Pneumonia of the Clinical Pulmonary Infection Score and the Physicians' Estimate of Clinical Probability of Pneumonia at Baseline and After Incorporating the Results of Respiratory Specimens Gram Stains

	Sensitivity (%)	Specificity (%)	Positive Predictive Value (%)	Negative Predictive Value (%)	Likelihood Ratio
Pretest clinical probability > 60%	50%	49%	58%	49%	1.19
n	20/40	19/39			
CPIS baseline > 6	60%	59%	60%	59%	1.46
n	24/40	23/39			
CPIS gram BAL > 6	85%	49%	63%	76%	1.67
n	34/40	19/39			
CPIS gram PTC > 6	78%	56%	65%	71%	1.77
n	31/40	22/39			

Note: The pretest probability was provided by attending physicians requesting respiratory tract samples, and its diagnostic accuracy was assessed taking a probability of ventilator-associated pneumonia (VAP) of more than 60% as suggestive of pneumonia. The clinical pulmonary infection score was calculated at baseline (*CPIS baseline*) and after gram stain results of the protected telescoping catheter (*CPIS gram PTC*) and of bronchoalveolar lavage (*CPIS gram BAL*), and likelihood ratios for a positive test (CPIS of more than 6) are shown in the *right-hand column.*

(Courtesy of Fartoukh M, Maître B, Honoré S, et al: Diagnosing pneumonia during mechanical ventilation: The clinical pulmonary infection score revisited. *Am J Respir Crit Care Med* 168:173-179, 2003.)

56%, respectively) of the clinical score; it increased the likelihood ratio for pneumonia of a score of more than 6 from 1.46 to 1.67 and 1.77 (Table 4).

Conclusion.—The CPIS has low diagnostic accuracy. Incorporation of Gram stain results into the score may aid clinical decision making in patients with clinically suspected VAP.

▶ This study demonstrates that the CPIS probably misclassifies as many as 50% of patients, based on clinical criteria alone. The specimen Gram stain is really a key component and when added, increases the diagnostic accuracy, and therefore the quality of the specimen becomes crucial. In the authors' hands, directed or nondirected specimens had the same diagnostic accuracy so either may be used, especially if bronchoscopy is not readily available. The authors only used senior clinicians or residents in the last year of their training, so the experience level was high, yet they urge caution in using the CPIS and suggest a need for further refinement in the diagnosis of this important entity.

D. R. Snydman, MD

Comparison of 8 vs 15 Days of Antibiotic Therapy for Ventilator-Associated Pneumonia in Adults: A Randomized Trial
Chastre J, for the PneumA Trial Group (Groupe Hospitalier Pitié-Salpêtrière, Paris; et al)
JAMA 290:2588-2598, 2003   14–2

Background.—The most effective length of antimicrobial treatment for ventilator-associated pneumonia (VAP) has not been established. Shortening treatment time may help restrict the emergence of multiresistant bacteria in ICUs. Whether 8 days of antibiotic therapy is as effective as 15 days in patients with microbiologically proved VAP was determined.

Methods.—Between May 1999 and June 2002, 51 French ICUs enrolled a total of 401 patients in a prospective, randomized, double-blind clinical trial. One hundred ninety-seven patients received an 8-day antibiotic regimen, determined by the treating physician, and 204 received a 15-day regimen.

Findings.—Mortality rates in the 8- and 15-day groups were 17.2% and 18.8%, respectively. Infections recurred in 26% and 28.9%, respectively. However, patients treated for 8 days had more mean antibiotic-free days than those treated for 15 days. The 2 groups did not differ in number of mechanical ventilation-free days, number of organ failure-free days, length of ICU stay, or 60-day mortality rate. Patients with VAP caused by nonfermenting gram-negative bacilli did not have better outcomes with 8 days of treatment, but they had a greater rate of pulmonary infection recurrence. Among those in whom infections recurred, multiresistant pathogens emerged less often when antibiotic therapy lasted only 8 days.

Conclusions.—The efficacy of an 8-day antibiotic regimen was comparable to that of a 15-day regimen in patients receiving appropriate initial empirical therapy for VAP, except possibly for patients with nonfermenting gram-negative bacillus infections. Antibiotic use was lower in the patients treated for 8 days than for those treated for 15 days.

▶ The length of therapy for most infections is based on very little data. In no entity is this more applicable than VAP. This group of French investigators, long known for the excellence of their work on ICU infections, especially pneumonia, have taken on the challenge of defining the length of therapy for VAP. Their findings are not that surprising; we tend to overtreat with respect to length of therapy. They show that 8 days is equivalent to 15 days for most patients with VAP. The patient population was quite ill but there were a number of exclusions, including immunocompromise and early-onset VAP. They were a highly pretreated group with almost 85% receiving antibiotics before the onset of pneumonia and the average duration of ventilation being almost 2 weeks before onset. Yet despite their severity of illness by virtually all measures, the group assigned to the 8-day regimen fared as well as the 15-day regimen. But the reader should take note that the mean days of antibiotic therapy in the 8-day group was almost 13 days anyway. The group of patients in whom shorter therapy had a greater proportion of relapses was the relapse and superinfection rate among the patients with nonfermenting gram-negative bacilli as the cause of infection.

D. R. Snydman, MD

Decision Analysis of Antibiotic and Diagnostic Strategies in Ventilator-Associated Pneumonia

Ost DE, Hall CS, Joseph G, et al (North Shore-Long Island Jewish Health System, Manhasset, NY; New York Univ; SUNY at Stony Brook, NY)
Am J Respir Crit Care Med 168:1060-1067, 2003   14–3

Background.—Authorities disagree on the most effective approach for treating ventilator-associated pneumonia (VAP). A decision analysis was performed to clarify the benefits and risks of different strategies.

Methods.—Strategies used in the decision analysis were antibiotic treatment with and without diagnostic testing. Tests included were endotracheal aspirates, bronchoscopy with protected brush or bronchoalveolar lavage, and nonbronchoscopic mini-bronchoalveolar lavage (mini-BAL). The outcomes generated were cost, antibiotic use, survival, cost-effectiveness, antibiotic use per survivor, and cost-antibiotic use per survivor.

Findings.—Initial coverage with 3 antibiotics was superior in survival and cost to expectant management or 1 or 2 antibiotic approaches. The former strategy was associated with a 66% survival compared with 54% for the latter approach. In addition, costs were decreased from $55,447 per survivor to $41,483 per survivor. Mini-BAL testing did not increase survival but reduced cost from $41,483 to $39,967. This testing also reduced antibiotic use from 63 to 39 antibiotic days per survivor.

Conclusions.—The most effective strategy for treating VAP appears to be the use of 3 antibiotic agents plus mini-BAL. This approach minimizes cost and antibiotic use and maximizes survival.

▶ Although there have been other decision analyses regarding the management of ventilator associated pneumonia, they did not take into account the likelihood of adequate antibiotic coverage and evidence that inadequate empiric coverage increases mortality rate and cost. Therefore, prior models have failed to take into account the strategy of initial empiric therapy with rapid taper based on subsequent clinical information. This model takes such clinical practice into account. The authors' conclusion codifies current clinical practice: the use of 3 drugs empirically, such as vancomycin to cover methicillin-resistant *Staphylococcus aureus*, and double coverage of gram-negative pathogens. They also suggest that mini-BAL should be part of the preferred strategy, but unfortunately this technique is still not widely used in many ICUs.

D. R. Snydman, MD

15 Human Immunodeficiency Virus

Determinants of Survival Following HIV-1 Seroconversion After the Introduction of HAART
Porter K, for the CASCADE Collaboration (MRC Clinical Trials Unit, London)
Lancet 362:1267-1274, 2003   15–1

Background.—The efficacy of highly active antiretroviral therapy (HAART), introduced in 1996, relies on several variables, such as uptake and time of treatment initiation, adherence, previous treatments, and the presence of coinfections. Thus, survival improvements associated with HAART may not be uniform in all infected groups. Changes in the risk of AIDS and death among HIV-1 infected individuals and the prognostic importance of demographic factors since the introduction of HAART were investigated.

Methods.—Twenty-two cohorts of individuals from Europe, Australia, and Canada who had seroconverted were analyzed with the use of Cox models to estimate the effect of calendar year on time to AIDS and death. The effects of age at seroconversion, exposure category, sex, and presentation during acute HIV-1 infection before 1997, before the introduction of HAART; in 1997 and 1998, when the use of HAART was limited; and in 1999 to 2001, when HAART use was widespread, were compared.

Findings.—Twenty-six percent of 7740 patients who had seroconverted died. Compared with pre-1997 data, the hazard ratio for death declined to 0.47 (95% CI, 0.39-0.56) in 1997 and to 0.16 (95% CI, 0.12-0.22) in 2001. The proportion of person-time receiving HAART rose from 22% to 57% between 1997 and 2001. Compared with the pre-HAART period, in the period from 1999 to 2001, injecting drug users had a significantly greater mortality than did men infected by sex with other men. Before 1997, the risk of AIDS was greater in individuals aged 45 years or older at seroconversion than in individuals aged 16 to 24 years. However, between 1999 and 2001, little evidence of a difference in risk by age was observed. No such attenuation in the effect of age on survival was present (Table 3).

TABLE 3.—Variation in the Hazard Ratio of Death Over Calendar Time

	Calendar Period			P*
	Pre-1997	1997-98	1999-2001	
Exposure category				
Men				
Sex between men	1·00	1·00	1·00	<0·0001
Injecting drug use	1·03 (0·87-1·21)	2·81 (1·99-3·95)	4·59 (3·11-6·77)	
Sex with women	0·92 (0·69-1·21)	1·49 (0·83-2·68)	1·42 (0·67-2·98)	
Other	1·09 (0·68-1·75)	3·07 (1·46-6·48)	3·37 (1·17-9·67)	
Women				
Injecting drug use	0·99 (0·81-1·20)	1·69 (1·07-2·67)	2·99 (1·82-4·91)	
Sex with men	0·63 (0·48-0·83)	1·04 (0·60-1·82)	1·37 (0·73-2·56)	
Other	1·41 (0·81-2·44)	1·09 (0·12-9·68)	1·95 (0·26-14·8)	
	p=0·01†	p<0·0001†	p<0·0001†	
Age at seroconversion (years)				
16-24	1·00	1·00	1·00	0·63
25-34	1·27 (1·12-1·44)	1·17 (0·87-1·57)	1·33 (0·95-1·87)	
35-44	1·83 (1·55-2·15)	1·72 (1·14-2·59)	2·46 (1·57-3·85)	
≥45	2·80 (2·29-3·43)	3·86 (2·36-6·31)	2·97 (1·55-5·67)	
	p<0·0001†	p<0·0001†	p=0·0003†	
Acute infection				
No	1·00	1·00	1·00	0·23
Yes	1·33 (1·10-1·62)	0·85 (0·48-1·49)	1·03 (0·58-1·82)	
	p=0·005†	p=0·56†	p=0·92†	
Calendar period	1·00	0·26 (0·18-0·37)	0·09 (0·06-0·14)	<0·0001
People at risk	6308	5122	5346	
Person-years at risk	31 788	9081	12 246	
Deaths	1548	253	199	

Results for multivariable model that includes main effects and interaction between calendar period and each of exposure category, age at seroconversion, sex, and presentation with acute infection, stratified by cohort. Data are hazard ratio (95% confidence interval), p, or n.
*For variation of effect over calendar period.
†For variation of effect within calendar period.
(Courtesy of Porter K, for the CASCADE Collaboration: Determinants of survival following HIV-1 seroconversion after the introduction of HAART. *Lancet* 362:1267-1274, 2003. Reprinted with permission from Elsevier Science.)

Conclusions.—Since the introduction of HAART in 1996, the predicted survival rate for individuals with HIV-1 has continued to increase. The importance of age and exposure category as determinants of progression seems to have altered.

▶ Survival time has increased substantially in the HAART era, and the relative importance of prognostic factors has changed rather dramatically. Injection drug users now have a much shorter survival time after HIV seroconversion compared with men who have sex with men. Factors presumably include coinfection with hepatitis C and resultant liver disease, and lack of access to HAART or noncompliance with therapy. The role of gender is less clear, although female injection drug users have better survival than their male counterparts. Age at seroconversion is much less important as a risk factor, which is somewhat surprising, since immune reconstitution seems to be less robust in older individuals. These data are extremely important and will require follow-up studies to assess ongoing trends.

D. R. Snydman, MD

Prognostic Importance of Initial Response in HIV-1 Infected Patients Starting Potent Antiretroviral Therapy: Analysis of Prospective Studies

Egger M, for the Antiretroviral Therapy (ART) Cohort Collaboration (Univ of Bern, Switzerland; et al)

Lancet 362:679-686, 2003   15-2

Introduction.—Among patients with HIV-1 who are initiating highly active antiretroviral therapy (HAART), the prognosis is strongly linked with the CD4 cell count at baseline. Earlier reports of the prognosis after an early response to therapy have been based on single cohorts in which few clinical events were evaluated or have consisted primarily of patients who had previously received antiretroviral therapy. Whether the initial virologic and immunologic response to HAART is prognostic in patients with HIV-1 was determined in the Antiretroviral Therapy (ART) Cohort Collaboration, which was established in 2000 and includes 13 cohort investigations.

Methods.—The 13 cohort investigations from Europe and North America included 9323 adult treatment-naive patients who initiated HAART with a

TABLE 3.—Progression to AIDS or Death and Death From 6 Months after Starting HAART

	AIDS or Death	Death
Age (years)		
17-29	1	1
30-39	1·03 (0·63-1·69)	1·30 (0·56-3·00)
40-49	1·05 (0·64-1·75)	1·47 (0·63-3·44)
≥50	1·69 (1·01-2·84)	2·68 (1·13-6·37)
Sex		
Men	1	1
Women	1·00 (0·74-1·34)	1·18 (0·78-1·76)
Risk factor for transmission		
Male homosexual contact	1	1
Injection-drug use	1·85 (1·41-2·43)	2·54 (1·75-3·68)
Heterosexual contact	0·92 (0·69-1·23)	0·77 (0·50-1·19)
Other	0·92 (0·63-1·35)	0·64 (0·34-1·19)
Clinical CDC stage		
A/B at 6 months	1	1
C at baseline	1·75 (1·38-2·22)	1·97 (1·39-2·79)
A/B at baseline and C at 6 months	1·63 (1·11-2·39)	3·00 (1·89-4·75)
6-month CD4 count (cells/µL)		
<25	1	1
25-49	0·55 (0·32-0·96)	0·69 (0·36-1·35)
50-99	0·62 (0·40-0·96)	0·46 (0·26-0·82)
100-199	0·42 (0·28-0·64)	0·31 (0·18-0·53)
200-349	0·25 (0·16-0·38)	0·22 (0·12-0·39)
≥350	0·18 (0·11-0·29)	0·13 (0·07-0·25)
6-month plasma HIV-1 RNA (copies/mL)		
≥100 000	1	1
10 000-99 999	0·59 (0·41-0·86)	0·45 (0·25-0·79)
501-9999	0·42 (0·29-0·61)	0·43 (0·25-0·74)
≤500 (undetectable)	0·29 (0·21-0·39)	0·41 (0·27-0·63)

Note: Values are hazard ratios (95% CI) adjusted for all variables listed, estimated with multivariable Weilbull models.

(Courtesy of Egger M, for the Antiviral Therapy (ART) Cohort Collaboration: Prognostic importance of initial response in HIV-1 infected patients starting potent antiretroviral therapy: Analysis of prospective studies. *Lancet* 362:679-686, 2003. Reprinted with permission from Elsevier Science.)

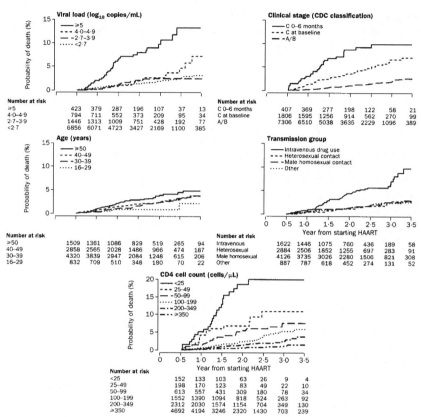

FIGURE 2.—Progression to death according to 6-month CD4 cell count, viral load, clinical stage, age, and exposure category. *Abbreviations: CDC*, Centers for Disease Control and Prevention; *HAART*, highly active antiretroviral therapy. (Courtesy of Egger M, for the Antiviral Therapy (ART) Cohort Collaboration: Prognostic importance of initial response in HIV-1 infected patients starting potent antiretroviral therapy: Analysis of prospective studies. *Lancet* 362:679-686, 2003. Reprinted with permission from Elsevier Science.)

combination of at least 3 drugs. Clinical progression was modeled from month 6 after initiation of HAART and incorporated the CD4 count and HIV-1 RNA level measured at both baseline and 6 months.

Results.—During 13,408 years of follow-up, 152 participants died and 874 subsequently had AIDS or died. When participants who had a 6-month CD4 count of less than 25 cells/μL were compared with the rest of the study group, adjusted hazard ratios for AIDS or death were 0.55 (95% CI, 0.32-0.96) for 25 to 49 cells/μL, 0.62 (95% CI, 0.40-0.96) for 50 to 99 cells/μL, 0.42 (95% CI, 0.28-0.64) for 100 to 199 cells/μL, 0.25 (95% CI, 0.16-0.38) for 200 to 349 cells/μL, and 0.18 (95% CI, 0.11-0.29) for 350 or more cells/ μL at 6 months. When participants who had a 6-month HIV-1 RNA level of 100,000 copies/mL or higher were compared with the rest of the study group, the adjusted hazard ratios for AIDS or death were 0.59 (95% CI, 0.41-0.86) for 10,000 to 99,999 copies/mL, 0.42 (95% CI, 0.29-0.61) for

500 to 9999 copies/mL, and 0.29 (95% CI, 0.21-0.39) for a 6-month HIV-1 RNA level of 500 copies/mL or lower (Table 3). The baseline CD4 count and HIV-1 RNA level were not linked with progression after an adjustment was made for 6-month concentrations. The probability of progression at 3 years ranged from 2.4% in participants in the lowest risk stratum to 83% in participants in the highest risk stratum (Fig 2).

Conclusion.—At 6 months after initiation of HAART, the current CD4 count and viral load, and not values at baseline, are strongly correlated with subsequent disease progression. This data should be used to inform guidelines on when to modify HAART.

▶ This very important study of a sizeable cohort of patients emphasizes the importance of the 6-month values for CD4 count and HIV viral load as a prognostic factor in those who start HAART and survive about 6 months. These data do have some limitations, namely, the lack of information about adherence, lack of information about cause-specific mortality, and the fact that the analysis did not look at the temporal relationships between the changing viral load and CD4 counts. Nevertheless, the data are quite compelling and provide a framework for clinicians to assess prognosis, and they underscore the fact that the 6-month data, not the baseline values or level of response, are the important independent prognostic indicators. Also, the data suggest that the absolute values of the CD4 count and the viral load at 6 months are important. Every CD4 cell counts, as does any diminution in the viral load. The authors can now demonstrate that progression is graded, that is, viral loads worsen the prognosis, depending on the level. However, absolute differences are small, unless viral loads exceed 100,000 copies.

D. R. Snydman, MD

Effect of Medication Adherence on Survival of HIV-infected Adults Who Start Highly Active Antiretroviral Therapy When the CD4$^+$ Cell Count Is 0.200 to 0.350 × 10^9 Cells/L
Wood E, Hogg RS, Yip B, et al (Univ of British Columbia, Vancouver, Canada)
Ann Intern Med 139:810-816, 2003   15–3

Background.—Whether delaying highly active antiretroviral therapy (HAART) is safe in HIV-infected patients with CD4$^+$ cell counts of less than 0.350 × 10^9 cells/L is not known. The effect on survival rates of baseline CD4$^+$ cell count and adherence to HAART was investigated.

Methods.—The prospective observational study included 1422 patients with HIV infection beginning HAART between August 1996 and July 2000. The patients were stratified by baseline CD4$^+$ cell count and adherence level and followed up through March 2002.

Findings.—Patients adhering to treatment and with CD4$^+$ counts of 0.200 × 10^9 cells/L or greater had no survival benefit from HAART. In adjusted analyses, nonadherent patients initiating HAART when CD4$^+$ cell counts were 0.200 to 0.349 × 10^9 cells/L had a significantly increased mor-

TABLE 2.—Probability of Survival 48 Months After the Initiation of Highly Active Antiretroviral Therapy According to Adherence and Baseline CD4$^+$ Cell Count

Adherence and CD4$^+$ Cell Count	Probability of Survival (95% CI), %*	P Value†
≥75% adherence		
≥0.350 × 10^9 cells/L	92.0 (88.7-95.2)	—
0.300-0.349 × 10^9 cells/L	94.7 (89.5-99.9)	>0.2
0.250-0.299 × 10^9 cells/L	91.0 (84.4-97.6)	>0.2
2.00-0.249 × 10^9 cells/L	93.2 (87.3-99.1)	>0.2
<0.200 × 10^9 cells/L	80.4 (76.0-84.8)	<0.001
≥95% adherence		
≥350 × 10^9 cells/L	95.5 (92.5-98.4)	—
300-349 × 10^9 cells/L	96.1 (90.6-100.0)	>0.2
250-299 × 10^9 cells/L	95.1 (89.7-100.0)	>0.2
200-249 × 10^9 cells/L	97.2 (93.3-100.0)	>0.2
<200 × 10^9 cells/L	86.5 (82.3-90.6)	<0.001

*For ≥75% adherence: accidents, suicides, and illicit drug overdoses included. For ≥95% adherence: accidents, suicides, and illicit drug overdoses were censored as nonevents.
†Log-rank P value comparing cumulative mortality rates between relevant strata less then 0.350 × 10^9 cells/L and the ≥0.350 × 10^9 cells/L reference category.
(Courtesy of Wood E, Hogg RS, Yip B, et al: Effect of medication adherence on survival of HIV-infected adults who start highly active antiretroviral therapy when the CD4$^+$ cell count is 0.200 to 0.350 × 10^9 cells/L. *Ann Intern Med* 139:810-816, 2003.)

tality rate compared with adherent patients initiating HAART at a CD4$^+$ cell count of 0.350 × 10^9 cells/L or higher. However, compared with adherent patients starting HAART at a CD4$^+$ cell count of 10^9 cells/L or higher, patients adhering to treatment and initiating HAART when the CD4$^+$ cell count was 0.2 to 0.349 × 10^9 cells/L had a comparable mortality rate (Table 2).

Conclusions.—Delaying HAART until CD4$^+$ cell counts decline to 0.200 × 10^9 cells/L does not increase the mortality rate among HIV-infected patients who adhere to treatment. However, the mortality rate increases if HAART is begun when CD4$^+$ cell counts are less than 0.200 × 10^9 cells/L. Nonadherent patients appear to have greater death rates than patients with similar counts who adhere to treatment. Medication adherence is the critical determinant of survival in patients with a CD4$^+$ cell count exceeding 0.200 × 10^9 cells/L.

▶ While there is no doubt about the benefits of HAART, the decision as to when to initiate therapy has been a difficult one for patients and physicians alike. Previous studies have shown that patients who initiate therapy when the CD4$^+$ count falls below 200 were at increased risk for death, regardless of the HIV viral load at the time of initiation. However, none of these studies adjusted for patient adherence. Despite the fact that there may be adherence classification bias in the study in that the first year of therapy was the defining time for adherence and follow-up was for 40 months, this bias would underestimate the effects of adherence. These data will be helpful in providing additional scientific data as the basis for guidelines.

D. R. Snydman, MD

Structured Treatment Interruption in Patients With Multidrug-Resistant Human Immunodeficiency Virus

Lawrence J, for the 064 Study Team of the Terry Beirn Community Programs for Clinical Research on AIDS (Univ of California, San Francisco; et al)

N Engl J Med 349:837-846, 2003   15–4

Background.—The best approach for treating multidrug-resistant HIV has not been established. Two strategies were compared.

Methods.—By random assignment, patients with multidrug-resistant HIV and HIV RNA levels of more than 5000 copies/mL received a 4-month structured interruption of treatment followed by a change in antiretroviral regimen or to immediate regimen change. One hundred thirty-eight patients were in the treatment interruption group and 132 in the control group. All patients underwent genotyping and phenotyping resistance testing.

Findings.—At the median 11.6-month follow-up, disease progression or death was documented for 22 patients in the treatment interruption group and 12 in the control group (Fig 1 and Table 2). The hazard ratio was 2.57 in the former group. Eight patients in each group died. Sixty-four percent of the patients in the treatment interruption group had complete or partial reversion to wild-type of the mutant HIV populations by 4 months. Compared with the control group, the treatment interruption group had a mean CD4 cell count 85 cells/mm³ lower in the first 4 months, 47 cells/mm³ lower in months 5 through 8, and 31 cells/mm³ lower after 8 months. The mean HIV RNA concentrations were 1.2 log copies/mL greater in the treatment interruption group in the first 4 months. However, these values did not differ sig-

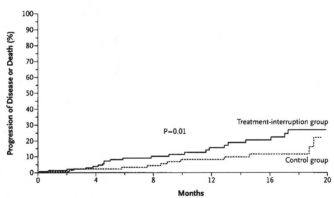

FIGURE 1.—Kaplan-Meier estimates of the cumulative incidence of progression of disease or death. The log-rank test was used to calculate the *P* value. (Reprinted by permission of *The New England Journal of Medicine* from Lawrence J, for the 064 Study Team of the Terry Beirn Community Programs for Clinical Research on AIDS: Structured treatment interruption in patients with multidrug-resistant human immunodeficiency virus. *N Engl J Med* 349:837-846, 2003. Copyright 2003 Massachusetts Medical Society. All rights reserved.)

TABLE 2.—Incidence of Progression of Disease or Death

Event	Treatment-Interruption Group		Control Group		Hazard Ratio (95% CI)*	P Value
	No. of Patients	Rate/100 Person-Yr	No. of Patients	Rate/100 Person-Yr		
Progression of disease or death	22	18.1	12	10.0	2.57 (1.2-5.5)	0.01
0-4 Mo	5	11.1	3	6.9		
5-8 Mo	7	8.0	2	2.3		
9-12 Mo	4	3.2	3	2.4		
13-20 Mo	6	5.3	4	3.4		
Death	8	6.1	8	6.5	1.44 (0.5-4.1)	0.50
Progression of disease	17	14.0	5	4.2	6.04 (1.8-20.8)	0.004

*Hazard ratios are for the treatment interruption group compared with the control group.
Abbreviation: CI, Confidence interval.
(Reprinted by permission of *The New England Journal of Medicine* from Lawrence J, for the 064 Study Team of the Terry Beirn Community Programs for Clinical Research on AIDS: Structured treatment interruption in patients with multidrug-resistant human immunodeficiency virus. *N Engl J Med* 349:837-846, 2003. Copyright 2003 Massachusetts Medical Society. All rights reserved.)

nificantly from those in the control group after the fourth month. The 2 groups had a comparable overall quality of life.

Conclusions.—Structured treatment interruption in patients with multidrug-resistant HIV was associated with a greater disease progression. This approach did not confer immunologic or virologic benefits and did not improve overall quality of life.

▶ Since treatment interruptions are being used more often in patients with disease refractory to therapy due to multiresistant virus, with the theory of limiting toxicity and allowing the emergence of wild-type virus that may be more sensitive, the authors undertook a study of the effects of such a treatment strategy. Unfortunately, disease progressed in the interruption group and although CD4 counts increased and responded to reinitiation of therapy, they never recovered to the level of the CD4 counts in the group that was not interrupted. These data lend credence to the management strategy that continuing treatment with an optimal regimen is the best option to prevent disease progression.

D. R. Snydman, MD

Tenofovir Disoproxil Fumarate in Nucleoside-Resistant HIV-1 Infection: A Randomized Trial
Cheng A, for the Study 907 Team (Univ of Southern California, Los Angeles; et al)
Ann Intern Med 139:313-320, 2003   15–5

Introduction.—Combination antiretroviral therapy has reduced mortality rates in patients with HIV-1 infection. However, resistance to antiretroviral agents continues to be a leading cause of treatment failure in patients infected with HIV-1. Tenofovir disoproxil fumarate (tenofovir DF), a novel, acyclic nucleotide analogue with in vitro activity against HIV-1 and HIV-2, was compared with placebo for efficacy and safety measures in patients with detectable viral replication, despite current antiretroviral therapy.

Methods.—Five hundred twenty-two HIV-1-infected adults who were receiving antiretroviral therapy and had stable HIV-1 RNA levels ranging from 400 to 10,000 copies per milliliter were assessed in a randomized, double-blind, placebo-controlled investigation through 24 weeks, after which all patients received open-label tenofovir DF for the remainder of the 48-week trial. Patients were randomly assigned in a 2-to-1 ratio to add 300 mg tenofovir DF or placebo to their existing antiretroviral regimen. Participants were from 75 North American, European, and Australian HIV clinics. Patients were followed up for their change in HIV-1 RNA level (time-weighted average from baseline through week 24), the proportion of patients with grade 3 or 4 laboratory abnormalities and adverse events, and genotypic HIV-1 resistance testing in a separate substudy at baseline, week 24, and week 48.

Results.—A statistically significant reduction in HIV-1 RNA levels through week 24 (the primary end point) was seen in the tenofovir DF versus the placebo group (-0.61 log_{10} copies per milliliter vs -0.03 log_{10} copies per milliliter, respectively, [$P < .001$]; difference, -0.58 log_{10} copies per milliliter [95% CI, -0.68 to -0.49 log_{10} copies per milliliter]). In a virologic substudy, 94% of 253 patients had plasma isolates that expressed reverse transcriptase mutations linked with nucleoside resistant mutations at baseline. Through week 24, the rate of adverse clinical events was similar in both treatment groups (14% placebo; 13% tenofovir DF). No evidence of tenofovir DF-associated toxic effects were observed through week 48.

Conclusion.—In treatment-experienced patients with suboptimal viral suppression, tenofovir DF significantly decreased HIV-1 RNA levels and had a safety profile similar to that of placebo.

▶ Tenofovir DF is an oral prodrug of tenofovir, a novel, acyclic nucleotide analogue with potent in vitro activity against HIV and hepatitis B. It is active in active and resting lymphoid cells and macrophages. It also has a very favorable safety profile and has considerable potential in HIV as well as hepatitis B therapy. This study confirms the antiviral efficacy and safety of this drug in patients with detectable HIV RNA, despite previous treatment with combination antiretroviral therapy.

D. R. Snydman, MD

16 Sepsis

Drotrecogin Alfa (Activated) Treatment of Older Patients With Severe Sepsis
Ely EW, Angus DC, Williams MD, et al (Vanderbilt Univ, Nashville, Tenn; Veterans Affairs Tennessee Valley Geriatric Research and Education Clinical Ctr, Nashville, Tenn; Univ of Pittsburgh, Pa; et al)
Clin Infect Dis 37:187-195, 2003   16–1

Background.—Sepsis associated with acute organ dysfunction, termed severe sepsis, has a mortality of 30% to 50% and its incidence increases dramatically in older patients. Recombinant human activated protein C, also called drotrecogin alfa (activated) (DAA), provides anti-inflammatory, antithrombotic, profibrinolytic therapy for the altered pathophysiology characteristic of severe sepsis. The result is reduced mortality, with the only concern an increased risk of adverse bleeding. The short- and long-term outcomes for older patients with severe sepsis who are given DAA were documented, with an analysis of the safety data accompanying DAA therapy.

Methods.—The 386 patients aged 75 years or older were enrolled in the Protein C Worldwide Evaluation of Severe Sepsis (PROWESS) trial, which was developed to assess the efficacy and safety of DAA treatment for severe sepsis. All patients had a known or suspected site of infection, at least 3 signs of systemic inflammation, and at least 1 sepsis-induced organ dysfunction whose duration was 48 hours or less. A placebo group and a treatment group were formed, with corresponding groups of patients aged 75 or older, or younger than 75. Mortality, morbidity, patient disposition, and serious adverse events were documented.

Results.—The older patients receiving DAA therapy had a reduction in the absolute risk for 28-day mortality (33.7%) of 15.5% and a reduction in in-hospital mortality (36.9%) of 15.6% compared with those receiving placebo (49.2% and 52.5%, respectively). The relative risk for 28-day mortality with DAA therapy was 0.68 for those aged 75 or older and 0.85 for those younger than 75; the in-hospital relative risks were 0.70 and 0.91, respectively.

During the 2-year follow-up, older patients receiving DAA had higher survival rates than those in the placebo group; a 284% increase was noted for the DAA group (Fig 2). The mean numbers of vasopressor-free days, ventilator-free days, ICU-free days, and hospital-free days were also significantly greater for those aged 75 or older who were receiving DAA than for the pla-

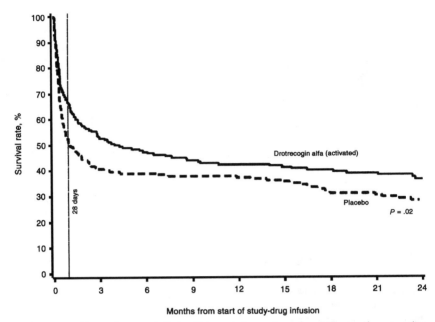

FIGURE 2.—Twenty-four–month Kaplan-Meir survival curves for patients ≥75 years of age, according to treatment group. Patients aged ≥75 years treated with drotrecogin alfa (activated; DAA) had significantly higher survival rates sustained throughout the 2-year follow-up period (*P* = .02). Older patients treated with DAA had an increase in the median duration of survival of approximately 3 months (88 days) (31 days for the placebo group vs 119 days for the DAA group). (Courtesy of Ely EW, Angus DC, Williams MD, et al: Drotrecogin alfa (activated) treatment of older patients with severe sepsis. *Clin Infect Dis* 37:187-195, 2003. Copyright 2003 by the Infectious Diseases Society of America. Reprinted by permission of the University of Chicago.)

cebo group (Fig 3). For the DAA group, 45% were discharged home, 9% were transferred to another hospital, and 44% were transferred to a nursing home; for the placebo group, 38% went home, 14% were transferred to another hospital, and 47% were transferred to a nursing home.

The incidences of serious bleeding occurring in patients aged 75 or older in the 28 days of the study were 3.9% for the older DAA group and 2.2% for the placebo group. These incidences were 3.4% and 2.0%, respectively, for patients younger than 75. Patients aged 75 or older receiving DAA had a reduction in thrombotic events compared wtih the placebo group. The placebo group also had higher rates of cardiac dysrhythmias and CNS-related events than the DAA group.

Conclusions.—Significant advantages were found at 28 days, during hospitalization, and 2 years after hospitalization with the use of DAA in older patients. DAA treatment was linked to a lower in-hospital mortality than placebo in patients aged 75 or older. Morbidity was similarly diminished in the DAA treatment group. A 1.7% higher rate of serious bleeding attended the use of DAA, but this is similar to the 1.4% increase noted in younger patients. Thus, DAA treatment could be considered for patients who are at

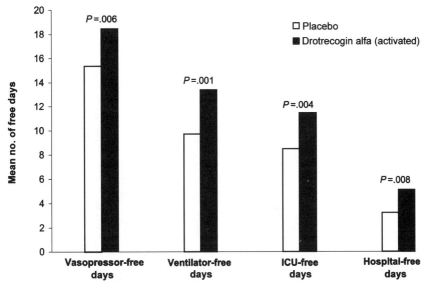

FIGURE 3.—Histogram showing resource use expressed as a "free-day analysis" (ie, days alive and free of the given measure) for patients aged ≥75 years, according to treatment group. Patients treated with drotrecogin alfa (activated) had significantly more vasopressor-, ventilator-, ICU-, and Hospital-free days, compared with the placebo group. (Courtesy of Ely EW, Angus DC, Williams MD, et al: Drotrecogin alfa (activated) treatment of older patients with severe sepsis. *Clin Infect Dis* 37:187-195, 2003. Copyright 2003 by the Infectious Diseases Society of America. Reprinted by permission of the University of Chicago.)

high risk of death from severe sepsis, for whom aggressive care is planned, and who have a favorable benefit-to-risk profile.

Systemic Host Responses in Severe Sepsis Analyzed by Causative Microorganism and Treatment Effects of Drotrecogin Alfa (Activated)

Opal SM, Garber GE, LaRosa SP, et al (Brown Univ, Providence, RI; Cleveland Clinic Foundation, Ohio; Univ of Wisconsin, Madison; et al)
Clin Infect Dis 37:50-58, 2003   16–2

Background.—In clinical studies of novel treatments for severe sepsis, patients appeared to respond differently depending on the causative microorganism. The impact of the infecting microorganism on the efficacy of recombinant human drotrecogin alfa (activated) (DrotAA) was investigated.

Methods and Findings.—Data from a large placebo-controlled trial of DrotAA were analyzed by type of causative microorganism for treatment-related differences in mortality, coagulopathy, and inflammatory response. Compared with placebo, DrotAA-related mortality rate was decreased consistently in each microorganism group, including those with gram-positive bacteria, gram-negative bacteria, mixed bacteria, fungi, other, and unknown microbial etiology (Table 2). The stratified relative risk was 0.8. The greatest mortality rate reduction was for *Streptococcus pneumoniae* infection, with a

TABLE 2.—Twenty-Eight-Day Mortality Rate, by Specific Causative Microorganism

Microorganism	Placebo Recipients ($n = 840$)		Drotrecogin Alfa (Activated) Recipients ($n = 850$)		Mortality Relative Risk (95% CI)
	No. (%) of Patients	Mortality, %*	No. (%) of Patients	Mortality, %*	
Gram-positive bacteria					
Staphylococcus aureus	110 (13.1)	30.0	108 (12.7)	27.8	0.93 (0.61-1.41)
Streptococcus pneumoniae	100 (11.9)	35.0	103 (12.1)	19.4	0.56 (0.35-0.88)
Enterococcus species†	49 (5.8)	28.6	50 (5.9)	32.0	1.12 (0.62-2.04)
Coagulase-negative staphylococci	15 (1.8)	26.7	16 (1.9)	12.5	0.47 (0.10-2.20)
Gram-negative bacteria					
Escherichia coli	134 (16.0)	20.2	123 (14.5)	17.1	0.85 (0.51-1.42)
Klebsiella species	59 (7.0)	42.4	40 (4.7)	32.5	0.77 (0.45-1.31)
Pseudomonas species	37 (4.4)	46.0	46 (5.4)	34.8	0.76 (0.45-1.28)
All other gram negative‡	139 (16.5)	26.6	155 (18.2)	25.2	0.95 (0.64-1.39)

Data for patients infected with more than 1 type of organism may be included more than once.
*Percentage of patients with specific microorganism infection who died within 28 days of study entry.
†The Clinical Evaluation Committee classification took into account all of the microorganisms isolated in the peritoneum in patients with peritonitis.
‡Other gram-negative microorganisms included *Enterobacter* species (n = 64), *Bacteroides* species (n = 58), *Haemophilus influenzae* (n = 50), *Neisseria meningitidis* (n = 19), *Legionella* species (n = 10), other enteric (n = 74), and other nonenteric organisms (n = 41).

(Courtesy of Opal SM, Garber GE, LaRosa SP, et al: Systemic host responses in severe sepsis analyzed by causative microorganism and treatment effects of drotrecogin alfa (activated). *Clin Infect Dis* 37:50-58, 2003. University of Chicago, publisher. © 2003 by the Infectious Diseases Society of America. All rights reserved.)

relative risk of 0.56. Levels of coagulation and inflammation biomarkers varied based on pathogen at study entry.

Conclusions.—Most patients in this large trial had evidence of a systemic host response with coagulopathy and inflammation apparently independent of the causative pathogen. When used as an adjunct to standard supportive care, including infective therapy, DrotAA can improve survival among patients with severe sepsis, regardless of the infecting organism and in the absence of a known causative agent. Identifying the causative microorganism is not essential to improve survival with DrotAA treatment after sepsis has progressed to include organ dysfunction.

▶ The 2 studies (Abstracts 16–1 and 16–2) of activated protein C (DrotAA) add to our information about management of sepsis. Older adults benefit to a greater extent than the population at large without an increase in toxicity. In addition, the second study, which assessed response by the causative organism, demonstrated the greatest effect from infections caused by *S pneumoniae.*

D. R. Snydman, MD

17 Viral Infections

Zoonotic Transmission of Hepatitis E Virus From Deer to Human Beings
Tei S, Kitajima N, Takahashi K, et al (Kasai City Hosp, Hyogo, Japan; Toshiba Gen Hosp, Tokyo)
Lancet 362:371-373, 2003   17–1

Background.—Some authorities have suggested that zoonosis is involved in the transmission of hepatitis E virus (HEV) infection. To date, this hypothesis has been based on indirect evidence. Direct evidence of zoonotic transmission of HEV is reported.

Methods.—In April 2003, a 44-year-old man sought medical attention for fever, nausea, and general malaise. Acute hepatitis was diagnosed on the basis of raised liver enzymes and bilirubin. One week later, the first patient's father reported similar symptoms. Within another week, the index patient's brother and a friend were also found to have hepatitis. On admission, all 4 patients were negative for serologic markers of hepatitis A, B, and C viruses. Later, all serum samples from these patients were positive for HEV RNA as well as immunoglobulins M and G antibodies to HEV. These findings led to the diagnosis of hepatitis E. The patients' histories revealed that all had eaten the meat of 2 wild-caught Japanese deer, uncooked, 3 times in the 7-week period preceding illness onset. A polymerase chain reaction analysis of a leftover portion of the meat demonstrated HEV RNA. The nucleotide sequence identified was that from the patients. The family members of the patients, who had eaten none or very little of the meat, were not infected.

Conclusions.—These patients became infected with HEV after eating raw meat from an infected deer, providing direct evidence of zoonotic transmission of HEV infection. The consumption of Sika deer should be added to the list of foods carrying a risk of HEV transmission.

▶ We have only begun to understand the epidemiology of HEV infection. There is a growing body of evidence that HEV may be a zoonosis. Antibodies can be found in a variety of animals, including swine. The authors report an outbreak with very strong epidemiologic evidence that deer meat, eaten raw or poorly cooked, was involved.

D. R. Snydman, MD

Management of Influenza in Adults Older Than 65 Years of Age: Cost-Effectiveness of Rapid Testing and Antiviral Therapy

Rothberg MB, Bellantonio S, Rose DN (Baystate Med Ctr, Springfield, Mass; Tufts Univ, Boston)

Ann Intern Med 139:321-329, 2003   17–2

Introduction.—A disproportionate number of the 20,000 deaths and 100,000 hospitalizations caused yearly in the United States by influenza virus infection occur among older adults. Influenza vaccination has been recommended for all persons 50 years and older. Amantadine and rimantadine are older drugs for treatment of influenza illness. They are not as efficacious

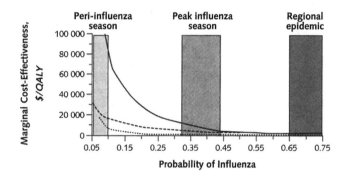

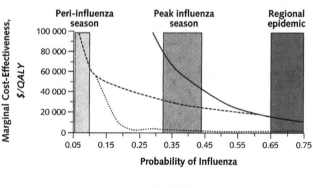

— Empirical
oseltamivir
--- Rapid test,
oseltamivir
···· Empirical
amantadine

FIGURE 3.—The cost-effectiveness of antiviral therapy or testing as a function of the probability of influenza. The *curves* represent the marginal cost-effectiveness of each strategy compared with the next best strategy for unvaccinated (**top**) and vaccinated (**bottom**) patients. The graphs are divided into 3 zones representing different probabilities of influenza: peri-influenza season, peak season, and regional epidemic. *Abbreviation: QALY,* Quality-adjusted life-year. (Courtesy of Rothberg MB, Bellantonio S, Rose DN: Management of influenza in adults older than 65 years of age: Cost-effectiveness of rapid testing and antiviral therapy. *Ann Intern Med* 139:321-329, 2003.)

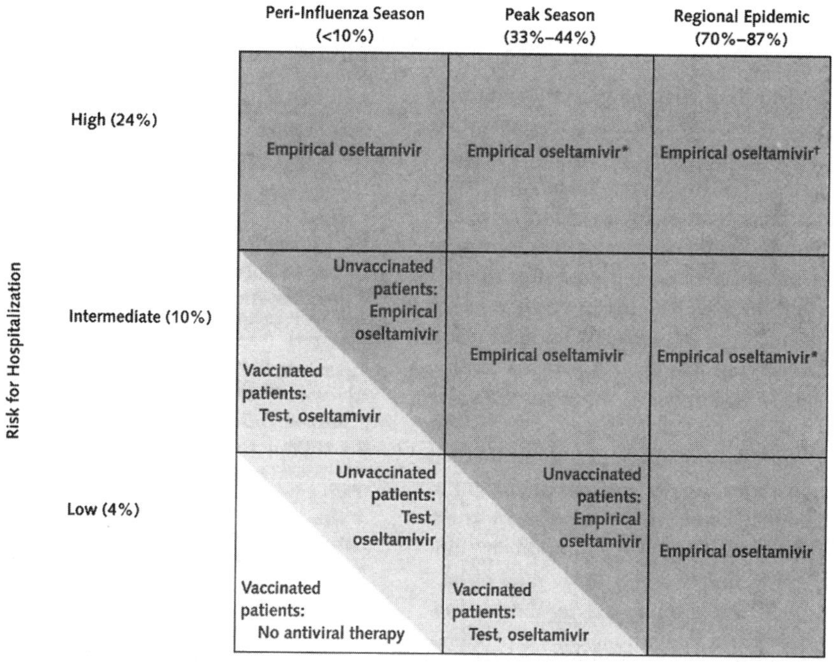

FIGURE 4.—Optimal influenza therapy based on risk, season, and vaccination status. The strategy providing the most quality-adjusted life-years at a marginal cost-effectiveness at or below $50,000 per quality-adjusted life-year saved. The *percentages* at the top of the figure are probabilities of influenza infection based on timing of presentation. Influenza season varies from year to year. Peak season is generally from December through February in the northern hemisphere; peri-influenza season months include October, November, March, and April; and "regional epidemic" denotes an area where influenza has recently been reported to be widespread. *Cost-saving in unvaccinated patients. †Cost-savings in all patients. (Courtesy of Rothberg MB, Bellantonio S, Rose DN: Management of influenza in adults older than 65 years of age: Cost-effectiveness of rapid testing and antiviral therapy. *Ann Intern Med* 139:321-329, 2003.)

or cost-effective as the recently released neuraminidase inhibitors, zanamivir and oseltamivir. Yet, cost-effectiveness in older adults is more dependent on reducing morbidity and mortality than on actual drug costs. A computer model was constructed to compare the cost-effectiveness of various testing and treatment strategies for older adults under various assumptions concerning the effect of antiviral therapy.

Methods.—A decision tree was constructed to compare 9 strategies: (1) no antiviral therapy; (2-5) empirical treatment with amantadine, rimantadine, oseltamivir, or zanamivir; and (6-9) rapid diagnostic testing followed by treatment with each of the antiviral drugs.

Results.—Compared with no intervention, empirically treating an unvaccinated 75-year-old patient with amantadine increased life expectancy by 0.0014 quality-adjusted life-years (QALYs) at a cost of $1.57, a cost-effectiveness ratio of $1129 per QALY saved. Compared with amantadine, rapid diagnostic testing followed by treatment with oseltamivir cost $5025 per QALY saved, whereas empirical treatment with oseltamivir cost $10,296 per QALY saved. Testing and treatment strategies were less cost-effective if the patient was vaccinated, and ranged from $2483 per QALY saved with amantadine to $70,300 per QALY saved with oseltamivir (Fig 3). The optimal strategy was defined as that which yields the most QALYs at the marginal cost-effectiveness ratio at or below $50,000 per QALY saved (Fig 4). Empirical treatment with oseltamivir is the optimal treatment strategy for all patients who are at high risk at any season and for every patient during regional epidemics.

Conclusion.—Community-based older adults benefit from antiviral therapy through an improvement in quality-adjusted life expectancy, if treatment is initiated within 48 hours of influenza-like illness. The optimal strategy depends on the patient's vaccination status, the probability that the patient has influenza, and the risk for hospitalization. The most cost-effective strategy is empirical treatment with oseltamivir when the likelihood of influenza or hospitalization is high. Rapid diagnostic testing followed by oseltamivir treatment is less effective than empirical treatment, yet is cost-effective in low-risk patients and vaccinated patients.

▶ As of this writing, the influenza season is making a significant public health impact. This cost-effectiveness analysis is very important since it establishes a framework for thinking about the use of empirical antiviral therapy or rapid diagnostic testing followed by antiviral therapy. Earlier cost-effectiveness analyses have focused on young healthy adults because this was the population in whom clinical trials of effectiveness were first undertaken. One important caveat to this analysis and take-home message is that the authors' analysis is predicated on data gleaned from observational studies, not data gathered from randomized trials. If the antiviral neuraminidase inhibitors do not prevent hospitalization, then the use of such agents would not be cost-effective. From this analysis it is clear that high-risk patients, regardless of the season, will benefit from empirical oseltamivir treatment.

D. R. Snydman, MD

Influenza- and Respiratory Syncytial Virus–Associated Morbidity and Mortality in the Nursing Home Population
Ellis SE, Coffey CS, Mitchel EF Jr, et al (Vanderbilt Univ, Nashville, Tenn; Tennessee Valley Healthcare System, Nashville; Univ of Alabama at Birmingham)
J Am Geriatr Soc 51:761-767, 2003   17–3

Background.—Seasonal outbreaks of influenza and respiratory syncytial virus (RSV)–associated illness often occur among nursing home residents, who are in close contact with one another and staff, facilitating the spread of these viruses. The attack rates during winter outbreaks can range from 10% to 40% for both viruses, and their case fatality rates are 2% to 20% for RSV and as high as 55% for influenza. A population-based survey was undertaken to estimate the viral-related morbidity and mortality among nursing home residents over 4 consecutive years.

TABLE 4.—Influenza and Respiratory Syncytial Virus–Attributable Deaths (Events) by Risk Group, Tennessee Medicaid Nursing Home Residents From 1995 to 1999

Risk Group	Rates, Events, and Person-Years by Season			Total Rates, Events, and Person-Years	Estimated Annual Events Attributable to Winter Viruses per 1,000 Person-Years* (95% Confidence Interval)		Percentage of Total Events Attributable to Winter Viruses†		
	Influenza	RSV	Non-Winter Viral		Influenza	RSV	Influenza	RSV	Both
No high risk									
Deaths per 1,000 person-years	201	175	143	165	6.2 (2.7-9.8)	16.3 (10.7-22.0)	3.8	9.9	13.7
Deaths	1,467	1,411	2,153	5,031					
Person-years	7,310	8,075	15,112	30,497					
High risk									
Deaths per 1,000 person-years	400	335	298	331	14.5 (11.0-18.1)	17.3 (11.5-23.3)	3.4	5.2	8.6
Deaths	4,582	4,661	7,767	17,010					
Person-years	11,459	13,901	26,029	51,389					

*Values are weighted averages of annual excess events for a population of 1000 persons within the specified age and risk group. The influenza excess events were calculated by multiplying the event rate difference between influenza and respiratory syncytial virus (RSV) by the proportion of overall study days in influenza season. The RSV excess events were calculated by multiplying the event rate difference between RSV and non–winter-viral season by the proportion of overall study days in RSV or influenza season (RSV circulated during both of these seasons). The weighted average difference in rates between influenza and RSV season and non–winter-viral season were calculated with stratum-specific person-years in all seasons as weights; strata were defined by study year, race, sex, and nursing home location.

†Percentage values are calculated by dividing the annual excess events attributable to influenza or RSV by the age and risk group specific total event rate.

(Courtesy of Ellis SE, Coffey CS, Mitchel EF Jr, et al: Influenza- and respiratory syncytial virus–associated morbidity and mortality in the nursing home population. *J Am Geriatr Soc* 51:761-767, 2003. Reprinted by permission of Blackwell Publishing.)

Methods.—A total of 381 Tennessee nursing homes were included, for 81,885 person-years of follow-up. The viral surveillance data delineated 3 seasons, identified as influenza when influenza and RSV cocirculated (23% of the person-years); RSV when RSV alone circulated (26%); and non–winter-viral when neither virus was circulating (51%). Estimates were made of annual hospitalizations, courses of antibiotics, and deaths attributable to influenza and RSV based on adjusted seasonal differences in the rates of cardiopulmonary hospitalizations, antibiotic prescriptions, and deaths over these 3 seasons.

Results.—A total of 1105 RSV culture or antigen-positive tests, 235 influenza culture or antigen-positive tests, and 77 parainfluenza-positive cultures were obtained over the 4 years. In the first year, cardiopulmonary hospitalizations were higher in RSV season than influenza or non–winter-viral seasons, but they were higher in the influenza season in all of the other years. Fifteen percent of the cardiopulmonary hospitalizations of persons with no other high-risk conditions and 7% of hospitalizations in high-risk cases were attributable to influenza and RSV. The highest rate of antibiotic prescriptions occurred when both influenza and RSV were circulating.

Combining those with high-risk conditions and those without, influenza and RSV accounted for 8% to 9% of all antibiotic courses. The seasonal death rates were higher during the influenza and RSV seasons than the non–winter-viral seasons, with a peak in each influenza season. RSV and influenza accounted for 14% of deaths among persons without other high-risk conditions and 9% of deaths among persons with high-risk conditions (Table 4).

Conclusion.—Hospitalization rates, antibiotic use, and deaths are markedly increased among elderly nursing home residents each winter as a result of influenza and RSV infections. The development and testing of RSV vaccines and the effective use of influenza vaccine coverage are important aspects in addressing this problem.

▶ The effect of influenza and RSV infection in the nursing home population is incompletely described. While it is known that there are winter outbreaks of RSV, with an attack rate as high as 20% to 40% and case fatality rates as high as 20% for RSV, the epidemiology of this virus in nursing home residents and the clinical impact is incompletely described. This population-based study attempts to quantify the relative importance of both RSV and influenza. It should be noted that these data infer from statewide surveillance the clinical impact and probably overestimate the contribution of RSV, and even influenza, but using their methodology, the authors show a considerable attributable risk from RSV. Unfortunately, the RSV is difficult to diagnose and treat. However, the data suggest that strategies which can reduce RSV transmission will have significant economic and clinical impact on the nursing home population.

D. R. Snydman, MD

Human Metapneumovirus Infection in the United States: Clinical Manifestations Associated With a Newly Emerging Respiratory Infection in Children

Esper F, Boucher D, Weibel C, et al (Yale Univ, New Haven, Conn)
Pediatrics 111:1407-1410, 2003   17–4

Background.—A newly identified human respiratory virus, human metapneumovirus (hMPV), has been reported in The Netherlands. Whether hMPV was circulating in the United States was investigated, and the clinical features associated with this virus were discussed.

Methods.—Respiratory specimens from 296 patients younger than 5 years were analyzed. The children had negative results for respiratory syncytial virus (RSV), influenza A and B, parainfluenza viruses 1 to 3, and adenovirus by direct fluorescent antibody testing. Specimens were screened for hMPV by reverse transcriptase-polymerase chain reactions.

Findings.—Nineteen (6.4%) patients showed evidence of hMPV infection. This virus was identified in children with upper and lower respiratory tract infection. Common clinical manifestations were wheezing, hypoxia, and abnormal chest radiographic findings. At least 1 patient had a nosocomial infection.

Conclusions.—These data show that hMPV is currently circulating in the United States. The virus is associated with respiratory tract disease in patients with respiratory illnesses not caused by RSV, influenza, parainfluenza viruses, and adenovirus. Further research is needed to determine the epidemiology and extent of this disease in the general population.

▶ Most physicians had never heard of hMPV infection prior to the SARS outbreak when it was implicated in some of the cases as a possible copathogen. However, investigators in The Netherlands, Australia and the United Kingdom detected this virus in 1999 and 2000. This investigation analyzes the clinical manifestations of hMPV infection in children in a single center in New Haven, Conn in 2001. What is apparent is that this virus behaves like RSV in children. It may cause both upper and lower respiratory tract infection. The authors did note coinfection with RSV in 1 patient and influenza A and cytomegalovirus in another. The nature of the surveillance for viral infection in this study does not allow for an assessment of prevalence, but it is clear that hMPV infection is common, and methods for detection will need to be developed.

D. R. Snydman, MD

Human Metapneumovirus Infections in Young and Elderly Adults

Falsey AR, Erdman D, Anderson LJ, et al (Univ of Rochester, NY; Ctrs for Disease Control and Prevention, Atlanta, Ga)
J Infect Dis 187:785-790, 2003   17–5

Introduction.—Human metapneumovirus (hMPV) is a newly identified human respiratory pathogen for which limited epidemiologic data are available. Cohorts of younger and older adults were prospectively assessed for hMPV infection during 2 winter seasons. Patients hospitalized for cardiopulmonary conditions during this period were also evaluated.

Methods.—As part of an ongoing investigation of hMPV and influenza virus infection, 4 cohorts of adults were assessed for hMPV infection during the 1999-2001 winter seasons. The research subjects included 305 healthy adults aged 65 years or older, 304 high-risk adults with underlying cardiopulmonary diseases, 195 healthy adults younger than 40 years of age, and 134 residents of a long-term care facility.

Results.—Overall, 44 illnesses (4.5%) were related to hMPV infection, and 9 (4.2%) of 217 asymptomatic persons were infected. There was a significant increase in the rates of hMPV illness between year 1 and year 2 (7/452 [1.5%] vs 37/532 [7.0%]; $P < .0001$). In year 2, 11% of hospitalized patients had evidence of hMPV infection. Infections occurred in all age groups; most frequently in young adults. Frail elderly patients with hMPV infection often sought medical attention.

Conclusion.—hMPV infection occurs in adults of all ages, both in the community and in nursing homes and may be responsible for a significant proportion of patients hospitalized with respiratory infections during some years.

▶ The authors used RT-PCR testing and serology to assess the impact of hMPV infection in young and elderly adults. Like the cohort of children cited above (Abstract 17–4) this surveillance study of healthy adults both below and above the age of 65 years, those with cardiopulmonary disease and residents of long-term care facilities were prospectively assessed. The symptoms resemble those described in children, with wheezing being prominent in older adults and hoarseness being seen in younger adults, and more frequently in comparison to respiratory syncytial virus in younger adults. However, none of these symptoms is unique to hMPV. One potential distinguishing feature is the absence of fever, which may help differentiate this infection clinically from influenza. As with all respiratory pathogens, seasonality was also demonstrated. These data underscore the fact that this pathogen can affect all ages and cause significant morbidity.

D. R. Snydman, MD

18 Bacterial Infections

Vancomycin-Intermediate *Staphylococcus aureus* With Phenotypic Susceptibility to Methicillin in a Patient With Recurrent Bacteremia
Naimi TS, Anderson D, O'Boyle C, et al (Minnesota Dept of Health, Minneapolis; Abbott Northwestern Hosp, Minneapolis; Ctrs for Disease Control and Prevention, Atlanta, Ga)
Clin Infect Dis 36:1609-1612, 2003   18–1

Background.—Vancomycin-intermediate *Staphylococcus aureus* (VISA) isolates and glycopeptides have emerged in several countries. A case of VISA infection in a patient undergoing hemodialysis, in whom VISA isolates were oxacillin susceptible despite the continued presence of the *mecA* gene, was reported.

Case Report.—Man, 59, had diabetes, hypertension, atrial fibrillation, peripheral vascular disease, and hepatitis C. In 1998, bacteremia caused by methicillin-resistant *S aureus* (MRSA) developed, associated with an infected foot ulcer. A year later, MRSA bacteremia again developed in association with an infected hemodialysis arteriovenous fistula. Several months later, MRSA bacteremia was diagnosed as a result of infection in a hemodialysis arteriovenous synthetic graft. Subsequently, a below-the-knee amputation was performed, followed by a 6-week course of vancomycin for MRSA bacteremia associated with an infected, nonhealing leg ulcer. In March, 2000, T11-T12 osteomyelitis and MRSA bacteremia were diagnosed, and treatment with vancomycin and gentamicin was reinitiated. Nafcillin was substituted for gentamicin, and the patient's bacteremia finally resolved. In June 2000, the patient died of heart failure and hemorrhagic stroke complications.

Discussion.—In this patient, who was undergoing hemodialysis and had received 26 weeks of vancomycin treatment, a significant inverse relationship was noted between the minimum inhibitory concentrations (MICs) of vancomycin and oxacillin in *S aureus* isolates. All isolates were *mecA* positive. They were indistinguishable by pulsed-field gel electrophoresis. The evolving susceptibility patterns of this strain complicate the detection and treatment of VISA infections.

▶ The evolution of the *S aureus* isolate in this patient under antibiotic pressure and the development of heteroresistance is striking and probably underappreciated. All the more remarkable is the loss of resistance to oxacillin or nafcillin despite the continued presence of the *mecA* gene. Suppression of *mecA* gene expressed vancomycin-resistant laboratory strains has been reported, as has an inverse relationship between vancomycin and oxacillin MICs. The clinical implications of this patient's isolate are that the data suggest that vancomycin-oxacillin combinations to treat MRSA might improve treatment efficacy and prevent the development of VISA resistance. These findings apply to VISA strains of MRSA, not VRSA strains of MRSA.

D. R. Snydman, MD

A Prospective Multicenter Study of *Staphylococcus aureus* Bacteremia: Incidence of Endocarditis, Risk Factors for Mortality, and Clinical Impact of Methicillin Resistance
Chang F, MacDonald BB, Peacock JE, et al (Univ of Pittsburgh, Pa; Veterans Affairs Med Ctr, Pittsburgh, Pa; Veterans Affairs Med Ctr, Houston)
Medicine 82:322-332, 2003   18–2

Background.—Antibiotic therapy for *Staphylococcus aureus* bacteremia is designed to eliminate bacteremia and prevent relapse or secondary infection of the heart valves or elsewhere. It is important that the presence of endocarditis be determined. Increasingly, cases of endocarditis are caused by methicillin-resistant *S aureus* (MRSA); knowing the clinical differences between disease caused by MRSA and that caused by methicillin-susceptible *S aureus* (MSSA) can be diagnostically useful. Answers were sought to the following questions: (1) What is the incidence of endocarditis in community-acquired, hemodialysis-related, or hospital-acquired *S aureus* bacteremia? (2) What are the clinical tests that can accurately differentiate *S aureus* bacteremia from *S aureus* endocarditis? (3) Could the endocarditis be caused by MRSA? and (4) What are the risk factors for mortality in endocarditis cases?

Methods.—The prospective observational study included 6 university teaching hospitals, involving 505 consecutive patients with *S aureus* bacteremia.

Results.—The prevalence of endocarditis was 21% in community-acquired *S aureus* bacteremia, 12% in hemodialysis patients, and 5% in hospital-acquired cases. MSSA caused infection in 69% of cases and MRSA in 31%. New endocarditis developed in 7 patients, usually via an intravascular catheter. Relapse occurred 17 to 87 days after ceasing antistaphylococcal antibiotics in 5 patients; bacteremia in 2 patients persisted for more than 7 days while on antibiotic therapy. Six had severe arteriosclerotic heart or valvular disease; all 7 received vancomycin therapy for less than 4 weeks. Risk factors

TABLE 4.—Factors Associated With Mortality (30 Days) in 64 Patients
With Endocarditis*

Parameter	Deaths (%)	P Value
Insulin-dependent diabetes	47	NS (.10)
Nondiabetic	26	
Transplant recipient	100	.03
No transplant	28	
Persistent bacteremia	59	.004[1]
No persistence	21	
MRSA	50	.03
MSSA	23	
Hemodialysis	55	NS (.08)
No hemodialysis	26	
AV block on EKG	100	.002
No AV block	29	

*No significant association was seen with sex, race, presence of prosthetic valve, history of prior endocarditis, hospital acquisition, or vital signs at onset of bacteremia.

Abbreviations: AV, Atrioventricular; *EKG*, electrocardiogram; *MRSA*, methicillin-resistant *S aureus*; *MSSA*, methicillin-sensitive *S aureus*; *NS*, not significant.

(Courtesy of Chang F, MacDonald BB, Peacock JE, et al: A prospective multicenter study of staphylococcus aureus bacteremia: incidence of endocarditis, risk factors for mortality, and clinical impact of methicillin resistance. *Medicine* 82:322-332, 2003.)

significant for endocarditis were valvular heart disease, previous endocarditis, IV drug use, community-acquired infection, no initially recognized portal of entry, and nonwhite race. MSSA endocarditis cases were community acquired more often than MRSA cases and were noted more often among IV drug users and persons with previous endocarditis. Hospitalized patients, older patients, and those with renal insufficiency or having hemodialysis were more likely to have MRSA endocarditis. Persistent bacteremia was seen significantly more in MRSA endocarditis. Renal insufficiency occurred significantly more in MRSA than MSSA endocarditis. Factors linked to persistent bacteremia were hemodialysis, creatinine level more than 2 mg/dL, total APACHE III score, IV drug use, and MRSA infection; multivariate analysis identified only MRSA as significant. The 30-day mortality rate was 31% and at 60 days, 34%. The mortality rate was significantly related to APACHE III score and persistent bacteremia (Table 4). The affected valve was resected in 6 patients and all survived, whereas 50% of patients only receiving medical therapy died.

Conclusions.—Risk factors for endocarditis were valvular heart disease, IV drug use, community acquisition, previous endocarditis, nonwhite race, and unknown source of infection. Persistent bacteremia after starting antibiotic therapy was a significant independent risk factor for both endocarditis and mortality. Of the community-acquired *S aureus* bacteremia cases, 21% had endocarditis. The mortality rate was significantly higher in patients with MRSA endocarditis than in those with MSSA disease. Repeated blood cultures are advised in all patients with *S aureus* bacteremia 3 days after starting therapy; endocarditis is strongly suspected when bacteremia persists, and requires stronger therapy. In hospital-acquired endocarditis with renal insufficiency, MRSA infection should be suspected and treated with appropriate antibiotics. Surgery improved survival rate and should also be considered.

▶ This is a very large prospective observational study of *S aureus* bacteremia in 6 university-affiliated hospitals. The study underscores the importance of persistent bacteremia at day 3 as a prognostic factor for mortality as well as the presence of AV block, infection with MRSA, and not unexpectedly, severity of illness. It is incumbent upon clinicians to prove sterility of blood cultures to determine optimal management. Of note, endocarditis was associated with approximately 12% of hemodialysis patients, and new onset endocarditis developed exclusively either in patients with hospital-acquired bacteremia, or in those on hemodialysis, and the intravascular catheter was the portal of entry in 71% of the patients. This high-risk subset must be kept in mind in determining treatment strategies and underscores the need to treat aggressively and for a long period. This study probably underestimates the overall incidence of endocarditis, since endocardiography was not performed in all patients. Therefore, the incidence of 21% is undoubtedly a minimal estimate.

D. R. Snydman, MD

Staphyloccus aureus **Bacteremia: Recurrence and the Impact of Antibiotic Treatment in a Prospective Multicenter Study**
Chang F, Peacock JE Jr, Musher DM, et al (Univ of Pittsburgh, Penn; Wake Forest Univ, Winston-Salem, NC; Veterans Affairs Med Ctr, Houston; et al)
Medicine 82:333-339, 2003   18–3

Background.—Bacteremia caused by *Staphylococcus aureus* recurs in 5% to 12% of patients even when antibiotics are given. The causes of this disease include endocarditis, distal septic complications, and a short duration of parenteral antibiotic therapy when the bacteremia is catheter-related. Patient morbidity and mortality rates increase when bacteremia recurs. Because methicillin-resistant organisms are commonly found and vancomycin is easy to administer, especially in patients with renal insufficiency, this agent has been used more often, assuming that it is as effective as β-lactam antibiotics, a belief that has not been proved. To assess the risk factors for *S aureus* bacteremia recurrence, a multicenter prospective observational study was done.

Methods.—The study included 505 consecutive patients who had *S aureus* bacteremia. Their conditions were monitored for 6 months, with a 3-year follow-up for patients with endocarditis. Recurrence was defined as a return of *S aureus* bacteremia after negative blood cultures were documented, clinical improvement was noted, or both, once the course of antistaphylococcal antibiotic therapy was completed; it was further described as reinfection or relapse on the basis of pulsed-field gel electrophoresis testing, which was conducted on all blood isolates obtained from cases of recurrent bacteremia.

Results.—Demographic data were obtained from 448 patients, 16 to 97 years old (mean age, 56.5 years), 132 of whom were female and 316 male. Methicillin-susceptible *S aureus* (MSSA) was the infecting agent in

298 patients, methicillin-resistant *S aureus* (MRSA) in 146 patients, and unknown susceptibility in 4 patients. Fifty-six cases of recurrent bacteremia were found in 42 patients, with relapses diagnosed in 26 patients and reinfections in 7. Native valve disease or endocarditis occurred significantly more often among patients with recurrence than among those without a recurrence. Excluding cases of endocarditis, a relapse of *S aureus* bacteremia was significantly related to the presence of cirrhosis of the liver; further analysis indicated relapse was also significantly associated with native valvular disease and cirrhosis. Six of the 8 patients who had multiple recurrences of bacteremia were infected by MSSA; all 8 were given vancomycin. Relapse occurred earlier than reinfection (median, 36 vs 99 days). Patients with endocarditis were significantly more likely to suffer relapse than those with a removable focus of infection. The type of therapy and its duration had no significant influence on relapse rates. Compared with those receiving vancomycin therapy, patients with MSSA bacteremia receiving nafcillin showed significantly higher rates for male sex, community-acquired infection, or IV drug use; they were less likely to have a catheter-related infection. Hemodialysis patients were more likely to be given vancomycin. All patients with MSSA bacteremia responded better to nafcillin therapy than to that with vancomycin, as demonstrated by no bacteriologic failures. Relapse was predictable on the basis of the presence of endocarditis and vancomycin treatment.

Conclusions.—When antistaphylococcal therapy was given, recurrences were noted in 9.4% of the patients with *S aureus* bacteremia; most were relapses. The type of antibiotic therapy was linked to the occurrence of relapse, with nafcillin proving superior to vancomycin in preventing relapse in patients with MSSA bacteremia.

▶ This study demonstrates the fact that vancomycin is not as good as an antistaphylococcal β-lactam in the management of *S aureus* bacteremia. Patients were less likely to have persistence if treated with an antistaphylococcal β-lactam, and were also less likely to have relapse (but the numbers were too small for a statistical power). In fact, vancomycin use instead of an antistaphylococcal β-lactam, was associated with an increased likelihood of relapse along with the presence of endocarditis.

D. R. Snydman, MD

19 Vaccines

Effectiveness of Pneumococcal Polysaccharide Vaccine in Older Adults
Jackson LA, for the Vaccine Safety Datalink (Group Health Cooperative, Seattle; Univ of Washington, Seattle; Veterans Affairs Puget Sound Health Care System, Seattle; et al)
N Engl J Med 348:1747-1755, 2003   19–1

Background.—An estimated 350,000 to 620,000 persons, 65 years and older, are hospitalized each year with community-acquired pneumonia. *Streptococcus pneumoniae* is the most common cause of community-acquired pneumonia in older adults. A vaccine that provides protection against pneumococcal pneumonia could reduce the risk of community-acquired pneumonia among the elderly population. However, most cases of pneumococcal pneumonia are not associated with bacteremia, so an effect of vaccination would likely only be noticeable if the vaccine provided protection against nonbacteremic pneumococcal pneumonia. At present it is unclear whether use of the pneumococcal polysaccharide vaccine changes the overall risk of community-acquired pneumonia. The effectiveness of the pneumococcal vaccine in a large population of older adults was assessed retrospectively.

Methods.—The study included 47,365 Group Health Cooperative members, 65 years or older, followed up for 3 years. The main outcome measures were hospitalization because of community-acquired pneumonia, pneumonia in patients who were not hospitalized, and pneumococcal bacteremia. Multivariate Cox proportional-hazards models were used to evaluate the association between pneumococcal vaccination and the risk of each outcome, with adjustments for age, sex, nursing-home residence or nonresidence, smoking status, medical conditions, and receipt or nonreceipt of influenza vaccine.

Results.—A total of 1428 study participants were hospitalized with community-acquired pneumonia; 3061 participants were diagnosed with outpatient pneumonia, and 61 were diagnosed with pneumococcal bacteremia. A significant reduction was noted in the risk of pneumococcal bacteremia in association with receipt of the pneumococcal vaccine (Table 3). However, the vaccination was also associated with a slightly increased risk of hospitalization for pneumonia. Pneumococcal vaccination had no effect on the risk of outpatient pneumonia or of any case of community-acquired pneumonia, regardless of whether hospitalization was required.

TABLE 3.—Risk of Pneumonia, Pneumococcal Bacteremia, and Death From Any Cause According to Pneumococcal-Vaccination Status Among Groups Defined by Immunocompetency, Presence of Chronic Lung Disease, and Receipt of Influenza Vaccine*

Outcome	Immunocompetent (N=38,207)	Immunocompromised (N=9158)	Immunocompetent with Chronic Lung Disease (N=3126)	Immunocompetent with Receipt of Influenza Vaccine Annually (N=20,806)
Hospitalization for community-acquired pneumonia verified by medical-record review				
No. of events	959	469	257	479
Multivariate-adjusted hazard ratio (95% CI)	1.14 (0.99-1.31)	1.14 (0.94-1.39)	1.04 (0.79-1.36)	1.05 (0.86-1.29)
P value for adjusted hazard ratio	0.07	0.19	0.79	0.65
Outpatient pneumonia				
No. of events	2310	751	407	1315
Multivariate-adjusted hazard ratio (95% CI)	1.02 (0.93-1.11)	1.18 (0.95-1.31)	1.01 (0.81-1.25)	0.94 (0.83-1.06)
P value for adjusted hazard ratio	0.73	0.17	0.95	0.34
Pneumococcal bacteremia				
No. of events	39	22	6	19
Multivariate-adjusted hazard ratio (95% CI)	0.46 (0.24-0.87)	0.78 (0.32-1.87)	0.19 (0.04-1.09)†	0.35 (0.14-0.87)
P value for adjusted hazard ratio	0.02	0.57	0.06	0.02
Hospitalization with a discharge diagnosis of pneumonia (ICD-9-CM codes 480 through 487.0)				
No. of events	1628	808	383	815
Multivariate-adjusted hazard ratio (95% CI)	1.05 (0.94-1.17)	1.09 (0.93-1.26)	1.11 (0.88-1.37)	0.93 (0.80-1.09)
P value for adjusted hazard ratio	0.39	0.29	0.39	0.37
Death from any cause				
No. of events	3613	2077	482	1875
Multivariate-adjusted hazard ratio (95% CI)	0.88 (0.83-0.95)	1.09 (0.99-1.19)	1.00 (0.82-1.22)	0.85 (0.77-0.93)
P value for adjusted hazard ratio	0.005	0.08	0.96	<0.001

*The hazard ratios are for vaccinated subjects as compared with unvaccinated subjects and were adjusted, where appropriate, for age (65 to 74, 75 to 84, or more than 84 years); sex; nursing-home residence or nonresidence; receipt or nonreceipt of influenza vaccine; smoking status (currently smoking, not currently smoking, or no data); presence or absence of coronary artery disease, diabetes mellitus, chronic lung disease, and dementia or stroke; number of outpatient visits in the year before study entry (fewer than 6, 6 to 12, or more than 12); and any hospitalization for pneumonia in the year before cohort entry. CI denotes confidence interval, and ICD-9-CM the *International Classification of Diseases, 9th Revision, Clinical Modification.*

†The hazard ratio was not adjusted for receipt or nonreceipt of influenza vaccine, sex, smoking status, presence or absence of dementia or stroke, and number of outpatient visits in the year before study entry because there were too few events to allow these variables to be estimated in the model.

Conclusions.—The effectiveness of the pneumococcal polysaccharide vaccine for the prevention of bacteremia is supported by these studies. However, it appears that alternative strategies are needed to prevent nonbacteremic pneumonia, which is the most common form of pneumococcal infection in persons 65 years or older.

▶ This large group health observational cohort study of individuals 65 years of age and older confirms that pneumococcal polysaccharide vaccine prevents bacteremic pneumococcal pneumonia. The magnitude of the reduction is about 40%. However, there was no reduction in rates of pneumococcal pneumonia, in fact pneumonia was a little more likely to occur within 6 months of vaccination. And there was no reduction in overall mortality rate among the victims. One might ask why? Since this is an observational trial and not an intervention trial, one can only speculate as to why these results were seen. The authors offer no answers. Subtle unrecognized biases may have entered into the cohort. Nevertheless, it is reassuring that the reduction in bacteremic disease in this cohort was confirmed. Improvements in the immunogenicity of pneumococcal vaccine may be necessary for this population to show reduced rates of all cause hospitalization for pneumonia, which has been shown with the protein conjugate vaccine in children. In fact, all forms of invasive pneumococcal disease have been reduced, especially that caused by vaccine and vaccine-related serotypes. Remarkably, disease rates have also declined among adults. The vaccine should have a similar impact on adults once clinical trials prove effectiveness and safety.

D. R. Snydman, MD

Decline in Invasive Pneumococcal Disease After the Introduction of Protein–Polysaccharide Conjugate Vaccine
Whitney CG, for the Active Bacterial Core Surveillance of the Emerging Infections Program Network (Ctrs for Disease Control and Prevention, Atlanta, Ga; et al)
N Engl J Med 348:1737-1746, 2003   19–2

Background.—A 7-valent protein-polysaccharide pneumococcal conjugate vaccine (Prevnar) was licensed in the United States in 2000 for use in infants and young children. Controlled trials have shown that the vaccine, when administered as a 4-dose regimen to infants, is highly effective against invasive disease and somewhat effective against otitis media and pneumonia. However, the efficacy of the vaccine in infants given less than 4 doses and in older children is not known. It is also unclear whether vaccination of young children will reduce carriage and subsequently affect disease in other age groups. Data from the Active Bacterial Core Surveillance of the Centers for Disease Control and Prevention (CDC) were analyzed in an effort to answer these questions.

Methods.—Population-based data from the CDCs Active Bacterial Core Surveillance were reviewed to detect changes in the burden of invasive dis-

TABLE 2.—Changes in Estimated Rates of Invasive Pneumococcal Disease Among Adults, According to Age Group, Year, and Serotype, From 1998 Through 2001*

Age and Serotype	Average for 1998 and 1999		2001		%Change in Estimated Rate (95% CI)‡	P Value§
	No. of Cases	Estimated Rate†	No. of Cases	Estimated Rate†		
		cases/100,000		cases/100,000		
20-39 Yr						
All vaccine serotypes	285.5	6.60	176	3.97	−40 (−49 to −29)	<0.001
4	86.5	2.00	50	1.13	−44 (−58 to −23)	<0.001
6B	19	0.44	18	0.41	−8 (−46 to +56)	0.74
9V	51.5	1.19	27	0.61	−49 (−66 to −24)	0.001
14	62	1.43	38	0.86	−40 (−58 to −16)	0.003
18C	19	0.44	12	0.27	−39 (−68 to +11)	0.13
19F	18.5	0.43	9	0.20	−53 (−76 to −4)	0.05
23F	29	0.67	22	0.50	−25 (−54 to +17)	0.23
All vaccine-related serotypes¶	60	1.39	48	1.08	−22 (−44 to +7)	0.14
All nonvaccine serotypes	138.5	3.21	114	2.57	−20 (−35 to −1)	0.04
40-64 Yr						
All vaccine serotypes	481.5	11.58	431	9.95	−14 (−23 to −4)	0.006
4	113.5	2.73	118	2.72	−1 (−19 to +23)	0.99
6B	54	1.30	44	1.02	−22 (−44 to +9)	0.17
9V	74.5	1.79	64	1.48	−17 (−38 to +8)	0.18
14	108.5	2.61	76	1.75	−33 (−48 to −14)	0.002
18C	28.5	0.69	40	0.92	+33 (−8 to +97)	0.16
19F	38	0.91	32	0.74	−19 (−45 to +19)	0.32
23F	64.5	1.55	57	1.32	−15 (−36 to +15)	0.29
All vaccine-related serotypes¶	103.5	2.49	103	2.38	−4 (−23 to +20)	0.74
All nonvaccine serotypes	310	7.46	321	7.41	−1 (−13 to +13)	0.93

≥65 Yr

All vaccine serotypes	511.5	33.43	374	23.91	−29 (−36 to −20)	<0.001
4	76.5	5.00	58	3.71	−26 (−44 to −1)	0.05
6B	66	4.31	57	3.64	−16 (−37 to +13)	0.28
9V	77.5	5.10	51	3.26	−36 (−52 to −13)	0.005
14	144	9.41	94	6.01	−36 (−48 to −20)	<0.001
18C	27	1.76	19	1.21	−31 (−58 to +12)	0.17
19F	34.5	2.25	34	2.17	−4 (−34 to +43)	0.95
23F	86	5.62	61	3.90	−31 (−47 to −9)	0.01
All vaccine-related serotypes¶	128.5	8.38	102	6.52	−22 (−38 to −4)	0.02
All nonvaccine serotypes	278	18.18	298	19.05	+5 (−8 to +20)	0.52

*The data are from the Active Bacterial Core Surveillance.

†The estimated rates were calculated on the assumption that the serotype distribution for cases with missing serotype data (12% of all cases) was the same as the distribution for cases with serotype data available.

‡CI denotes confidence interval.

§The P value was calculated by a chi-square test or Fisher's exact test that compared the estimated number of cases and noncases (the total surveillance population minus the number of estimated cases) in 2001 with the same figures for 1998 and 1999 combined. The estimated number of cases and totals were calculated on the assumption that the serotype distribution for cases with missing serotype data was the same as the distribution for cases with serotype data available. Repeated analysis with only cases with serotype data available. The estimated number of cases with known serotypes included rather than the estimated number of cases did not change the results.

¶Types 6A, 9A, 9L, 9N, 18A, 18B, 18F, 19A, 19B, 19C, 23A, and 23B are included.

ease, which was defined by isolation of *Streptococcus pneumoniae* from a normally sterile site. Serotyping and susceptibility testing of isolates were performed, and trends were assessed by evaluation of data from 7 geographic areas with continuous participation from 1998 through 2001 (population, 16 million).

Results.—A decline was noted in the rate of invasive disease, from an average of 24.3 cases per 100,000 persons in 1998 and 1999 to an average of 17.3 per 100,000 persons in 2001. The decrease in the rate of invasive disease was greatest in children less than 2 years old; in this age group, the rate of disease was 69% less in 2001 than the baseline rate. The rates of disease caused by vaccine and vaccine-related serotype decreased by 78% and 50%, respectively. Declines were also noted in disease rates for adults (Table 2). The rate of disease from penicillin-resistant strains was 35% less in 2001 than the rate in 1999.

Conclusions.—The use of the pneumococcal conjugate vaccine is preventing pneumococcal disease in young children and may also be reducing the rate of disease in adults.

Assessing Pneumococcal Revaccination Safety Among New York State Medicare Beneficiaries
Shih A, Quinley J, Lee T-K, et al (IPRO, Lake Success, NY; State Univ of New York, Stony Brook)
Public Health Rep 117:164-173, 2002   19–3

Background.—The safety of pneumococcal revaccination, especially at intervals of less than 5 years, has not been studied adequately. Revaccination safety was investigated by determining whether such revaccination is associated with a greater use of health care resources after revaccination than that after initial vaccination.

Methods.—The study included data from a cohort of 119,990 New York State Medicare beneficiaries, 65 years and older. All had received pneumococcal vaccinations between February 1, 1999, and December 17, 1999. Of the total cohort, 23,663 (20%) had had previous pneumococcal vaccination, including 13,466 (57%) for whom the revaccination interval was less than 5 years. The primary outcome measures were emergency department (ED) visits, hospitalizations, and office visits in the 2 weeks after vaccination.

Findings.—After adjustment for demographic and comorbidity factors, revaccination within 5 years of initial vaccination correlated with greater rates of ED visits in the 2 weeks after vaccination (odds ratio [OR], 1.17), and of office visits (OR, 1.13), compared with the same rates after initial vaccination. Several ICD-9-CM codes suggesting reactions to vaccination were documented more often for persons undergoing revaccination than for the comparison group.

Conclusions.—Medicare beneficiaries receiving pneumococcal revaccination less than 5 years after initial vaccination have higher rates of ED and office visits in the 2 weeks after vaccination than do beneficiaries after an initial vaccination. These data have important public health implications, which warrant further study.

▶ Although this study has limitations, including the facts that (1) it is an analysis of a Medicare data base; (2) not all claims of pneumococcal vaccination enter the Medicare data base; (3) such claims may be underrepresented and even miscoded from other vaccinations; such misclassification would have actually reduced the difference in outcomes. Nevertheless, the data underscore the fact that Medicare beneficiaries who receive pneumococcal vaccination at an interval of less than 5 years, have higher rates of ED and office visits within 14 days post vaccination than those whose immunization is the first. Even rates of subsequent hospitalization approach significance. The data support continued pneumococcal revaccination at intervals of longer than 5 years after initial vaccination, and they do not contradict this recommendation. However, revaccination must be carefully considered, documented, and the potential for some adverse event must be weighed against the risk of not revaccinating.

D. R. Snydman, MD

20 Parasitic Disease

Delayed Onset of Malaria—Implications for Chemoprophylaxis in Travelers
Schwartz E, Parise M, Kozarsky P, et al (Tel Aviv Univ, Israel; Ctrs for Disease Control and Prevention, Atlanta, Ga; Public Health Service, Atlanta, Ga; et al)
N Engl J Med 349:1510-1516, 2003   20-1

Background.—Most antimalarial agents for travelers act on the parasite's blood stage. Thus, they do not prevent late-onset disease, especially that from species causing relapsing malaria. The extent of this problem was investigated in Israeli and American travelers.

Methods and Findings.—Malaria surveillance data from Israel and the United States were analyzed. Between 1994 and 1999, 300 Israeli travelers returning home had malaria in which one species of plasmodium was identified. In 44.7% of these patients, illness developed more than 2 months after return. Almost all these cases were caused by infection with *Plasmodium vivax* or *P ovale*. Eighty-one percent of these patients had used an antimalarial regimen following national guidelines. Among American travelers, 2822 returned home with malaria in which the cause could be determined between 1992 and 1998. Thirty-five percent had late-onset illness. Infection was caused by *P vivax* in 811 travelers, *P ovale* in 66, *P falciparum* in 59, and *P malariae* in 51. Sixty-two percent of the travelers with late-onset disease had appropriately used an effective antimalarial agent.

Conclusions.—Illness developed more than 2 months after return in more than one third of these travelers contracting malaria. Commonly used, effective blood schizonticides do not prevent such late-onset disease. For better prevention of malaria in travelers, agents that act on the liver phase of malaria parasites are needed.

▶ Although malaria prophylaxis is quite effective, this study serves as a reminder that late-onset malaria following prophylaxis does occur, although rarely. The astute clinician should recognize this entity in the returned traveler, most of which is *P malariae* or *P vivax*. Currently, primaquine or atovaquone-proguanil are able to eliminate the liver stage; although for vivax, studies of the use for treatment or prophylaxis are lacking.

D. R. Snydman, MD

Tolerability of Malaria Chemoprophylaxis in Non-immune Travelers to Sub-Saharan Africa: Muliticentre, Randomised, Double Blind, Four Arm Study

Schlagenhauf P, Tschopp A, Johnson R, et al (Univ of Zurich, Switzerland)

BMJ 327:1078-1081, 2003   20–2

Background.—Approximately 50 million people annually travel to places where malaria is endemic, such as sub-Saharan Africa. Recommendations vary greatly regarding the best prophylactic treatment. The lack of consensus about the best regimen is primarily caused by disagreement about the tolerability of antimalarial agents in nonimmune, healthy travelers. The tolerability of malaria chemoprophylaxis regimens were compared in such travelers.

Methods.—Six hundred twenty-three nonimmune travelers to sub-Saharan Africa were included. One hundred fifty-three persons received doxycycline, mefloquine, or combined chloroquine and proguanil. Another 164 were given fixed combination atovaquone and proguanil. All patients underwent placebo run-in.

Findings.—A large percentage of patients reported adverse events, even during placebo run-in. None of these events was serious. The occurrence of mild to moderate adverse events was highest in the patients receiving chloroquine and proguanil, at 45%. This percentage was 42% in the mefloquine group, 33% in the doxycycline group, and 32% in the atovaquone and proguanil group. The highest percentage of more severe events occurred in the mefloquine group, at 12%, and in the combined chloroquine and proguanil group, at 11%. The combined atovaquone and proguanil group, as well as the doxycycline group, had the lowest proportion of more severe events, at 7% and 6%, respectively. The occurrence of moderate to severe neuropsychologic adverse events was greatest in the mefloquine group, especially in women, at 37%. Moderate to severe skin problems occurred in 12.8% of the chloroquine and proguanil group, 3% in the doxycycline group, in 2% of the atovaquone and proguanil group, and in 1% of the mefloquine group (Table 2).

Conclusions.—The combination of atovaquone and proguanil as well as doxycycline monotherapy are well-tolerated antimalarial treatments. Broader experience with these agents is needed to identify rare adverse effects.

▶ This is a very nicely done randomized trial that also used a placebo during a run-in period and also during a washout phase in 2 arms. The findings confirm that neuropsychologic events occurred in about 50% of women given mefloquine. The best-tolerated regimens were doxycycline or atovaquone and proguanil. Surprisingly, skin reactions were not that common in the doxycycline arm. However, some kind of mild adverse event was common in all groups when assessed as a whole, occurring in at least a third of all participants.

D. R. Snydman, MD

TABLE 2.—Proportion of Participants in Each Antimalarial Prophylaxis Arm Reporting Adverse Events, by Type and Severity

Type of Adverse Event	Mefloquine Group (n=153)	Chloroquine and Proguanil Group (n=153)	Doxycycline Group (n=153)	Atovaquone and Proguanil Group (n=164)	P Value
Neuropsychological*:					
Severe	8 (5, 2 to 9)	6 (4, 1 to 7)	1 (1, 0 to 2)	5 (3, 0 to 6)	0.139
Moderate	56 (37, 29 to 44)	46 (30, 23 to 37)	36 (24, 17 to 30)	32 (20, 13 to 26)	0.003
All events	118 (77, 70 to 84)	107 (70, 63 to 77)	105 (69, 61 to 76)	109 (67, 60 to 74)	0.187
Gastrointestinal†:					
Severe	6 (4, 1 to 7)	9 (6, 2 to 10)	3 (2, 0 to 4)	5 (3, 0 to 6)	0.312
Moderate	24 (16, 10 to 22)	31 (20, 14 to 27)	14 (9, 5 to 14)	26 (16, 10 to 22)	0.058
All events	89 (58, 50 to 66)	93 (61, 53 to 69)	81 (53, 45 to 61)	88 (54, 46 to 61)	0.451
Skin‡:					
Severe	1 (1, 0 to 2)	2 (1, 0 to 3)	3 (2, 0 to 4)	1 (1, 0 to 2)	0.635
Moderate	2 (1, 0 to 3)	12 (8, 4 to 12)	5 (3, 1 to 6)	4 (2, 0 to 5)	0.013
All events	36 (24, 17 to 30)	40 (26, 19 to 33)	36 (24, 17 to 30)	34 (21, 15 to 27)	0.730
Skin and vaginal§:					
Severe	2 (1, 0 to 3)	2 (1, 0 to 3)	4 (3, 0 to 5)	1 (1, 0 to 2)	0.509
Moderate	5 (3, 1 to 6)	13 (9, 4 to 13)	9 (6, 2 to 10)	4 (2, 0 to 5)	0.058
All events	45 (29, 22 to 37)	45 (29, 22 to 37)	42 (28, 20 to 35)	40 (24, 18 to 31)	0.717
Other:					
Severe	3 (2, 0 to 4)	5 (3, 0 to 6)	4 (3, 0 to 5)	2 (1, 0 to 3)	0.644
Moderate	12 (8, 4 to 12)	16 (11, 6 to 15)	12 (8, 4 to 12)	12 (7, 3 to 11)	0.748
All events	46 (30, 23 to 37)	47 (31, 23 to 38)	48 (31, 24 to 39)	36 (22, 16 to 28)	0.201

Values are numbers (percentages, 95% confidence intervals) unless otherwise stated
*Symptoms include headache, strange or vivid dreams, dizziness, anxiety, depression, sleeplessness, and visual disturbance.
†Nausea, diarrhea, mouth ulcers.
‡Itching, abnormal reddening of skin.
§Itching, abnormal discharge.
(Courtesy of Schlagenhauf P, Tschopp A, Johnson R, et al: Tolerability of malaria chemoprophylaxis in non-immune travelers to Sub-Saharan Africa: Multicentre, randomized, double blind, four arm study. BMJ 327:1078-1081, 2003. Copyright 2003 with permission from the BMJ Publishing Group.)

21 Miscellaneous

Effects of a Multivitamin and Mineral Supplement on Infection and Quality of Life: A Randomized, Double-blind, Placebo-controlled Trial

Barringer TA, Kirk JK, Santaniello AC, et al (Univ of North Carolina, Charlotte; Wake Forest Univ, Winston-Salem, NC)
Ann Intern Med 138:365-371, 2003   21–1

Background.—The use of multivitamins and mineral supplements is widespread in the United States. However, few well-designed studies on the benefits of these agents have been published. The effects of a daily multivitamin and mineral supplement on infection and well-being were investigated in a randomized, double-blind, placebo-controlled trial.

Methods.—One hundred thirty community-dwelling adults were enrolled in the study. The participants were stratified by age and diabetes status. Treatment consisted of a daily multivitamin and mineral supplement or placebo for 1 year. The physical and mental health subscales of the Medical Outcomes Study 12-Item Short Form were used to assess outcomes.

Findings.—More placebo recipients reported having an infectious illness during the study year than did recipients of multivitamin and mineral supplements: 73% and 43%, respectively. Fifty-seven percent of the placebo group reported infection-related absenteeism compared with 21% of the active treatment group. Among diabetic participants, 93% of those receiving placebo had an infection compared with 17% of those receiving supplements (Table 3). The 2 groups did not differ significantly in their Medical Outcomes Study 12-Item Short Form scores.

Conclusions.—In this series, the use of a multivitamin and mineral supplement decreased the incidence of participant reports of infection and related absenteeism. Patients with type 2 diabetes appeared especially to benefit from multivitamin and mineral supplements. Further research is needed.

▶ We recommend that patients take multivitamin and mineral supplements, but this is one of the few studies to demonstrate a benefit in the reduction of the incidence of infection and infection-related absenteeism. However, the benefit was solely seen in those individuals older than 65 years with type 2 diabetes. The explanation of the effects demonstrated remains somewhat speculative since the authors did not examine patients for vitamin deficiency. They also did not examine the impact of vitamin supplementation on the immune system. The authors did assess each individual's nutritional status with

TABLE 3.—Effect of a Multivitamin and Mineral Supplement on Infection Incidence and Infection-Related Absenteeism According to Diabetes Status and Age

Variable	Participants	Infection Incidence				Infection-Related Absenteeism*			
	n	Placebo Group	Treatment Group	Relative Risk (95% CI)	*P* Value	Placebo Group	Treatment Group	Relative Risk (95% CI)	*P* Value
		%	%			%	%		
Main effect									
Overall study group	130	73	43	0.59 (0.43-0.81)	<0.001	57	21	0.36 (0.21-0.62)	<0.001
Stratified analysis†									
Age					>0.2				>0.2
<65 y	97	78	43	0.55 (0.38-0.78)		58	21	0.37 (0.20-0.67)	
≥65 y	33	59	44	0.74 (0.38-1.47)		53	19	0.35 (0.12-1.08)	
Diabetes status					<0.001				0.002
No diabetes	79	60	59	0.98 (0.68-1.41)		35	33	0.95 (0.52-1.76)	
Type 2 diabetes mellitus	51	93	17	0.18 (0.07-0.44)		89	0	0	

*Absenteeism was used as the marker for severity of infection and was calculated as the percentage of participants who had any days during which planned activities could not be performed because of infection-related illness.

†χ² test for relative risk calculated within groups. A Mantel-Haenszel test of homogeneity was computed to test for differences according to age groups and diabetes status. Statistically significant differences were seen only between participants with and those without diabetes. Age group comparisons were not statistically significant.

(Courtesy of Barringer TA, Kirk JK, Santaniello AC, et al: Effects of a multivitamin and mineral supplement on infection and quality of life: A randomized, double-blind, placebo-controlled trial. *Ann Intern Med* 138:365-371, 2003.)

a 3-day food diary. They did find a trend toward a greater proportion of nutritional deficiency in the placebo arm.

D. R. Snydman, MD

High Rates of *Trichomonas vaginalis* Among Men Attending a Sexually Transmitted Diseases Clinic: Implications for Screening and Urethritis Management
Schwebke JR, Hook III EW (Univ of Alabama, Birmingham; Jefferson County Department of Health, Birmingham, Ala)
J Infect Dis 188:465-468, 2003   21–2

Background.—*Trichomonas* is known to cause nongonococcal urethritis (NGU). In the past, a lack of sensitive diagnostic techniques hindered the study of the prevalence of this infection in men. Current evidence shows that a polymerase chain reaction–based diagnostic test is significantly more sensitive than culture in diagnosing *T vaginalis* in men. This assay was used to determine the prevalence and clinical spectrum of trichomoniasis in men attending an urban sexually transmitted disease clinic.

Methods and Findings.—Three hundred men fulfilling study criteria were included in the case series study. DNA amplification enabled the assessment of infection. The prevalence of chlamydial and gonorrhea infections in these men was 19.6% and 17.7%, respectively. The prevalence of *T vaginalis* was 17%. Forty-two percent of the men were infected with at least 1 of these diseases. In this subgroup, 13.4% were coinfected with gonorrhea and chlamydia: 9.4% with gonorrhea and trichomonas, 11% with chlamydia and trichomonas, and 4.7% with all 3. Trichomonas was detected in 19.9% of men with NGU.

Conclusions.—These findings have implications for treating NGU as well as controlling trichomoniasis. Further research is needed on how *T vaginalis* relates to NGU in men.

► Earlier studies using culture techniques demonstrated that *T vaginalis* was found in 6% of men seeking care in a clinic for sexually transmitted diseases. There was also a strong association with a sexual partner with NGU or a sexually transmitted disease. This study, which used molecular techniques, showed that trichomoniasis is as common as chlamydia or *Neisseria gonorrhea*. This very important study underscores the need to consider this coinfection and perhaps to institute empiric therapy directed at *Trichomonas* for men who are symptomatic or have a sex partner with NGU.

D. R. Snydman, MD

Incidence of Serious Side Effects From First-Line Antituberculosis Drugs Among Patients Treated for Active Tuberculosis

Yee D, Valiquette C, Pelletier M, et al (McGill Univ, Montreal; Montreal Chest Inst)

Am J Respir Crit Care Med 167:1472-1477, 2003   21–3

Background.—The adverse reactions associated with antituberculosis agents can compromise treatment regimens for patients with tuberculosis (TB). The incidence of and risk factors for major side effects from first-line anti-TB drugs in a group of patients treated for active TB were determined. *Methods and Findings.*—The study included data from 430 patients treated between 1990 and 1999. The incidence of all major adverse effects was 1.48 per 100 person-months of exposure to pyrazinamide, 0.49 for isoniazid, 0.43 for rifampin, and 0.07 for ethambutol. The occurrence of any major adverse event correlated with being female, being older than 60 years, being born in Asia, and being HIV positive. Side effects associated with pyrazinamide correlated with being older than 60 years and being born in Asia. Adverse events associated with rifampin correlated with being older than 60 years and being HIV positive (Table 4). The incidence of hepatotoxicity and rash during pyrazinamide treatment for active TB was markedly more than with other first-line anti-TB agents and greater than previously believed.

TABLE 4.—Adjusted Hazard Ratios for Side Effects to Specific Drugs, in Association With Patient Characteristics

	INH		RIF		PZA	
Characteristics (Comparison)	HR*	95% CI	HR*	95% CI	HR*	95% CI
Female sex (versus male)	2.5	0.96 to 6.6	2.2	0.8 to 6.1	2.2	0.96 to 4.8
Age, yr						
35-59 (versus < 35)	3.4	**1.1 to 10.3**	2.3	0.6 to 8.7	1.1	0.4 to 3.0
60+ (versus < 35)	1.9	0.5 to 8.1	3.9	**1.02 to 14.9**	2.6	**1.01 to 6.6**
From Asia (versus all others)	2.1	0.8 to 5.6	2.8	0.9 to 8.4	3.4	**1.4 to 8.3**
Method of detection passive (versus active)	—†	—	—	—	1.5	0.5 to 4.1
Smear positive (versus smear negative)	1.2	0.5 to 3.3	0.8	0.2 to 2.5	1.5	0.7 to 3.5
Drug resistant (versus pansensitive)	3.4	**1.1 to 10.9**	1.4	0.3 to 6.6	1.9	0.7 to 5.3
Abnormal baseline LFTs (versus normal)‡	0.5	0.1 to 4.1	1.7	0.4 to 8.1	2.2	0.7 to 6.6
HIV-positive (versus -negative or NA)	2.4	0.3 to 19.5	8.0	**1.5 to 43**	2.1	0.3 to 17.1

Note: Boldface entries indicate statistically significant associations.
*Hazard ratio and 95% confidence interval estimated from Cox multivariate proportional hazards modeling.
†Insufficient numbers, so estimates unstable.
‡Before anti-TB therapy the liver transaminases were above the upper limit of normal.
Abbreviations: CI, Confidence interval; *HIV,* human immunodeficiency virus; *HR,* hazard ratio; *LFT,* liver function test; NA, not available.
(Courtesy of Yee D, Valiquette C, Pelletier M, et al: Incidence of serious side effects from first-line antituberculosis drugs among patients treated for active tuberculosis. *Am J Respir Crit Care Med* 167:1472-1477, 2003. Official Journal of the American Thoracic Society. Copyright 2003, American Lung Association.)

Conclusions.—Serious adverse reactions to anti-TB agents are common. Female, older, HIV-infected, and Asian-born patients are at increased risk for such adverse effects. Better-tolerated treatments for TB are needed.

▶ Adverse reactions to rifampin and ethambutol have been well described; however, the assessment of side effects and risk factors with the addition of pyrazinamide have not been well analyzed when this drug is added to tuberculosis treatment regimens.

This study, although single center, has enough power to alert clinicians about the rate of side effects and risk factors associated with such side effects. Pyrazinamide-associated events were the most common, and are more than 3-fold more common than any of the other agents.

D. R. Snydman, MD

Myopericarditis Following Smallpox Vaccination Among Vaccinia-Naive US Military Personnel

Halsell JS, and the Department of Defense Smallpox Vaccination Clinical Evaluation Team (Univ of Virginia, Charlottesville; et al)
JAMA 289:3283-3289, 2003
21–4

Background.—The estimated incidence of myocarditis in the US population is 1 to 10 per 1,000,000 annually. One percent to 5% of patients with acute viral infections have myocardial involvement. Myopericarditis is a rare event after vaccination with the currently used strain of vaccinia virus. Cases of probable myopericarditis after smallpox vaccination among US military personnel are discussed.

Methods.—Cases were identified through sentinel reporting to US military headquarters surveillance or to the Vaccine Adverse Event Reporting System. Affected persons had been vaccinated between December 2002, and March 2003. The primary outcome measures were increased serum levels of creatinine kinase, troponin I, and troponin T, usually associated with ST-segment elevation on electrocardiogram and wall motion abnormalities on echocardiogram.

Findings.—Eighteen cases of probable myopericarditis after smallpox vaccination were reported among 230,734 primary vaccines, an incidence of 7.8 per 100,000 during 30 days. None of the 95,622 persons previously vaccinated were affected by myopericarditis after vaccination. All persons affected were white men, 21 to 33 years old, who manifested acute myopericarditis 7 to 19 days after vaccination. The rate of myopericarditis among primary vaccines was 3.6-fold greater than that expected among nonvaccinated personnel.

Conclusions.—Myopericarditis occurred in 1 per 12,819 US military personnel vaccinated primarily against smallpox. Thus, this adverse event should be expected after smallpox vaccination. The diagnosis of myopericarditis should be considered in patients reporting chest pain 4 to 30 days after smallpox vaccination. Clinicians must also report this adverse event.

▶ The close temporal relationship with vaccination, the occurrence only in vaccinees who were at risk for primary infection, and the absence of other etiologies, suggest a causal relationship with smallpox vaccine. Although the implications for older individuals, or those with preexisting cardiac diseases are unclear, the occurrence of such cases has essentially eliminated the smallpox vaccine programs among civilians. Fortunately, all the cases recovered clinically from their illness. But long-term consequences must be evaluated further.

The finding of a rare and unexpected side effect with mass vaccination in the context of a potential new public health threat has historical similarity to the Guillain-Barré syndrome that occurred among swine flu vaccine recipients in 1976. When this occurred, it was also very rare. It is still poorly understood and has not occurred subsequently; however, it halted a major public health initiative.

D. R. Snydman, MD

Diagnosis and Management of Adults With Pharyngitis: A Cost-Effectiveness Analysis
Neuner JM, Hamel MB, Phillips RS, et al (Med College of Wisconsin, Milwaukee; Beth Israel Deaconess Med Ctr, Boston)
Ann Intern Med 139:113-122, 2003   21–5

Background.—An estimated 18 million US patients sought care for a sore throat in 1996, and 4 to 6 times as many with sore throat did not seek care. The chief organisms causing sore throat are group A β-hemolytic streptococcus (GAS), nongroup A streptococcus, *Mycoplasma pneumoniae, Chlamydia pneumoniae*, and various respiratory viruses. No compelling data support the treatment of pharyngitis not caused by GAS, a condition that occurs in about 10% of adults who see a physician; however 75% of these patients seeking care are given antibiotics. GAS is sensitive to penicillin, yet broad-spectrum antibiotics are most often prescribed. When no definitive randomized clinical trials provide direction concerning the choice of strategies for treatment, cost-effectiveness and decision analyses incorporating medical costs can be used to assess management approaches. To evaluate 5 common approaches to testing and treating suspected GAS pharyngitis, a cost-utility analysis was used.

Methods.—The 5 strategies analyzed were (1) observation without testing or treatment; (2) empirical treatment with penicillin; (3) throat culture with a two-plate selective culture technique; (4) optical immunoassay (OIA), followed by culture to confirm negative OIA test results; and (5) OIA only. Measurements included the cost per lost quality-adjusted life-days, which were converted to life-years when appropriate, and the incremental cost-effectiveness. Base-case and sensitivity analyses were performed.

TABLE 2.—Cost-effectiveness of Baseline Pharyngitis Management Strategies*

Strategy	Average Cost, $†	Average Effectiveness, *lost quality-adjusted life-days*	Incremental Cost-Effectiveness
Culture	6.66	0.2668	—
Observation	9.84	0.2752	Dominated
OIA alone	11.73	0.2717	Dominated
Empirical therapy	12.74	0.4083	Dominated
OIA culture	15.15	0.2716	Dominated

*"Dominated" indicates that the strategy is less effective and more costly. For explanation of strategies, see the Methods section.
†In 2000 US dollars.
Abbreviation: OIA, Optical immunoassay.
(Courtesy of Neuner JM, Hamel MB, Phillips RS, et al: Diagnosis and management of adults with pharyngitis: A cost-effectiveness analysis. *Ann Intern Med* 139:113-122, 2003.)

Results.—In the base-case analysis the culture strategy was dominant, with the OIA-culture, OIA alone, and observation strategies producing similar results, but with the empirical therapy considerably less effective (Table 2). The cost of OIA-culture was twice as much per patient as the least expensive strategy. In the sensitivity analyses, when GAS pharyngitis had a prevalence of more than 20%, the OIA-culture strategy was the most effective, while a prevalence of less than 6% made observation the least costly option. For prevalences between 6% and 20%, culture was both more effective and less expensive than the other methods. Empirical treatment was the least expensive when the prevalence exceeded 71%. The OIA-culture strategy was most effective with a probability of analysis approximately half of the baseline probability, but observation was the most effective at a probability 1.6 times that of baseline. OIA alone was only less expensive than culture when the OIA cost was less than half of baseline.

Conclusions.—Observation, culture, and the 2 strategies involving rapid antigen tests proved to be reasonable and cost-effective for diagnosing and treating adults with suspected GAS pharyngitis. Empirical therapy was reasonable only when the probabilities approached 70%, which would only be the case in an epidemic of streptococcal infection or when streptococcal pharyngitis is being spread between family members or patients.

▶ Pharyngitis is among the most common complaints and reasons for patients to seek medical care, yet strategies to diagnose and treat group A, β-hemolytic streptococcal pharyngitis in adults are still debated and analyzed. Expert panels have traditionally recommended culture as the gold standard, although recent recommendations have included the use of rapid office-based tests, which have improved in sensitivity and specificity. In this clinical decision analysis, culture is still marginally the most cost-effective strategy, assuming a baseline likelihood of group A streptococcus prevalence of about 9.7%. Empirical therapy is the least cost-effective. Interestingly, all strategies but empiric treatment have similar clinical utilities and cost effectiveness results. This is not surprising since one can make a clinical argument for any of the strategies. In a sense, these results mirror the confusion as to how best manage such patients. The dilemmas are the fact that culture, the traditional gold standard, cannot be provided as a point-of-care test, and may be falsely positive due to the presence of the carriage of streptococci in the throat. The data from this study do not provide support for the current American College of Physicians guidelines for the management of pharyngitis in the adult and underscore the lack of compelling data in choosing one strategy over another. The major take-home message from this study is that empirical treatment of pharyngitis with penicillin is not warranted in the absence of an outbreak.

D. R. Snydman, MD

Community-Acquired Febrile Urinary Tract Infection in Diabetics Could Deserve a Different Management: A Case-control Study
Horcajada JP, Moreno I, Velasco M, et al (Hosp Clinic Universitari-IDIBAPS, Barcelona, Spain)
J Intern Med 254:280-286, 2003   21–6

Background.—Patients with diabetes tend to have a higher incidence of urinary tract infections (UTIs) and to suffer severe complications, including emphysematous pyelonephritis and the formation of abscesses. Differences in clinical presentation may also be present. Whether relevant differences are seen in the clinical course, microbiological spectrum, and outcome characteristics of community-acquired UTI with fever in patients with diabetes compared with the same factors in those patients without diabetes was investigated.

Methods.—The study included 108 patients, half of whom had either type 1 or type 2 diabetes, were matched for age (mean, 67.9 years) and sex. All had been admitted to a university-affiliated hospital with febrile UTI. Analyzed were the clinical, analytical, microbiological, and outcome variables of the 2 groups by means of the McNemar test or the Wilcoxon matched pairs signed rank test.

Results.—The group with diabetes had a significantly more frequent occurrence of urinary incontinence than the control group and were more likely to have fever without focal symptoms (27% vs 9%) and a diminished consciousness level (25% vs 10%). Shock was present on admission in 1 patient with diabetes and in 2 patients without diabetes. All nondiabetic patients and 45 of the 54 patients with diabetes had *Escherichia coli* grow in urine cultures, with *Klebsiella pneumoniae, Citrobacter* spp., *Proteus mirabilis, Staphylococcus aureus,* and *Streptococcus agalactiae* seen in other patients (Table 2). Quinolone-resistant bacteria were found in 17% of patients with diabetes and in only 3.7% of those without diabetes. Bacteremia was found in 32 diabetic patients and in 23 nondiabetic patients (59% vs 43%, respectively). Patients with diabetes continued to have fever for 1.75 days, whereas nondiabetic patients had fever for 1.5 days. But the length of hospitalization for patients with diabetes was 5.2 days, and that for nondiabetic patients was 3.9 days.

TABLE 2.—Analytical, Microbiological, and Outcome Data in the Studied Population

	Diabetes ($n = 54$)	Nondiabetes ($n = 54$)	P Values*
Serum creatinine (mg dL^{-1}), mean (SD)	1 (0.32)	1.1 (0.43)	0.83
Leucocyte count ($\times 10^9$ L^{-1}), mean (SD)	13365 (5385)	14412 (7139)	0.75
Blood immature forms (%), mean (SD)	8.8 (4.9)	8.4 (7.5)	0.79
C-reactive protein (mg dL^{-1}), mean (SD)	14 (10.5)	15 (8.7)	0.55
Erythrocyte sedimentation rate (mm h^{-1}), mean (SD)	78 (33.4)	66 (27.9)	0.05
Non-*E. coli* in the urine culture*, *n* (%)	9 (17)	0 (0)	0.004
Quinolone resistant uropathogens, *n* (%)	9 (17)	2 (3.7)	0.07
Bacteraemia, *n* (%)	32 (59)	23 (43)	0.09
Duration of fever after antibiotic was started (days), mean (SD)	1.75 (1)	1.5 (1.1)	0.17
Duration of low urinary tract symptoms after antibiotic was started (days), mean (SD)	1.2 (1.6)	1.4 (1.1)	0.54
Duration of lumbar tenderness, mean (SD)	1.1 (1.3)	1.2 (1.1)	0.94
Hospital stay (days), mean (SD)	5.2 (3.3)	3.9 (2.6)	0.006
Bacteriological recurrence 1 month later, *n* (%)†	15 (41)	9 (21)	0.22
Clinical recurrence 1 month later, *n* (%)†	5 (14)	4 (9)	0.21

Klebsiella pneumoniae (n = 3), *Citrobacter* spp. (n = 2), *Proteus mirabilis* (n = 2), *Staphylococcus aureus* (n = 1), and *Streptococcus agalactiae* (n = 1).
†Calculated over 33 pairs.
(Courtesy of Horcajada JP, Moreno I, Velasco M, et al: Community-acquired febrile urinary tract infection in diabetics could deserve a different management: A case-control study. *J Intern Med* 254:280-286, 2003. Reprinted by permission of Blackwell Publishing.)

Conclusions.—Diabetic patients with fever but no localizing symptoms should be suspected of having a UTI. In addition, the empirical antibiotic therapy for diabetic patients with febrile UTI should differ from that of those without diabetes because of the frequent involvement of non-*E coli* uropathogens and the trend toward more quinolone-resistant organisms, particularly when quinolone-resistant *E coli* strains are widely found in the community. Thus, diabetic patients with febrile UTI have both clinical and microbiological findings that differ from nondiabetic patients and require adjustment in determining the diagnosis and choosing therapy.

▶ UTIs are often quite complex in diabetic patients. An analysis of hospitalized patients confirmed what was suspected: urinary tract infections in diabetic patients tend to be associated with some subtleties, namely, a decreased likelihood of focal symptoms, and a greater likelihood of being infected with an organism other than *E coli*. Moreover, they are more likely to be infected with organisms resistant to the quinolones. The implications are that when confronted with fever in the diabetic patient, the urinary tract should be considered a potential focus even in the absence of symptoms that might be suggestive of a UTI. In addition, diabetic patients are more likely to have bacteremia. They are also more likely to have bacteriologic relapse or clinical recurrence, although the power to detect a difference for these 2 variables in this study was insufficient. One problem with this study was that it did not prospectively follow treatment. For some patients, it might be argued that the

2-week course of therapy was not sufficient for someone with a complex UTI; therefore, the differences in outcome in relation to therapy were not assessed, and all patients were hospitalized, selecting presumably the more severely ill diabetic patients as well as the control subjects who had a UTI.

D. R. Snydman, MD

PART THREE

HEMATOLOGY AND ONCOLOGY
PATRICK J. LOEHRER, SR, MD

22 Cancer Prevention

Incidence of Cancer and Mortality Following α-Tocopherol and β-Carotene Supplementation: A Postintervention Follow-up
Virtamo J, for the ATBC Study Group (Natl Public Health Inst, Helsinki; et al)
JAMA 290:476-485, 2003   22–1

Objective.—Epidemiologic data have linked low intake of antioxidants to an increased cancer risk. Results of the Alpha-Tocopherol, Beta-Carotene Cancer Prevention (ATBC) Study found a significant reduction in the incidence of prostate cancer among subjects receiving α-tocopherol supplementation but a significant increase in lung cancer and total mortality among those receiving β-carotene. Additional follow-up was performed to clarify the effects of these antioxidants on cancer risk and mortality rate.

Methods.—The postintervention follow-up study included 25,563 Finnish men who participated in the ATBC study. Cancer incidence and cause-specific death were analyzed on the basis of 6-year follow-up data and total mortality rate on the basis of 8-year follow-up data. In the study, more than 29,000 male smokers aged 50 to 69 years were randomly assigned to receive α-tocopherol, β-carotene, both antioxidants, or placebo for 5 to 8 years. Outcomes were assessed by using national cancer and death registry data, with confirmation of all cases of cancer.

Results.—The increase in lung cancer incidence among men receiving β-carotene was nonsignificant on posttrial follow-up: relative risk was 1.06 (95% confidence interval, 0.94 to 1.20). There was also no significant reduction in prostate cancer incidence among men receiving β-carotene: relative risk was 0.88 (95% confidence interval, 0.76 to 1.03). There were no late preventive effects on other types of cancers and no difference in relative mortality risk. The excess risk observed for patients assigned to β-carotene resolved within 4 to 6 years and was mainly attributed to cardiovascular diseases.

Conclusions.—Both the positive and negative effects of antioxidant supplementation reported in the ATBC Study disappear with longer follow-up. Neither α-tocopherol nor β-carotene is effective in preventing cancer. The results still suggest that β-carotene supplementation may be harmful to smokers—total mortality rate is 8% higher among men assigned to β-carotene versus placebo.

▶ This is a follow-up from an important prevention trial. With time the results have been muted a bit, but smokers should still avoid β-carotene. We need to be vigilant in advising our patients regarding potential risks of supplemental treatments. Data like this help.

P. J. Loehrer, Sr, MD

High Prognostic Value of _p16_^{INK4} Alterations in Gastrointestinal Stromal Tumors

Schneider-Stock R, Boltze C, Lasota J, et al (Otto-von-Guericke Univ, Magdeburg, Germany; Armed Forces Inst of Pathology, Washington, DC)

J Clin Oncol 21:1688-1697, 2003   22–2

Background.—Gastrointestinal stromal tumors (GISTs) are a distinctive but histologically heterogeneous group of neoplasms and are the most common mesenchymal tumors of the gastrointestinal tract. The malignant potential of these tumors is often uncertain. Immunohistochemically, GISTs are defined as KIT (CD117, stem cell factor receptor)-positive tumors. A cyclin-dependent kinase 4 inhibitor (_p16_^{INK4}) gene located at 9p21 has been shown to be inactivated in a variety of tumors by homozygous deletions, point mutations, or de novo methylation of its promoter region. The prognostic relevance of _p16_^{INK4} alterations in GISTs was determined by investigation of a larger group of GISTs and correlation of the genetic findings with clinicopathologic factors and patient survival.

Methods.—A total of 43 GISTs in 39 patients were evaluated for methylation status of the promoter by methylation-specific polymerase chain reaction (PCR), the presence of mutations by PCR-SSCP-sequencing, the loss of heterozygosity at the _p16_^{INK4} locus, and the immunohistochemical expression of _p16_^{INK4} protein.

Results.—Alterations of _p16_^{INK4} were identified in 25 of 43 GISTs (58.1%), with no differences in the type and frequency of alterations among benign, borderline, or malignant GISTs. _p16_^{INK4} alterations were correlated with a loss of _p16_^{INK4} protein expression. Patients with tumors with _p16_^{INK4} alterations had a poorer prognosis compared with patients with tumors that had no _p16_^{INK4} alterations. In terms of clinical outcome, a high predictive value for _p16_^{INK4} alterations was found only in patients with benign and borderline GISTs. Univariate Cox proportional hazard regression analysis showed a strong correlation between _p16_^{INK4} alterations, tumor size, mitotic index, and overall survival rate. However, multivariate analysis showed that only _p16_^{INK4} alterations were an independent prognostic factor.

Conclusions.—The evaluation of _p16_^{INK4} alteration status in patients with gastrointestinal stromal tumors is a helpful prognostic tool, particularly in patients with benign and borderline tumors.

▶ There is more to know about GISTs than the presence of _c-kit_ mutations. Patients in this series with _p16_^{INK4} alterations have strikingly different outcomes. This provides critical prognostic information and serves as further focus of research in this modern model of treatable malignancies.

P. J. Loehrer, Sr, MD

A Controlled Trial of a Human Papillomavirus Type 16 Vaccine

Koutsky LA, for the Proof of Principle Study Investigators (Univ of Washington, Seattle; et al)
N Engl J Med 347:1645-1651, 2002   22–3

Background.—Approximately 20% of adults acquire human papillomavirus type 16 (HPV-16) infections, most of which are benign. In some patients, however, infection progresses to anogenital cancer. Therefore, a vaccine that decreases the incidence of HPV-16 infection may have an important impact on public health.

Methods.—A total of 2392 women (aged 16-23 years) were included in a randomized double-blind study. The women were assigned to 3 doses of placebo or HPV-16 viruslike-particle vaccine, 40 µg, at baseline and at months 2 and 6. Genital samples were obtained periodically. The median follow-up period was 17.4 months after completing the vaccination regimen.

Findings.—The incidence of persistent HPV-16 infection per 100 person years at risk was 3.8 in the placebo group and 0 in the vaccinated group. All 9 women with HPV-16–related cervical intraepithelial neoplasia had been given placebo.

Conclusions.—This HPV-16 vaccine decreases the incidence of HPV-16 infection and HPV-16–related cervical intraepithelial neoplasia. Immunizing HPV-16–negative women may ultimately decrease the incidence of cervical cancer.

▶ This double-blind placebo-controlled study by Koutsky et al evaluated the efficacy of a vaccine against HPV-16 in preventing persistent HPV-16 infection in women between the ages of 16 and 23 years. The data suggest a significant reduction in the rate of persistent infection and raise the possibility of future reduction in the incidence of cervical carcinoma by the use of an HPV vaccine. This may represent an exciting breakthrough in the control of cervical carcinoma.

J. T. Thigpen, MD

2001 Consensus Guidelines for the Management of Women With Cervical Intraepithelial Neoplasia

Wright TC Jr, for the 2001 ASCCP-Sponsored Consensus Workshop (Columbia Univ, New York; et al)
Am J Obstet Gynecol 189:295-304, 2003   22–4

Background.—Evidence-based guidelines for the management of cervical intraepithelial neoplasia (CIN) developed with the support of the American Society for Colposcopy and Cervical Pathology are presented.

Participants.—The guidelines were developed by an independent panel of 121 experts in professional organizations, federal agencies, national and international health organizations, and other groups. Guidelines were drafted by working groups based on formal literature reviews and an Internet-based bulletin board. The final version was approved by consensus in September 2001.

Management of CIN Grade 1.—Patients with biopsy-confirmed CIN-1 and a satisfactory colposcopic examination can be monitored without treatment or treated with ablation or excision. Under the first option, patients should undergo repeat cervical cytologic testing at 6 and 12 months or human papillomavirus (HPV) testing at 12 months. Colposcopy should be repeated if cytologic results reveal atypical squamous cells or greater risk or if high-risk types of HPV DNA are present. Annual cytologic screening can resume when cytologic findings are negative twice in a row or the 12-month HPV DNA test is negative. Alternatively, patients can be monitored with a combination of repeat cytologic testing and colposcopy at 12 months. Women with regression during follow-up should undergo repeat cytologic testing at 12 months. Acceptable treatment options include cryotherapy, laser ablation, and a loop electrosurgical excision procedure. Before ablation of CIN-1, endocervical sampling should be performed. If CIN-1 recurs after ablative therapy, excision should be performed. For patients whose colposcopic examination is unsatisfactory, a diagnostic excisional procedure is recommended. Follow-up alone may suffice for these patients, however, if they are pregnant, immunosuppressed, or adolescents.

Management of CIN Grades 2 and 3.—For patients with CIN-2 or CIN-3 and a satisfactory colposcopic examination, excision and ablation are both acceptable. Excision is preferred, however, for patients with recurrent CIN-2 or CIN-3. If the colposcopy examination is unsatisfactory, a diagnostic excisional procedure should be performed. Hysterectomy cannot be recommended as primary therapy for CIN-2 or CIN-3. After treatment, patients should be monitored with cytologic testing (with or without colposcopy) every 4 to 6 months until at least 3 cytologic results are negative, with annual cytologic testing thereafter. As with CIN-1, if cytologic testing reveals atypical squamous cells or greater risk, the patient should be referred for colposcopy. Alternatively, these patients may be monitored with HPV DNA testing at least 6 months after treatment. In this setting, annual cytologic exam is sufficient when HPV DNA test results are negative; however, colposcopy is recommended if high-risk types of HPV DNA are found. A single positive HPV test is not sufficient for performing a hysterectomy or repeat conization.

When CIN is identified at the margins of a diagnostic excisional procedure or in a postprocedure endocervical sample, endocervical sampling and colposcopy should be repeated 4 to 6 months later. A repeat diagnostic excisional procedure is acceptable in this setting, and hysterectomy can be performed if repeat diagnostic excision is not feasible or if CIN-2 or CIN-3 recurs or persists. Adolescents with CIN-2 whose colposcopic examinations are satisfactory and whose endocervical samples are negative should undergo colposcopy and cytologic testing every 4 to 6 months for 1 year. Adolescents with CIN-3 should undergo ablation or excision.

▶ This article summarizes the results of a consensus conference looking at the management of cervical intraepithelial neoplasia and provides guidelines for the management of these patients. It should be a useful guide for those involved in the management of preinvasive disease of the cervix.

J. T. Thigpen, MD

Systematic Review of the Effectiveness of Stage Based Interventions to Promote Smoking Cessation
Riemsma RP, Pattenden J, Bridle C, et al (Univ of York, England; Univ of the West of England, Bristol; Univ of Aberdeen, Scotland)
BMJ 326:1175-1177, 2003   22–5

Background.—In 1997, more than 11 million adults in the United Kingdom were regular smokers. In the ensuing 5 years, the proportion of smokers in the population has stabilized or may even be increasing; more recent data indicate that about 25% of 15-year-olds are regular smokers. The risk of disease is reduced after smoking cessation, and several cessation methods are used: pharmacologic methods (nicotine replacement therapy or antidepressants), hypnotherapy, and exercise-based interventions. Behavioral approaches include stage-based interventions, which propose that interventions that account for the current stage of the individual will be more effective and efficient than "one size fits all" interventions. These stage-based models are widely used, yet there is limited evidence of the effectiveness of this approach. The effectiveness of stage-based interventions in effecting positive change in smoking behavior was evaluated.

Methods.—This systematic review used 35 electronic databases, catalogs, and Internet resources. Bibliographies of references were scanned for relevant publications, and authors were contacted where necessary.

Results.—A total of 23 randomized controlled trials were reviewed, including 2 that reported details of an economic evaluation. Eight trials reported effects supportive of stage-based interventions, 3 trials reported mixed results, and 12 trials found no statistically significant difference between a stage-based intervention and a non–stage-based intervention or no intervention. A stage-based intervention was compared with a non–stage-based intervention in 11 trials, and 1 trial reported statistically significant effects for the stage-based intervention. Two studies reported mixed effects, and 8 reported no statistically significant differences between groups. The methodologic quality of the trials was inconsistent, and few of the studies reported any validation of the instrument used to assess participants' stage of change.

Conclusions.—The overall findings of this systematic review indicate that there is limited evidence in support of the effectiveness of stage-based interventions in altering smoking behavior.

▶ A popular method for smoking cessation in the United Kingdom is "stage-based intervention," in which individuals are separated into 5 stages (precontemplation, contemplation, preparation, action, and maintenance). Progression through the stages is sequential, and interventions are stage-specific.

Stage of change needs to be reassessed frequently, as individuals can relapse to an earlier stage or progress to a later one, and interventions adapt in response to the individual's movement through the stages of change.

Despite the fact that this model is commonly practiced and taught in the United Kingdom, there has been relatively little evidence that this approach is effective. Unfortunately, this systematic review did not find any evidence to support this model system over non–stage-based or no interventions in changing smoking behavior. The authors do admit that the methodologic quality of the reviewed trials was mixed, and only 2 of the 23 trials used a previously validated instrument. This review illustrates the need for more rigorous intervention studies that address the effectiveness of different cessation strategies.

J. H. Schiller, MD

Continued Cigarette Smoking by Patients Receiving Concurrent Chemoradiotherapy for Limited-Stage Small-Cell Lung Cancer Is Associated With Decreased Survival

Videtic GMM, Stitt LW, Dar AR, et al (Harvard Med School, Boston; London Regional Cancer Centre; Kingston Regional Cancer Centre, Ont, Canada; et al)
J Clin Oncol 21:1544-1549, 2003   22–6

Background.—For patients with some types of cancers (eg, stage III/IV head and neck, renal, bladder, and glottic cancers), continuing to smoke during radiotherapy is associated with decreased survival compared with patients who stop smoking during treatment. Whether continuing smoking during concurrent chemotherapy and radiotherapy affects survival in patients with limited-stage small cell lung cancer (SCLC) was retrospectively examined.

Methods.—The participants were 186 patients (112 men and 74 women, most aged ≥60 years) with limited-stage SCLC who underwent chemotherapy (6 cycles of cyclophosphamide, doxorubicin, and vincristine alternating every 3 weeks with etoposide and cisplatin) and radiotherapy (during etoposide and cisplatin therapy). All patients were smokers at the start of the study. Survival was compared between the 79 patents (42.5%) who continued smoking during treatment and the 107 patients (57.5%) who stopped smoking during treatment. The incidence of toxicity (defined as a break during radiotherapy because of hematologic or locoregional toxicity, or both) was also compared between the 2 groups.

Results.—The median follow-up period for the 186 patients was 14.8 months. During radiotherapy, 38 patients (20.5%) experienced toxicity and required a break in treatment (median, 5 days). With respect to causes of death, 71 of 75 deaths (94.9%) in patients who continued smoking during treatment were cancer related, compared with 81 of 96 deaths (84.4%) in patients who quit smoking during treatment. The 5-year actuarial survival was significantly better in patients who had stopped smoking during treatment than in patients who continued smoking during treatment (8.9% vs 4%, respectively). The incidence of toxicity did not differ significantly between the

2 groups (42.5% in those who continued smoking vs 57.5% in those who quit). Survival was best in patients who quit smoking and had no treatment breaks (median, 23 months), and worse in patients who continued smoking and who developed toxicity during treatment (median, 13.4 months).

Conclusion.—Patients with limited-stage SCLC who continue to smoke during concurrent chemotherapy and radiotherapy have poorer survival rates than patients who stop smoking during treatment. Smoking status did not affect the incidence of treatment interruptions caused by toxicity. Physicians should urge their patients with limited-stage SCLC who smoke to stop smoking during chemotherapy and radiotherapy.

▶ Continued smoking has been associated with poorer outcome in patients with a variety of cancers, although results in SCLC have been conflicting. In this study, Videtic and coworkers retrospectively review 186 smokers with limited-stage SCLC treated over 10 years with concurrent chemo-radiotherapy, and conclude that patients who continue to smoke have a poorer survival than patients who quit during treatment. The reasons for this are unclear, but do not appear to be caused by an increase in breaks in radiotherapy because of toxicities or comorbid conditions, such as respiratory or cardiovascular events, in the patients who continue to smoke.

Limitations of the study include the fact that the investigators did not quantitate the amount of cigarette use at the beginning of the study, verify smoking status during treatment, determine how many patients who quit smoking resumed after treatment, or how long they quit. Nevertheless, these findings raise some interesting questions, particularly given the magnitude of the differences in survival observed (a doubling of 5-year survival, from 4% to 8.9%). The magnitude of this difference (a doubling of long-term survival) is better than that observed in most "positive" clinical therapeutic trials. Is the negative impact on survival from smoking caused by an increased resistance to radiotherapy from hypoxia, or would it be observed in patients treated with chemotherapy as well? Is this observation generalizable to non–small cell lung cancer? And if true, should we be stratifying patients with limited SCLC based on smoking status?

J. H. Schiller, MD

23 Thoracic Cancers

Lung Cancer Rates Convergence in Young Men and Women in the United States: Analysis by Birth Cohort and Histologic Type
Jemal A, Travis WD, Tarone RE, et al (American Cancer Society, Atlanta, Ga; Armed Forces Inst of Pathology, Washington, DC; Natl Cancer Inst, Bethesda, Md)
Int J Cancer 105:101-107, 2003   23–1

Background.—Largely because of differences in patterns of cigarette smoking between men and women, age-specific lung cancer rates have been consistently greater for U.S. men than women. In recent birth cohorts, however, these sex differences have decreased. Recent studies suggest that women may be more susceptible to the carcinogenic effects of smoke than men. Population-based incidence and mortality data were analyzed to determine trends in age-specific lung cancer rates by birth cohort according to sex, ethnic group, and histologic findings.

Methods and Findings.—Rates of death from lung cancer were found to converge between men and women born after 1960, especially among whites. Among whites, the male-to-female mortality ratio among 35- to 39-year-olds declined from 3.0 for the 1915 birth cohort to 1.1 in the 1960 birth cohort. Among blacks, it declined from 4.0 in the 1925 birth cohort to 1.5 in the 1960 birth cohort. Incidence rates for white women and men converged rapidly for adenocarcinoma, small cell carcinoma, and large cell carcinoma. Less convergence was seen for squamous cell carcinoma. Cigarette smoking among white men and women aged 24 years was comparable in cohorts born after 1960. However, smoking in these cohorts continued to be greater among black men than among black women.

Conclusions.—Lung cancer death rates have converged among men and women born after 1960. These data suggest that men and women are equally susceptible to lung cancer from a given amount of cigarette smoking.

▶ A number of studies published in the 1990s suggested that women are more susceptible to the carcinogenic effects of tobacco smoke, even when corrected for amount of nicotine exposure. The authors postulate that if so, lung cancer mortality should be the same between the 2 sexes, particularly since smoking prevalence was about equal in white men and women born after 1960. Using data from the SEER database, they examined trends in age-specific rates of lung cancer by birth cohort. Although there were slight differences in terms of histology (squamous cell carcinoma) and race (black men vs black women), they found that the lung death rate was about equal between young white men and women born after 1960, suggesting that men and women are equally susceptible to the development of lung cancer from a given amount of cigarette smoking.

J. H. Schiller, MD

Staging of Non–Small-Cell Lung Cancer With Integrated Positron-Emission Tomography and Computed Tomography

Lardinois D, Weder W, Hany TF, et al (Univ Hosp of Zurich, Switzerland; Univ of Zurich, Switzerland)
N Engl J Med 348:2500-2507, 2003   23–2

Background.—Integrated positron emission CT (PET-CT) scanners have been introduced recently. The accuracy of integrated PET-CT was compared with that of other imaging modalities in staging non–small cell lung cancer (NSCLC).

Methods.—Fifty patients with proved or suspected NSCLC underwent integrated PET-CT scanning. In addition, CT alone, PET alone, and visually correlated PET and CT were done. Tumor-node-metastasis staging was assigned on the basis of image analysis.

Findings.—In 41% of the patients, integrated PET-CT provided additional information beyond that available with visual correlation of PET and CT. The diagnostic accuracy of integrated PET-CT was greater than that of the other modalities. In addition, tumor staging was significantly more accurate with integrated PET-CT than with CT alone, PET alone, or visual PET-CT correlation. Node staging was also significantly more accurate with integrated PET-CT than with PET alone. In 2 of 8 patients undergoing staging of metastasis, integrated PET-CT increased diagnostic certainty.

Conclusions.—When integrated PET-CT becomes more widely available, it will be the preferred modality for determining disease stage in patients with NSCLC. If further research verifies the current findings, integrated PET-CT may become the new standard for imaging lung cancer.

▶ Accurate staging is the key to appropriate management of lung cancer. Radiologic exams such as CT or PET yield both false-positive and false-negative results. As a result, many clinicians use both to improve diagnostic accuracy. However, whereas CT provides good anatomic detail, it is neither very specific nor sensitive; PET, on the other hand, although more specific and sensitive, is not precise on the exact location of possible abnormalities. Even when PET and CT are visually correlated, the precise location of lesions is sometimes difficult to determine. This study compared the diagnostic accuracy of CT alone, PET alone, and visual correlation of PET and CT with the information obtained with the new PET-CT scanners.

Integrated PET-CT was significantly more accurate in tumor staging than visual PET alone, CT alone, or visual correlation of PET-CT. Integrated PET-CT was also more accurate than visual correlation of PET and CT in staging the mediastinum. PET was more accurate than CT in detecting metastases; integrated PET-CT detected their location in 2 patients where visual correlation could not.

It should be noted, however, that PET or integrated PET-CT is unable to pick up micrometastases; 3 such lesions were missed in this study. Thus, a negative scan does not mean there is no need for mediastinal staging by mediastinoscopy. In addition, false-positives continue to occur, particularly in the mediastinum. One patient classified as having a positive N3 node was found to have inflammatory changes, and 2 patients classified as having N1 disease had hilar extension of the tumor.

Thus, does PET-CT obviate the need for surgical staging of the mediastinum? Apparently not. It does, however, allow for more accurate anatomic location of possible lesions. In addition, PET appears to have a major role in detecting unsuspected extrathoracic metastases (16% in this study). PET detected the location of these in 6 of 8 patients and PET-CT in all 8.

J. H. Schiller, MD

Observation-Only Management of Early Stage, Medically Inoperable Lung Cancer: Poor Outcome
McGarry RC, Song G, des Bosiers P, et al (Indiana Univ, Indianapolis)
Chest 121:1155-1158, 2002   23–3

Background.—The risk of developing a bronchogenic carcinoma is estimated at 1 in 12 for men and at 1 in 18 for women; lung cancer is the most frequent cause of cancer death among individuals in North America. Records of patient with early stage non–small cell lung carcinoma were retrospectively drawn from the Richard L. Roudebush VA Medical Center tumor registry between 1994 and 1999. The treatments that each received and the outcomes were assessed.

Methods.—A total of 128 male patients were identified, ranging in age from 54 to 85 years (average age, 70.8 years). Therapeutic interventions were noted, and the results of management were reviewed. The probability of survival from the time of diagnosis was calculated.

Results.—Forty-nine patients received no treatment, 36 received radiotherapy only, and 43 patients had primary surgery. The presence of chronic obstructive pulmonary disease was the most common medical reason for not treating a patient. For those not receiving treatment, the mean size of the lung mass was 3.1 cm at diagnosis, and pulmonary function as determined by forced expiratory volume in 1 second (FEV_1) was 0.42 to 2.4 L. The median survival time was 14.2 months, and patients with stage I and stage IIA disease had essentially the same survival times. Fifty-three percent of patients died of lung cancer; 30% died of other causes. Four patients were alive at final follow-up. Those receiving radiotherapy alone had a mean lung mass size at diagnosis of 4.0 cm and a mean FEV_1 of 1.7 L on referral. Twenty different fractional schemes were used, and no significant differences in survival rates were produced by radiotherapy of curative versus palliative intent. Forty-three percent of these patients died of their cancer, and 5% died of other causes; 8 patients were still alive at last follow-up. Of the 43 patients having curative resection with lobectomy, the average size of the resected tumors was 3.04 cm, and the patients' mean FEV_1 was 2.09 L. The median survival time was 46.2 months.

Conclusions.—A significant number of patients who had no therapy died of their cancer. Those receiving radiotherapy had better survival rates, but the best results were achieved when curative resection with lobectomy was used.

▶ This is an interesting article on stage I and II non–small cell lung cancer that focuses largely on the results of observation only in patients with medically inoperable disease. Some patients who had surgery and some who had radiotherapy were also included. The patients who received surgery had their disease pathologically staged (ie, the authors only included those patients who had node-negative disease). How many patients had unsuspected mediastinal nodal disease is not given because their disease was no longer thought to be stage I or II. The patients who had no treatment and the patients who received radiotherapy had their disease clinically staged only, and no striking difference was found in their median survival times. At the same time, many of the patients who received radiotherapy received only palliative doses to relieve symptoms, so no real attempt was made to treat the disease aggressively. Sometimes, these symptoms can be caused by bronchial obstruction, in which case modest local treatment may improve the exchange of air and a patient's performance status. On the other hand, such focused intervention is not likely to have an impact on the long-term outcome.

I think this article is interesting largely in light of the standpoint of those who have argued in recent years that early stage lung cancer may include a subset of patients with a very favorable outcome. I assume that they are extrapolating from patients who have prostate cancer. I do not think I have ever seen lung cancer with a favorable outcome in terms of its natural history. To ignore intervention for a patient with lung cancer at an early stage is counterintuitive in my mind.

E. Glatstein, MD

Phase II Study of Pemetrexed With and Without Folic Acid and Vitamin B₁₂ as Front-Line Therapy in Malignant Pleural Mesothelioma

Scagliotti GV, Shin D-M, Kindler HL, et al (Univ of Turin, Torino, Italy; Univ of Pittsburgh, Pa; Univ of Chicago; et al)
J Clin Oncol 21:1556-1561, 2003   23–4

Background.—Malignant pleural mesothelioma (MPM) usually presents at an advanced stage and has no accepted therapy. Patients usually receive only supportive care. Pemetrexed is a newer antifolate with broad antitumor acivity. The efficacy of pemetrexed as a treatment for patients with advanced MPM was examined in a multicenter phase II study.

Study Design.—The study group consisted of 64 treatment-naive patients with advanced MPM. Participants received 500 mg/m^2 of pemetrexed IV every 3 weeks. After December 10, 1999, the protocol was changed so that study participants received folic acid and vitamin B$_{12}$ supplementation during their therapy to improve safety. The primary outcome was tumor response. Secondary outcomes included response duration, survival, time to disease progression, time to treatment failure, quality of life, and pulmonary function.

Findings.—A partial response to pemetrexed therapy was observed in 14% of patients. The Kaplan-Meier estimate of median overall survival was 10.7 months. The median overall survival was 13 months for patients who received vitamin supplementation and 8 months for patients without supplementation. Patients who received vitamin supplementation completed more cycles of chemotherapy. Grade 3/4 neutropenia occurred in 23.4% of patients, and grade 3/4 leukopenia occurred in 18.8%. The incidence of toxicity was also lower in supplemented patients.

Conclusions.—Pemetrexed treatment of patients with advanced MPM resulted in a moderate response rate and a median overall survival of 10.7 months. Survival was increased and toxicity reduced in those patients who received folic acid and vitamin B$_{12}$ supplementation. Patients with MPM may be able to benefit from pemetrexed therapy. A recently completed phase III study should help to answer this question.

▶ Treatment options for mesothelioma have been limited. For those with localized disease, surgery remains the treatment of choice. Chemotherapy has been largely ineffective with only anecdotal responses reported. Pemetrexed is a new multitargeted antifolate that has at least 3 enzymatic targets, including thymidylate synthase, dihydrofolate reductase, and glycinamide ribonucleotide formyl transferase. Not only did this trial confirm a modest response rate with pemetrexed, but it also demonstrated that supplementation with folate acid and vitamin B$_{12}$ improved the toxicity with an apparent improvement of survival.

P. J. Loehrer, Sr, MD

Malignant Thymoma in the United States: Demographic Patterns in Incidence and Associations With Subsequent Malignancies
Engels EA, Pfeiffer RM (Natl Cancer Inst, Rockville, Md)
Int J Cancer 105:546-551, 2003   23–5

Background.—The cause of thymoma has not been established. To date, there have been no population-based studies of demographic patterns of thymoma incidence. Previous research has associated thymoma with diverse subsequent malignancies, but these relations remain uncertain. The incidence of malignant thymoma in the United States between 1973 and 1998 was determined.

Methods.—Data were obtained from the Surveillance, Epidemiology and End Results data to determine malignant thymoma incidence by sex, age, and race. These data were also analyzed to compare malignancies after a thymoma diagnosis with those expected in the general population.

Findings.—Overall, the incidence of malignant thymoma was 0.15 per 100,000 person-years. A total of 849 cases were identified. The incidence of thymoma increased by decade of life until the eighth decade, then declined. The incidence was greater in men than women. It was highest in Asians and Pacific Islanders, who had an incidence of 0.49 per 100,000 person-years. Sixty-six malignancies were documented after the diagnosis of thymoma. An excess risk was observed for non-Hodgkin's lymphoma, with a standardized incidence ratio (SIR) of 4.7. An excess was also noted for digestive system cancers, with an SIR of 1.8, and soft tissue sarcomas, with an SIR of 11.1. No other cancers occurred with increased frequency.

Conclusions.—Malignant thymoma is rare. The incidence of this disease appears to peak in late adulthood. The documented variation in incidence by race suggests that genetic factors play a role. There appears to be no broadly increased risk for malignancies after thymoma.

▶ Thymoma is one of the most rare malignancies. Despite this, the association with a variety of paraneoplastic syndromes, including myasthenia gravis, pure red cell aplasia, hypohemoglobinemia, and other autoimmune diseases, makes this a unique tumor. This is an excellent article that highlights one of the other observations associated with thymoma—the association of secondary malignancies. Highest in incidence are non-Hodgkin lymphoma, soft tissue sarcomas, and gastrointestinal cancers. This article only addresses malignancies after the diagnosis of thymoma. As this is an indolent tumor, many cases of malignancies antedate the diagnosis of thymic malignancies. The epidemiologic background of thymoma is well discussed in this article.

P. J. Loehrer, Sr, MD

24 Breast Cancer

High Prevalence of Premalignant Lesions in Prophylactically Removed Breasts From Women at Hereditary Risk for Breast Cancer
Hoogerbrugge N, Bult P, de Widt-Levert LM, et al (Univ Med Ctr Nijmegen, The Netherlands)
J Clin Oncol 21:41-45, 2003   24–1

Background.—Many women with a hereditary predisposition for breast cancer consider prophylactic mastectomy to avoid the extremely high risk of invasive breast carcinoma that is associated with this hereditary predisposition. However, the utility of mastectomy for breast cancer prevention is a matter of debate. Whether women at high hereditary risk for breast cancer have high-risk histopathologic lesions was determined, as well as the variables related to, and predictive for, the presence of such high-risk lesions.

Methods.—This prospective study examined breast specimens from 67 women at extremely high genetic risk of breast cancer, with or without previous breast cancer, who had undergone prophylactic mastectomy. Two thirds of these women were carriers of a *BRCA1* or *BRCA2* mutation. Breast specimens were studied by radiographic and macroscopic examination of 5-mm tissue slices. Histologic analysis involved suspicious lesions and random samples from each quadrant of the breast and the nipple area.

Findings.—One or more different types of high-risk histopathologic lesions were present in 57% of the women. One woman had a 4-mm invasive ductal carcinoma with ductal carcinoma in situ. None of these lesions had been detected by palpation or mammography. The presence of high-risk lesions was independently related to age older than 40 years (odds ratio, 6.6; $P = .01$) and to bilateral oophorectomy before prophylactic mastectomy (odds ratio, 0.2; $P = .02$).

Conclusions.—Many women at high risk of hereditary breast cancer have high-risk histopathologic lesions develop, particularly after age 40 years. These high-risk histopathologic lesions are not detected by surveillance.

▶ The ductal epithelium of the breast undergoes a series of changes from simple hyperplasia to hyperplasia with atypia to in situ carcinoma that are associated with increasing levels of risk for the development of invasive breast cancer. This study of prophylactic mastectomy specimens in women with genetic risk for the development of breast cancer indicates that a high proportion (57%) of high-risk women have histologic risk lesions that are clinically silent.

The likelihood of these lesions increases with increasing age, suggesting a time-dependent element in their development. In addition, the frequency of risk lesions was decreased in women who had undergone oophorectomy, an intervention known to decrease risk in gene mutation carriers. These findings suggest that the identification of high-risk lesions through epithelial sampling techniques such as random fine-needle aspiration or ductal lavage could further stratify risk in women with a genetic predisposition to breast cancer and might influence the timing of chemoprevention or prophylactic surgery. Since this study was limited to women at a high genetic risk for breast cancer development, its application to women at risk on the basis of other factors is uncertain, but worthy of study.

M. Morrow, MD

Twenty-Year Follow-up of a Randomized Trial Comparing Total Mastectomy, Lumpectomy, and Lumpectomy Plus Irradiation for the Treatment of Invasive Breast Cancer
Fisher B, Anderson S, Bryant J, et al (Natl Surgical Adjuvant Breast and Bowel Project, Pittsburgh, Pa; Univ of Pittsburgh, Pa)
N Engl J Med 347:1233-1241, 2002   24–2

Background.—Previous results from the National Surgical Adjuvant Breast and Bowel Project (NSABP) B-06 trial of breast-conserving surgery for women with stage I or II breast cancer have suggested similar survival outcomes for women undergoing total mastectomy, lumpectomy with postoperative breast irradiation, or lumpectomy alone. However, the risk of recurrence in the operated breast was lower in women undergoing lumpectomy plus irradiation than in those undergoing lumpectomy alone. The 20-year results of the B-06 trial were reported.

Methods.—Between 1976 and 1984, a total of 2163 women with stage I or II breast cancer and tumor diameters of 4 cm or less were randomly assigned to undergo total mastectomy, lumpectomy alone, or lumpectomy with postoperative breast irradiation. At follow-up in 2002, complete data including lymph node status were available on 1851 patients. Survival and tumor recurrence rates were compared among the 3 groups.

Results.—The tumor recurrence rate in the ipsilateral breast was 39.2% in the lumpectomy-only group versus 14.3% in the lumpectomy plus irradiation group. All survival outcomes continued to be similar among the 3 groups, including disease-free survival, distant-disease–free survival, and overall survival. Compared with the mastectomy group, hazard ratios for death were nonsignificant in both lumpectomy groups. On analysis of women undergoing lumpectomy who had tumor-free resection margins, the risk of death was not significantly different between those who did and those who did not undergo irradiation. Women receiving radiation had a marginally significant reduction in the risk of death from breast cancer, with some increase in death from other causes.

Conclusions.—The 20-year follow-up data continue to show similar survival rates for women with early stage breast cancer treated with mastectomy or with lumpectomy. For women undergoing lumpectomy, postoperative irradiation is associated with a significant reduction in the risk of tumor recurrence in the ipsilateral breast. As long as the resection margins are tumor free, and the cosmetic results are satisfactory, lumpectomy plus irradiation is an appropriate choice of treatment for breast cancer. The findings underscore the need for long-term follow-up after breast cancer treatment, since many events occur after 5 years.

▶ The results of the National Surgical Adjuvant Breast and Bowel Project (NSABP) B-06 trial comparing total mastectomy with lumpectomy alone or lumpectomy with breast irradiation have been published before. This 20-year follow-up is important because of the long natural history of breast cancer. No survival benefit for mastectomy is seen. In addition, there is no evidence of an increase in the risk of contralateral breast cancer in the women who received radiotherapy. The incidence of local recurrence after lumpectomy and irradiation is surprisingly low; 14.3% at 20 years, in spite of the fact that women were entered into NSABP B-06 between 1976 and 1984. During this period, the extent of mammographic evaluation before surgery was limited compared with the diagnostic workups done today, and US and MR were not routinely used. The low rate of local recurrence in patients selected by mammography alone should serve as a cautionary note for those who advocate the routine use of other imaging modalities to identify multicentric cancer, which is then considered an indication for mastectomy. Clearly, much of this subclinical disease is controlled by radiotherapy. In contrast, the incidence of local failure without breast irradiation was 39.2%, suggesting that improved imaging techniques might allow identification of a subset of women who require radiation only to the quadrant of the breast in which the primary tumor is located. Finally, this study emphasizes the importance of lifelong surveillance of the breast cancer patient. Eleven percent of all recurrences, including 9% of local recurrences, 7% of regional recurrences, and 13% of distant recurrences, were detected more than 10 years after diagnosis. In addition, 32% of contralateral breast cancer occurred more than 10 years after diagnosis. This study clearly demonstrates that breast conservation with radiotherapy is a safe and effective treatment that allows the majority of women to preserve their breasts, even with long-term follow-up.

M. Morrow, MD

25 Ovarian Cancer

Phase III Randomized Trial of 12 Versus 3 Months of Maintenance Paclitaxel in Patients With Advanced Ovarian Cancer After Complete Response to Platinum and Paclitaxel-based Chemotherapy: A Southwest Oncology Group and Gynecologic Oncology Group Trial
Markman M, Liu PY, Wilczynski S, et al (Cleveland Clinic Found, Ohio; Ohio State Univ, Columbus; Southwest Oncology Group Statistical Ctr, Seattle; et al)
J Clin Oncol 21:2460-2465, 2003   25–1

Background.—Standard initial treatment for ovarian cancer generally includes 5 to 6 courses of a platinum/taxane regimen. Limited randomized study data show no advantage of additional treatment or a consolidation strategy in ovarian cancer or other malignant tumors. However, findings of nonrandomized studies suggest that more protracted treatment with paclitaxel may benefit patients with ovarian cancer. An effort was made to determine whether continuing paclitaxel for an extended period prolongs progression-free survival (PFS) and improves survival in women with advanced ovarian cancer who had obtained a clinically defined complete response to a platinum/paclitaxel–based chemotherapy.

Methods and Findings.—By random assignment, 277 patients received 3 or 12 cycles of single-agent paclitaxel every 28 days. Fifty-four PFS events occurred in 222 patients during follow-up. The regimens did not differ significantly in toxicity except for peripheral neuropathy. The median PFS was 21 months in the 3-cycle group and 28 months in the 12-cycle group. The Cox model–adjusted 3-cycle progression hazard ratio compared with the 12-cycle progression was 2.31. These findings resulted in trial discontinuation. As of the date of study termination, overall survival did not differ between groups.

Conclusions.—A 12-cycle course of single-agent paclitaxel significantly prolongs PFS in women with advanced ovarian cancer who attain a clinically defined complete response to initial platinum/paclitaxel–based chemotherapy.

▶ With few exceptions, maintenance therapy has not proved to be useful in malignant disease. In general, patients "win or lose" in the early phases of treatment. This was a relatively straightforward article in which patients who achieved a remission with 5 or 6 cycles of a platinum/paclitaxel regimen were randomly assigned to 3 additional cycles or 12 additional cycles of paclitaxel and cisplatin. The discussion in the article by Dr Markham and the accompanying editorial by Tate Thigpen clearly delineates the problems with this study. The study was terminated early by a Data Monitoring Safety Committee when the relapse-free survival was found to be highly significant statistically. Overall survival may show a difference but has not yet done so. The article does not produce a paradigmship for the treatment of ovarian cancer, but it should lead to points of discussion between physicians and those patients who achieve a complete remission after induction chemotherapy with cisplatin and paclitaxel. With longer follow-up, this may indeed become the standard of care.

P. J. Loehrer, Sr, MD

Phase III Trial of Carboplatin and Paclitaxel Compared With Cisplatin and Paclitaxel in Patients With Optimally Resected Stage III Ovarian Cancer: A Gynecologic Oncology Group Study
Ozols RF, Bundy BN, Greer BE, et al (Fox Chase Cancer Ctr, Philadelphia; Roswell Park Cancer Inst, Buffalo, NY; New York Presbyterian Hosp-Cornell Med Ctr; et al)
J Clin Oncol 21:3194-3200, 2003   25–2

Background.—In the United States, standard therapy for advanced epithelial ovarian cancer is cisplatin plus paclitaxel, on the basis of trials performed by the Gynecologic Oncology Group (GOG). Carboplatin is an analogue of cisplatin with less hematologic toxicity. GOG 158 was designed as a noninferiority study comparing the efficacy and toxicity of carboplatin plus paclitaxel with cisplatin plus paclitaxel for treatment of small-volume stage III ovarian cancer.

Study Design.—The study group consisted of 792 women with stage III epithelial ovarian cancer, no prior therapy, and no residual disease greater than 1.0 cm in diameter after surgery. These women were randomly assigned to receive either cisplatin and paclitaxel or carboplatin and paclitaxel. These 2 groups were similar in terms of prognostic factors. Analysis was by intention to treat. Outcomes included overall survival (OS), progression-free survival (PFS), and adverse effects.

Findings.—Gastrointestinal, renal, and metabolic toxicity and grade 4 leukopenia were significantly more common among patients treated with cisplatin plus paclitaxel. Grade II or more thrombocytopenia was significantly more common among patients treated with carboplatin plus paclitaxel. Neurologic toxicity was similar for both treatments. The median PFS was 19.4 months and OS was 48.7 months for those in the cisplatin arm and 20.7 and 57.4 months, respectively, for those in the carboplatin arm.

Conclusions.—For patients with advanced ovarian cancer, chemotherapy with carboplatin plus paclitaxel was less toxic, easier to administer, and not inferior to chemotherapy with cisplatin plus paclitaxel. Because more than 70% of patients will have recurrence with a median progression time of less than 2 years, more effective therapies are still needed. GOG is currently participating in an international, randomized clinical trial of new 3-drug and sequential combinations. For the present, carboplatin and paclitaxel continue to be the standard therapy for ovarian cancer.

A Randomized Clinical Trial of Cisplatin/Paclitaxel Versus Carboplatin/ Paclitaxel as First-Line Treatment of Ovarian Cancer

du Bois A, et al for the Arbeitsgemeinschaft Gynäkologische Onkologie (AGO) Ovarian Cancer Study Group (Dr-Horst-Schmidt-Kliniken, Wiesbaden, Germany; et al)
J Natl Cancer Inst 95:1320-1330, 2003   25–3

Purpose.—OVAR-3, a randomized, phase III, noninferiority trial, was designed to compare the safety and efficacy of cisplatin-paclitaxel (PT) to carboplatin-paclitaxel (TC) in patients with advanced ovarian cancer.

Study Design.—The study group consisted of 798 adult women with FIGO stage IIB to IV ovarian cancer who had undergone radical debulking surgery within the previous 6 weeks. Patients were randomly assigned to receive TC or PT. The primary end point was the proportion of patients without disease progression at 2 years. Secondary end points included toxicity, quality of life (QOL), overall survival (OS), progression-free survival (PFS), and treatment response. Survival curves were calculated with the Kaplan-Meier method and hazard ratios were estimated by the Cox proportional hazards model.

Findings.—In the patients without disease progression, the median PFS and median OS were not significantly different between the 2 treatment groups. TC therapy was associated with greater hematologic toxicity but lower gastrointestinal and neurologic toxicity than PT therapy. The mean global QOL scores were significantly better for the TC patients.

Conclusions.—Therapy with TC was as effective as therapy with PT but was better tolerated and associated with better QOL. The use of carboplatin instead of cisplatin may be better for the patient and should be considered a first-line treatment option for patients with advanced ovarian cancer and for use in clinical trials.

▶ The current standard chemotherapy regimen for advanced ovarian carcinoma, paclitaxel plus a platinum compound, is based on 2 independent studies (GOG Protocol 111 and a European-Canadian study OV-10) that compared cyclophosphamide/cisplatin to PT and found the PT regimen to be superior in terms of response rate, clinical complete response rate, PFS, and OS. By far the more common regimen used in the United States, however, is TC on the basis of prior studies suggesting that carboplatin had similar activity to that of cisplatin but a more favorable therapeutic index. This is an assumption, however, that is potentially incorrect since it does not account for the fact that paclitaxel and carboplatin clearly interact with each other. This interaction results in a marked decrease in the amount of myelosuppression observed with the combination compared with single-agent carboplatin. Since the mechanism of this bone marrow protection is not clear, it could not be stated with confidence that the interaction did not also protect the tumor.

These concerns led to 2 large trials comparing TC to PT to determine whether the 2 regimens were equivalent. DuBois et al (Abstract 25–3) evaluated the 2 regimens in patients with stages IIB to IV disease and used an area under the curve of 6 for carboplatin. This trial showed no significant difference in efficacy but small trends favoring the cisplatin regimen. Ozols et al (Abstract 25–2) studied the regimens in patients with small-volume residual stage III disease and used an area under the curve of 7.5 for carboplatin. This trial also produced no significant difference in efficacy, but there were strong trends favoring the carboplatin regimen.

Taken together, the 2 trials suggest that the 2 regimens are equivalent (at almost 800 eligible patients, each study had, in round figures, a 90% probability of detecting a 30% difference in survival). The trends, however, raise some interesting concerns about the dose of carboplatin. If in fact the interaction between carboplatin and paclitaxel does affect antitumor effect, the 2 studies suggest that the higher dose of carboplatin used in the GOG trial is needed to overcome that interaction and optimize therapeutic results. While this issue is important since the increased carboplatin dose causes more neuropathy, no trials are underway to evaluate this. Such studies seem unlikely to evolve in light of the large number of promising new agents available for testing.

For now, it would seem prudent for the physician to initiate chemotherapy for advanced ovarian carcinoma at the higher carboplatin dose of area under the curve of 7.5 and to reduce the dose in subsequent courses as required by toxicity.

J. T. Thigpen, MD

26 Gastrointestinal Cancer

A Randomized Trial of Aspirin to Prevent Colorectal Adenomas
Baron JA, Cole BF, Sandler RS, et al (Dartmouth-Hitchcock Med Ctr, Lebanon, NH; Dartmouth Med School, Hanover, NH; Univ of North Carolina, Chapel Hill; et al)
N Engl J Med 348:891-899, 2003   26-1

Introduction.—Epidemiologic studies, experimental studies in animals, and randomized trials in patients at risk for the development of colorectal adenomas provide evidence of the anticarcinogenic effects of nonsteroidal anti-inflammatory drugs (NSAIDs). A group of patients with a recent history of colorectal adenomas participated in a randomized, double-blind trial to determine the anti-neoplastic effect of aspirin in the large bowel.

Methods.—The study group included 1121 patients, 372 assigned to placebo, 377 to 81 mg of aspirin, and 372 to 325 mg of aspirin daily. All patients underwent a complete colonoscopy within 3 months of recruitment and had no known remaining colorectal polyps. Excluded were individuals with a history of familial colorectal cancer syndrome, invasive large-bowel cancer, or malabsorption syndromes. At follow-up, patients were advised to avoid aspirin and other NSAIDs; acetaminophen was distributed for treatment of minor pain and fever. A complete surveillance colonoscopy was performed 34 to 40 months after the qualifying examination.

Results.—Follow-up data were available for 1084 randomly assigned patients (96.7%). Reports of compliance were excellent and similar in the aspirin and placebo groups. A majority of patients avoided nonprotocol use of aspirin and other NSAIDs. Six hundred seventy patients had a total of 1812 polyps. At least 1 colorectal adenoma was diagnosed in 47.1% of patients in the placebo group, 38.3% of patients in the 81-mg aspirin group, and 45.1% in the 325-mg aspirin group. Colorectal cancer was diagnosed in 1, 2, and 3 patients, respectively, in these 3 treatment groups. The risks of death and serious bleeding were similar among groups. For advanced neoplasms, the relative risks (as compared with the placebo group) were 0.59 in the 81-mg aspirin group and 0.83 in the 325-mg group.

Conclusion.—Aspirin, taken daily at a low dose (81 mg), had a moderate effect in reducing the risk of recurrent adenoma among patients with a recent history of adenoma. The risk reduction was greater for advanced lesions than for all lesions combined, suggesting that the effects of aspirin may be more important in later stages of the adenoma-carcinoma sequence.

▶ Aspirin remains one of the most effective drugs in use today for a variety of disease entities. This is a large prospective randomized trial that documents the use of low doses of aspirin as a chemopreventive agent. Would all patients benefit from aspirin? Clearly, no, but perhaps with better molecular markers, we may be able to target those that might.

P. J. Loehrer, Sr, MD

▶ In addition to prevention of colorectal carcinoma (CRC) through screening modalities, optimally with colonoscopy, is the use of chemopreventive agents. The most frequently utilized chemopreventive agent is aspirin. Its mechanism of action is presumed to be inhibition of cyclo-oxygenase-2, which is found in CRC. Most CRC develops from adenomatous polyps; therefore, in the interest of being able to complete a study, most end points are polyps (size- and number-related). Initially, sulindac—and recently celecoxib—have reduced the number and size of polyps in patients with familial adenomatous polyposis.

Baron et al reported a randomized, double-blind, placebo-controlled trial on the efficacy of aspirin to prevent the development of colorectal adenomas. They utilized 2 dosages, comparing daily intake of 81 mg and 325 mg of aspirin with placebo. Their primary end point was the detection of polyps in a group of more than 1000 patients who, within 3 months of the initiation of the study, had undergone colonoscopy with removal of their polyps. They found that after approximately 3 years of treatment, there was a moderately reduced risk of recurrent adenomas with ASA. The reduction in the risk of advanced lesions (those with villous features, size greater than 1 cm, and/or dysplasia or cancer) was greater, with a 40% reduction in the group ingesting 81 mg ASA. Interestingly, but unexplained, is that the 325-mg dose did not significantly reduce the rate of recurrence.

J. S. Barkin, MD

Results of Repeat Sigmoidoscopy 3 Years After a Negative Examination
Schoen RE, for the Prostate, Lung, Colorectal, and Ovarian Cancer Screening Trial Group (Univ of Pittsburgh, Pa; et al)
JAMA 290:41-48, 2003   26–2

Background.—Several trials using tandem colonoscopy or colonoscopy by 1 practitioner followed immediately by a second colonoscopy by a second practitioner have demonstrated that adenomas, particularly small adenomas, are easily missed. The extent of adenomas and cancer in the distal colon as detected by repeat flexible sigmoidoscopy (FSG) 3 years after a negative examination was reviewed in the Prostate, Lung, Colorectal, and Ovarian Cancer Screening Trial (PLCO), a randomized, controlled, community-based investigation assessing the effectiveness of cancer screening tests on site-specific mortality rates.

Methods.—The mean patient age was 65.7 years at trial entry (1993-1995); 61.6% were men. Participants underwent screening FSG at baseline and at 3 years as part of the protocol and were referred to their personal physicians for further assessment of screen-identified abnormalities. Results from subsequent diagnostic examinations were tracked using a standardized method. Of 11,583 participants who were eligible for repeat screening FSG 3 years after an initial negative examination, 9317 (80.4%) returned for follow-up. The primary outcome measures were a polyp or mass identified in the distal colon at year 3 repeat FSG; the incidence of adenoma or cancer in the distal colon at year 3 follow-up; determination of reason for detection (increased depth of insertion or improved preparation at the 3-year examination, or detection in a previously inspected area).

Results.—A total of 1292 returning participants (13.9%) had a polyp or mass that was identified by FSG 3 years after the initial examination. In the distal colon, of 9317 participants, 292 (3.1%) had an adenoma or cancer. The incidence of advanced adenoma (n = 72) or cancer (n = 6) identified at the year 3 examination was 78 (0.8%) of 9317. Among participants with advanced distal adenomas identified at the 3-year examination, 58 of 72 (80.6%) had lesions identified in a portion of the colon that had been sufficiently examined at the initial sigmoidoscopy.

Conclusion.—Repeat FSG 3 years after a negative examination will identify advanced adenomas and distal colon cancers at a rate of 0.8%. The overall percentage with identifiable abnormalities is modest, but these data raise concerns about the impact of a prolonged screening interval after a negative FSG examination.

▶ The Prostate, Lung, Colorectal, and Ovarian Cancer Screening Trial is a prospective, randomized, community-based study that evaluates several screening tests on specific cancer mortality. This article reports the effectiveness of FSG examined 3 years after a prior negative examination. Approximately 1 in 7 such patients had a polyp or mass detected on repeat examination. Were these polyps missed on the initial examination, or did they develop in the interim? By the authors' evaluation, most were thought to be new neoplasms. The proper interval for undergoing an FSG remains unclear, but many recommendations currently are at the 5-year interval. Should colonoscopy be used in place of FSG? It is estimated from this and other articles that about 1% to 2% of new malignancies occur in the proximal colon and are not reached by FSG.[1,2] A colleague described the use of a FSG as similar to obtaining a screening mammogram in one breast only. Perhaps virtual colonoscopy will supplant conventional colonoscopy, but ultimately it should be recognized that endoscopy is both a screening and therapeutic modality. Optimal uses of these modalities are important on a cost-effective basis for this to be useful.

P. J. Loehrer, Sr, MD

References

1. Lieberman DA, Weiss DG, Bond JH, et al: Use of colonoscopy to screen asymptomatic adults for colorectal cancer: Veterans Affairs Cooperative Study Group 380. *N Engl J Med* 343:162-168, 2000.
2. Imperiale TF, Wagner DR, Lin CY, et al: Risk of advanced proximal neoplasms in asymptomatic adults according to the distal colorectal findings. *N Engl J Med* 343:169-174, 2000.

Tumor Microsatellite-Instability Status as a Predictor of Benefit From Fluorouracil-Based Adjuvant Chemotherapy for Colon Cancer
Ribic CM, Sargent DJ, Moore MJ, et al (Univ of Toronto; Mayo Found, Rochester, Minn; Queen's Univ, Kingston, Ontario, Canada; et al)
N Engl J Med 349:247-257, 2003   26–3

Background.—Colon cancers with high-frequency microsatellite instability manifest clinical and pathologic features that can be used to differentiate them from microsatellite-stable tumors. The usefulness of microsatellite-instability status as a predictor of the benefits of adjuvant chemotherapy with fluorouracil in patients with stage II and stage III colon cancer was evaluated.

Methods.—Specimens were obtained from 570 patients with colon cancer who were enrolled in randomized trials of fluorouracil-based adjuvant chemotherapy. Mononucleotide and dinucleotide markers were used to assess microsatellite instability.

Results.—Of the 570 specimens evaluated, 95 (16.7%) showed high-frequency microsatellite instability. Among 287 patients who did not receive adjuvant therapy, patients with tumors that demonstrated high-frequency microsatellite instability had a better 5-year rate of overall survival than patients with tumors that exhibited microsatellite stability or low-frequency instability. Among the remaining patients who received adjuvant chemotherapy, no correlation was found between high-frequency microsatellite instability and increased overall survival. Benefits of treatment were significantly different according to the microsatellite-instability status. On multivariate analysis adjusted for stage and grade, overall survival was improved by adjuvant chemotherapy in patients with microsatellite-stable tumors or tumors that demonstrated low-frequency microsatellite instability. However, there was no benefit of adjuvant chemotherapy among patients with high-frequency microsatellite instability.

Conclusions.—Fluorouracil-based adjuvant chemotherapy provided benefits to patients with stage II or stage III colon cancer with microsatellite-stable tumors or tumors exhibiting low-frequency microsatellite instability, but not patients with tumors that demonstrated high-frequency microsatellite instability.

▶ The Prostate, Lung, Colorectal, and Ovarian Cancer Screening Trial is a prospective, randomized, community-based study that evaluates several screening tests on specific cancer mortality. This article reports the effectiveness of FSG examined 3 years after a prior negative examination. Approximately 1 in 7 such patients had a polyp or mass detected on repeat examination. Were these polyps missed on the initial examination, or did they develop in the interim? By the authors' evaluation, most were thought to be new neoplasms. The proper interval for undergoing an FSG remains unclear, but many recommendations currently are at the 5-year interval. Should colonoscopy be used in place of FSG? It is estimated from this and other articles that about 1% to 2% of new malignancies occur in the proximal colon and are not reached by FSG.[1,2] A colleague described the use of a FSG as similar to obtaining a screening mammogram in one breast only. Perhaps virtual colonoscopy will supplant conventional colonoscopy, but ultimately it should be recognized that endoscopy is both a screening and therapeutic modality. Optimal uses of these modalities are important on a cost-effective basis for this to be useful.

P. J. Loehrer, Sr, MD

References

1. Lieberman DA, Weiss DG, Bond JH, et al: Use of colonoscopy to screen asymptomatic adults for colorectal cancer: Veterans Affairs Cooperative Study Group 380. *N Engl J Med* 343:162-168, 2000.
2. Imperiale TF, Wagner DR, Lin CY, et al: Risk of advanced proximal neoplasms in asymptomatic adults according to the distal colorectal findings. *N Engl J Med* 343:169-174, 2000.

Prognostic Value of Thymidylate Synthase, Ki-67, and *p53* in Patients With Dukes' B and C Colon Cancer: A National Cancer Institute–National Surgical Adjuvant Breast and Bowel Project Collaborative Study

Allegra CJ, Paik S, Colangelo LH, et al (NIH, Bethesda, Md; Natl Surgical Adjuvant Breast and Bowel Project, Pittsburgh, Pa; Belfast City Hosp, Northern Ireland)
J Clin Oncol 21:241-250, 2003   26–4

Background.—Colorectal cancer is the third most common cancer in the United States. Approximately 60% of all patients diagnosed with colorectal carcinoma will present with locally advanced disease. For these patients, appropriate therapeutic decision making is dependent primarily on the depth of penetration of the primary tumor and malignant involvement of the regional lymph nodes. Under present guidelines, many patients will receive chemotherapy unnecessarily, yet other patients who might benefit from it are not recommended to receive chemotherapy. The value of thymidylate synthase (TS), Ki-67, and *p53* as prognostic markers in patients with stage II and III colon cancer was defined.

Methods.—A retrospective analysis was conducted of the prognostic value of TS, Ki-67, and *p53* in 706 patients with Duke's B (291 patients) or Dukes' C (415 patients) colon carcinoma who were treated with either surgery alone (275 patients) or surgery plus fluorouracil-leucovorin chemotherapy (431 patients) in National Surgical Adjuvant Breast and Bowel Project protocols C01-C03. Immunohistochemical techniques were used to analyze these 3 markers. Five years of follow-up data were used for this analysis.

Results.—This retrospective analysis found an association between the intensity of TS, Ki-67, and *p53* for recurrence-free survival and overall survival. High TS intensity levels and positive *p53* staining were associated with a worse outcome. Patients with tumors that contained a high percentage of Ki-67–positive cells enjoyed an improved outcome compared with patients with tumors containing relatively few positive cells. No interaction with treatment was identified for any marker.

Conclusions.—These findings show that TS, Ki-67, and *p53* staining each had significant prognostic value in patients with Dukes' B and C colon carcinoma. However, none of these markers demonstrated sufficient power to clearly discern groups of patients who could be predicted to obtain greater or lesser benefit from the use of adjuvant chemotherapy.

▶ We are getting closer, but not quite there yet. This is a very elegant paper by Dr Allegra that attempts to correlate several markers to define a treatment algorithm. As expected, overexpression of TS and mutated *p53* was associated with a decreased relapse-free survival and overall survival. What is difficult to understand is that higher proliferative indices (as measured by Ki67) were associated with a better outcome. In total, these factors categorize those patients with a relatively good prognosis (80% vs 51% for relapsed-free survival). Unfortunately, this paper does not yet tease out the treatment-related outcomes as to whether those patients with poor expectations would benefit from specific therapy. This is a good start, however.

P. J. Loehrer, Sr, MD

The Continuing Increase in the Incidence of Hepatocellular Carcinoma in the United States: An Update
El-Serag HB, Davila JA, Petersen NJ, et al (Houston Veterans Affairs Med Ctr; Baylor College of Medicine, Houston; Natl Cancer Inst, Bethesda, Md; et al)
Ann Intern Med 139:817-823, 2003 26–5

Background.—A previous study has reported an increase in the incidence and mortality rates of hepatocellular carcinoma in the United States. However, there are several possible alternative explanations for this observed increase in hepatocellular carcinoma, including changes in the demographic structure of the underlying populations, resulting in an increasing number of persons at high risk for hepatocellular carcinoma, better detection of the disease as a result of improved diagnostic testing, or an increase in high-risk sex or racial or ethnic groups of the population residing in one or a few high-risk geographic regions. Temporal trends in the incidence of hepatocellular carcinoma were examined.

Methods.—Data for this study were obtained from population-based registries of the Surveillance, Epidemiology, and End Results program. The study population included persons given a diagnosis of hepatocellular carcinoma between 1975 and 1998. A linear Poisson multivariate regression model, with adjustment for differences in age, sex, race or ethnicity, and geographic region, was calculated among patients with hepatocellular carcinoma in the underlying population.

Results.—There was an increase in the overall age-adjusted incidence rates of hepatocellular carcinoma from 1.4 per 100,000 from 1975 to 1977 to 3.0 per 100,000 from 1996 to 1998. A 25% increase occurred during the last 3 years compared with the preceding 3 years. Age groups older than 40 years were most affected by this increase, with the greatest increase in incidence occurring in the 45- to 49-year-old age group. Men had the greatest increase (31%) in the last time period (1996 to 1998) compared with 1993 to 1995. The Poisson regression model confirmed the findings of a nearly 2-fold increase in the incidence rate ratio for hepatocellular carcinoma between 1975 and 1977 and 1996 and 1998.

Conclusions.—There has been a rapid increase in the incidence of hepatocellular carcinoma in the United States, with the fastest increase in rates occurring in white men aged 45 to 54 years. The findings of this study are consistent with a true increase in incidence. It is likely that the incidence of hepatocellular carcinoma will continue to increase in the near future because persons infected with the hepatitis C virus ultimately have cirrhosis develop unless there is improvement in the secondary prevention of hepatocellular carcinoma.

▶ Hepatocellular carcinoma is one of the most common cancers worldwide. It is associated with chronic liver disorders (eg, hepatitis B, alcoholic and non-alcoholic cirrhosis). Hepatitis C virus (HCV) leads to chronic hepatitis in approximately 80% of exposed individuals, despite antibodies to the virus. This study highlights a disturbing picture of the rapid rise of a very malignant disease. The findings are consistent with HCV infections acquired 30 to 40 years ago. As treatment options for advanced malignancies are limited, increased secondary measures to prevent HCV exposure and infection are clearly needed.

P. J. Loehrer, Sr, MD

27 Genitourinary

A Randomized, Placebo-controlled Trial of Zoledronic Acid in Patients With Hormone-Refractory Metastatic Prostate Carcinoma
Saad F, for the Zoledronic Acid Prostate Cancer Study Group (Centre Hospitalier de l'Université de Montréal; et al)
J Natl Cancer Inst 94:1458-1468, 2002   27–1

Background.—Prostate carcinoma is 1 of the most common cancers in men, and a preferred metastatic site is bone. Patients with hormone-refractory metastatic prostate cancer are especially prone to progressive bone disease. Biphosphonates, pyrophosphate analogues that inhibit bone destruction, may be useful in the treatment of these patients. The effectiveness and safety of a new biphosphonate, zoledronic acid, in reducing skeletal events associated with metastatic bone disease in men with hormone-refractory prostate cancer was analyzed in a randomized, placebo-controlled, double-blind phase III trial.

Study Design.—The study group included 643 men with hormone-refractory prostate cancer and bone metastases who were randomly assigned to receive either 4 or 8 mg of zoledronic acid or placebo once every 3 weeks for 15 months. The 8-mg treatment arm was reduced to 4 mg because of renal toxicity. All patients also received calcium and vitamin D supplementation. The primary efficacy variable was the proportion of patients with at least 1 skeleton-related event, defined as pathologic bone fractures, spinal cord compression, bone surgery, bone radiotherapy, or a change in antineoplastic therapy to treat bone pain. Secondary efficacy variables included time to first skeleton-related event, skeletal morbidity rate, time to disease progression, objective bone lesion response, bone biochemical markers, and quality of life. All analyses were performed on an intention-to-treat basis. Safety was assessed by serial laboratory tests and adverse events.

Findings.—A greater proportion of patients who received placebo had skeleton-related events than those who received zoledronic acid. The median time to first skeleton-related event was 321 days for placebo patients and was not reached for patients receiving 4 mg of zoledronic acid. Urinary markers of bone resorption were significantly decreased in patients receiving zoledronic acid. Pain and analgesic scores were higher in placebo patients. No differences in disease progression, performance status, or quality-of-life scores were noted between placebo and treatment patients. Zoledronic acid was well tolerated at 4 mg, but the 8-mg dose was associated with renal toxicity.

Conclusions.—Patients with metastatic prostate cancer who received 4 mg of the biphosphonate, zoledronic acid, every 3 weeks tolerated it well and had fewer skeleton-related events than those who received placebo. The optimal role of zoledronic acid in the treatment of patients with metastatic prostate cancer is still being defined.

► Patients with prostate cancer experience develop skeletal complications from both malignant and nonmalignant causes. Androgen ablative therapy, which is being used more frequently and earlier in the course of prostate cancer, contributes significantly to osteoporosis. This article by Saad et al describes a landmark trial that proved to be the basis of approval of zoledronic acid by the FDA. The population studied was that of patients with hormonally refractory disease and known bone metastases. This incidence of skeleton-related events was significantly better for patients treated with zoledronic acid at 8 mg. Interestingly, the arm that initially used a higher dose of zoledronic acid and later cut back to 4 mg was not significantly different from the placebo arm. When we look back at the prestudy characteristics between the 3 treatment groups we find that the 4-mg group did have the fewest incidents of prestudy-related skeletal events and the shortest time from diagnosis to treatment (the latter suggesting a shorter exposure to androgen ablative therapy). This is clearly an important trial; however, the impact of zoledronic acid in previously untreated patients with prostate cancer needs to be defined.

P. J. Loehrer, Sr, MD

Update on Late Relapse of Germ Cell Tumor: A Clinical and Molecular Analysis
George DW, Foster RS, Hromas RA, et al (Indiana Univ Med Ctr, Indianapolis; Ohio State Univ, Columbus)
J Clin Oncol 21:113-122, 2003   27–2

Background.—Germ cell tumor (GCT), though rare, is the most common malignancy to develop in men aged 15 to 35 years. The cure rate for early stage testicular cancer is 95% to 100% with modern cisplatin-based chemotherapy and appropriate surgery. The cure rate for advanced disease is 70%. However, cancer relapses in up to 10% of men who become free of disease with initial chemotherapy. The clinical characteristics, outcomes, and molecular and cytogenetic features of patients with late relapses of GCT were reported.

Methods.—The review included 83 patients seen at 1 center from 1993 through 2000 for GCT relapse occurring more than 2 years after initial treatment. Some specimens were available for analysis for expression of the transcription regulator FoxD3 and apurinic/apyrimidinic endonuclease. The presence of chromosome 12 abnormalities was also investigated in these specimens.

Findings.—The median length of time between initial presentation and relapse was 85 months. Of 49 patients with late relapse undergoing surgery, 43 achieved disease-free status. Twenty of this subgroup (46.5%) remained disease free. Of 32 patients given chemotherapy, only 6 (18.8%) achieved complete remission, 5 of whom remained disease free. Three of these 5 had not previously had chemotherapy. Eighteen of the 32 patients undergoing chemotherapy achieved disease-free status after postchemotherapy surgery, 12 of whom remained disease free. Overall, 85.2% of the 81 treated patients ultimately obtained disease-free status, with 46.9% remaining continuously free of disease at a median follow-up of 24.5 months. Another 9 patients are currently disease free after treatment for subsequent relapses. No definitive conclusions could be drawn from molecular and cytogenetic analyses.

Conclusions.—Lifetime follow-up is mandatory for men with GCT. Surgical resection alone continues to be the authors' preferred treatment for late relapse.

▶ The reality of late relapses in germ cell tumors has emerged during the last few years. Contraintuitively, patients who relapse greater than 2 years from initial diagnosis are less likely to be cured with chemotherapy alone than patients with earlier relapses. This study reviews a single institution's experience. The characteristics of patients with late relapses point out the findings that the vast majority have had prior nonseminomatous disease and on relapse are associated with elevated alphafetoprotein. Complete surgical resection of localized disease remains the primary treatment approach.

P. J. Loehrer, Sr, MD

Neoadjuvant Chemotherapy Plus Cystectomy Compared With Cystectomy Alone for Locally Advanced Bladder Cancer
Grossman HB, Natale RB, Tangen CM, et al (MD Anderson Cancer Ctr, Houston; Cedars-Sinai Comprehensive Cancer Ctr, Los Angeles; Southwest Oncology Group Statistical Ctr, Seattle; et al)
N Engl J Med 349:859-866, 2003   27–3

Background.—Patients with locally advanced cancer of the bladder are at a significant risk for metastases despite aggressive local therapy. A previous study by the Southwest Oncology Group showed that radiation therapy before radical cystectomy provided no improvement in outcome. Because of this finding, systemic chemotherapy has been explored in both neoadjuvant and adjuvant settings. The ability of neoadjuvant chemotherapy for improving outcome in patients with locally advanced bladder cancer who were treated with radical cystectomy was evaluated.

Methods.—A total of 307 patients with muscle-invasive bladder cancer (stage T2 to T4a) were randomly assigned to either surgery alone (154 patients) or combination of methotrexate, vinblastine, doxorubicin, and cisplatin followed by radical cystectomy (153 patients). The patients were stratified according to age (younger than 65 years vs 65 years or older) and stage (superficial muscle invasion vs more extensive disease). Analysis was by intention to treat.

Results.—Intention-to-treat analysis showed that the median survival among patients assigned to surgery alone was 46 months, whereas that of patients assigned to combination therapy was 77 months. Improved survival in both groups was associated with the absence of residual cancer in the cystectomy specimen. Significantly more patients in the combination-therapy group than in the cystectomy group had no residual disease (38% vs 15%).

Conclusions.—Among patients with locally advanced bladder cancer, the use of neoadjuvant methotrexate, vinblastine, doxorubicin, and cisplatin followed by radical cystectomy, in comparison with radical cystectomy alone, increased the likelihood of eliminating residual cancer in the cystectomy specimen. This combination therapy is associated with improved survival compared with cystectomy alone.

▶ Approximately 50% of patients with invasive bladder cancer will succumb to their disease despite surgical resection. As such, adjuvant therapy would appear logical. This study represents one of the first large trials demonstrating a therapeutic advantage with neoadjuvant methotrexate, vinblastine, doxorubicin, and cisplatin chemotherapy. Data from Europe using a cisplatin-based regimen before surgery or radiation therapy also show a survival advantage in a much larger population.[1] The authors are to be congratulated on their diligence in the completion of these trials. For patients with good performance status and organ function, this trial finally supports a role for systemic therapy.

P. J. Loehrer, Sr, MD

Reference

1. Hall RR: Updated results of a randomized controlled trial of neoadjuvant cisplatin (C), methotrexate (M) and vinblastine (V) chemotherapy for muscle-invasive bladder cancer [abstract]. *Prog Proc Am Soc Clin Oncol* 21:178a, 2002.

28 Hematologic

A Phase 2 Study of Bortezomib in Relapsed, Refractory Myeloma
Richardson PG, Barlogie B, Berenson J, et al (Dana-Farber Cancer Inst, Boston; Univ of Arkansas, Little Rock; Cedars-Sinai Med Ctr, Los Angeles; et al)
N Engl J Med 348:2609-2617, 2003   28–1

Background.—The boronic acid dipeptide bortezomib is a novel proteasome inhibitor. Preclinical and phase I studies have shown that bortezomib has antimyeloma activity. The effects of bortezomib were investigated in patients with relapsed, refractory myeloma.

Methods.—Two hundred two patients were enrolled in the multicenter, open-label, nonrandomized trial. All had relapsed myeloma refractory to most recent treatment. Treatment consisted of bortezomib, 1.3 mg/m² of body surface area, twice weekly for 2 weeks, followed by 1 week with no therapy, for up to 8 cycles. Oral dexamethasone was added to the treatment regimen of patients with a suboptimal response to bortezomib alone. At the end of the study, 193 patients were evaluable.

Findings.—Ninety-two percent of the evaluable patients had received 3 or more of the major classes of agents for myeloma. The bortezomib response rate was 35%. Among the responders were 7 patients in whom myeloma protein became undetectable and 12 in whom this protein was detected only by immunofixation. Overall, the median survival was 16 months. The median duration of response was 12 months. Fourteen percent of patients had grade 4 adverse events. Grade 3 events included thrombocytopenia in 28%, fatigue in 12%, peripheral neuropathy in 12%, and neutropenia in 11%.

Conclusions.—In this series of patients with relapsed, refractory myeloma, the novel proteasome inhibitor bortezomib was able to induce a clinically significant response with manageable toxic effects. Currently, an international, randomized, phase III trial is underway comparing bortezomib with high-dose dexamethasone in this patient population.

► Multiple myeloma is a complex hematologic disorder with limited available therapies. Front-line therapy typically consists of chemotherapy followed by high-dose chemotherapy with stem cell rescue. Even with this aggressive therapy, there is no cure for multiple myeloma. Recent studies have demonstrated that the class of drugs known as proteasome inhibitors has activity in multiple myeloma and may have use in the setting of relapsed and refractory disease. This phase II trial represents a large single-arm experience with the proteasome inhibitor bortezomib. The agent, administered twice weekly for 2 weeks followed by a week off, was able to induce objective responses in 35% of the 193 evaluable patients. Among these responders were 7 patients who attained complete responses with disappearance of their myeloma protein. The median overall survival in this heavily pretreated group was approximately 16 months. The agent was well tolerated, with mild myelosuppression as its principle toxicity. This study is critical for a number of reasons; first, it defines the activity of this agent in a significantly unmet need. Second, it represents the first evidence of activity for a new class of drugs, the proteasome inhibitors, and provides a rationale for further investigation of these agents in other malignancies. A phase III trial comparing bortezomib with standard pulse dexamethasone has been completed and the results are pending.

M. S. Gordon, MD

Imatinib Compared With Interferon and Low-Dose Cytarabine for Newly Diagnosed Chronic-Phase Chronic Myeloid Leukemia
O'Brien SG, Guilhot F, Larson RA, et al (Univ of Newcastle, England; Centre Hospitalier Universitaire de Poitiers, France; Univ of Chicago; et al)
N Engl J Med 348:994-1004, 2003   28–2

Background.—Imatinib is a selective inhibitor of the BCR-ABL tyrosine kinase. Research has shown that it yields high response rates in patients with chronic-phase chronic myeloid leukemia (CML) who did not respond to interferon-α. The efficacy of imatinib and interferon-α combined with low-dose cytarabine in patients with newly diagnosed chronic-phase CML were investigated.

Methods and Findings.—By random assignment, 1106 patients received imatinib or interferon-α plus low-dose cytarabine, with crossover to the alternative treatment permitted. The median patient follow-up was 19 months. The estimated rate of a major cytogenetic response at 18 months was 87.1% in imatinib recipients and 34.7% in combination therapy recipients. Estimated rates of complete cytogenetic response in the 2 groups were 76.2% and 14.5%, respectively. The estimated rate of freedom from progression to accelerated-phase or blast-crisis CML at 18 months was 96.7% and 91.5% in the imatinib and combined treatment groups, respectively. Patients given imatinib tolerated treatment better than those receiving the combination.

Conclusions.—On several measures, imatinib has advantages over interferon-α plus low-dose cytarabine as first-line therapy in patients with newly diagnosed chronic-phase CML. Imatinib was superior in hematologic and cytogenetic response, tolerability, and the likelihood of progression to accelerated-phase or blast-crisis CML.

▶ The signal transduction inhibitor imatinib has revolutionized the care and management of patients with CML. Having already demonstrated the ability to induce responses in patients with CML who are intolerant of interferon, the next critical question was whether or not imatinib should replace interferon and low-dose cytarabine as the front-line standard therapy. To this end, this randomized trial was initiated. Patients with newly diagnosed CML in chronic phase were randomly assigned to standard interferon-α with low-dose cytarabine versus imatinib. More than 1100 patients were randomized and crossover was allowed. With a median follow-up of more than 1.5 years, the imatinib arm demonstrated a statistically significant improvement in major and complete cytogenetic responses as well as a significant decrease in migration from chronic phase to either accelerated phase or blast-crisis phase. This study establishes imatinib as the new standard for the first-line therapy of CML.

M. S. Gordon, MD

Randomized Comparison of ABVD and MOPP/ABV Hybrid for the Treatment of Advanced Hodgkin's Disease: Report of an Intergroup Trial
Duggan DB, Petroni GR, Johnson JL, et al (State Univ of New York, Syracuse; Univ of Rochester, NY; Duke Univ, Durham, NC; et al)
J Clin Oncol 21:607-614, 2003   28-3

Purpose.—In patients with Hodgkin's disease, research has identified both the combination chemotherapy regimens of doxorubicin, bleomycin, vinblastine, and dacarbazine (ABVD) and mechlorethamine, vincristine, procarbazine, prednisone, doxorubicin, bleomycin, and vinblastine (MOPP/ABV) as effective. Because treatment-related toxicities may not develop for many years after the end of treatment, long-term assessment of the risks and benefits of these regimens is essential. The ABVD and MOPP/ABV regimens were compared as initial chemotherapy for Hodgkin's disease.

Methods.—Eight hundred fifty-six adult patients with advanced Hodgkin's disease, stage III$_2$A or higher, were randomly assigned to receive ABVD or MOPP/ABV. Responses, survival, and toxic effects were analyzed at a median follow-up of 6 years.

Results.—Response and survival outcomes were similar between the 2 regimens. Complete remission rates were 76% with ABVD and 80% with MOPP/ABV. Five-year failure-free survival was 63% and 66%; overall survival was 82% and 81%, respectively. Patients receiving MOPP/ABV had higher rates of clinically significant acute pulmonary and hematologic toxic effects, whereas cardiac toxicity was similar between groups. Of 24 treatment-related deaths, 9 occurred in the ABVD group and 15 in the MOPP/ABV group. Numbers of second malignancies were 18 and 28, respectively. Eleven of thirteen cases of myelodysplasia or acute leukemia occurred in the MOPP/ABV group. The other 2 patients were initially assigned to ABVD but later received MOPP chemotherapy and radiotherapy.

Conclusions.—The results confirm that both ABVD and MOPP/ABV are effective first-line chemotherapy regimens for Hodgkin's disease. However, MOPP/ABV may carry a higher risk of acute toxic effects, myelodysplasia syndrome, and leukemia. Thus, ABVD is the initial treatment of choice for advanced Hodgkin's disease.

▶ MOPP was the prototypical combination chemotherapy regimen in medical oncology. Over the past several decades, several randomized trials have strongly evolved to look at improved and less toxic therapy. This trial should finally put to rest this old and faithful battleship. Improvement over ABVD is our next challenge and is discussed well in an accompanying editorial by Dr Volker Diehl.[1]

P. J. Loehrer, Sr, MD

Reference

1. Diehl V: Advanced Hodgkin's disease: ABVD is better, yet is not good enough [editorial]! *J Clin Oncol* 21:583-585, 2003.

Second Malignant Neoplasms Among Long-term Survivors of Hodgkin's Disease: A Population-Based Evaluation Over 25 Years

Dores GM, Metayer C, Curtis RE, et al (Natl Cancer Inst, Bethesda, Md; Univ of Iowa, Iowa City; Univ of Toronto, Ont; et al)
J Clin Oncol 20:3484-3494, 2002   28–4

Background.—Successful treatment for Hodgkin's disease (HD) has permitted more patients to survive longer and to have second cancers develop. The absolute excess risk and relative site-specific risk for second cancers was investigated among a large group of long-term HD survivors.

Study Design.—This study group consisted of 32,591 HD survivors, of whom 2861 had survived at least 20 years. Cancer registries were searched for second malignant neoplasms that developed at least 1 year after HD diagnosis. The risk of second cancer was stratified by sex, age, elapsed time, and initial treatment.

Findings.—The average age at diagnosis was 37 years. Second malignancies developed in 2153 of these survivors, including 1726 solid tumors. The most common types of cancers in this patient group were lung, digestive tract, and female breast. The actuarial risk of a solid tumor developing was 21.9% after 25 years. The relative risk of a solid neoplasm developing decreased with increasing age at HD diagnosis. Patients aged 51 to 60 years at HD diagnosis had the highest cancer burden. There was a progressive increase in relative risk and absolute excess risk for solid tumors with time after diagnosis until after 25 years, when there appeared to be a decrease. Temporal and treatment group cancer distribution suggested a radiogenic effect.

Conclusions.—Patients who survive HD appear to be at risk for second cancers, especially those of the lung, digestive tract, and breast. This risk is increased with time elapsed since diagnosis for 25 years, after which it appears to decline.

▶ HD represents one of a number of highly curable malignancies. Even after relapse from initial therapy, salvage with radiation standard to high-dose chemotherapy is associated with significant cure rates. Treatment for HD has traditionally incorporated significant doses of alkylator-based therapy and, hence, the risk of second malignancy in this setting can be significant. Dores et al review more than 32,000 HD patients in long-term follow-up to assess the incidence of second malignancies in this patient population. The study indicates a significantly high risk for second solid tumor malignancy, with common tumors such as lung and breast cancer being particularly prevalent. The risk of solid tumors in radiation therapy ports appeared to be significantly increased, suggesting the increased risk of combined modality therapy. The maximum risk for second tumors appears to be at approximately 15 years, with a decrease beyond 25 years. In addition, the risk of second malignancies was higher in patients diagnosed with HD at a younger age, suggesting that time at risk is an important contributor. Vigilant monitoring of patients with HD after successful treatment is critical for early identification of second tumors. Whether more aggressive screening strategies need to be utilized is not yet defined.

M. S. Gordon, MD

29 Head and Neck

An Intergroup Phase III Comparison of Standard Radiation Therapy and Two Schedules of Concurrent Chemoradiotherapy in Patients With Unresectable Squamous Cell Head and Neck Cancer

Adelstein DJ, Li Y, Adams GL, et al (Cleveland Clinic Found, Ohio; Arthur G James Cancer Hosp, Columbus, Ohio; Dana-Farber Cancer Inst, Boston; et al)

J Clin Oncol 21:92-98, 2003   29–1

Background.—Radiation therapy has been standard care for patients with unresectable squamous cell head and neck cancer. Unfortunately, overall survival after radiation has been less than 25%. The Head and Neck Intergroup reported a phase III randomized study of the benefits of adding chemotherapy to radiation in this patient population.

Methods.—Two hundred ninety-five patients were enrolled in the trial between 1992 and 1999. Patients were assigned randomly to 1 of 3 arms. Arm A, the control group, received single daily fractionated radiation at 70 Gy at 2 Gy/d. Arm B received identical radiation therapy with concurrent bolus cisplatin on days 1, 22, and 43. Arm C received a split course of single daily fractionated radiation plus 3 cycles of a concurrent infusional fluorouracil and bolus cisplatin chemotherapy, 30 Gy administered with the first cycle and 30 to 40 Gy given with the third cycle. Surgical resection was done if possible after the second chemotherapy cycle in patients assigned to arm C. If necessary, salvage therapy was performed in all groups.

Findings.—Toxicity of grade 3 or higher occurred in 52% of patients in arm A, 89% of those in arm B, and 77% of those in arm C. The median follow-up was 41 months. The 3-year projected overall survival rate for arm A patients was 23%, compared with 37% for arm B patients. The projected overall survival rate for arm C patients was 27%, not significantly different from that for arm A.

Conclusion.—Concurrent high-dose, single-agent cisplatin with conventional single daily fractionated radiation increases toxicity but also significantly improves survival. Splitting the radiation course resulted in a loss of efficacy that was not offset by multiagent chemotherapy or the possibility of midcourse surgery.

▶ Head and neck cancer is one of the most challenging diseases to treat. It clearly represents one of the models for multimodality therapy with surgery, radiation, and chemotherapy. The optimal treatment for unresected squamous cell carcinoma of the head and neck has been poorly defined. It has been suggested that cisplatin-based chemotherapy plus concurrent radiation therapy was superior to radiation therapy alone, but this has not been proven through phase III studies.

This is a nicely performed phase III trial evaluating 3 popular approaches for the treatment of stage III or IV (without evidence of distant hematogenous metastases) disease. Cisplatin plus radiotherapy, though more toxic, was associated with the best 3-year overall survival and disease-specific survival. Arm C of the study actually had 2 variables (the addition of 5-FU and use of split course radiotherapy) but was no better than the other 2 arms. Debate may continue regarding the role of fluoropyrimidine therapy, but, as of now, cisplatin plus radiation appears to be the optimal therapy.

P. J. Loehrer, Sr, MD

30 Supportive Care and Miscellaneous

Influenza Vaccination in Elderly Patients With Advanced Colorectal Cancer
Earle C (Harvard Med School, Boston)
J Clin Oncol 21:1161-1166, 2003   30–1

Background.—Yearly influenza vaccination is recommended for people aged 65 years and older, especially those with underlying immunosuppressive disorders. There is debate over the use of influenza vaccine in patients with cancer, reflecting concerns about the resulting antibody response or possible immunosuppression. The outcomes of influenza vaccination in older adults with advanced colorectal cancer were analyzed.

Methods.—The National Cancer Institute's Survival, Epidemiology, and End Results registry was used to identify Medicare patients treated for stage IV colorectal cancer between 1993 and 1998. All patients had survived at least 4 months with colorectal cancer and were alive during the fall months, making them potentially eligible for influenza vaccination. Medicare data were used to determine whether the patients received influenza vaccination and to assess their subsequent outcomes. A total of 1225 patients met the study criteria, receiving chemotherapy over a total of 1577 person-years of observation.

Results.—The rate of influenza vaccination was 39.7% overall, increasing from 26% to 43% in the years studied. More than two thirds of vaccinated patients received the vaccine from their primary care physician. Factors associated with influenza vaccination included white race, higher socioeconomic status, and increased comorbidity. During treatment, vaccinated patients were less likely to be diagnosed as having influenza or pneumonia. Vaccination was also associated with a lower rate of chemotherapy interruptions and an increased chance of survival to the start of fall the next year (hazard ratio, 0.88). Vaccinated patients also had a slight reduction in health care resource utilization.

Conclusions.—For elderly patients with advanced colorectal cancer, the benefits of influenza vaccination appear comparable to those of cancer-free older adults. Vaccination rates are relatively low in this population, particularly for minority and lower income patients. Oncologists should advocate yearly influenza vaccinations for patients being treated for advanced cancer.

▶ This year will mark one of the most severe influenza seasons in this country. Oncologists become the primary care providers for many patients diagnosed with cancer. As physician caretakers, responsibility for other typically noncologic medical needs falls to us. This study is a reminder.

P. J. Loehrer, Sr, MD

Sensitivity of a Blood Culture Drawn Through a Single Lumen of a Multilumen, Long-term, Indwelling, Central Venous Catheter in Pediatric Oncology Patients

Robinson JL (Univ of Alberta, Edmonton, Canada)
J Pediatr Hematol Oncol 24:72-74, 2002   30–2

Background.—Bacteremia is common among pediatric oncology patients; blood cultures drawn from these patients because of fever will be positive in approximately 10% of cases. These blood cultures are often drawn from long-term, indwelling, central venous catheters because this prevents the need for venipuncture; however, these cultures may have a higher sensitivity than do peripheral blood cultures. In many centers, it has become common practice to draw simultaneous blood cultures from all lumens when long-term, indwelling, central venous catheters have multiple lumens. This practice increases the incidence of contaminated blood cultures, yet it may also increase the detection rate of true bacteremias. The sensitivity of a blood culture drawn from only 1 lumen of a multilumen, long-term, indwelling, central venous catheter was assessed in pediatric oncology patients.

Methods.—Records of a microbiology laboratory were used to conduct a retrospective review of all positive blood cultures obtained from pediatric oncology patients admitted to 1 center from January 1994 through March 1999. Episodes of positive findings on blood culture were included only if cultures were sent simultaneously from multiple lumens of a long-term, indwelling, central line and if the culture was thought to represent a true bacteremia.

Results.—Discordant findings occurred in 13 (32%) of 41 episodes of blood cultures drawn simultaneously from different lumens. The estimated sensitivity of a culture obtained from a single lumen was 84%, which is lower than the minimum acceptable standard of 95%.

Conclusions.—It is recommended that blood cultures should be drawn from all lumens in patients with central venous catheters with multiple lumens because the sensitivity of a blood culture from a single lumen in a pediatric patient with a long-term, indwelling, venous catheter appears to be lower than the minimum acceptable sensitivity of 95%. Drawing blood cultures from multiple lumens increases the risk of obtaining a contaminated blood culture and can introduce infections, but the failure to recognize bacteremia or a delay in making the diagnosis increases the risk of septic shock and secondary seeding and may increase the need for removal of the line or prolongation of hospital stay.

▶ The issue of where to draw blood cultures from patients with central venous catheters that have single or multiple lumens is addressed in this study. Importantly, the results demonstrate a 32% discordance in cultures drawn simultaneously from different lumens. The sensitivity of a culture from a single lumen was 84%. While the volume of blood drawn is also known to affect the sensitivity of blood cultures, the results of this study would argue for sampling all lumens of multilumen catheters to increase the sensitivity of detecting bacteremia.

R. J. Arceci, MD, PhD

Overweight, Obesity, and Mortality from Cancer in a Prospectively Studied Cohort of U.S. Adults
Calle EE, Rodriguez C, Walker-Thurmond K, et al (American Cancer Society, Atlanta, Ga)
N Engl J Med 348:1625-1638, 2003   30–3

Background.—An increasing number of Americans are overweight or obese, and the health risks from overweight and obesity are frequently topics in the popular media. The relationship between excess body weight and mortality not only from all causes but also from cardiovascular disease are well established. It has been known for some time that excess weight is also a significant factor in death from cancer, but there are only limited data on the magnitude of this relationship, both for all cancers and for cancers at individual sites, and the public health effect of excess weight in regard to total mortality is unclear. Previous studies have consistently shown associations between adiposity and increased risk of cancers of the endometrium, kidney, gallbladder (in women), and colon (particularly in men). The relationships between body mass index (BMI) and the risk of death from cancer at specific sites were determined.

Methods.—This prospective study enrolled more than 900,000 adults (404,576 men and 495,477 women) who were cancer-free at enrollment in 1982. There were 57,145 deaths from cancer during 16 years of follow-up. This study examined the relationship between BMI in 1982 and the risk of death from all cancer and from cancers at individual sites. Multivariate proportional hazards models were used to control for other risk factors. The proportion of all deaths from cancer that was attributable to overweight and obesity in the US population was calculated on the basis of risk estimates from the current study and national estimates of the prevalence of overweight and obesity in the US adult population.

Results.—The members of this cohort with a BMI of 40 had death rates from all cancers combined that were 52% higher for men and 62% higher for women, than the rates in men and women of normal weight. BMI was also significantly associated in both men and women with higher rates of death from cancer of the esophagus, colon and rectum, liver, gallbladder, pancreas, and kidney. This was also true for death from non-Hodgkin's lymphoma and multiple myeloma. Significant trends of increasing risk with higher BMI values were noted for death from cancers of the stomach and prostate in men and death from cancer of the breast, uterus, cervix, and ovary in women. It was estimated from these findings that current patterns of overweight and obesity in this country are responsible for 14% of all deaths from cancer in men and 20% of cancer deaths in women.

Conclusions.—This prospective study in a large population cohort of adults in the United States found that increased body weight was associated with increased death rates from all cancers combined as well as cancers at multiple specific sites.

▶ This is an exhaustive study that points at another reason why obesity is bad for you. The findings are even more impressive when the breadth of diversity of malignant diseases is noted even among those patients who are nonsmokers. The preclinical explanation for obesity-related carcinogenesis is largely unknown. One can even take the extreme and ask whether cancer-related cachexia is a natural response to fight cancer. All of this is worth further study; but until then, eat well and exercise.

P. J. Loehrer, Sr, MD

▶ Obesity is increasing in frequency in the United States. Frank obesity (BMI >30) is estimated to affect up to one third of our population. This population has associated increased morbidity and mortality, primarily resulting from cardiovascular disease. It is suggested that in the gastrointestinal tract, colon cancer and adenocarcinoma of the esophagus are increasing. Calle et al conducted a prospective study of an incredibly large population of 107,030 men and 276,564 women to determine the relations between BMI and the risk of death from cancer at specific sites. Six of the cancers that were found to have increased were in the gastrointestinal tract.

This study confirmed the previous association noted with overweight and obesity—both for colon and esophageal adenocarcinoma. The increased rate of esophageal adenocarcinoma may be related to increased BMI predisposing to gastroesophageal reflux. The authors also found an increased risk of gallbladder cancer, which may be explained by the increased risk of gallstones found in obesity that increases the risk of gallbladder cancer. Pancreatic and liver cancer risks are increased in patients with a high BMI. Liver cancer may result from cirrhosis, which is found in patients with nonalcoholic steatohepatitis. The mechanism predisposing obese patients to pancreatic cancer is unclear.

J. S. Barkin, MD

PART FOUR

KIDNEY, WATER, AND ELECTROLYTES

SAULO KLAHR, MD

31 Glomerular Disease

Introduction

The chapter's initial article by Praga et al (Abstract 31–1) is the first to show, in a prospective and randomized design, a clearly beneficial effect of enalapril (an angiotensin-converting enzyme [ACE] inhibitor) on the long-term outcome of patients with immunoglobulin A nephropathy (IgAN) with proteinuria equal or exceeding 0.5 g per day. Proteinuria decreased significantly in the ACE-treated group. In this study, the beneficial effect of enalapril appeared to be largely independent of its antihypertensive effect.

In 8 patients with idiopathic membranous nephropathy and lasting persistent proteinuria, Ruggenenti et al (Abstract 31–2) used the IV infusion of the anti-CD20 monoclonal antibody (rituximab) and achieved a 60% reduction in proteinuria. The 8 patients (3 men) aged 52.8 ± 19.6 years had heavy proteinuria, hypoalbuminemia, mild to moderate renal insufficiency, and hypercholesterolemia.

IgAN was first described by Berger[1] in France in 1969. A retrospective study by Geddes et al (Abstract 31–3) from 4 centers (Glasgow, Helsinki, Sydney, and Toronto) included 711 adults with biopsy-proven IgAN and achieved a 60% reduction in proteinuria.

A study by Hoang et al (Abstract 31–4) was an effort to elucidate the mechanism of aging associated with glomerular filtration rate depression.

Markowitz et al (Abstract 31–5) suggests that C1q nephropathy falls within the clinical-pathologic spectrum of focal segmental glomerulosclerosis (FSGS) and minimal-change disease (MCD).

Saulo Klahr, MD

Reference

1. Berger J: IgA glomerular deposits in renal disease. *Transplant Proc* 1:939-944, 1969.

Treatment of IgA Nephropathy With ACE Inhibitors: A Randomized and Controlled Trial

Praga M, Gutiérrez E, González E, et al (Hosp 12 de Octubre, Madrid)
J Am Soc Nephrol 14:1578-1583, 2003   31–1

Background.—Progressive renal insufficiency develops in 40% to 60% of patients with IgA nephropathy (IgAN), which is predicted on the basis of impaired renal function, high blood pressure (BP), and proteinuria exceeding 1 g/d. IgAN patients tend to have a slow rate of progression: end-stage renal failure develops in 20% of cases after 10 years and in 30% after 20 years. The suggestion that the progression of IgAN may be positively influenced by angiotensin-converting enzyme (ACE) inhibitors, specifically, enalapril, was subjected to a prospective controlled investigation.

Methods.—The study included 44 patients who had biopsy-proven IgAN, proteinuria of at least 0.5 g/d, and serum creatinine (SCr) levels of 1.5 mg/dL or less. The patients were randomly assigned to a group receiving enalapril (n = 23) or to a control group (n = 21) where BP was regulated by means of non-ACE inhibitor antihypertensive agents. The main outcome sought was renal survival as estimated by a 50% increase in the baseline SCr determination. In addition, the presence of a SCr level more than 1.5 mg/dL at the final visit and the evolution of proteinuria were assessed.

Results.—At baseline, the mean proteinuria values were 2 g/d in those receiving enalapril and 1.7 g/d in the control group. Seventeen percent of the treatment group and 4% of the control group had proteinuria in the nephrotic range. Three patients who were given enalapril and 12 control patients reached the 50% SCr increase point. The probability of renal survival was significantly improved in those receiving enalapril when compared to that of the control group 4 years after the study began, with 100% survival rate for those with the enalapril treatment and only a 70% survival rate among the control patients. At 7 years, these rates were 92% and 55%, respectively. Only treatment with enalapril and reduced proteinuria within 1 year were statistically related to renal survival on univariate analysis and only enalapril treatment on multivariate analysis. The SCr was less than 1.5 mg/dL in 3 enalapril patients and 11 control patients at the last visit, and proteinuria was significantly less in the enalapril group but tended to increase among the control patients.

Conclusions.—The renal survival of patients with proteinuric IgAN with normal or moderately reduced renal function was significantly better when they received treatment with enalapril than with BP control with non-ACE inhibitor agents. Because of these findings, ACE inhibitors could form the first line of intervention for IgAN patients with persistent proteinuria.

▶ IgAN is a glomerular disease defined by the mesangial deposition of IgA. Diffuse mesangial IgA is the defining hallmark. IgA and C3, and less commonly IgM, may also be found in the same distribution. IgA also occurs sometimes along a capillary loop. The range of presentations of IgAN includes recurrent macroscopic hematuria, asymptomatic microscopic hematuria with or without proteinuria, the nephrotic syndrome, acute renal failure due to tubular occlusion and chronic renal failure.

Several studies have demonstrated that ACE inhibitors have a significant renoprotective effect in chronic proteinuric nephropathies. However, a prospective and controlled study of ACE on the progression of IgAN has not been done. Praga et al designed a prospective and randomized study that was in a single center from September of 1990 to September of 1995. Forty-four adult patients were eligible for the trial. From the 44 patients with biopsy-proven IgAN, 23 received ACE inhibitors, and the other 21 did not receive ACE inhibitors (control group). Most of the patients were less than 40 years old and most of them were men. The mean proteinuria was 2 g/d in the patients that were to be given ACE. The patients in the control group had proteinuria of 1.7 g/d.

This study is the first to show, in a prospective and randomized design, a clearly beneficial effect of enalapril (an ACE inhibitor) on the long-term outcome of IgAN patients with proteinuria equal or exceeding 0.5 g/d. Proteinuria decreased significantly in the ACE inhibitor-treated group. In this study, the beneficial effect of enalapril appeared to be largely independent of its antihypertensive effect.

In conclusion, ACE inhibitors, such as enalapril, decrease proteinuria in patients with IgAN with normal or moderately reduced kidney function.

S. Klahr, MD

Rituximab in Idiopathic Membranous Nephropathy: A One-Year Prospective Study
Ruggenenti P, Chiurchiu C, Brusegan V, et al (Mario Negri Institute for Pharmacological Research, Bergamo, Italy; Azienda Ospedaliera, Bergamo, Italy)
J Am Soc Nephrol 14:1851-1857, 2003   31–2

Background.—The treatment of idiopathic membranous nephropathy (IMN) has relied on steroids and immunosuppresant drugs, which are not fully specific and may have severe toxic effects. Currently available monoclonal antibodies against the B-cell surface antigen CD20 have been used to investigate whether specific inhibition of B cells might improve the outcome of IMN and avoid the side effects of steroids and immunosuppressants. The 1-year outcome of patients with IMN treated with a course of rituximab infusions was evaluated in a prospective, observational study.

Methods.—The study group included 8 patients (3 men) aged 52.8 ± 19.6 years and with known IMN for 29.7 ± 13.5 months. All the patients had biopsy-proved IMN, heavy proteinuria, hypoalbuminemia, mild to moderate renal insufficiency, and hypercholesterolemia. Their blood pressure was well controlled. Main baseline clinical and laboratory characteristics of the patients are provided in Table 1. The patients were treated with 4 weekly IV infusions of rituximab (375 mg/m^2).

Results.—At 3 and 12 months, proteinuria decreased significantly from a mean ($\pm$SD) of 8.6 ± 4.2 to 4.3 ± 3.3 (-51%) and 3.0 ± 2.5 (-66%) g/24 hours (Fig 1). Albumin fractional clearance decreased from 2.3 ± 2.1 to $1.2 \pm$

TABLE 1.—Main Clinical and Laboratory Characteristics at Study Entry (Month 0) of Individual Patients With Idiopathic Membranous Nephropathy (IMN)

	Patient							
Parameter	1	2	3	4	5	6	7	8
Age (yr)	55	70	28	75	69	24	40	59
Gender (male/female)	F	F	F	M	F	F	M	M
Disease duration (mo)	14	35	46	24	24	13	33	49
Histology stage (1-4)	2	2	1	2	1	2	2	2
Urinary protein excretion (g/24 h)	16.0	7.0	4.8	5.6	5.7	9.1	14.1	6.7
Serum creatinine (mg/dl)	1.7	1.6	1.0	3.7	1.1	0.9	0.9	1.2

(Courtesy of Ruggenenti P, Chiurchiu C, Brusegan V, et al: Rituximab in idiopathic membranous nephropathy: A one-year prospective study. *J Am Soc Nephrol* 14:1851-1857, 2003.)

1.7 (−47%) and 0.5 ± 0.6 (−76%), and serum albumin concentration increased from 2.7 ± 0.5 to 3.1 ± 0.23 (+21%) and 3.5 ± 0.4 (+41%) mg/dL. At 12 months, proteinuria decreased to 0.5 g/24 hours or less, or 3.5 g/24 hours or less in 2 and 3 patients, respectively. Proteinuria decreased in the remaining patients by 74%, 44%, and 41%, respectively. There were progressive reductions in body weight, diastolic blood pressure, and serum cholesterol in parallel with an improvement of edema in all patients. Renal function stabilized, and CD20 B lymphocytes decreased below normal ranges through the end of the study. There were no major drug-related events or major changes in other laboratory parameters.

Conclusions.—Rituximab safely promotes sustained disease remission in patients who would otherwise progress to end-stage renal disease. The long-term risk-benefit profile of rituximab appears to be significantly more favorable compared with that of the commonly used immunosuppressive drugs.

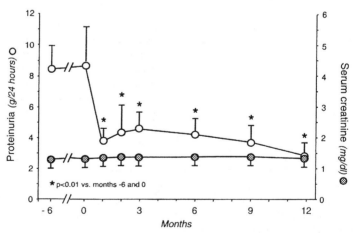

FIGURE 1.—Time course of serum creatinine concentration and 24-h urinary protein excretion rate in eight patients with idiopathic membranous nephropathy (IMN) from 6 mo before rituximab administration to study end (month 12). (Courtesy of Ruggenenti P, Chiurchiu C, Brusegan V, et al: Rituximab in idiopathic membranous nephropathy: A one-year prospective study. *J Am Soc Nephrol* 14:1851-1857, 2003.)

▶ Membranous glomerulonephritis is a well-defined cause of the nephrotic syndrome. Its salient features include diffuse glomerular basement membrane thickening, characteristic glomerular basement membrane "spikes" on silver-stained sections, and diffuse deposition of IgG and complement. About two thirds of membranous glomerulonephritis is idiopathic, and one third is associated with underlying disease or drugs. Eighty percent or 90% of cases occur in patients older than 30 years.

In 8 patients with IMN and lasting persistent proteinuria, Ruggenenti et al used the IV infusion of the anti-CD20 monoclonal antibody (rituximab) and achieved a 60% reduction in proteinuria. Table 1 depicts the main clinical and laboratory findings at study entry. The 8 patients (3 males) aged 52.8 ± 19.6 years had heavy proteinuria, hypoalbuminemia, mild to moderate renal insufficiency, and hypercholesterolemia. Fig 1 depicts the course of serum creatinine and the 24-hour urinary protein excretion.

At this point (July 2003), no major drug-related side effects or major adverse events have been reported in patients given rituximab for immune-mediated diseases. In the 8 patients with membranous glomerulonephritis, rituximab infusion reduced proteinuria and prevented disease progression, and the drug was well tolerated. The effect of rituximab was probably mediated by specific drug-related effects on autocrine B-cell clones.

Randomized trials with longer follow-up are needed to verify the long-term tolerability of rituximab therapy.

S. Klahr, MD

A Tricontinental View of IgA Nephrology

Geddes CC, Rauta V, Gronhagen-Riska C, et al (Western Infirmary, Glasgow, Scotland; Univ of Helsinki; Univ of Toronto; et al)
Nephrol Dial Transplant 18:1541-1548, 2003   31–3

Background.—The most common primary glomerulopathy is immunoglobulin A (IgA) nephropathy (IgAN), which was originally believed to have a benign outcome but has since been noted to produce end-stage renal failure in up to 43% of patients within 10 years. Data were collected from 4 large IgAN databases covering 4 countries on 3 continents concerning the long-term outcome of IgAN and identifying any geographic variables that may predict outcome independent of clinical and laboratory findings at diagnosis.

Methods.—Seven hundred eleven adults who had biopsy-proven IgAN were included. There were 112 from Glasgow, Scotland; 204 from Helsinki, Finland; 121 from Sydney, Australia; and 274 from Toronto, Canada. Age, gender, 24-hour urine protein excretion (UP_0), mean arterial pressure (MAP_0), and creatinine clearance ($CrCl_0$) were documented from the initial presentation to a nephrologist, with outcomes determined by the slope of CrCl and renal survival data.

Results.—The lowest median UP_0, lowest MAP_0, and highest $CrCl_0$ were recorded for patients from Helsinki, which suggested milder cases of IgAN

TABLE 1.—Clinical Characteristics of Patients With Biopsy-Proven Immunoglobulin A Nephropathy at Presentation

	Glasgow ($n = 112$)	Helsinki ($n = 204$)	Sydney ($n = 121$)	Toronto ($n = 274$)	P
All subjects					
Median year of presentation (range)	1989 (77-95)	1987 (80-95)	1985 (59-93)	1984 (63-97)	—
Median follow up (months)	86	123	73	53	<0.001*
Mean age (years)	37.3	34.9	33.9	37.0	0.05†
Male:female ratio	4.6	1.7	1.5	1.8	<0.001‡
Median serum creatinine (μmol/l)	118	90	110	115	<0.001*
Mean CrCl (ml/min)	79.1	98.7	82.6	74.2	<0.001†
Median urine protein (UP) excretion (g/day)	1.72	0.64	1.28	1.75	<0.001*
Proportion with UP <0.5 g/day	22.9%	46.4%	26.2%	5.8%	<0.001‡
Mean of mean arterial blood pressure (mmHg)	105	94.0	103	105	<0.001†
Subjects presenting CrCl < 75 ml/min					
Number (%)	52 (46.4)	34 (16.7)	51 (42.1)	132 (48.2)	<0.001‡
Mean age (years)	45.3	47.6	37.7	39.1	<0.001†
Mean CrCl (ml/min)	44.1	55.8	52.1	52.2	0.003†
Median urine protein (UP) excretion (g/day)	2.24	1.28	1.28	2.2	0.006*
Mean of mean arterial blood pressure (mmHg)	107	102	109	108	0.223†

*Kruskal-Wallis test of variance.
†Test of analysis of variance.
‡4×2 χ^2 test.
(Courtesy of Geddes CC, Rauta V, Gronhagen-Riska C, et al: A tricontinental view of IgA nephrology, *Nephrol Dial Transplant* 18:1541-1548, 2003. By permission of Oxford University Press.)

than were seen in other centers (Table 1). Renal survival overall was 77.8% at 10 years, 69.8% at 15 years, and 55.3% at 20 years. However, the various centers differed significantly on this measure, ranging from a high of 95.7% in Helsinki to a low of 61.6% in Toronto, with Sydney having a renal survival of 87.0% and Glasgow, 63.9%. Gender was the only variable assessed that did not have a significant impact on renal survival. Significant independent variables predicting reduced renal survival were younger age at presentation, increased UP_0, and decreased $CrCl_0$.

Patients from Helsinki and Sydney had significantly longer renal survival than those from Toronto, regardless of age at presentation. The greatest impact on renal survival was exerted by $CrCl_0$. The median slope of CrCl was -1.24 mL/min/y in Helsinki; it was -3.99 mL/min/y in Toronto, with Glasgow and Sydney having intermediate values. Patients from Glasgow and Toronto appeared to have more severe disease, based on their $CrCl_0$ and UP_0 levels.

A significantly slower rate of deterioration was noted for patients from Helsinki that was independent of other factors on presentation. In addition, slower deterioration was noted with older age at diagnosis, higher $CrCl_0$, and lower UP_0. Analysis of 269 patients whose $CrCl_0$ was less than 75 mL/min yielded no independent center effect.

Conclusion.—Geographic variability in the long-term outcome for IgAN was substantiated. The basis for this effect includes lead time bias and the inclusion of milder cases in centers that have apparently good outcomes, but the effect of other factors—such as genetics, diet, or treatment differences—was not excluded.

▶ IgAN was first described by J. Berger in France in 1969. This retrospective study from 4 centers (Glasgow, Scotland; Helsinki, Finland; Sydney, Australia; and Toronto, Canada) included 711 adults with biopsy-proven IgAN (see Table 1).

The cohort included subjects presenting between 1959 and 1997. The overall 10-, 15-, and 20-year actuarial survivals were 77.8%, 69.8%, and 55.3% respectively. This study describes the long-term natural history of the largest cohort of patients with IgAN reported to date. The size of the cohort and the length of follow-up allow meaningful comparison of factors at presentation affecting long-term outcome. Poor kidney function at presentation and marked proteinuria at presentation were adverse risk factors for the development of end-stage renal failure.

Previous single-center studies have suggested geographic variability in the long-term outcome of IgAN. This was confirmed in this study of Geddes et al. There was a 10-year renal survival ranging from 99.3% in Helsinki to 61.4% in Toronto. The potential for bias in this study is highlighted by the observation that in the 2 centers with the shortest kidney survival and most negative slope of creatinine (Toronto and Glasgow), the proportion of patients with a creatinine slope less than 75 mL/min implies more severe disease than patients from Helsinki and Sydney. Another table shows the Cox proportional hazards at presentation and subsequent renal survival.

Further studies should determine if these geographical differences may also relate to genetic factors, environmental factors, or differences in subsequent medical management.

S. Klahr, MD

Determinants of Glomerular Hypofiltration in Aging Humans
Hoang K, Tan JC, Derby G, et al (Stanford Univ, Calif)
Kidney Int 64:1417-1424, 2003   31–4

Background.—The inverse relationship between the glomerular filtration rate (GFR) and age was first demonstrated more than 50 years ago. The technique used at that time was the urinary clearance of inulin, which continues to be the gold standard for determination of GFR. Since that first study in men, the negative correlation of GFR with age has also been demonstrated in women. Evidence that renal plasma flow (RPF) declines in parallel with the GFR has suggested a possible hemodynamic basis for the hypofiltration associated with aging. The extent to which GFR is depressed in healthy aging research subjects was confirmed, and the mechanism of this hypofiltration was identified.

Methods.—A total of 159 healthy volunteers aged 18 to 88 years underwent determination of GFR, RPF, afferent oncotic pressure, and arterial pressure. Glomeruli in 33 renal biopsy specimens of healthy kidney transplant donors aged 23 to 69 years underwent morphological analysis to determine glomerular hydraulic permeability and filtration surface area. The GFR determinants were then subjected to mathematical modeling to determine the glomerular ultrafiltration coefficient (K_f) for 2 kidneys and individual glomeruli.

Results.—The GFR was significantly depressed (22%) in aging research subjects (55 years or older) compared with youthful subjects (40 years or younger). Corresponding with this decline in GFR with aging were reductions in RPF by 28%, 2-kidney K_f by 21% to 53%, glomerular hydraulic permeability by 14%, and the single-nephron K_f by 30% (Table 2). No significant differences were seen between aging and youthful subsets for afferent oncotic pressure and filtration surface area per glomerulus.

TABLE 2.—Glomerular Morphometry

	Age ≤40 Years (N = 16)	Age ≥55 Years (N = 7)	P Value
Glomerular volume $\mu m^3 \times 10^5$	2.4 ± 0.9	2.3 ± 0.5	NS
Filtration surface density $\mu m^2/\mu m^3$	0.13 ± 0.04	0.10 ± 0.01	0.01
Filtration slit frequency *slits/mm*	1272 ± 182	1110 ± 97	<0.05
Glomerular basement membrane width *nm*	417 ± 61	461 ± 81	NS
Fractional interstitial area %	14.1 ± 4.3	13.4 ± 4.6	NS

(Courtesy of Hoang K, Tan JC, Derby G, et al: Determinants of glomerular hypofiltration in aging humans. *Kidney Int* 64 (4):1417-1424, 2003. Reprinted by permission of Blackwell Publishing.)

Conclusions.—A reduction in the overall, 2-kidney K_f seems to contribute to depression of the GFR in aging research subjects. It is suggested that this is a result, at least in part, of structural changes that lower the single-nephron K_f and a result, in part, of the reduction in the actual number of functioning glomeruli that has been demonstrated in previous autopsy studies.

▶ This study by Hoang et al was an effort to elucidate the mechanism of aging-associated GFR depression. In this study, 192 healthy individuals (age range, 18-88 years) were divided into 2 groups: one with 159 volunteers, of which 94 were men, and the other with 33 transplant donors, 27 of whom were living, related donors.

The term *renal senescence* refers to a series of structural and physiologic alterations that decrease renal functioning in aging individuals. Table 1 (in the original article) depicts the dynamics of filtration, including glomerular filtration, RPF, filtration fraction, plasma oncotic pressure, and mean arterial pressure. It is clear from this table that individuals 40 years or younger (N = 110) have a greater GFR than individuals 55 years or older (N = 27).

The finding of a parallel fall in RPF and GFR with advancing age (Fig 2 in the original article) has been demonstrated by other investigators using para-aminohippuric acid clearance[1,2] or the xenon washout technique.[3]

An important finding in this study is the alteration in glomerular structure with aging that lowers the K_f at the level of individual, patent glomeruli. This is a consequence of a decline in both filtration surface density and hydraulic permeability (see Table 2).

In conclusion, the authors propose that "a reduction in the size and capacity of the renocortical vascular bed and an ensuing glomerulopenia are more likely to account for the low RPF in aging humans than altered vasomotor tone."

S. Klahr, MD

References

1. Davies DF, Shock NW: Age changes in glomerular filtration rate, effective renal plasma flow, and tubular excretory capacity in adult males. *J Clin Invest* 29:496-507, 1950.
2. Wesson LG Jr: Renal hemodynamics in physiological states, in *Physiology of the Human Kidney.* New York, Grune and Stratton, 1969, pp 96-108.
3. Hollenberg NK, Adams DF, Solomon HS, et al: Senescence and the renal vasculature in normal man. *Circ Res* 34:309-316, 1974.

C1q Nephropathy: A Variant of Focal Segmental Glomerulosclerosis
Markowitz GS, Schwimmer JA, Stokes MB, et al (Columbia Univ, New York)
Kidney Int 64:1232-1240, 2003
31–5

Background.—C1q nephropathy, an entity with distinctive immuno-pathologic features, is poorly understood. A large case series was reported to better define the clinical-pathologic spectrum of C1q nephropathy.

Methods.—Among 8909 native kidney biopsies performed between 1994 and 2002, 19 (0.21%) biopsies were identified as having C1q nephropathy. The defining criteria were dominant or codominant immunofluorescence staining for C1q, mesangial electron dense deposits, and no clinical or serologic evidence of systemic lupus erythematosus (SLE).

Findings.—African Americans comprised 74% percent of the patients, and 74% were female. Patients were from 3 to 42 years old (mean, 24.2 years). Initial evaluation revealed nephritic range proteinuria in 78.9% of the patients, nephritic syndrome in 50%, renal insufficiency in 27.8%, and hematuria in 22.2%. None of the patients had hypocomplementemia or evidence of underlying autoimmune or infectious disorders. Renal biopsy demonstrated focal segmental glomerulosclerosis (FSGS) in 17 patients and minimal-change disease (MCD) in 2. Codeposits of IgG were documented in all biopsies, with IgM in 84.2%, IgA in 31.6%, and C3 in 52.6%. Foot process effacement ranged from 20% to 100%. Of 16 patients with available follow-up data, 12 (75%) received immunosuppressive treatment. Proteinuria remission was complete in 1 patient and was partial in 6. Four patients with FSGS pattern had progressive renal insufficiency, including 2 progressing to endstage renal disease. The median length of time between biopsy and end-stage disease was 81 months. In a multivariate analysis, the degree of tubular atrophy and interstitial fibrosis were the strongest correlates of renal insufficiency at biopsy and follow-up.

Conclusions.—C1q nephropathy is within the clinicopathologic spectrum of MCD-FSGS. C1q deposition may be a nonspecific marker of increased mesangial trafficking in patients with glomerular proteinuria. Further research is needed to determine the pathologic mechanism of C1q deposition.

▶ In their initial description of C1q nephropathy, Jennette and Hipp[1] described a wide spectrum of pathologic findings. Microscopic evaluations were available in 13 cases and revealed no significant glomerular abnormality (2 cases), mesangial proliferation (3 cases), focal proliferative glomerulonephritis (5 cases), and diffuse proliferative glomerulonephritis (3 cases).

All cases stained positively by immunofluorescence for C1q with a mean intensity of 3.6 (range, 0.5-4). In this study from Columbia Presbyterian Medical Center from 1994 to 2002, 8909 renal biopsies were reviewed retrospectively for the diagnosis of C1q nephropathy. This entity was defined by (1) the presence of mesangial immune deposits that stain for C1q; (2) corresponding mesangial electron dense deposits by electron microscopy; (3) negative antinuclear antibody (ANA); and (4) absence of clinical evidence of systemic lupus erythematosus (SLE). The authors reviewed 17 cases of C1q nephropathy.

This study suggests that C1q nephropathy falls within the clinical-pathologic spectrum of FSGS and MCD. Similar to primary FSGS, it is an idiopathic condition most common in young adults and children, and exhibits an African American racial predominance. Patients present with heavy proteinuria, often accompanied by the nephrotic syndrome, in the absence of systemic disease or hypocomplementemia. Although mesangial hypercellularity is common, the histologic manifestations are predominantly those of FSGS, including collapsing and cellular variants.

Additional studies are needed to determine the specificity and pathologic mechanisms of C1q deposition in this condition and to define optimal therapy.

S. Klahr, MD

Reference

1. Jennette JC, Hipp CG: C1q nephropathy: A distinct pathologic entity usually causing nephrotic syndrome. *Am J Kidney Dis* 6:103-110, 1985.

32 Other Diseases of the Kidney

Introduction

Morii et al (Abstract 32–1) suggested that heavy proteinuria itself might contribute to renal tubular damage by increasing the expression of monocyte chemoattractant protein-1 (MCP-1) in renal tubuli and consequently accelerate the progression of diabetic nephropathy.

Nephropathy due to contrast medium remains one of the most clinically important complications of the use of iodinated contrast medium. A report by Aspelin and colleagues (Abstract 32–2) is a randomized, prospective, double-blind, multicenter study comparing the nephrotoxicity of iodixanol with that of iohexol in patients with stable diabetes mellitus and impaired kidney function who underwent coronary or aortofemoral angiography.

McCreath et al (Abstract 32–3) show the retrospective evidence that port access mitral valve surgery is associated with less acute renal injury than conventional techniques. Findings suggest that a port access approach to mitral valve surgery may be indicated for patients at high risk of perioperative acute renal dysfunction.

Magistroni et al (Abstract 32–4) demonstrate significant renal disease variability among the patients with the same *PKD2* mutations. Within individual families, the authors observed elderly patients with very mild renal disease and younger patients with end-stage renal disease.

Markowitz et al (Abstract 32–5) ascertain that tubular renal injury may occur after the administration of drugs or diagnostic agents such as amphotericin B, cisplatin, the aminoglycoside antibiotics, and radiocontrast agents. The pathology in these cases reveals widespread tubular degenerative changes in the absence of glomerular pathology, interstitial nephritis, or vascular disease.

In a study by Perkins et al (Abstract 32–6), lower levels of glycosylated hemoglobin (less than 8%), a low systolic blood pressure (less than 115 mm Hg), and low levels of cholesterol and triglycerides (less than 198 mg/dL and 145 mg/dL, respectively) were independently associated with regression of microalbuminuria.

Han et al (Abstract 32–7) reviewed outpatient charts of all patients with a diagnosis of antineutrophil cytoplasmic autoantibody (ANCA)–associated vasculitis that were followed serially at Massachusetts General Hospital between January 1, 1990, and February 1, 2001. The most important question arising from the study is whether preemptive treatment of patients for ANCA titer rises during remission provides more benefit—by preventing relapses—than harm as a result of undesirable side effects of immunosuppression.

Wolf et al (Abstract 32–8) have focused on the mechanisms involved in the hypertrophic effect of angiotensin on proximal tubular cells. Angiotensin II induces the protein expression of $p27^{Kip1}$ in proximal tubular cells in vitro and in vivo.

Approximately 500,000 Americans suffer yearly from kidney stones. The estimated cost for treatment exceeds $4 million per 1000 patients treated per year.

Kramer et al (Abstract 32–9) used data from a cohort of 51,529 male health care professionals to investigate prospectively the independent association between gout and incident kidney stones.

A study by Zhang et al (Abstract 32–10) shows that diabetic nephropathy can develop rapidly in patients with specific baseline patterns despite good metabolic control. By contrast, patients with type 1 diabetes who have poor metabolic control can remain free from the complication for a long time, depending on their demographic and clinical status at baseline.

Wei et al (Abstract 32–11) show in their study that angiotensin-converting enzyme inhibition before the onset of severe kidney insufficiency offers major renoprotective benefits.

The main observation of a study by Langston et al (Abstract 32–12) is that a decreased hematocrit and chronic kidney disease are usually frequent among elderly patients with a myocardial infarction admitted to community hospitals and are independently associated with increased mortality after discharge.

In a study from Italy by Marenzi et al (Abstract 32–13), 114 consecutive patients with chronic renal failure who were to have coronary angiography or an elective percutaneous coronary intervention were studied between January 1, 2000, and October 31, 2001. It appears that prophylactic hemofiltration in the ICU appears to be an effective and safe strategy for the prevention of contrast-agent–induced acute renal dysfunction in patients who are undergoing percutaneous coronary interventions.

The aim of the study by Pozzi et al from Italy (Abstract 32–14) was to investigate the pathological and clinical correlates of light chain deposition disease (LCDD) systematically, focusing on their impact on renal disease and patient prognosis.

Saulo Klahr, MD

Association of Monocyte Chemoattractant Protein-1 With Renal Tubular Damage in Diabetic Nephropathy

Morii T, Fujita H, Narita T, et al (Akita Univ, Japan)
J Diabetes Complications 17:11-15, 2003

32–1

Background.—The increased excretion of protein in the urine appears to aggravate lesions of the renal tubulointerstitium and accelerate the progression of diabetic nephropathy. Monocyte chemoattractant protein-1 (MCP-1) mediates inflammation of the renal interstitium, tubular atrophy, and interstitial fibrosis, recruiting monocytes/macrophages into the renal tubulointerstitium. MCP-1 expression is increased when there is increased leakage of plasma protein from glomerular capillaries into tubular fluid. An overload of protein in the renal tubular cells upregulates the MCP-1 gene and its protein expression; the increased expression of MCP-1 in renal tubules may produce further damage to the renal tubules and accelerate the progression of diabetic nephropathy. To obtain information on the urinary MCP-1 levels in patients with diabetic nephropathy without the use of an enzyme-linked immunosorbent assay (ELISA), an immunoradiometric assay (IRMA) was developed to provide measures of urinary excretion levels of MCP-1 in type II diabetic patients in various stages of nephropathy. The contribution of MCP-1 to renal tubular damage in patients with diabetic nephropathy was assessed.

Methods.—The levels of MCP-1 and a sensitive marker of renal tubular damage, specifically, N-acetylglucosaminidase (NAG), excreted in the urine were measured in patients with type II diabetes, 29 of whom had normoalbuminuria, 25, microalbuminuria, and 18, macroalbuminuria.

Results.—The prevalence of hypertension was increased in patients with microalbuminuria and macroalbuminuria compared with that of patients with normoalbuminuria. Serum levels of creatinine in the macroalbuminuria group were significantly higher than those found in the other 2 groups. All patients had very low serum MCP-1 levels, below the detection limit of the IRMA. The median urinary excretion levels of MCP-1 for the groups were 159.6 ng/g creatinine for the normoalbuminuria group, 193.9 ng/g for the microalbuminuria group, and 394.4 ng/g for the macroalbuminuria group (Fig 1). Significant correlations were noted between urinary excretion levels of MCP-1 and albumin levels and between urinary excretion of MCP-1 and NAG levels in all participants.

Conclusions.—All MCP-1 levels were very low as determined by IRMA. The urinary excretion levels of MCP-1 were significantly increased in the macroalbuminuria group compared to that of the other 2 groups. In addition, urinary MCP-1 levels were notably higher than serum MCP-1 levels in patients who had established diabetic nephropathy, indicating that the increased urinary excretion of MCP-1 most likely results from an enhanced production of MCP-1 in the renal tubules, probably because of excessive exposure to plasma protein filtered from the damaged glomeruli. Thus, heavy

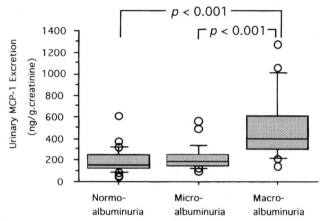

FIGURE 1.—Urinary MCP-1 excretion in three patient groups with normoalbuminuria, microalbuminuria, and macroalbuminuria. (Courtesy of Morii T, Fujita H, Narita T, et al: Association of monocyte chemoattractant protein-1 with renal tubular damage in diabetic nephropathy. *J Diabetes Complications* 17:11-15, 2003.)

proteinuria contributes to renal tubular damage by increasing the expression of MCP-1 and accelerating the progression of diabetic nephropathy.

▶ Proteinuria is an independent mediator in the progression of renal disease. Diabetic nephropathy is characterized histologically by glomerular changes, such as capillary basement membrane thickening and mesangium expansion. An increase in urinary protein excretion seems to aggravate renal tubulointerstitial lesions and accelerates the progression of nephropathy.

MCP-1 is produced by mesangial cells and tubular epithelial cells. MCP-1 plays an important role in the recruitment of monocytes-macrophages into the tubulointerstitium and is a mediator of renal interstitial inflammation tubular atrophy, and interstitial fibrosis. Morii et al suggested that increased expression of MCP-1 in tubules may increase the leakage of plasma protein from glomerular capillary to tubular fluid and may contribute to the progression of diabetic nephropathy.

The authors recruited 29 patients without diabetes, 25 patients with incipient diabetic nephropathy and 18 patients with established diabetic nephropathy. As depicted in Fig 1, the patients with a greater excretion of MCP-1 in the urine had more macroalbuminuria. The authors suggested that heavy proteinuria itself may contribute to renal tubular damage by increasing the expression of MCP-1 in renal tubuli and consequently accelerate the progression of diabetic nephropathy.

S. Klahr, MD

Nephrotoxic Effects in High-Risk Patients Undergoing Angiography
Aspelin P, for the NEPHRIC Study Investigators (Huddinge Univ Hosp, Stockholm; et al)
N Engl J Med 348:491-499, 2003   32–2

Background.—In less than 2% of cases in the general population, nephropathy may result from the use of low-osmolar contrast medium. However, among patients with renal impairment and diabetes, the risk is increased, leading to a significantly higher incidence—specifically, 12% to 50% of cases. Iodixanol is a nonionic dimeric contrast medium that is iso-osmolar to blood at all concentrations and has a lower level of general toxicity than other low-osmolar contrast media. Its nephrotoxicity in high-risk patients was investigated.

Methods.—A randomized, double-blind, prospective, multicenter trial was conducted on 129 patients to compare the nephrotoxic effects of iodixanol (64 patients) to those of iohexol (65 patients), a low-osmolar, nonionic, monomeric contrast medium. The 129 patients studied had diabetes, with serum creatinine concentrations of 1.5 to 3.5 mg/dL; all were undergoing either coronary or aortofemoral angiography. The investigation was continued to the primary end point of the peak increase in creatinine concentration from baseline during the 3 days after the angiography. Increases in creatinine concentration from 0.5 mg/dL to 1.0 mg/dL or more, and the total change in creatinine concentration from initiation until day 7 were also determined.

Results.—Patients who received iodixanol had significantly lower creatinine concentration increases than those who received iohexol. The mean peak increase in creatinine from day 0 to 3 was 0.13 mg/dL among those receiving iodixanol and 0.55 mg/dL among those receiving iohexol. Only 3% of the iodixanol patients had creatinine concentration increases of 0.5 mg/dL or greater, whereas this level occurred in 26% of those receiving iohexol. Ten iohexol patients had increases of 1.0 mg/dL in creatinine concentration, but no patients receiving iodixanol reached this level. For the iodixanol group the mean change in creatinine concentration from day 0 to 7 was 0.07 mg/dL; for the iohexol group the change was 0.24 mg/dL.

Conclusions.—The increase in creatinine concentration was significantly less when patients received iodixanol than when they were given iohexol. A significantly lower peak increase in serum creatinine concentration occurred during days 0 to 3 with the use of iodixanol, and a significant difference was also noted at day 7. The odds of nephrotoxicity were 11 times higher with iohexol than with iodixanol. No iodixanol patients experienced an increase of serum creatinine concentration of 1.0 mg/dL or more, whereas 15% of those in the iohexol group did.

▶ Nephropathy due to contrast medium remains one of the most clinically important complications of the use of iodinated contrast medium. The incidence of nephropathy induced by low-osmolar contrast medium is low in the general population and has been calculated to be less than 2%. Patients at increased risk include those with impaired kidney function and those with diabetes. In such patients, the incidence is significantly higher—in the range of 12% to 50%. Several clinical studies and meta-analyses have indicated that the use of low-osmolar contrast medium substantially reduces the risk of nephropathy in high-risk patients as compared with the risk resulting from the use of high-osmolar contrast medium.

A randomized prospective, double blind, multicenter study compared the nephrotoxicity of iodixanol with that of iohexol in patients with stable diabetes mellitus and impaired kidney function who underwent coronary or aortofemoral angiography. The study included 17 centers in 5 European countries (Denmark, France, Germany, Spain, and Sweden). It was designed to compare the renal effects of a nonionic, iso-osmolar, dimeric contrast medium iodixanol (320 mg of iodine/mL with 290 mOsm per kg of water), with those of the nonionic, low-osmolar, monomeric contrast medium iohexol (350 mg of iodine/mL with 780 mOsm per kg of water).

This study found that the use of iodixanol resulted in a significantly smaller increase in the serum creatinine concentration than did the use of iohexol. The peak increase in the serum creatinine concentration between day 0 and day 3 was significantly lower in the iodixanol group than in the iohexol group. The difference was also significant at day 7. An increase in the serum creatinine concentration of 1.0 mg/dL did not occur in any of the patients in the iodixanol group but did occur in 15% of the patients receiving iohexol.

S. Klahr, MD

Mitral Valve Surgery and Acute Renal Injury: Port Access Versus Median Sternotomy
McCreath BJ, Swaminathan M, Booth JV, et al (Duke Univ, Durham, NC)
Ann Thorac Surg 75:812-819, 2003   32–3

Background.—Patients who undergo cardiac surgery and then develop acute renal dysfunction, seen in 7% of cases, face increased risks for morbidity, mortality, and higher costs. Minimally invasive cardiac surgery and minimally invasive cardiopulmonary bypass systems have been developed to reduce risks and improve outcomes. Whether the minithoracotomy port access technique (Port) used in mitral valve surgery is associated with acute perioperative renal injury (as well as the degree of injury) was assessed in comparison with conventional surgery with median sternotomy (MS) incisions.

Methods.—Data were collected and retrospectively reviewed from all of the isolated mitral valve operations performed between 1990 and 2000 by a single surgeon, yielding 90 MS patients and 227 Port patients. A secondary assessment was carried out for all mitral valve surgeries done by MS or Port approaches from 1996 to 2002; these latter covered 93 MS and 240 Port patients. Statistical analysis focused on relationships between surgical technique and peak postoperative creatinine ($Cr_{max}Post$) and peak postoperative fractional change in creatinine (%ΔCr), with a *P* value under .05 deemed significant.

Results.—The serum creatinine and estimated creatinine clearance values were similar in all groups, but postoperatively the Port and MS patients differed significantly with respect to Cr_{max}Post, ΔCr, and %ΔCr. Surgical approach and %ΔCr were highly significantly correlated, showing that MS surgery is associated with a higher risk of acute renal injury. The date of surgery did not significantly predict %ΔCr. With the use of the time-concurrent analysis of %ΔCr, MS surgery again was shown to be highly significantly associated with a greater risk of acute renal injury. Major adverse outcomes were also more frequently seen with MS surgery.

Conclusion.—The retrospective review of data collected for Port and conventional surgery showed that acute renal injury was more likely when MS was performed. MS also was linked to a higher incidence of major adverse outcomes than the Port approach to mitral valve surgery. Thus, patients at high risk for perioperative acute renal dysfunction should undergo Port rather than median sternotomy.

▶ Acute renal dysfunction after cardiac surgery is associated with marked increases in morbidity, mortality, and cost. The incidence of this postoperative complication exceeds 7%, and renal replacement therapy is necessary in 1% to 2% of patients. Despite advances in dialytic technology, the mortality rate for patients requiring dialysis after cardiac surgery is greater than 60%. Even minor kidney injury reflected by a serum creatinine rise that never exceeds the normal range is linked to adverse outcomes. In the absence of effective pharmacologic interventions to prevent or treat acute renal injury, it is vital to minimize the risk of sustaining kidney damage during cardiac surgery.

The authors tested the hypothesis that mitral valve surgery with Port and conventional surgery with an MS incision are associated with different degrees of acute renal injury. A total of 333 patients met the defined selection criteria. Demographic and renal function data were collected for all patients with femoral artery cannulation (patient group PortFem) (n = 81), ascending aorta (PortA) (n = 146), and MS (n = 90) during this study.

Postoperative serum creatinine and estimated creatinine clearance were similar between patients groups. However, postoperative markers of renal function were significantly different between Port and MS patients with regard to Cr_{max}Post (104.3 ± 36.3 vs 127.2 ± 84.0 µmol/L; *P* = .02), ΔCr (15.4 ± 25.3 vs 33.6± 67.8 µmol/L; *P* = .02), and %ΔCr (18.5 ± 28.8 vs 35.4% ± 58.3%; *P* = .01).

A total of 333 patients underwent isolated mitral valve surgery between May 1996 and March 2002. Eight surgeons performed 93 MS surgeries and 240 Port procedures for mitral valve repair.

This study presents retrospective evidence suggesting that Port is associated with less perioperative acute renal injury than conventional techniques. In the absence of prospective randomized trials, this is the first comparison of perioperative organ injury between unselected patient cohorts undergoing mitral valve surgery by Port and traditional surgical techniques. In addition, we have confirmed the association of previously known perioperative variables with the development of acute renal injury after mitral valve surgery. The technical feasibility of Port has been well established, but our data suggesting that this surgical approach is associated with reduced renal risk relative to traditional techniques require prospective validation.

The retrospective evidence that Port is associated with less acute renal injury than conventional techniques. A trend toward reduced major adverse outcomes was also observed. The findings suggest that a Port approach to mitral valve surgery may be indicated for patients at high risk of perioperative acute renal dysfunction.

S. Klahr, MD

Genotype-Renal Function Correlation in Type 2 Autosomal Dominant Polycystic Kidney Disease

Magistroni R, He N, Wang K, et al (Univ Health Network, Toronto; Univ of Colorado, Denver; Mem Univ, St John's, Newfoundland, Canada; et al)
J Am Soc Nephrol 14:1164-1174, 2003   32–4

Background.—Autosomal dominant polycystic kidney disease (ADPKD) occurs in about 1 in 1000 live births and is found in 5% to 8% of cases of end-stage renal disease (ESRD). Cases are associated with mutations in 2 genes, with 80% to 85% involving mutations of the *PKD1* gene and 10% to 15% mutations of the *PKD2* gene. The degree of renal disease varies significantly both within and between families. For example, *PKD1* families generally have a significantly earlier onset of ESRD than those with *PKD2*-type mutations. It has been suggested that allelic heterogeneity may influence the severity of the renal disease. The correlation between genotype and renal function was evaluated in 461 individuals from 71 ADPKD families who had known germline *PKD2* mutations.

Methods.—An analysis was carried out of the clinical and genetic data for the 461 individuals. The 50 different mutations identified ranged from exon 1 to 14 of *PKD2*. The renal disease outcomes were ESRD—defined as severe chronic renal failure with serum creatinine values of 500 μM or the requirement of renal replacement therapy—and chronic renal failure (CRF)—defined as moderately severe chronic renal failure having a calculated creatinine clearance of 50 mL/min/1.73m² or less.

Results.—ESRD was found in 117 patients; 47 patients died without ESRD (Fig 1). Sixty-five patients had CRF, but 232 had neither CRF nor ESRD at final follow-up. ESRD and CRF developed later among female patients than among male patients. The age of onset of ESRD did not correlate with the location of *PKD2* mutations, but patients with splice site mutations tended to have milder forms of disease than those who had mutations at other sites. Renal disease characteristics were extremely variable among the affected individuals with the same mutations of the *PKD2* gene.

Conclusion.—The correlation of genotype with renal function was evaluated in families with known mutations of the *PKD2* gene and revealed that there was a late age of onset of ESRD and CRF and gender disparity in renal

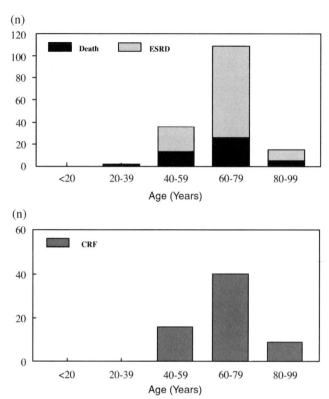

FIGURE 1.—Frequency distribution of age at onset of end stage renal disease (*ESRD*), death (without ESRD), and chronic renal failure (*CRF*) in the study patients. Typical of type 2 autosomal dominant polycystic kidney disease, the mode of distribution of these events occurred at a relatively late age (age range, 60-79 years). However, considerable renal disease variability (age range of onset of ESRD, 40-88 years) was also evident between individual patients. (Courtesy of Magistroni R, He N, Wang K, et al: Genotype-renal function correlation in type 2 autosomal dominant polycystic kidney disease. *J Am Soc Nephrol* 14:1164-1174, 2003.)

disease severity among the individuals studied. The mutations were found between exons 1 and 14 and covered the entire spectrum of *PKD2* mutations known currently. Significant variability in the clinical manifestations of renal disease were noted among patients with the same *PKD2* mutations.

▶ ADPKD is caused by an abnormality on the short arm of chromosome 16 in about 85% of the classic form of the disease. A gene on chromosome 4 accounts for the remaining cases (15%; ARPKD2). This entity accounts for 5% to 8% of ESRD. Polycystin 1 and 2, the gene products of PKD1 and PKD2, are transmembrane proteins that share sequence homology and are currently thought to be part of novel signaling pathways that regulate intracellular calcium.

This study encompasses 461 individuals affected by the disease from 71 ADPKD families. The *PKD2* mutations in 50 families have been previously described. The diagnosis of ADPKD in the patients and at risk individuals from each study was established using US-based criteria. The authors analyzed the clinical and genetic data of 461 ADPKD subjects (44.2% male and 55.8% female). Overall, 117 of these affected individuals (25.4%) had ESRD; 47 died without ESRD (10.2%) (see Fig 1).

This study demonstrates significant renal disease variability among the patients with the same *PKD2* mutations. Within individual families, the authors observed elderly patients with very mild renal disease and younger patients with ESRD. This is consistent with the finding of significant renal disease variability within families with *PKD1* linkage and among patients with the same *PKD1* mutations. Several population-based studies have examined the polymorphic variants of the angiotensin-converting enzyme and endothelial nitric oxide synthase genes as modifiers of renal disease progression in ADPKD. New studies will be required to dissect the individual components of this modifier effect.

S. Klahr, MD

Toxic Acute Tubular Necrosis Following Treatment With Zoledronate (Zometa)
Markowitz GS, Fine PL, Stack JI, et al (Columbia College of Physicians & Surgeons, New York; Morristown Mem Hosp, NJ; Community Med Ctr, East Toms River, NJ)
Kidney Int 64:281-289, 2003   32–5

Background.—Renal failure and toxic acute tubular necrosis may occur after exposure to a variety of therapeutic or diagnostic agents. Zoledronate is a new, powerful biphosphonate used in the treatment of hypercalcemia of malignancy. Deterioration in renal function is a poorly characterized complication of treatment with zoledronate. The first clinical-pathologic study of nephrotoxicity associated with zoledronate was reported.

Methods.—The study group consisted of 6 patients (4 men and 2 women) with a mean age of 69.2 years. Five patients received bisphosphonate therapy for multiple myeloma, and one patient received the same therapy for Paget disease. Zoledronate was administered to all patients at a dose of 4 mg IV monthly, infused over at least 15 minutes. The mean duration of therapy was 4.7 months, with a range of 3 to 9 months.

Results.—Renal failure developed in all patients, with an increase in serum creatinine from a mean baseline level of 1.4 mg/dL to 3.4 mg/dL. Renal biopsy revealed the presence of toxic acute tubular necrosis, which was characterized by tubular cell degeneration, loss of brush border, and apoptosis. Immunohistochemical staining showed a significant increase in cell cycle–engaged cells (Ki-67 positive) and derangement in tubular Na^+,K^+-ATPase expression. All the patients had been treated with pamidronate before zoledronate therapy, but none of the biopsy specimens demonstrated the characteristic pattern of collapsing focal segmental glomerulosclerosis seen in pamidronate nephrotoxicity. After renal biopsy, treatment with zoledronate was discontinued. All the patients experienced an improvement in renal function, with a mean final serum creatinine of 2.3 mg/dL at 1 to 4 months of follow-up.

Conclusions.—The close temporal relationship between zoledronate administration and the onset of renal failure, and the partial recovery of renal function after withdrawal of zoledronate strongly suggest a role for this drug in the development of toxic acute tubular necrosis.

▶ Tubular renal injury may occur after the administration of drugs or diagnostic agents such as amphotericin B, cisplatin, the aminoglycoside antibiotics, and radiocontrast agents. The pathology in these cases reveals widespread tubular degenerative changes in the absence of glomerular pathology, interstitial nephritis, or vascular disease.

Zoledronate is a new, potent bisphosphonate that is used for the treatment of hypercalcemia of malignancy. Markowitz et al reported the occurrence of renal failure secondary to toxic acute tubular necrosis after treatment with zoledronate. The clinical features of 6 patients with kidney failure after treatment with zoledronate are shown in Table 1 (see original article).

The course of renal failure after treatment with zoledronate was primarily subacute, occurring over a period of months. Although the mean duration of zoledronate therapy before the development of renal failure was 4.7 months, this constituted a mean of only 4.7 administration, since the drug is given once per month. A small increase in serum creatinine level was noted as early as 1 month in patient 4 (from 1.4 to 1.6 mg/dL) and in patient 6 (from 1.0 to 1.4 mg/dL).

Proteinuria was noted in these patients. The authors suspected that proximal tubular dysfunction might be the source of the proteinuria.

It is known that after reaching the systemic circulation, zoledronate is predominantly excreted unchanged via the kidneys. Renal clearance of bisphosphonates exceeds glomerular filtration rate, indicating active renal transport and secretion.

Thus, the list of etiologies of renal failure in patients with multiple myeloma should include zoledronate-associated acute tubular necrosis.

S. Klahr, MD

Regression of Microalbuminuria in Type 1 Diabetes
Perkins BA, Ficociello LH, Silva KH, et al (Joslin Diabetes Ctr, Boston; Harvard Med School, Boston; Massachusetts Gen Hosp Biostatistics Ctr, Boston; et al)
N Engl J Med 348:2285-2293, 2003   32–6

Background.—Three landmark studies in the early 1980s suggested an ominous prognosis for patients with type 1 diabetes with minute elevations of urinary albumin excretion, or microalbuminuria. It was posited that microalbuminuria conferred a 60% to 85% risk of the development of overt proteinuria within 6 to 14 years. In this model of diabetic nephropathy, microalbuminuria in type 1 diabetes signaled an inexorable progression to overt proteinuria. The frequency of a significant reduction in urinary albumin excretion in patients with type 1 diabetes and microalbuminuria, and factors affecting this reduction were determined.

Methods.—Included in the study were 386 patients with type 1 diabetes and persistent microalbuminuria, as indicated by repeated measurements of urinary albumin excretion in the range of 30 to 299 µg/min during an initial 2-year evaluation period. Subsequent measurements were grouped into 2-year periods during the next 6 years. These measurements were averaged and analyzed for regression of microalbuminuria, which was defined as a 50% reduction in urinary albumin excretion from one 2-year period to the next.

Results.—There was frequent regression of microalbuminuria, with a 6-year cumulative incidence of 58%. The use of angiotensin-converting enzyme (ACE) inhibitors was not associated with the regression of microalbuminuria. However, short-duration microalbuminuria, salutary levels of glycosylated hemoglobin (<8%), low systolic blood pressure (<115 mm Hg), low cholesterol levels (<198 mg/dL), and low triglyceride levels (<145 mg/dL) were independently associated with the regression of microalbuminuria. The hazard ratio for regression in patients with salutary levels of all modifiable factors was 3.0, compared with patients with no salutary levels of any modifiable factor.

Conclusions.—The frequent regression of microalbuminuria in patients with type 1 diabetes indicates that microalbuminuria is more likely to subside to normal levels than to progress to overt proteinuria. Thus, the evolution of early diabetic nephropathy may not be confined to a single pathway leading to progression to proteinuria.

▶ Microalbuminuria in patients with type 1 diabetes has been considered the first sign toward progression to proteinuria and renal failure. Persistent elevation of albumin in the urine above 30 µg/min is rare in the general population. However, in patients with type 1 diabetes, the lifetime risk of such elevation is about 60%. Early studies of microalbuminuria indicated that the risk of a progressive increase in albumin excretion to overt proteinuria within 6 to 14 years was 60% to 85%.

It has been shown that the use of ACE inhibitors retards the increase of albumin excretion in short-term clinical trials. ACE inhibitors prevent the progression of microalbuminuria to proteinuria.

In the present study by Perkins et al, lower levels of glycosylated hemoglobin (less than 8%), a low systolic blood pressure (less than 115 mm Hg), and low levels of cholesterol and triglycerides (less than 198 mg/dL and 145 mg/dL, respectively) were independently associated with regression of microalbuminuria.

It can be hypothesized that a very low systemic blood pressure attenuates shear stress and permits the recovery of glomerular integrity. However, whether pharmacologic intervention that results in a very low systemic blood pressure is effective in reducing urinary albumin excretion remains to be determined.

Clinical trials that assess the optimal target level of albumin excretion as well as the optimal levels of other factors (blood pressure, glycosylated hemoglobin, use of ACE inhibitors) are warranted.

S. Klahr, MD

▶ The authors of this important and essentially encouraging article begin their Discussion by saying, "Microalbuminuria in patients with type 1 diabetes has been considered the first step toward proteinuria and renal failure, yet our results indicate that microalbuminuria is more likely to subside to normal levels than to progress to overt proteinuria." That microalbuminuria in type 1 diabetes is just as likely to regress than progress over a 4- to 6-year period is good news indeed, but whether it really means, as the authors imply, that previous views on the significance of microalbuminuria were incorrect is surely questionable. Microalbuminuria is the first step toward more serious renal damage and eventual renal failure—the fact that it may regress does not negate that view. Nor do the results of this observational study, in which patients were presumably receiving 1990s "standard of care" treatment, throw into question the findings and implications of the studies that originally established microalbuminuria as an early marker for diabetic nephropathy in type 1 diabetes.[1-3] My fear is that the emphasis put on the difference between their findings and those of earlier studies—and the "spin" that this yields possible new insights into pathophysiology rather than that it reflects the success of 1990s versus 1970s management—could lead the less-discerning reader to conclude that microalbuminuria is not as important as we have grown to believe. If so, that would have the opposite effect to what I am sure the authors intended.

This study confirms the importance of glycemic control and blood pressure as determinants of progression or regression of microalbuminuria. By the end of the study, approximately 50% of all the patients were on ACE-inhibitors and/or other antihypertensive drugs. These are unsurprising findings, though the implication that achieving a low systolic blood pressure may be more important than the class of antihypertensive used may be considered controversial. Perhaps the most interesting finding is the association between low levels of serum cholesterol and triglycerides and the regression of microalbuminuria, which, as the authors suggest, provides a rationale for pharmacologic intervention with lipid-lowering agents in type 1 diabetes even if overt dyslipidemia is not present—something that could be relatively easily tested in a prospective randomized study.

L. Kennedy, MD, FRCP

References

1. Viberti GC, Hill RD, Jarrett RJ, et al: Microalbuminuria as a predictor of clinical nephropathy in insulin-dependent diabetes mellitus. *Lancet* 1:430-432, 1982.
2. Parving H-H, Oxenbøll B, Svendsen PA, et al: Early detection of patients at risk of developing diabetic nephropathy: A longitudinal study of urinary albumin excretion. *Acta Endocrinologica (Copenh)* 100:550-555, 1982.
3. Mogensen CE, Christensen CK: Predicting diabetic nephropathy in insulin-dependent patients. *N Engl J Med* 311:89-93, 1984.

Serial ANCA Titers: Useful Tool for Prevention of Relapses in ANCA-Associated Vasculitis
Han WK, Choi HK, Roth RM, et al (Harvard Med School, Boston)
Kidney Int 63:1079-1085, 2003   32–7

Background.—Vasculidites can be associated with circulating antineutrophil cytoplasmic autoantibodies (ANCA), particularly antiproteinase-3 (PR3) and antimyeloperoxidase antibodies. Treatment of vasculitis requires aggressive immunosuppression with steroids in combination with other agents. This treatment is associated with toxic side effects. Therefore, as soon as remission is achieved, therapy is tapered, which is then followed by relapse. The usefulness of serial ANCA titers in assessing disease activity and guiding treatment was evaluated in this retrospective study of patients with ANCA-associated vasculitis.

Study Design.—The study group consisted of 48 patients who were diagnosed with ANCA-associated vasculitis and followed serially from January 1990 to February 2001 (Table 1). Patients had ANCA tests and titers performed at 2- to 3-month intervals. Titers were compared with the lowest level after immunosuppression and a 4-fold increase was considered as necessitating a change in treatment. Disease activity was scored with the Disease-Specific Activity Index for Wegener's Granulomatosis: Modification of the Birmingham Vasculitis Activity Score. Those who experienced 4-fold titer increases without increased immunosuppression (group 1) were compared with those who received increased immunosuppression (group 2).

Findings.—Of the 48 patients with ANCA-associated vasculitis, 17 went into complete remission after initial immunosuppressive therapy. Among these 17 patients, there were 21 episodes of at least 4-fold increases in ANCA titers. Among those who did not receive increased immunosuppressive therapy (group 1), all had relapses after each episode. Among group 2 patients who did receive increased immunosuppressive therapy, only 2 relapses occurred. This difference was highly significant. For the other 31 patients, changes in ANCA titers were used to govern changes in immunosuppressive therapy. The overall outcome in the entire group of 48 patients was favor-

TABLE 1.—Characteristics of the 48 Patients in the Study

Gender *M/F*	25/23
PR3/MPO-ANCA	27/21
Mean age	60.4 ± 18.2
Mean follow-up *months*	46.4 ± 29.1
Mean CrCl at diagnosis *mL/min*	67.3 ± 38.9
Mean BVAS/WG at entry	6.0 (range, 2 to 12)
Mean interveral between ANCA tests *months*	2.3 ± 0.8

Abbreviations: CrCl, plasma creatinine clearance estimated by (140 − age)/creatinine; *PR3-ANCA*, antineutrophil cytoplasmic antibodies against proteinase 3; *MPO-ANCA*, antineutrophil cytoplasmic antibodies against myeloperoxidase; *BVAS/WG*, Birmingham Vasculitis Acitivity Score for Wegener's Granulomatosis.
(Courtesy of Han WK, Choi HK, Roth RM, et al: Serial ANCA Titers: Useful tool for prevention of relapses in ANCA-associated vasculitis. *Kidney Int* 63:1079-1085, 2003. Reprinted by permission of Blackwell Publishing.)

able, with 46 alive at the end of the study. Two patients died of unrelated causes.

Conclusions.—This retrospective study examined the use of serial ANCA titers to assist in the management of ANCA-associated vasculitis. This study indicates that the benefits of preemptive immunosuppressive therapy appear to outweigh the risks. A prospective randomized trial is necessary to confirm these results.

▶ Wegener's granulomatosis, microscopic polyangiitis, and polyarteritis nodosa are the systemic vasculitides, which are frequently managed by nephrologists. They are members of a spectrum of clinical syndromes. The site and size of blood vessels involved, as well as the presence or absence of either accompanying granulomata or aneurysms classified them morphologically. Only 2 types of ANCA, PR3 and antimyeloperoxidase antibodies, account for this association and they are highly specific markers for these vasculitides.

In this study by Han et al, the authors reviewed the outpatients charts of all patients with a diagnosis of ANCA-associated vasculitis who were followed serially at the Massachusetts General Hospital between January 1, 1990, and February 1, 2001. Only patients who had entered remission after induction of immunosuppression were included. Forty-eight patients met the criteria and were monitored for a mean of 46.2 months, with ANCA titers determined at intervals on average of 2 to 3 months. The course of the disease in the 48 patients was evaluated, using measurements of relapses, progression to end-stage renal disease, death, and complications. Table 1 depicts the characteristics of the 48 patients in the study.

The present study confirms and extends several reports that describe the value of PR3-ANCA titer rises in predicting relapses.

The most important question arising from the study is whether preemptive treatment of patients for ANCA titer rises during remission provides more benefit, by preventing relapses, than harm, as a result of undesirable side effects of immunosuppression. The authors propose that the benefits of preemptive increased immunosuppressive treatment largely outweigh the risks. The evidence for this conclusion should be evaluated in a prospective randomized trial.

S. Klahr, MD

Angiotensin II-Induced Hypertrophy of Proximal Tubular Cells Requires p27[Kip1]
Wolf G, Jablonski K, Schroeder R, et al (Univ of Hamburg, Germany; Univ of Washington, Seattle)
Kidney Int 64:71-81, 2003   32–8

Background.—These authors and others have previously shown that angiotensin II (Ang II) stimulates hypertrophy of cultured proximal tubules. This hypertrophy is associated with posttranscriptional induction of the cyclin-dependent kinase (CDK) inhibitor p27[Kip1]. To understand the role of

$p27^{Kip1}$ in Ang II-induced hypertrophy, proximal tubular cell cultures were established from wild-type and from $p27^{Kip1}$ $-/-$ mice.

Methods.—Proximal tubule cell cultures were established from $p27^{Kip1}$ $+/+$ and $-/-$ mice. Western blotting was used to detect $p27^{Kip1}$ and Ang II protein expression. An inducible vector system was set up to reconstitute $p27^{Kip1}$ expression. Cell proliferation and hypertrophy were analyzed.

Results.—Incubation of proximal tubular cell cultures with Ang II induced cell cycle arrest and hypertrophy of wild-type cells. In $p27^{Kip1}$ $-/-$ cell cultures, Ang II facilitated cell cycle progression without inducing hypertrophy. The hypertrophic phenotype could be restored by reconstituting the $p27^{Kip1}$ expression using an inducible expression system. Ang II did not induce apoptosis in either wild-type or knockout cell lines.

Conclusions.—A culture of $p27^{Kip1}$ knockout proximal tubule cells was used to demonstrate that $p27^{Kip1}$ is required for Ang II-mediated hypertrophy.

▶ Several investigators have demonstrated that Ang II induces hypertrophy of proximal tubular cells through activation of AT_1 receptors. In chronic renal diseases, hypertrophy of proximal tubules is an adaptive process to compensate for the loss of nephrons.

The authors of this study have focused on the mechanisms involved in the hypertrophic effect of angiotensin on proximal tubular cells. Ang II induces the protein expression of $p27^{Kip1}$ in proximal tubular cells in vitro and in vivo.

A functional role for $p27^{Kip1}$ in Ang II-induced hypertrophy has not completely been established. The availability of the p27 null mouse has overcome this problem. Treatment with Ang II causes cell cycle arrest and induces hypertrophy in primary cultures of $p27^{Kip1}$ $+/+$ proximal tubular cells.

These findings indicate that $p27^{Kip1}$ is required for Ang II-induced hypertrophy of proximal tubular cells. However, other factors induced by Ang II contribute to this hypertrophy.

Liu and Preisig[1] have demonstrated that cell cycle-dependent hypertrophy of tubules is not limited to the cell culture conditions. They reported that compensatory growth of proximal tubular cells induced in mice by uninephrectomy is hypertrophic and depends on downregulation of CDK2/cyclin as E kinase activity, whereas CDK4/cyclin D kinase remains activated.

Because local Ang II concentrations are enhanced in the remnant kidney, one may speculate that this peptide is induced as the likely mediator of cell arrest and compensatory tubular hypertrophy in vivo.

S. Klahr, MD

Reference

1. Liu B, Preisig PA: Compensatory renal hypertrophy is mediated by a cell cycle-dependent mechanism. *Kidney Int* 62:1650-1658, 2002.

The Association Between Gout and Nephrolithiasis in Men: The Health Professionals' Follow-up Study
Kramer HJ, Choi HK, Atkinson K, et al (Loyola Univ, Maywood, Ill; Massachusetts Gen Hosp, Boston; Harvard Med School, Boston; et al)
Kidney Int 64:1022-1026, 2003   32–9

Introduction.—Gout has been linked to kidney stone disease in several earlier trials. Data from a cohort of 51,529 male health care professionals participating in the Health Professionals' Follow-up (HPFS) Study were prospectively assessed to determine the independent relationship between gout and incident kidney stones.

Methods.—The age range of the HPFS cohort was 40 to 75 years in 1986. Data were gathered concerning diet, medical history, and medication use from questionnaires mailed biennially to HPFS participants. After as many as 6 mailings of the biennial questionnaire, the follow-up was above 90%. Data concerning gout and kidney stones were also gathered by the biennial questionnaires. Cases of gout were considered verified if participants reported 6 or more of 11 gout criteria. To verify the validity of self-report of kidney stones, the medical records were obtained from a random sample of 60 cases; kidney stone was verified in 97%.

Results.—In a cross-sectional analysis of gout and kidney stone disease reported on the 1986 baseline questionnaire, the prevalence of kidney stone disease was nearly 2-fold higher in men with than in those without a history of gout (15% vs 8%). After adjusting for age and body mass index, a history of gout remained significantly correlated with kidney stone disease (odds ratio, 1.88; 95% confidence interval [CI], 1.68-2.11). The risk of incident kidney stones was prospectively examined in men with and without verified gout after excluding men who reported a history of kidney stone disease in the baseline questionnaire. A verified diagnosis of gout increased the multivariate relative risk (RR) of incident kidney stones (RR, 2.12; 95% CI, 1.22-3.68). A history of kidney stone disease was not linked with increased risk of gout (RR, 1.05; 95% CI, 0.54-2.07).

Conclusion.—A history of gout independently increases the risk for incident kidney stones in men. Physicians should provide patients with gout with dietary counseling (including increased fluid intake and reduced salt consumption) and alert them to risk factors (including a family history of kidney stones) to diminish the likelihood of stone formation.

▶ Approximately 500,000 Americans suffer yearly from kidney stones. The estimated cost for treatment exceeds $4 million per 1000 patients treated per year. This study used data from a cohort of 51,529 male health care professionals to investigate prospectively the independent association between gout and incident kidney stones.

In this prospective study of men, a history of gout increased the risk of incident kidney stone disease by almost 2-fold, even after controlling several parameters such as age, dietary factors, body mass index, and thiazide. The authors noted no association between history of kidney stone disease and risk of incident gout. The authors suggest that no previous studies have prospectively investigated the association between gout and kidney stone disease.

Patients with gout usually have persistent acid urine due to a defect in the production of ammonia by the kidney. This may be inherent or secondary to damage of tubules due to urate crystal deposition. Gout may increase the risk for calcium oxalate stone formation, which is the most common of kidney stones. In this study, among 1258 patients with primary gout, 22% reported a history of kidney stones, which is higher than the 12% lifetime risk reported in the general population.

Among several limitations of this study is the lack of an association between kidney stone and risk of incident gout, which may have been because of the small number of incident gout cases among men with kidney stones diagnosed after 1986. This limits the power of this study to examine this association. Also due to the older age of the cohort, it is possible that the exclusion of patients who reported kidney stone disease or gout on the baseline 1986 questionnaire may have led to a selection bias. In conclusion, this study shows that men with gout have a 2-fold increased risk for developing incident kidney stones, compared with men without gout.

S. Klahr, MD

Factors Predictive of Nephropathy in DCCT Type 1 Diabetic Patients With Good or Poor Metabolic Control

Zhang L, Krzentowski G, Albert A, et al (Univ of Liège, Belgium; Univ Hosp of Charleroi, Belgium)
Diabetic Med 20:580-585, 2003
32–10

Introduction.—The Diabetes Control and Complications Trial (DCCT) reported a substantial reduction in the development and progression of diabetic neuropathy in intensively treated patients versus patients who received conventional therapy (mean HbA_{1c} level about 7% vs about 9%). The time-related risk of diabetic neuropathy (albumin excretion rate [AER] 40 mg/24 h or greater) from baseline covariates in patients with type 1 diabetes with either good or poor metabolic control (MC) was assessed.

Methods.—With the use of material from the DCCT, 1441 patients were considered to be under good or poor MC if their HbA_{1c} mean level up to the last visit dropped in the lowest (6.9% or less) or highest (9.5% or greater) quintile of the overall HbA_{1c} distribution, respectively. Prevalence cases of nephropathy were not included. Survival and Cox regression analyses were performed.

Results.—Among 277 patients with good MC, 15% had nephropathy develop by final follow-up. In 268 patients with poor MC, the proportion without the complication was 52%. When adjusting for MC, time to diabetic nephropathy was associated with gender ($P < .01$) and baseline determinations of age ($P < .0001$), AER ($P < .001$), duration of diabetes ($P < .005$), and body mass index ($P < .005$). Patients who had upper normal range AER levels, longer duration of diabetes, and lower body mass index were at increased risk, regardless of MC. The adverse effect of younger age on diabetic nephropathy was more striking in good versus poor MC. Females tended to have the complication more often under good MC, but they seem to be better protected under poor MC.

Conclusion.—Diabetic nephropathy can develop quickly in patients with specific baseline patterns, despite good MC. In contrast, patients with type 1 diabetes with poor MC can remain free of the complication for a long period, depending on their demographic and clinical status at baseline.

▶ Diabetic nephropathy is a frequent complication of diabetes and a major cause of end-stage kidney disease. The DCCT, which focused on patients with type 1 diabetes, demonstrated a marked reduction in the development and progression of diabetic nephropathy in intensively treated patients (mean HbA_{1c} level, about 7%) when compared with patients receiving conventional therapy, where the mean Hb Aκ level was about 9%.

The DCCT recruited 1441 type 1 diabetes patients during the period 1983 to 1989. Follow-up was on average 6.5 ± 1.6 years, including a 2-year feasibility study (phase II) to assess specific operational objectives before launching the full-scale clinical trial (phase III). In patients with good MC (HbA_{1c} of 6.9% or less) the proportion of nephropathy cases over 9 years was 15%, confirming that such patients do not necessarily escape the complication. In patients with poor MC (HbA_{1c}, 9.5% or greater), an estimated proportion of 52% was free from diabetic nephropathy at the end of the study period.

Thus, patients with poor MC can escape the complication for a long period of time. More importantly, after accounting for MC, Cox regression analysis revealed that baseline AER, age, gender, body mass index, and duration of diabetes were independent risk factors associated with time to diabetic nephropathy.

In conclusion, this study shows that diabetic nephropathy can develop rapidly in patients with specific baseline patterns despite good MC. By contrast, type 1 diabetic patients with poor MC can remain free from the complication for a long time period, depending on their demographic and clinical status at baseline.

S. Klahr, MD

Long-term Renal Survival in HIV-Associated Nephropathy With Angiotensin-Converting Enzyme Inhibition

Wei A, Burns GC, Williams BA, et al (Saint Vincent's Hosp, New York; New York Med College, Valhalla; Albert Einstein Med Ctr, Philadelphia)
Kidney Int 64:1462-1471, 2003

32–11

Background.—Among patients with HIV-1 infection, HIV-associated nephropathy (HIVAN) is the commonest cause of end-stage renal disease (ESRD). Highly active antiretroviral therapy has not influenced the incidence of HIVAN, which has been increasing dramatically since 1991. A short-term benefit has been achieved by using angiotensin-converting enzyme (ACE) inhibitors. The long-term effects of this therapy on renal survival for HIVAN patients were assessed.

Methods.—Forty-four patients with biopsy-proven HIVAN agreed to participate before developing severe renal insufficiency, defined as having a serum creatinine level of 2.0 mg/dL or less. Fosinopril, 10 mg/day, was given to 28 patients, while 16 served as control subjects. ESRD and death were the end points defined for the study, which lasted for 1890 days, or 5.1 years. Survival was defined as the absolute median number of days. The impact of treatment on survival was assessed by Kaplan-Meier product-limit estimates.

Results.—No significant differences were found between the 2 groups with respect to age, significant exposure to antiretroviral therapy (2 or more antiviral drugs for at least 30 consecutive days), CD4 lymphocyte count, initial median serum creatinine concentration, or degree of proteinuria. All of the untreated controls progressed to ESRD, but only 1 of the patients receiving ACE inhibitor therapy developed ESRD. The median renal survival for control subjects was 146.5 days, while that for treated patients was 479.5 days. The ACE inhibitor reduced the relative risk of renal failure, with a relative risk of 0.003 ($P < .0001$).

The effect of the ACE inhibitor therapy was independent of nephrotic range proteinuria, CD4 cell count, antiretroviral therapy exposure, or the presence of moderate to severe chronic interstitial changes. The survival rate for the ACE inhibitor group was 87.5%, and that for the control group was 21.4% ($P < .001$).

Conclusion.—A positive effect on long-term renal survival was produced by the use of ACE inhibitor therapy for patients with HIVAN before they developed severe renal insufficiency. Thus, patients whose clinical status suggests HIVAN should be diagnosed early so that treatment can begin and renal survival can be prolonged.

▶ Between 1993 and 1997, patients seen in the Saint Vincent's Hospital with HIV were screened by dipstick for urinary protein. Patients positive for proteinuria had measurements of 24-hour urinary protein excretion and serum creatinine concentrations obtained. Proteinuria of more than 500 mg/d was confirmed on 3 separate measurements within a 10-day period. During this time (1993-1997), 75 HIV-positive patients underwent renal biopsy for tissue diagnosis of the nephropathy. Of this group, 44 patients met the following criteria: clinical and pathologic characteristics indicative of HIVAN, serum creatinine of 2 mg/dL or less, normal blood pressure, normal serum potassium, normal blood sugar, no prior renal disease, no IV drug use, and no laboratory evidence of sickle-cell disease. There were 37 African Americans (84.1%), 5 Hispanics (11.4%), and 2 Asians (4.5%). Of the 44 patients, 41 were male (93.2%) and 3 were female (6.8%).

Prolonged kidney function is seen with the administration of ACE inhibitors in a variety of proteinuric nephropathies. This study by Wei et al shows the renoprotective effects of ACE inhibition in patients with HIVAN. Patients in the treated group had a preservation of renal function with a median follow-up of serum creatinine of 1.85 mg/dL from an initial creatinine of 1.95 mg/dL. Untreated controls progressed from an initial serum creatinine of −2 mg./dL to 9.30 mg dL at the end of follow-up. The median 24-hour proteinuria of treated patients decreased from 4.4 to 1.5 g compared with an increase of proteinuria from 6.2 to 10.2 g in the cohort not treated. This study shows that ACE inhibition prior to the onset of severe kidney insufficiency offers major renoprotective benefits.

S. Klahr, MD

Renal Insufficiency and Anemia Are Independent Risk Factors for Death Among Patients With Acute Myocardial Infarction
Langston RD, Presley R, Flanders WD, et al (Georgia Med Care Found, Atlanta; Emory Univ, Atlanta, Ga)
Kidney Int 64:1398-1405, 2003   32–12

Background.—Patients with coronary artery disease are at an increased risk for death when they also have chronic kidney disease (CKD). This increased risk of death has been observed in patients with coronary artery disease after noncardiac and cardiac surgery, coronary angioplasty, and acute myocardial infarction. The Heart Outcomes and Prevention Evaluation (HOPE) study found that CKD was associated with a 40% increased risk of myocardial infarction, stroke, and death due to cardiovascular disease. Some population-based studies (but not all) have found an association between renal insufficiency and risk of all-cause and cardiovascular disease (CVD)–associated death.

The factors associated with CKD that may increase the risk of mortality in patients with cardiovascular disease have not been well defined. Anemia is known to be associated with increased mortality in patients with end-stage renal disease and may also increase the risk among patients with cardiovascular disease. The combined role of anemia and CKD in the mortality risk after an acute myocardial infarction was described.

Methods.—The study group consisted of a random sample of patients admitted to hospital in 1 state with a primary diagnosis of acute myocardial infarction. A total of 559 patients with a mean age of 73.8 years were followed up after hospital discharge.

Results.—CKD was found in 60% of patients. A hematocrit of 40% or greater was found in 46% of patients; a hematocrit between 36% and 39% was found in 26% of patients; a hematocrit between 30% and 35% in 21.8% of patients; and a hematocrit of less than 30% in 5.9% of patients. The 1-year mortality rate among patients with CKD was 31.7%, compared with a rate of 10.4% among patients without CKD. Mortality at 1 year was 18.6% for patients with a hematocrit of 40% or greater; 23.5% for patients with a hematocrit of 36% to 39%; 30.7% for patients with a hematocrit of 30% to 35%; and 35.8% for patients with a hematocrit of less than 30%. Hematocrit and serum creatinine level were independently associated with an increased risk of death during follow-up after controlling for other patient factors.

Conclusion.—Chronic kidney disease and anemia occur frequently in older patients hospitalized for acute myocardial infarction and are independent predictors of subsequent risk of death.

▶ The main observation of this study by Langston et al is that a decreased hematocrit and CKD are usually frequent among elderly patients with a myocardial infarction admitted to community hospitals, and are independently associated with increased mortality after discharge. The risk of death in patients with anemia after hospitalization for acute myocardial infarction could encompass several factors. Anemia may increase hypoxia associated with intermittent episodes of angina pectoris.

This study included 709 patients admitted to community hospitals with acute myocardial infarction. The mean age of the cohort was 73.8 years, with a range of 32 to 97 years. Forty-nine percent were female and 82% were white. A history of prior myocardial infarction was found in 35% of the patients. Hypertension was present in 71% of the patients and diabetes in 33%. History of a previous stroke was reported for 19% and heart failure was reported in 23% of patients.

The authors found a high prevalence of a decreased hematocrit and CKD among elderly patients discharged alive from the hospital after an acute myocardial infarction. It is clear that both anemia and CKD are independent predictors of death during follow-up.

The authors suggest that anemia should be identified in CKD patients with ischemic heart disease. Decreased hemoglobin should be restored with a target goal between 11g/dL and 12g/dL. Partial correction of renal-related anemia should improve quality of life, cognitive status, exercise tolerance, and functional status in patients with CKD.

S. Klahr, MD

The Prevention of Radiocontrast-Agent–Induced Nephropathy by Hemofiltration
Marenzi G, Marana I, Lauri G, et al (Univ of Milan, Italy)
N Engl J Med 349:1333-1340, 2003   32–13

Background.—Radiocontrast agent–induced nephropathy is a potential complication of percutaneous coronary interventions and is associated with significant in-hospital and long-term morbidity and mortality. Most of the patients who develop contrast agent–induced nephropathy have risk factors for this condition, and patients with preexisting renal failure are at a particularly high risk. The role of hemofiltration in comparison with isotonic saline hydration in the prevention of contrast agent–induced nephropathy was investigated in patients with renal failure.

Methods.—A total of 114 consecutive patients were studied. All of the patients had chronic renal failure and were undergoing coronary interventions. The patients were randomly assigned to either hemofiltration in an ICU (58 patients) at a mean ($\pm$SD) serum creatinine concentration of 3.0 ± 1.0 mg/dL or isotonic saline hydration at a rate of 1 mL/kg body weight per hour, administered in a step-down unit (56 patients). Hemofiltration and saline hydration were initiated 4 to 8 hours before the coronary intervention and were continued for 18 to 24 hours after completion of the procedure.

Results.—An increase in serum creatinine concentration of greater than 25% above baseline after the coronary intervention occurred less frequently in patients in the hemofiltration group than in patients in the isotonic saline control group (5% vs 50%). Temporary renal replacement therapy was required in 25% of patients in the isotonic saline group compared with 3% of patients in the hemofiltration group. The rate of in-hospital events was 9% in the hemofiltration group and 52% in the isotonic saline group. The hemofiltration group also had a lower in-hospital mortality rate (2%) than the isotonic saline control group (14%). Cumulative 1-year mortality was 10% in the hemofiltration group and 30% in the isotonic saline group.

Conclusion.—It appears that periprocedural hemofiltration in an ICU setting is effective in preventing the deterioration of renal function caused by contrast agent–induced nephropathy in patients with chronic renal failure who are undergoing percutaneous coronary interventions. The practice is associated with improved in-hospital and long-term outcomes in these patients.

▶ The use of radiocontrast agents is a frequent cause of renal failure. This event can range from a transient increase of the serum creatinine concentration to permanent renal failure requiring dialysis. It has been reported that 9% of such nephropathy occurs in patients with preexisting kidney failure.

Contrast-induced nephropathy is a partially preventable event. However, several current strategies, such as hydration and the use of mannitol, furosemide, calcium antagonists, acetylcysteine, fenoldopam, or other renoprotective agents, have been shown to have no benefit or to reduce the incidence of this occurrence. Only in patients with mild kidney impairment and exposure to a low volume of contrast agents is a benign outcome observed.

In this study from Italy by Marenzi et al, 114 consecutive patients with chronic renal failure who were to have coronary angiography or an elective percutaneous coronary intervention were studied between January 1, 2000, and October 31, 2001. Eligible patients were those with a serum creatinine concentration more than 2 mg/dL, and a creatinine clearance rate of less than 5 mL/min. A nonionic, low osmolality contrast agent (Iopentol, Nycomed Imaging) was used in all patients. Of the 114 patients included in the study, 58 were randomly assigned to the control group. The relative risk of death within 1 year in the control group, as compared with the hemofiltration group, was 1.16 ($P =$ .11) among patients with a baseline serum creatinine concentration of less than 4 mg/dL and 3.53 (95% confidence interval, 1.08-11.20; $P =$ .002) among those with a baseline serum creatinine concentration of 4 mg/dL or higher.

It appears that prophylactic hemofiltration in the ICU appears to be an effective and safe strategy for the prevention of contrast-agent–induced acute renal dysfunction in patients who are undergoing percutaneous coronary interventions. In addition, in-hospital and 1-year clinical outcomes were also significantly improved in the hemofiltration group, as compared with the control group.

S. Klahr, MD

Light Chain Deposition Disease With Renal Involvement: Clinical Characteristics and Prognostic Factors
Pozzi C, D'Amico M, Fogazzi GB, et al (A Manzoni Hosp, Lecco, Italy; IRCCS Maggiore Hosp, Milan, Italy; San Carlo Borromeo Hosp, Milan, Italy; et al)
Am J Kidney Dis 42:1154-1163, 2003   32–14

Background.—Light chain deposition disease (LCDD) is a systemic disease characterized by deposition of immunoglobulin light chains. The clinical picture is heterogeneous but is dominated by kidney involvement. Renal insufficiency appears in all patients and can lead to uremia. The pathologic and clinical correlates of LCDD were examined in a cohort of 63 patients in a multicenter restrospectic study.

Study Design.—The 63 patients were from 5 nephrologic centers in northern Italy. They were diagnosed with LCDD between 1978 and 2002. All patients had renal biopsy specimens processed for light microscopy and immunofluorescence. Electron microscopy was also performed.

Findings.—The patients were aged 28 to 94 years, with a slight preponderance of males and of κ–light chain deposition (Table 1). Multiple myeloma was diagnosed in 65% of patients, lymphoproliferative disease in 3%, and idiopathic LCDD in 32%. Renal insufficiency was detected at pre-

---

TABLE 1.—Clinical Characteristics at Renal Biopsy

Variable	
No. of patients	63
Age (y)	58 ± 14.2
Sex (M/F %)	63.5/36.5
Type of LC (κ/λ %)	68/32
Underlying disease (%)	
Idiopathic LCDD	32
MM	65
Lymphoproliferative disorders	3
Renal function (%)	
Acute/rapidly progressive renal insufficiency	52
Chronic renal insufficiency	44
Normal	4
Serum creatinine (mg/dL)	3.8 (25th, 75th percentiles: 2.3, 7)
Proteinuria (%)	
>3.5 g/d	40
1-3.5 g/d	44
<1 g/d	16
Proteinuria (g/d)	2.7 (25th, 75th percentiles: 1.5, 5.2)

Note: To convert serum creatinine in milligrams per deciliter to μmoles per liter, multiply by 88.4.
Abbreviations: LC, Light chain; *LCDD*, light chain deposition disease.
(Courtesy of Pozzi C, D'Amico M, Fogazzi GB, et al: Light chain deposition disease with renal involvement: Clinical characteristics and prognostic factors. *Am J Kidney Dis* 42:1154-1163, 2003. Copyright 2003 National Kidney Foundation.)

sentation in 96% of these patients and proteinuria in 84%. During follow-up, the incidence rate of uremia was 24/100 patient-years, and the mortality rate was 18/100 patient-years. Factors independently associated with worse prognosis were age and serum creatinine at presentation. Factors independently associated with patient survival were age and extra-renal light chain deposition. Histologic parameters were not predictive of prognosis. Survival of dialysis patients was similar to that of patients without uremia.

Conclusion.—LCDD is usually seen with renal insufficiency and proteinuria. Both immunofluorescence and electron microscopy are necessary for accurate diagnosis. Patients who develop uremia should be treated with dialysis, as they do just as well as those patients who do not develop uremia. LCDD is progressive and does not have a good prognosis.

▶ LCDD is a systemic disorder characterized by the deposition of monotypical immunoglobulin light chains in various organs. The clinical manifestations depend on which tissues or organs are involved in the light chain deposition and the dysfunction of the organ affected. The clinical picture is usually very heterogenous and can simulate a number of other diseases. The aim of this study from Italy was to investigate the pathologic and clinical correlates of LCDD systematically in a cohort of LCDD patients, focusing on their impact on renal disease and patient prognosis.

Sixty-three cases of LCDD were identified. The clinical characteristics at renal biopsy are reported in Table 1. Multiple myeloma was diagnosed in 65% of the patients and lymphoproliferative disorders (chronic lymphatic leukemia) in 3%. Also, 32% of the patients did not meet the criteria for the diagnosis of any hematologic diseases. Ninety-six percent of the patients presented with renal insufficiency at kidney biopsy. The median serum creatinine level was 3.8 mg/dL. Forty percent of the patients had nephrotic proteinuria greater than 3.5 g/d at presentation, 44% had proteinuria of 1 to 3.5 g/d, and 16% had proteinuria of less than 1 g/d.

This study showed that LCDD usually presents with renal insufficiency associated with proteinuria in patients with plasma cell dyscrasias and/or serum or urinary monoclonal proteins. Immunofluorescence and electron microscopy are necessary to avoid misdiagnosing of LCDD. In this study, the only factors affecting the progression of renal insufficiency to uremia were advanced age and the degree of renal insufficiency at presentation. The histologic parameters evaluated in this study did not correlate with renal prognosis as has been reported by Lin et al.[1] These negative findings may indicate that renal prognosis is not affected by factors other than severity of renal damage at the beginning. Another explanation may be a lack of power of the study or the fact that patients may have died prior to reaching uremia.

S. Klahr, MD

Reference

1. Lin J, Markowitz GS, Valeri AM, et al: Renal monoclonal immunoglobulin deposition disease: The disease spectrum. *J Am Soc Nephrol* 12:1482-1492, 2001.

33 Chronic Renal Failure

Introduction

Hebert et al (Abstract 33–1) tested the hypothesis that fluid intake is significantly associated with glomerular filtration rate decline during follow-up in the Modification of Diet in Renal Disease (MDRD) study. Patients with and without polycystic kidney disease (PKD) were analyzed separately because of evidence from experimental models of renal disease that high fluid intake might increase progression in patients with PKD but decrease progression in patients without PKD.

In the study by Borgmann et al (Abstract 33–2), the genetic linkage of ANCA-associated vasculitides with allelic frequencies of interleukin 1 (IL-1), a proinflammatory cytokine, was investigated. Genes of the IL-1 family encode 3 structurally and functionally related polypeptides, IL-1a, IL-1B, and IL-1 receptor antagonist (IL-1ra).

The study by Merjanian et al (Abstract 33–3) was a cross-sectional study of patients with type 2 diabetes mellitus and diabetic renal disease not on dialysis. Nondiabetic controls were also on dialysis.

About 2 million patients have chronic kidney disease in the United States. A study by Jafar et al (Abstract 33–4) used data of 11 randomized controlled trials to compare the efficacy of antihypertensive regimens with and without angiotensin-converting enzyme inhibitors in patients with kidney disease that was not due to diabetes.

Chronic kidney disease is highly prevalent and is an important predictor of mortality in patients with coronary artery disease. A total of 4584 patients were included in an analysis by Reddan et al (Abstract 33–5). Coronary artery revascularization has worse outcomes among patients with chronic kidney disease.

The study by Prinsen et al (Abstract 33–6) evaluated whether albumin and fibrinogen synthesis are part of a hepatic response in patients with chronic renal failure with the use of endogenous labeling with ^{13}C-valine.

Saulo Klahr, MD

High Urine Volume and Low Urine Osmolality Are Risk Factors for Faster Progression of Renal Disease

Hebert LA, Greene T, Levey A, et al (Ohio State Univ, Columbus; Cleveland Clinic Found, Ohio; New England Med Ctr, Boston; et al)
Am J Kidney Dis 41:962-971, 2003   33–1

Background.—In studies of animals, increased intake of fluids slows the progression of renal disease and in humans, fluid intake is encouraged for patients with chronic renal insufficiency. It was hypothesized that in patients with chronic renal insufficiency, a significant relationship exists between urine volume, urine osmolality (Uosm), or both and glomerular filtration rate (GFR) decline. This hypothesis was tested in a retrospective study.

Methods.—Data were collected from the Modification of Diet in Renal Disease (MDRD) Study A cohort and included 139 patients with polycystic kidney disease (PKD) and 442 patients without PKD. The GFR slope in relation to mean 24-hour urine volume and Uosm during follow-up (mean, 2.3 years) were the main outcome measures.

Results.—With the use of the regression of GFR slope on mean follow-up 24-hour urine volume adjusted for body surface area and MDRD diet and blood pressure measurements, it was found that higher urine volumes were linked to a faster GFR decline regardless of whether the patient had PKD. Patients without PKD whose mean follow-up 24-hour urine volume was 2.4 L had a difference in GFR slope of -1.01 mL/min per year; patients with PKD and like measurements had a difference in GFR slope of -1.20 mL/min per year. A similar, although inverse, relationship between GFR decline and mean 24-hour Uosm was found for both patient groups. The results were significant even when there were adjustments for 13 relevant baseline and follow-up covariables.

Conclusions.—For patients with chronic renal insufficiency, both sustained high urine volume and low Uosm were found to be independent risk factors for an accelerated decline in GFR. Increased fluid intake would therefore not retard the progression of renal disease in humans. Patients with PKD may be at increased risk for this effect and should not be advised to maintain a generous fluid intake, but only drink as guided by their thirst.

▶ The present study used the MDRD study database to examine retrospectively the relationship between fluid intake (reflected by 24-hour urine volume and Uosm) and renal disease progression (decline in GFR). The authors tested the hypothesis that fluid intake is significantly associated with GFR decline during follow-up in the MDRD study. Patients with and without PKD were analyzed separately because of evidence from experimental models of renal disease that high fluid intake might increase progression in patients with PKD but decrease progression in patients without PKD.

The authors found that for patients with and without PKD, there was a significant association between mean 24-hour urine volume and GFR decline during follow-up in the MDRD study. The higher the mean 24-hour urine volume, the greater the GFR decline. The mean 24-hour urine volume was significantly and inversely related to the mean 24-hour Uosm. Thus, a significant but inverse association existed between mean Uosm and GFR decline during follow-up in the MDRD study in patients with and without PKD.

The authors conclude that there are 2 principal hypotheses that can explain the association of high daily urine volume and low Uosm with faster GFR decline. Hypothesis 1 stated that high urine volume with low Uosm causes faster renal disease progression. In this scenario, excess fluid intake causes nephron damage (and cyst growth in patients with PKD). Hypothesis 2 stated that high urine volume with low Uosm is the result of faster renal disease progression. This scenario was explained in 2 ways: (1) faster progression of renal disease directly caused increased urine volume and decreased Uosm by causing greater tubular injury (urinary concentrating defect and/or salt wasting), or (2) faster progression of renal disease indirectly causes increased urine volume by directly increasing thirst.

In summary, high fluid intake that results in increased urine volume and low Uosm is not associated with slower renal disease progression. Indeed, high fluid intake might promote progression of renal disease, although this cannot be proved from this retrospective analysis. The authors suggest the most prudent interpretation of their findings is that until better data becomes available, patients with chronic renal insufficiency should not be encouraged to ingest a high fluid intake unless it is needed to manage such specific problems as nephrogenic or central diabetes insipidus or urolithiasis. Avoidance of excess fluid intake might be particularly important for those patients with PKD.

S. Klahr, MD

Proinflammatory Genotype of Interleukin-1 and Interleukin-1 Receptor Antagonist Is Associated With ESRD in Proteinase 3-ANCA Vasculitis Patients
Borgmann S, Endisch G, Hacker UT, et al (Univ of Tübingen, Germany; Klinikum Innenstadt, Germany; Univ of Munich; et al)
Am J Kidney Dis 41:933-942, 2003   33–2

Background.—The small-vessel vasculitides, such as Wegener's granulomatosis, are linked to antineutrophil cytoplasmic antibodies (ANCAs), which are diagnostic markers and correlate with disease activity. Myeloperoxidase (MPO) is the principal antigen for perinuclear ANCAs; cytoplasmic ANCAs are targeted for the most part against proteinase 3 (PR3). The clinical course of small-vessel, relapsing vasculitides is heterogeneous, with wide variations in disease severity. Interleukin 1 (IL-1) family genes encode for 3 polypeptides, specifically, IL-1α, IL-1β, and IL-1 receptor antagonist (IL-1ra). It was hypothesized that 2 cytokine polymorphisms in the IL-1β and IL-1ra genes were associated with clinical manifestations and the outcome of ANCA-associated vasculitides.

Methods.—Through polymerase chain reaction and restriction fragment-length polymorphism analyses, 79 patients with PR3-ANCA, 30 patients with MPO-ANCA vasculitis, and 196 healthy controls were evaluated. The specific targets were polymorphisms in the IL-1β and IL-1ra genes of these individuals.

Results.—The allelic frequencies of the IL-1β and IL-1ra polymorphisms were similar between the control and PR3-ANCA groups and between the reference population and patients with MPO-ANCA. Patients with PR3-ANCA and end-stage renal disease had significantly increased frequencies of both high secretion levels of IL-1β and low secretion levels of IL-1ra, constituting the so-called proinflammatory genotype.

Conclusion.—The polymorphisms of IL-1β and IL-1ra were not linked with disease occurrence, but they were found to be contributing factors in the course of PR3-ANCA–associated vasculitis. Patients with MPO-ANCA vasculitis did not exhibit this carrier genotype. Thus, anti-inflammatory therapy targeted at antagonizing the proinflammatory effect of IL-1β may prove useful in treating patients with such small-vessel vasculitides as Wegener's granulomatosis with renal manifestations.

▶ In this study by Borgmann et al, they investigated the genetic linkage of ANCA-associated vasculitides with allelic frequencies of IL-1, a proinflammatory cytokine. Genes of the IL-1 family encode 3 structurally and functionally related polypeptides: IL-1α, IL-1β, and IL-1ra.

In this study, genetic linkage of ANCA-associated vasculitides with allelic frequencies of IL-1β and IL-1ra gene polymorphisms was investigated. The authors found that although these polymorphisms are not associated with disease occurrence, they contribute to the course of PR3-ANCA–associated vasculitis. It is usually accepted that the kidney is affected in patients with MPO-ANCA, whereas in patients with PR3-ANCA carrying the proinflammatory genotype, early treatment of the disease would be most beneficial.

The different inflammation patterns between patients with PRC-ANCA and MPO-ANCA vasculitis might result from different expression of proinflammatory cytokines because greater expression rates of IL-1β (and tumor necrosis factor α and IL-2 receptor) have been observed in kidney biopsy specimens of patients with Wegener's granulomatosis compared with those with microscopic polyangiitis.

This study contributes to better understanding of the clinical course of disease in patients with ANCA vasculitis carrying the proinflammatory genotype. It is possible that early use of anti-inflammatory drugs may prevent the loss of kidney function in such patients.

S. Klahr, MD

Coronary Artery, Aortic Wall, and Valvular Calcification in Nondialyzed Individuals With Type 2 Diabetes and Renal Disease
Merjanian R, Budoff M, Adler S, et al (Harbor-Univ of California, Torrance)
Kidney Int 64:263-271, 2003   33–3

Background.—Electron beam CT studies have found a high prevalence of coronary artery and valvular calcification in patients with end-stage renal

TABLE 1.—Characteristics of Individuals in the 3 Study Cohorts

	Diabetic Renal Disease	Diabetic Controls	Nondiabetic Controls
Number	32	18	95
Age *years*	57 ± 1.5	58.2 ± 1.9	57 ± 0.9
Gender *male/female*	13/19	11/7	39/56
Ethnicity			
Hispanic	20 (62%)	12 (67%)	59 (62%)
African American	8 (25%)	2 (11%)	24 (25%)
Caucasian	2 (6%)	4 (22%)	6 (6%)
Asian	2 (6%)	0	6 (6%)
Dyslipidemia	24 (75%)	15* (88%)	73 (77%)
Hypertension	28† (90%)	10 (56%)	70 (74%)
Known coronary artery disease	15 (47%)	6 (33%)	57 (60%)

*N = 17.
†N = 31.
(Courtesy of Merjanian R, Budoff M, Adler S, et al: Coronary artery, aortic wall, and valvular calcification in nondialyzed individuals with type 2 diabetes and renal disease. *Kidney Int* 64:263-271, 2003. Reprinted by permission of Blackwell Publishing.)

disease (ESRD). It is not known at what stage this calcification develops, but it may well be related to the high cardiovascular morbidity and mortality among ESRD patients. To understand the development of these calcifications, the prevalence of calcification was investigated in those with diabetic renal disease, those with normoalbuminuric diabetes, and matched nondiabetic controls in this cross-sectional case-control study.

TABLE 2.—Subgroup Analyses of the Prevalence and Severity of Coronary Artery Calcification in Individuals With Diabetic Renal Disease and Nondiabetic Controls

	Prevalence, % Patients		Severity, Median Score	
	Diabetic Renal Disease	Nondiabetic Controls	Diabetic Renal Disease	Nondiabetic Controls
Overall	94%* (N = 32)	59% (N = 95)	238* (55-789)	10 (0-90)
Gender				
Male	92% (N = 13)	67% (N = 39)	619† (82-972)	18 (0-168)
Female	95%† (N = 19)	54% (N = 56)	232* (52-470)	6 (0-61)
Dyslipidemia				
Present	92%† (N = 24)	55% (N = 73)	224* (49-789)	6 (0-89)
Absent	100% (N = 8)	73% (N = 22)	506† (171-679)	27 (0-111)
Hypertension				
Present	96%† (N = 28)	67%§ (N = 70)	238* (64-789)	17§ (0-155)
Absent	67% (N = 3)	36% (N = 25)	4 (2-470)	0 (0-18)
Known coronary artery disease				
Present	100%† (N = 15)	60% (N = 57)	543*‡ (232-894)	16 (0-93)
Absent	88% (N = 17)	58% (N = 38)	74† (14-257)	7 (0-97)

Note: The numbers in parentheses associated with the coronary artery calcification scores are interquartile ranges in each designated subgroup.
*$P < .001$ for difference between diabetic renal disease individuals and controls.
†$P < .05$ for difference between diabetic renal disease individuals and controls.
‡$P < .004$ for difference between diabetic renal disease individuals with and without known coronary artery disease.
§$P < .01$ for difference between diabetic renal disease individuals with and without hypertension.
(Courtesy of Merjanian R, Budoff M, Adler S, et al: Coronary artery, aortic wall, and valvular calcification in nondialyzed individuals with type 2 diabetes and renal disease. *Kidney Int* 64:263-271, 2003. Reprinted by permission of Blackwell Publishing.)

Study Design.—The study group consisted of 32 patients with diabetic renal disease, 18 diabetic controls, and 95 nondiabetic controls, with no renal disease. Controls were matched for age, gender, ethnicity, and the presence of dyslipidemia, hypertension, and coronary artery disease (CAD) (Table 1). All participants had electron beam CT studies performed to assess calcification.

Findings.—The presence and severity of coronary artery calcification was significantly higher among those with diabetic renal disease than nondiabetic controls or diabetic controls (Table 2). There was also significantly greater prevalence of aortic and mitral valve calcification among those with diabetic renal disease than among controls. Mutivariate analysis identified age and diabetic renal disease as independent predictors for calcification.

Conclusions.—Patients with diabetic renal disease who have never had dialysis still have a significantly higher prevalence and severity for vascular and valvar calcification than matched nondiabetic controls with normal renal function or normoalbuminuric diabetics. These findings reveal that calcification begins before ESRD and dialysis. This calcification may be associated with atherosclerosis.

▶ Studies that used electron beam CT have discovered a high prevalence of coronary artery calcification in patients with ESRD.

This study by Merjanian et al was a cross-sectional study in patients with type 2 diabetes mellitus and diabetic renal disease not on dialysis. Nondiabetic controls were also on dialysis. Nondiabetic controls were also studies (see Table 1 for the characteristics of the individuals in the 3 study cohorts).

The 32 diabetic renal disease individuals, the 18 diabetics without renal disease, and the 95 nondiabetics were studied. The 32 diabetic controls were well matched for age, gender, ethnicity, and presence/absence of dyslipidemia (Table 1).

Coronary artery disease was reported in 94% of the patients with diabetic renal disease compared with all the diabetic controls and 59% of nondiabetic controls ($P < .001$) compared with diabetic renal disease (Table 2).

A total of 44% of patients with diabetic renal disease had calcification of at least 1 of the 2 valves. Aortic and mitral valve calcification were, respectively, present in 23% and 25% of patients with diabetic renal disease compared with 11% and 11% of diabetic controls and 6% and 2% of nondiabetic controls.

This study demonstrated a significantly higher prevalence of valvular calcification in diabetic kidney disease compared with controls.

Several studies in patients without kidney disease have demonstrated correlations between valvular calcification and the traditional risk factors for cardiovascular disease and the presence of atherosclerotic disease at other sites.

S. Klahr, MD

Progression of Chronic Kidney Disease: The Role of Blood Pressure Control, Proteinuria, and Angiotensin-Converting Enzyme Inhibition: A Patient-Level Meta-analysis

Jafar TH, for the AIPRD Study Group (Tufts-New England Med Ctr, Boston; et al)

Ann Intern Med 139:244-252, 2003   33–4

Introduction.—Angiotensin-converting enzyme (ACE) inhibitors decrease blood pressure and urine protein excretion and slow the progression of chronic kidney disease. A patient-level meta-analysis was performed by using data from the ACE Inhibition in Progressive Renal Disease (AIPRD) Study Group database to determine the levels of blood pressure (BP) and urine protein excretion associated with the lowest risk for progression of chronic kidney disease during antihypertensive therapy with and without ACE inhibitors.

Methods.—The MEDLINE database was searched for English language trials published between 1977 and 1999. The AIPRD Study group database included 1860 patients with nondiabetic kidney disease who were enrolled in 11 randomized controlled trials of ACE inhibitors used to decrease the progression of kidney disease. The progression of kidney disease was considered to be the doubling of the baseline serum creatinine level or the onset of kidney failure. Multivariable regression analysis was performed to determine the correlation between systolic and diastolic BP and urine protein excretion with kidney disease progression from 22,610 patient visits.

Results.—The mean follow-up was 2.2 years. Three hundred eleven patients had kidney disease progression. Systolic BP of 110 to 129 mm Hg and urine protein excretion below 2.0 g/d were linked with the lowest risk for kidney disease progression. The ACE inhibitors remained beneficial after adjusting for BP and urine protein excretion (relative risk, 0.67; 95% confidence interval, 0.53-0.84). The increased risk for kidney progression at higher systolic BP levels was higher in patients with urine protein excretion in excess of 1.0 g/d ($P < .006$).

Conclusion.—Reverse causation cannot be excluded with certainty. A systolic BP goal between 110 and 129 mm Hg may be beneficial for patients with urine protein excretion higher than 1.0 g/d. Systolic BP below 110 mm Hg may be linked with a higher risk for kidney disease progression.

▶ About 2 million patients have chronic kidney disease in the United States. This study by Jafar et al used data from 11 randomized controlled trials which compared the efficacy of antihypertensive regimens with and without ACE inhibitors in patients with kidney disease not due to diabetes.

The findings of Jafar et al in the meta-analysis confirm that higher systolic BP and protein excretion levels lead to adverse outcomes of kidney function. The higher levels of protein excretion in the urine and higher levels of systolic BP require more aggressive management than in patients with lower levels of protein excretion. Jafar et al found that follow-up systolic BP less than 110 mm Hg was associated with increased risks for worsening renal disease.

Several lessons can be extracted from this meta-analysis. Proteinuria is a risk factor. Reducing proteinuria is an important factor in preserving kidney function, not only in patients with diabetes but also in nondiabetic patients with hypertension. It would be important to perform dipstick urine testing periodically to detect proteinuria in patients with hypertension. In patients with proteinuria, it is important to reduce the levels of proteinuria to less than 1 to 2 g per day.

In patients with chronic kidney disease and proteinuria, the systolic BP should be maintained between 110 and 130 mm Hg. Also target systolic and not diastolic blood pressures. The finding that systolic BP is more strongly associated with kidney disease progression than is diastolic BP was also observed in a recent analysis of data from the Systolic Hypertension in the Elderly Program.[1] Due to the high risk for cardiovascular disease in patients with chronic kidney disease, the National Kidney Foundation Task Force recommends an upper limit of systolic BP of 130 mm Hg in patients with decreased kidney function.

S. Klahr, MD

Reference

1. Young JH, Klag MJ, Muntner P, et al: Blood pressure and decline in kidney function: Findings from the Systolic Hypertension in the Elderly Program (SHEP). *J Am Soc Nephrol* 13:2776-2882, 2002.

Chronic Kidney Disease, Mortality, and Treatment Strategies Among Patients With Clinically Significant Coronary Artery Disease
Reddan DN, Szczech LA, Tuttle RH, et al (Duke Univ, Durham, NC; Baxter Healthcare, Gurnee, Ill)
J Am Soc Nephrol 14:2373-2380, 2003   33–5

Introduction.—Cardiovascular disease is a major cause of mortality among patients with chronic kidney disease (CKD). The correlation between CKD, cardiac revascularization strategies, and mortality was examined among patients with CKD and cardiovascular disease.

Methods.—All patients undergoing cardiac catheterization between 1995 and 2000 with documented stenosis of 75% or greater of at least 1 coronary artery and available creatinine data were included. The CKD was staged by means of creatinine clearance (CrCl) derived from the Cockcroft-Gault formula (normal, 90 mL/min or greater; mild, 60 to 89 mL/min; moderate, 30 to 59 mL/min; severe, 15 to 29 mL/min). The Cox proportional-hazard regression model was used to estimate the association between clinical variables, including CrCl and percutaneous coronary artery intervention (PCI), coronary artery bypass grafting (CABG), medical management, and patient survival.

Results.—A total of 4584 patients were included (Table 1); 24% had CrCl below 60 mL/min. Each 10-mL/min decrement in CrCl was linked with an increase in mortality (hazard ratio, 1.14; $P < .0001$). Coronary artery bypass

TABLE 1.—Demographics and Clinical Characteristics for 4584 Patients Stratified by Renal Function

Characteristic	Normal (n = 1945)	Mild (n = 1546)	Moderate (n = 917)	Severe (n = 107)	ESRD (n = 69)	Overall (n = 4584)
Age (yr)	54 (48, 61)	66 (59, 72)	74 (68, 79)	77 (70, 81)	60 (53, 69)	63 (54, 71)
White (%)	80.4	77.0	76.1	62.6	37.3	77.4
Female (%)	21.6	33.6	52.3	77.6	47.8	33.5
History of (%)						
hypertension	55.4	60.1	71.3	86.0	97.1	61.5
hyperlipidemia	56.0	52.0	49.8	44.9	46.4	53.0
cerebrovascular disease	6.3	11.3	17.8	26.2	18.8	10.9
peripheral vascular disease	9.3	11.1	19.3	13.1	29.0	12.3
congestive heart failure	14.3	20.6	31.0	44.3	49.3	21.0
diabetes mellitus	31.5	24.3	27.5	43.9	68.1	29.1
myocardial infarction	55.0	47.8	48.1	46.7	39.1	50.8
smoking	72.7	63.8	52.0	40.2	60.9	64.6
mild valvular disease	0.8	1.4	2.7	5.6	0.0	1.5
Ejection fraction	55.9 (45.8, 63.9)	55.9 (45.3, 65.2)	54.2 (39.9, 64.4)	50.0 (35.3, 60.4)	48.7 (29.2, 64.2)	55.2 (44.0, 64.4)
Ventricular gallop (%)	2.0	4.1	5.3	9.4	5.8	3.6
CHF severity (%)						
no CHF	86.7	81.2	71.4	57.3	53.9	80.6
NYHA class I	2.5	4.5	6.3	6.8	6.2	4.1
NYHA class II	4.5	4.6	6.1	8.7	10.8	5.0
NYHA class III	3.5	6.1	10.3	14.6	12.3	6.1
NYHA class IV	2.9	3.7	5.9	12.6	16.9	4.2
Number of diseased vessels (%)						
1	44.4	35.7	28.1	19.6	18.8	37.3
2	29.0	29.9	30.4	19.6	29.0	29.4
3	26.6	34.4	41.4	60.8	52.2	33.4
Left main disease* (%)	4.8	8.9	9.7	11.2	4.4	7.3
Severe coronary disease† (%)	27.8	36.6	43.0	60.8	53.6	34.9
Systolic blood pressure (mmHg)	136 (120, 152)	141.5 (123, 160)	150 (130, 172)	156 (133, 180)	152 (135, 172)	140 (122, 160)
Diastolic blood pressure (mmHg)	79 (70, 88)	78 (68, 86)	78 (67, 86)	76 (70, 85)	78 (67, 86)	78 (68, 87)
Treatment						
medical	25.0	29.2	37.6	51.4	58.0	30.1
PCI	47.6	35.7	26.7	15.9	14.5	38.2
CABG	27.4	35.1	35.7	32.7	27.5	31.8

Note: Continuous variables are presented as median (25th and 75th percentile). Categorical or dichotomous variables are presented as percentages.
*Defined as stenosis of the left main coronary artery of 75% or greater.
†Defined as either left main coronary artery stenosis of 75% or greater or significant stenoses in 3 coronary arteries.
Abbreviations: CHF, Congestive heart failure; NYHA, New York Heart Association; PCI, percutaneous coronary artery intervention; CABG, coronary artery bypass grafting.
(Courtesy of Reddan DN, Szczech LA, Tuttle RH, et al: Chronic kidney disease, mortality, and treatment strategies among patients with clinically significant coronary artery disease. *J Am Soc Nephrol* 14:2373–2380, 2003.)

grafting was correlated with a survival benefit among both patients with normal renal function and those with CKD versus patients managed medically. In patients with normal renal function, CABG was not correlated with survival benefit over PCI. In patients with CKD, CABG was linked with improved survival.

Percutaneous artery intervention was correlated with a survival benefit, compared to medical management of patients with normal or mildly or moderately impaired renal function. In patients with severe CKD, PCI was not correlated with improved patient survival. CABG was linked with a greater decrease in mortality than PCI in patients with severe CKD.

Conclusion.—Patients with more advanced CKD experienced a survival benefit from CABG versus medical management. The benefit associated with PCI did not remain significant as renal function declined to the most severe range. CABG was correlated with improved survival, compared with PCI in patients who had advanced CKD.

▶ CKD is highly prevalent and is an important predictor of mortality in patients with coronary artery disease. Usually, patients with advanced CKD have an increased frequency of comorbidities, including severe cardiac disease (severe left ventricular dysfunction and worse coronary artery disease).

A total of 4584 patients were included in this analysis by Reddan et al. Of these, 923 patients were excluded because they did not have a serum CrCl available. Compared with individuals with normal kidney function, patients with CKD were, in general, older; more often black; more often female; and more likely to have comorbidities such as hypertension, diabetes, cerebrovascular disease, peripheral vascular disease, and congestive heart failure (see Table 1).

Coronary artery revascularization has worse outcomes among patients with CKD. Patients with end-stage renal disease who undergo PCI have almost doubled the rate of restenosis and have a greater mortality risk after CABG than patients with normal renal function. It is estimated that more than 6 million Americans have CKD. Because of the striking prevalence and impact of cardiac disease in this population, the treatment of coronary artery disease represents a critical intervention to improve survival.

The conclusions of this study should be interpreted in the setting of certain limitations. Bias may affect the results of any observational study in that the indication for treatment may affect the outcomes. To be enrolled in this study, patients had to be referred for cardiac catheterization. If referral for catheterization is affected by the presence of CKD because of concerns such as the risk of acute renal failure due to contrast nephrotoxicity, the generalizability of these results to the entire population of patients with concurrent renal and cardiac disease may be affected. Future research should focus on the mechanism for the differential effects of coronary artery revascularization strategy based on renal function.

S. Klahr, MD

Increased Albumin and Fibrinogen Synthesis Rate in Patients With Chronic Renal Failure

Prinsen BH, Rabelink TJ, Beutler JJ, et al (Univ Med Ctr, Utrecht, The Netherlands; Jeroen Bosch Medicentrum, Den Bosch, The Netherlands; Univ of California-Davis, Mather; et al)

Kidney Int 64:1495-1504, 2003

33–6

Background.—Hypoalbuminemia is strongly predictive of mortality and morbidity in patients with chronic renal failure (CRF). The long-term survival rate in dialysis is low, and half of patients die of cardiovascular complications. Low levels of nutritional indices such as albumin, prealbumin, and creatinine have been associated with poor survival in patients undergoing dialysis. Multivariate analysis has shown that a low plasma albumin concentration is correlated most strongly with markers of inflammation and peritoneal albumin loss. Hyperfibrinoginemia has also been associated with an increased prevalence of coronary heart disease, both in the normal situation and in patients undergoing dialysis. However, the mechanisms responsible for hypoalbuminemia and hyperfibrinoginemia in CRF are unknown. Whether albumin and fibrinogen synthesis are part of a coordinated upregulated hepatic response in patients with CRF was determined with the use of endogenous labeling with ^{13}C-valine.

Methods.—Albumin and fibrinogen kinetics were measured in vivo in 6 predialysis patients, in 7 patients undergoing peritoneal dialysis, and in 8 control subjects with the use of L-[1-^{13}C]-valine.

Results.—Plasma albumin concentrations were significantly lower in patients undergoing peritoneal dialysis than in control subjects. A significant increase was seen in plasma fibrinogen concentrations in both predialysis patients and patients undergoing peritoneal dialysis when compared with control subjects. Unlike albumin, fibrinogen is only lost in peritoneal dialysate and not in urine. Patients undergoing peritoneal dialysis showed increased absolute synthesis rates of albumin and fibrinogen compared with control subjects. Albumin synthesis is strongly correlated with fibrinogen synthesis. The hypoalbuminemia observed in the patients undergoing peritoneal dialysis in this study could not be explained by malnutrition, inadequate dialysis, inflammation, metabolic acidosis, or insulin resistance. It is thought that peritoneal albumin loss has relevance.

Conclusions.—The synthesis rate of albumin and fibrinogen are upregulated in a coordinated manner, and both albumin and fibrinogen are lost in peritoneal dialysis fluid. Albumin synthesis is upregulated in an effort to compensate for protein loss, but the response in patients undergoing peritoneal dialysis, unlike predialysis patients, does not fully correct plasma albumin concentrations. The increased synthesis of fibrinogen is an independent risk factor for atherosclerosis in patients with CRF because the plasma fibrinogen pool is enlarged.

▶ A major decrease in albuminemia is a strong predictor of morbidity in patients with CRF. The survival rate of patients in dialysis is low (less than 5 years), and half of the patients die of cardiovascular complications. In these patients, low levels of nutritional indices such as albumin, prealbumin, and creatinine have been associated with poor survival rates.

Using endogenous labeling with ^{13}C-valine, Prinsen et al tested the hypothesis that albumin and fibrinogen synthesis are part of a hepatic response in patients with CRF. Table 1 (in the original article) shows the clinical data of the patients and control subjects.

The authors showed that both albumin synthesis and fibrinogen synthesis were increased in patients with CRF. Fibrinogen synthesis was increased in the peritoneal dialysis group. The authors hypothesized that fibrinogen synthesis is increased as part of a coordinated response of liver proteins, such as occurs in the nephrotic syndrome. Of 13 patients, 11 were prescribed medication, consisting of a β-blocker, an angiotensin-converting enzyme inhibitor, or a combination of both drugs. Both drugs are known to reduce plasma fibrinogen levels, yet fibrinogen levels remained elevated. In contrast to albumin, fibrinogen is lost in peritoneal dialysis fluid but not in the urine.

This study demonstrated that albumin synthesis is 20% higher in predialysis patients and 35% higher in peritoneal dialysis patients. Renal failure per se does not reduce the albumin synthesis rate.

Malnutrition, inadequate dialysis, inflammation, metabolic acidosis, or insulin resistance did not explain the hypoalbuminemia in the peritoneal dialysis patients. Because fibrinogen synthesis is positively correlated with the plasma fibrinogen concentration, this linkage may contribute to the risk of cardiovascular disease in patients with renal failure.

S. Klahr, MD

34 Hypertension

Introduction

The study by Baigent and Landry (Abstract 34–1) compared ezetimibe/simvastatin with placebo among 9000 patients with chronic kidney disease (approximately 6000 of whom will be predialysis and 3000 undergoing dialysis), with treatment scheduled to continue for at least 4 years. The primary aim was to assess the effects of lowering low-density lipoprotein cholesterol on the time to a first "major vascular event" (defined as nonfatal myocardial infarction or cardiac death, nonfatal or fatal stroke, or revascularization).

Nicod et al (Abstract 34–2) compared the frequency of 2 linked CYP11B2 polymorphisms in 141 patients with hypertension. Supine aldosterone-to-renin ratio (ARR) was normal in 104 patients and raised in 37 patients.

In Japan, Izawa et al (Abstract 34–3) performed a large study of 33 single nucleotide polymorphisms of 27 candidates' genes and hypertension. Their aim was to predict the genetic risk for hypertension.

A study from Scuteri et al (Abstract 34–4) shows that inhibition of nitric oxide by asymmetric dimethyl arginine contributes to the increase in blood pressure during high-salt intake in normotensive postmenopausal women not receiving estrogen.

Saulo Klahr, MD

Study of Heart and Renal Protection (SHARP)
Baigent C, Landry M (Clinical Trial Service Unit, Oxford, England)
Kidney Int 63 Supplement 84:S207-S210, 2003   34–1

Background.—For patients with preexisting coronary heart disease, decreasing low-density lipoprotein cholesterol (LDL-C) concentration by approximately 1 mmol/L for 4 to 5 years produces a 25% reduction in the risk of experiencing coronary events and stroke. However, patients who have established chronic kidney disease (CKD) carry a higher risk of vascular disease, leading to the hypothesis that a similar reduction in LDL-C concentration may also prove advantageous. Most trials have excluded patients with CKD; thus, this hypothesis is untested and may prove unfounded because some trials have found a negative association between blood total cholesterol and mortality rates. Only about 25% of the cardiac mortality rate in CKD patients is attributable to acute myocardial infarction and therefore may be amenable to cholesterol-lowering effects. In addition, the safety of reducing cholesterol in CKD patients is unknown.

Methods.—The Study of Heart and Renal Protection (SHARP) is a large-scale randomized trial that is designed to assess the effects of lowering cholesterol on major vascular events and on the rate of progression to end-stage renal disease (ESRD) in patients with CKD. Two pilot studies were undertaken to establish parameters regarding safety and the biochemical efficacy of decreasing cholesterol levels in patients with CKD, and to assess the feasibility of designing a large-scale study around patients with CKD.

Results.—In the first United Kingdom Heart and Renal Protection (UK-HARP-I) study, simvastatin, 20 mg daily, reduced LDL-C by 26% from baseline in patients with CKD, which is similar to the results obtained in patients without CKD. However, it was found that the statin doses required by CKD patients increased the risk of muscle toxicity, so that patients with CKD were given a combination of ezetimibe (a cholesterol absorption inhibitor), 10 mg daily, plus simvastatin, 20 mg daily, with the result that reductions in mean LDL-C were about one fifth those of simvastatin alone but with lower toxicity. In the UK-HARP-II study, the ezetimibe-simvastatin combination will be evaluated for 6 months in 203 patients with CKD to assess the effects of ezetimibe on tolerance, markers of safety, and biochemical efficacy. Preliminary results note good tolerance and proportional reductions in LDL-C. The SHARP study, scheduled to begin in mid 2003, is designed to evaluate the effects of decreased LDL-C levels on the time to a first major vascular event, which includes nonfatal myocardial infarction or cardiac death, nonfatal or fatal stroke, or revascularization. In addition, the effects of ezetimibe-simvastatin on the progression to ESRD, various causes of death, major cardiac events, stroke, and hospitalization will also be assessed. The SHARP study will include more than 200 hospitals in 10 countries.

Conclusions.—The SHARP study will attempt to determine whether substantial reductions in LDL-C can decrease the risk of major vascular events in patients with CKD. The specific agents to be used are ezetimibe-simvastatin, and approximately 9000 patients will be evaluated.

► Patients with ESRD have a high risk of cardiovascular disease. In the general population, most heart mortality is attributable to atheromatous coronary heart disease, but in dialysis patients, most of the cardiac mortality appears to be caused by cardiomyopathy, leading to arrhythmia or congestive heart failure.

In prospective observational studies among predialysis patients, for example, about one third of those with moderate reduction in glomerular filtration rate (GFR) equivalent to CKD Stage 3 (GFR, 60-89 mL/min per 1.73 m²) have a history of overt cardiovascular disease.

This study compared ezetimibe-simvastatin combination versus placebo among 9000 patients with CKD (approximately 6000 of whom will be predialysis, and 3000 undergoing dialysis), with treatment scheduled to continue for at least 4 years. The primary aim of this study was to assess the effects of decreasing LDL-C on the time to a first "major vascular event" (defined as nonfatal myocardial infarction or cardiac death, nonfatal or fatal stroke, or revascularization). Secondary aims of this study included an assessment of the effects of ezetimibe-simvastatin on progression to ESRD (among predialysis patients), various causes of death, major cardiac events (defined as nonfatal MI or cardiac death), stroke, and hospitalization for angina. The effects on major vascular events will also be examined among particular subgroups of patients.

The SHARP study is an investigator-initiated study conducted by an international collaboration of nephrologists and clinical researchers in over 200 hospitals in about 10 countries. This study should begin in mid 2003.

It is currently unclear whether dyslipidemia in patients with CKD contributes to an increased risk of cardiovascular disease in such patients. In particular, there is a lack of epidemiologic evidence supporting such an association, and it remains unclear what proportion of cardiac disease is atherosclerotic and, hence, potentially avoidable by lowering cholesterol. In the coming years, SHARP (and also other studies in patients with renal disease) should help to answer these outstanding uncertainties by providing clear information about whether substantial reductions in LDL-C can reduce the risk of major vascular events in patients with CKD.

S. Klahr, MD

A Biallelic Gene Polymorphism of CYP11B2 Predicts Increased Aldosterone to Renin Ratio in Selected Hypertensive Patients
Nicod J, Bruhin D, Auer L, et al (Univ of Berne, Switzerland)
J Clin Endocrinol Metab 88:2495-2500, 2003   34–2

Background.—There has been increased interest in recent years in the role of a primary activation of the aldosterone axis in the pathogenesis of essential hypertension. It is estimated that about one third of patients with hypertension have low renin levels, with a higher proportion of low renin among blacks than among whites. In addition, up to 15% of unselected hypertensive patients have a raised aldosterone-to-renin ratio (ARR) in plasma. In most of these patients, plasma aldosterone is only partially suppressible on salt loading, which is the current diagnostic criterion for primary aldosteronism.

Measurements of ARR are important because they are predictive of the blood pressure response to spironolactone. The enzyme aldosterone synthase is the key rate-limiting enzyme in the final stages of aldosterone biosynthesis. Recent reports have suggested that altered control of expression of the aldosterone synthase gene (CYB11B2) may modulate the secretion of aldosterone. Supporting this view is the elevated ARR in some patients with essential hypertension. The distribution of the 2 linked polymorphic loci at the CYB11B2 gene was investigated in 2 groups of hypertensive patients stratified in relation to their ARR.

Methods.—The frequency of 2 linked CYP11B2 polymorphisms, 1 in the steroidogenic factor-1 (SF-1) binding site and the other in an inotronic conversion (Int2) were compared in relation to ARR in 141 patients with hypertension. The patients were divided into groups with either normal or high supine AR; a cutoff threshold of 145 pmol/L per ng/L was used.

Results.—Supine ARR was normal in 104 patients and elevated in 37 patients. The 2 polymorphisms were in strong linkage disequilibrium. The SF-1 T and Int2 C alleles were more prevalent among patients with high ARR (46% and 43%, respectively) than those with normal ARR (22% and 17%, respectively). The odds ratio for raised ARR in patients with a homozygous SF-1 T and Int2 C haplotype was 6.1 in comparison with the contrasting haplotype. Linear modeling of individual postural changes in renin and aldosterone demonstrated a maximal achievable aldosterone increase of 110 pmol/L with no mutated haplotype and 500 pmol/L with 2 mutated haplotypes.

Conclusion.—The finding in this study support the concept of a molecular basis for the regulation of aldosterone production.

▶ Angiotensin II is the principal stimulator of aldosterone production. The enzyme aldosterone synthase is the key rate-limiting enzyme in the final steps of aldosterone biosynthesis. Recent reports in the last 3 years (1999-2002) suggest that variations at the aldosterone synthase gene (CYP11B2) are associated with essential hypertension and may influence aldosterone secretion. One of these CYP11B2 polymorphisms (-344 C/T SF-1) is located in the promoter region and influences binding of the transcriptional regulatory protein SF-1. Another is a gene conversion in intron 2, so that most of the intron has a sequence corresponding to CYP11B1, the gene encoding for the 11b-hydroxylase, the enzyme involved in the final step of cortisol synthesis.

Nicod et al compared the frequency of 2 linked CYP11B2 polymorphisms in 141 hypertensive patients. The supine ARR was normal in 104 patients and raised in 37 patients. In 13 patients, supine plasma aldosterone concentration exceeded 500 (781 ±213) pmol/L and the ARR was greater than 145 (460 ± 235). Among these patients, they had a supine plasma aldosterone greater than 800 (964 ±142) pmol/L. A unilateral adrenal mass was demonstrated in all of them by MRI. Hypertension was cured by surgical removal of the tumor in all the subjects.

The findings of this study support the view that the regulation of aldosterone production has a strong genetic component. A single ARR may lead to an overestimation of the true prevalence of abnormal aldosterone regulation. The CC genotype is predictive of a normal ARR in 94% of the selected patients with normal supine and upright AAR.

S. Klahr, MD

Prediction of Genetic Risk for Hypertension

Izawa H, Yamada Y, Okada T, et al (Nagoya Univ, Japan; Gifu Internatl Inst of Biotechnology, Mitake, Japan; Nagoya Daini Red Cross Hosp, Japan)

Hypertension 41:1035-1040, 2003   34–3

Background.—Hypertension is a multifactorial disease that is believed to result from an interaction of genotype and environment. Because hypertension is a major risk factor for coronary artery disease, stroke, and chronic renal failure, prevention is an important public health goal. The identification of disease susceptibility genes would be useful in this regard. A large association study in Japan of 33 single nucleotide polymorphisms (SNPs) of 27 candidate genes and hypertension is described.

Study Design.—Public databases were searched to obtain 27 candidate genes suggested to be associated with hypertension and 33 SNPs of these genes that could be expected to affect expression or function. The study group consisted of 1067 participants with hypertension and 873 controls with normal blood pressure (BP). Venous blood was collected from each participant and DNA extracted. SNP genotypes were determined with fluorescence- or colorimetry-based allele-specific DNA primer-probe assays. Multivariate logistic regression analysis was used to adjust for risk factors, including age, body mass index, smoking, diabetes mellitus, hypercholesterolemia, and hyperuricemia.

Findings.—Multivariate logistic regression analysis, with adjustments, revealed 2 polymorphisms significantly associated with hypertension in men: 825C→T in the G protein subunit β3 subunit gene and 190G→A in the CC chemokine receptor 2 gene. One polymorphism was significantly associated with hypertension in women, −238G→A in the tumor necrosis factor α gene.

Conclusions.—Logistic regression analysis indicated 2 polymorphisms significantly associated with hypertension in men and 1 significantly associated with hypertension in women in a large cohort in Japan. Genotyping may be useful in the prediction of hypertension risk.

▶ Because hypertension is a major factor for stroke, coronary artery disease, and chronic kidney failure, prevention of hypertension is an important health goal. One of the approaches to prevent the development of hypertension is to identify disease susceptibility genes.

In Japan, Izawa et al have performed a large study of 33 SNPs of 27 candidates' genes and hypertension. Their aim was to predict the genetic risk for hypertension.

The study examined 1940 Japanese individuals, including 1067 patients with hypertension (514 men and 493 women) and 873 controls (533 men and 340 women). The authors identified 3 different SNP_2, 2 in men and 1 in women that were closely associated with hypertension. For men, the 825C→TSNP of the G protein β3 subunit gene and the 1906-ASM of the CC chemokine receptor 2 gene were significantly associated with hypertension. Siffert et al[1] previously showed that the 825C-TSNP in exon 10 of the G protein was associated with hypertension. Several studies have examined the relation between gene polymorphisms and hypertension. Most studies, however, remain controversial mainly because of the limited size of the populations examined.

S. Klahr, MD

Reference

1. Siffert W, Rosskopf D, Siffert G, et al: Association of a human G-protein beta3 subunit variant with hypertension. *Nat Genet* 18:45-48, 1988.

Nitric Oxide Inhibition as a Mechanism for Blood Pressure Increase During Salt Loading in Normotensive Postmenopausal Women
Scuteri A, Stuehlinger MC, Cooke JP, et al (NIH, Baltimore, Md; Stanford Univ, Calif)
J Hypertens 21:1339-1346, 2003   34–4

Background.—Young and middle-aged men in all racial groups tend to have higher blood pressure (BP) than women of similar age. However, after menopause, hypertension is more prevalent among women than among men. The reasons for gender differences in the age-associated rise in BP are not known. It has been suggested that estrogen is one of the factors responsible for the lower BP in younger women than in men, likely through the stimulation of nitric oxide (NO) production. The sensitivity of BP to sodium has also been reported to increase with age. One hypothesis states that the salt sensitivity of BP in normotensive research subjects and the subsequent development of hypertension are related to an abnormal pattern of vascular reactivity. However, the mechanism responsible for this abnormality has not been clearly defined. Asymmetric dimethylarginine (ADMA) is an endogenous inhibitor of NO, which plays an important role in natriuresis. Whether changes in endothelium-dependent vasodilation (EDD) and plasma ADMA are predictive of changes in BP after salt loading was determined in normotensive postmenopausal women.

Methods.—The study group was composed of 15 normotensive postmenopausal women aged 50 to 60 years who were not receiving estrogen. Ambulatory 24-hour BP and plasma lipid and ADMA levels were measured after 4 days of a low-salt diet (70 mEq/d) and after 7 days of high-salt intake (260 mEq/d). US was used to measure the brachial artery diameter at rest, during reactive hyperemia (ie, EDD), and after administration of sublingual nitroglycerin (non-EDD). The 24-hour urinary NO metabolite was measured by Griess reaction. Plasma ADMA was measured by high-pressure liquid chromatography.

Results.—The 24-hour BP levels during the low-salt diet averaged 121 ± 11 and 69 ± 7 mm Hg for systolic and diastolic blood pressure, respectively. After salt loading, the average 24-hour BP increases were 7.6 mm Hg for systolic, 2.2 mm Hg for diastolic, and 5.5 mm Hg for pulse pressure. A direct correlation was present between increases in systolic BP and 24-hour pulse pressure after salt loading and changes in ADMA. In addition, an inverse

TABLE 1.—24-Hour Blood Pressure (BP), Vasoreactivity, NOx, and ADMA During Low- and High-Salt Conditions

	Low-Salt	High-Salt	*P*
24-h SBP (mmHg)	121 ± 11.3	128.7 ± 14.1	0.04
24-h DBP (mmHg)	68.6 ± 7.0	70.8 ± 6.7	0.22
24-h MBP (mmHg)	85.9 ± 6.5	89.9 ± 6.6	0.03
24-h PP (mmHg)	52.4 ± 12.1	57.9 ± 15.3	0.20
24-h heart rate (bpm)	68.2 ± 6.6	65.6 ± 6.3	0.14
Daytime SBP (mmHg)	123.9 ± 10.2	131.7 ± 11.1	0.02
Daytime DBP (mmHg)	72.1 ± 8.4	75.1 ± 7.2	0.10
Daytime MBP (mmHg)	89.2 ± 7.1	93.8 ± 5.3	0.01
Daytime PP (mmHg)	51.9 ± 11.9	56.6 ± 14.7	0.20
Daytime heart rate (bpm)	71.8 ± 8.2	70.5 ± 8.8	0.32
Night-time SBP (mmHg)	114.7 ± 14.9	123.8 ± 19.8	0.08
Night-time DBP (mmHg)	62.4 ± 7.1	63.9 ± 7.3	0.24
Night-time MBP (mmHg)	79.7 ± 8.1	83.6 ± 9.5	0.08
Night-time PP (mmHg)	52.3 ± 13.7	59.9 ± 18.5	0.12
Night-time heart rate (bpm)	61.2 ± 6.4	58.1 ± 4.5	0.06
Brachial artery diameter (mm)	3.75 ± 0.71	4.50 ± 0.72	0.0001
EDD (%)	6.9 ± 3.4	4.6 ± 3.9	0.07
NonEDD (%)	13.0 ± 5.7	7.7 ± 6.2	0.05
24-h urinary Na (mEq)	38.9 ± 11.8	138.5 ± 48.6	0.001
24-h urinary NOx (μmol/l)	256.1 ± 102.3	492.5 ± 313.1	0.02
24-h urinary NOx/creatinine (μmol/mg per l)	5.4 ± 2.7	10.1 ± 5.8	0.007
Plasma ADMA (μmol/l)	2.7 ± 1.0	2.7 ± 0.8	0.70

Abbreviations: SBP, Systolic blood pressure; *DBP*, diastolic blood pressure; *MBP*, mean blood pressure; *PP*, pulse pressure; *EDD*, brachial artery endothelium-dependent dilation; *NonEDD*, brachial artery non–endothelium-dependent dilation; *NOx*, nitric oxide metabolites; *ADMA*, asymmetric dimethylarginine.

(Courtesy of Scuteri A, Stuehlinger MC, Cooke JP, et al: Nitric oxide inhibition as a mechanism for blood pressure increase during salt loading in normotensive postmenopausal women. *J Hypertens* 21:1339-1346, 2003.)

correlation of salt loading with changes in EDD was found, after adjustment for age and cholesterol level (Table 1).

Conclusions.—The increase in BP during high-salt intake in normotensive postmenopausal women not receiving estrogen may be attributable to the inhibition of NO bioavailability by ADMA and a subsequent reduction in EDD.

▶ Young and middle-aged men tend to have higher BP than women of a similar age. After menopause, however, hypertension is more prevalent among women than among men.

It has been suggested that estrogen is one of the factors responsible for the lower BP in younger women than in younger men, likely through stimulation of NO production.

Scuteri et al studied a total of 15 healthy normotensive (<140/90 mm Hg) women, aged 50 to 60 years, whose last menses was at least 1 year before the participation in the study. Exclusion criteria were the use of estrogen or other steroids within the past year, smoking, a history of surgically induced menopause, use of drugs that affect cardiovascular functioning, elevate serum cholesterol levels, or affect CNS functioning, or a history of cardiovascular, respiratory, renal, or hepatic disorders, or diabetes mellitus.

The mean age of the 15 normotensive postmenopausal women was 55.5 ± 3.1 years. All of them were white. Baseline average 24-hour BP values (day 0) were 123.2 ± 12 mm Hg for systolic pressure and 71.0 ± 8.0 mm Hg for diastolic pressure. The effects of salt loading on BP are shown in Table 1.

Inhibition of NO by ADMA contributes to the increase in BP during high-salt intake in normotensive postmenopausal women not receiving estrogen.

Previous studies indicated that NO production in response to a high-salt intake might be impaired in hypertensive patients. Also, salt loading attenuates the conversion of L-arginine to NO in the endothelium of the renal vasculature in salt-sensitive patients with hypertension.

S. Klahr, MD

35 Proteinuria

Introduction

In this article by Ruggenenti et al (Abstract 35–1), the authors conclude that the long-term favorable impact of short-term reduction in proteinuria was particularly strong in patients with higher levels of baseline urinary protein excretion rate. These findings imply that any treatment targeted at effectively reducing urinary protein excretion rate would possibly have a long-term beneficial effect on disease progression, particularly in patients with heavy proteinuria.

Saulo Klahr, MD

Retarding Progression of Chronic Renal Disease: The Neglected Issue of Residual Proteinuria

Ruggenenti P, for the Investigators of the GISEN Group (Mario Negri Inst for Pharmacological Research, Bergamo, Italy; et al)
Kidney Int 63:2254-2261, 2003   35–1

Background.—Early changes in proteinuria have been linked to long-term glomerular filtration rate (GFR) reduction, indicating that proteinuria is a major factor in the progression of chronic renal disease. Whether proteinuria makes a specific, independent contribution to the progression of chronic renal disease and whether its reduction ameliorates the outcome were investigated via measurements of the change in GFR (ΔGFR).

Methods.—Participants were part of the Ramipril Efficacy In Nephropathy (REIN) study and were randomly assigned to receive either ramipril or placebo and conventional therapy. Protein levels were determined at baseline and after 3 months. Residual proteinuria also was determined at 3 months, and the percent changes were assessed for their ability to predict ΔGFR in 273 patients with proteinuric chronic nephropathies. Follow-up extended for 24.5 to 50.3 months (median, 31.3 months).

Results.—During the first 3 months, 24-hour proteinuria showed a significant decrease in patients receiving ramipril and an increase in those receiving placebo (Tables 1, 2, and 3). After 3 months, the GFR had decreased from 46.6 to 44.6 mL/min per 1.73 m² in those taking ramipril and from 42.3 to 40.2 mL/min per 1.73 m² in those receiving placebo. GFR-corrected proteinuria declined significantly in both groups. However, the ΔGFR was

TABLE 1.—Main Basal Clinical Characteristics of the Study Patients as a Whole (Overall) and According to Randomization to Ramipril or Conventional Treatment and to Basal Proteinuria 1 to 3 g/24 Hours (Stratum 1) or ≥3 g/24 Hours (Stratum 2)

	Overall	Ramipril	Conventional	Stratum 1	Stratum 2
Age *years*	48.7 ± 0.8	47.3 ± 1.1	50.2 ± 1.2	49.3 ± 1.1	47.9 ± 1.3
Gender *M/F*	204/69	108/31	96/38	121/43	83/26
Disease *glomerular/other*	143/130	80/59	63/71	73/91	70/39*
Mean arterial pressure *mm Hg*	107.9 ± 0.7	107.1 ± 1.03	108.6 ± 1.05	107.2 ± 1.0	108.9 ± 1.0
Glomerular filtration rate *mL/min/1.73 m²*	44.5 ± 1.1	46.6 ± 1.7	42.3 ± 1.5	47.6 ± 1.4	39.8 ± 1.7
Proteinuria *g/24 hours*	3.2 ± 0.2	3.3 ± 0.2	3.1 ± 0.2	1.7 ± 0.1	5.4 ± 0.3†
Glomerular filtration rate–corrected proteinuria *g/24 hours/mL/min/1.73 m²*	0.09 ± 0.01	0.09 ± 0.01	0.09 ± 0.01	0.04 ± 0.00	0.16 ± 0.01†

*P < .01.
†P < .0001 vs stratum 1.
(Courtesy of Ruggenenti P, for the Investigators of the GISEN Group: Retarding progression of chronic renal disease: the neglected issue of residual proteinuria. *Kidney Int* 63:2254-2261, 2003. Reprinted by permission of Blackwell Publishing.)

TABLE 2.—Main Clinical Characteristics at 3 Months After Randomization of the Study Patients as a Whole (Overall) and According to Randomization to Ramipril or Conventional Treatment and to Basal Proteinuria 1 to 3 g/24 Hours (Stratum 1) or ≥3 g/24 Hours (Stratum 2)

	Overall	Ramipril	Conventional	Stratum 1	Stratum 2
Mean arterial pressure *mm Hg*	103.3 ± 0.7	100.7 ± 0.9	105.9 ± 0.9*	101.8 ± 0.9	105.5 ± 1.0†
Glomerular filtration rate *mL/min/1.73 m²*	42.5 ± 1.1	44.6 ± 1.7	40.2 ± 1.6	46.3 ± 1.4	36.7 ± 1.8‡
Proteinuria *g/24 hours*	3.0 ± 0.2	2.5 ± 0.2	3.4 ± 0.3§	1.7 ± 0.1	4.8 ± 0.3‡
Glomerular filtration rate–corrected proteinuria *g/24 hours/mL/min/1.73 m²*	0.09 ± 0.01	0.08 ± 0.01	0.11 ± 0.01§	0.04 ± 0.00	0.17 ± 0.01*

*P < .0001 vs ramipril.
†P < .001.
‡P < .0001 vs stratum 1.
§P < .001.
(Courtesy of Ruggenenti P, for the Investigators of the GISEN Group: Retarding progression of chronic renal disease: the neglected issue of residual proteinuria. *Kidney Int* 63:2254-2261, 2003. Reprinted by permission of Blackwell Publishing.)

TABLE 3.—Main Clinical Characteristics on Follow-up (Data Averaged From 6 Months to Study End) of the Study Patients as a Whole (Overall) and According to Randomization to Ramipril or Conventional Treatment and to Basal Proteinuria 1 to 3 g/24 Hours (Stratum 1) or ≥3 g/24 Hours (Stratum 2)

	Overall	Ramipril	Conventional	Stratum 1	Stratum 2
Mean arterial pressure *mm Hg*	103.1 ± 0.5	101.0 ± 0.7	105.1 ± 0.8*	102.1 ± 0.7	104.8 ± 0.8†
GFR *mL/min/1.73 m²*	38.4 ± 1.2	41.3 ± 1.7	35.2 ± 1.5‡	43.2 ± 1.5	30.9 ± 1.7§
Proteinuria *g/24 hours*	2.9 ± 0.1	2.5 ± 0.2	3.2 ± 0.2*	1.9 ± 0.1	4.6 ± 0.3§
GFR-corrected proteinuria *g/24 hours/mL/min/1.73 m²*	0.10 ± 0.01	0.09 ± 0.01	0.12 ± 0.01*	0.06 ± 0.00	0.19 ± 0.02§

*$P < .001$ vs ramipril.
†$P < .05$.
‡$P < .01$.
§$P < .0001$ vs stratum 1.
(Courtesy of Ruggenenti P, for the Investigators of the GISEN Group: Retarding progression of chronic renal disease: the neglected issue of residual proteinuria. *Kidney Int* 63:2254-2261, 2003. Reprinted by permission of Blackwell Publishing.)

significantly slower for patients who had a short-term reduction than for those who had no short-term reduction in proteinuria, regardless of whether they received ramipril or placebo. The ΔGFR was predicted significantly by the 3-month percent changes in proteinuria and by actual mean arterial pressure (MAP) values and proteinuria levels at 3 months and at follow-up. Regardless of therapy, patients' specular short-term changes in proteinuria correlated with significantly different ΔGFR values. Similar changes in proteinuria produced differing ΔGFR values between the 2 therapies, with a mean value in the ramipril group of 0.39 mL/min per 1.73 m²/month and a mean value in the conventional therapy group of 0.74 mL/min per 1.73 m²/month. These values were 7-fold higher in patients with basal proteinuria of 3 g/24 h or more than in those with basal proteinuria of 1 to 3 g/24 h.

Conclusions.—Regardless of blood pressure control and a randomly selected treatment, reliable predictions about long-term disease progression could be obtained with the use of measures of short-term changes in proteinuria and actual levels of residual proteinuria. Predictability was maximized when these changes were considered in combination with and after correction for the accompanying GFR values. Patients with higher levels of baseline urinary protein excretion rates had a greater long-term favorable impact of the short-term reduction in proteinuria. Thus, treatment focused on reducing urinary protein excretion rate can have a long-term beneficial effect on the progression of disease, especially among patients with greater levels of proteinuria.

▶ Studies in relatively small series of patients with diabetic or nondiabetic renal disease suggest that early reduction of proteinuria predicts less progression in the long term. More recently, the Modification of Diet in Renal Disease (MDRD) study found in a remarkably larger number of patients that a reduction in arterial blood pressure and proteinuria were both accompanied by a better-preserved GFR throughout the whole study period. However, between reduction in blood pressure and reduction in proteinuria, the actual determinant of improved long-term outcome was unresolved.

Recently, the REIN study provided indirect evidence that in nondiabetic chronic nephropathy proteinuria predicted disease progression and that proteinuria reduction obtained with angiotensin-converting enzyme (ACE) inhibitor therapy was renoprotective.

This trial compared the rate of GFR decline and the risk of progression to end-stage renal disease in 2 groups of patients with proteinuria chronic nephropathies randomly allocated to the same degree of blood pressure control (diastolic blood pressure < 90 mm Hg) achieved with ACE inhibitor ramipril or with placebo, plus non-ACE inhibitor antihypertensives as appropriate. A total of 273 patients followed up for a median (interquartile range) of 31.3 (24.5 to 50.3 months) were available for outcome analyses (see Tables 1, 2, and 3).

The authors conclude that the long-term favorable impact of short-term reduction in proteinuria was particularly strong in patients with higher levels of baseline urinary protein excretion rate. These findings would imply that any treatment targeted at effectively reducing urinary protein excretion rate would possibly have a long-term beneficial effect on disease progression, particularly in patients with heavy proteinuria.

S. Klahr, MD

36 Transplantation

Introduction

The majority of kidney transplants fail because of chronic allograft nephropathy. Radermacher et al (Abstract 36–1) tested whether a renal arterial resistance index of less than 80 was predictive of the long-term survival of the transplanted kidney.

In an article by Ojo et al (Abstract 36–2), the authors report an analysis of kidney outcomes in almost 70,000 recipients of non-kidney organ transplants such as heart, lung, both heart and lung, and liver and intestine in the United States between 1990 and 2000.

A study by Bunnapradist et al in Los Angeles (Abstract 36–3) used analyses data from living-donor kidney transplant patients registered with the United Network for Organ Sharing (UNOS) Renal Transplant Registry to compare 2-year graft survival between the 2 commonly used immunosuppression regimens, tacrolimus or cyclosporine, in conjunction with mycophenylate mofetil and steroids.

Venstrom et al (Abstract 36–4) examined the survival of patients who received simultaneous pancreas-kidney transplants and of patients with preserved kidney function who received pancreas transplants alone or pancreas after kidney transplants, compared with patients who remained on the waiting list for those procedures.

The study by Nankivell et al from Australia (Abstract 36–5) evaluated the natural history of chronic allograft nephropathy of 120 recipients with type 1 diabetes—all but one of whom received kidney-pancreas transplants.

Saulo Klahr, MD

The Renal Arterial Resistance Index and Renal Allograft Survival
Radermacher J, Mengel M, Ellis S, et al (Hannover Med School, Germany; Humboldt Univ of Berlin)
N Engl J Med 349:115-124, 2003   36–1

Background.—Eighty percent of renal transplant failures are attributable to chronic allograft nephropathy or death of the transplant recipient. However, no reliable predictors of long-term outcome in renal allograft have been identified. It was reported recently that a renal arterial index of 80 or higher is predictive of a poor outcome of treatment after correction of renal artery stenosis, as well as worsening renal function or death in patients with renal disease other than renal artery stenosis. Whether a renal arterial resistance index of less than 80 is predictive of long-term allograft survival was investigated.

Methods.—The study group comprised 601 patients who underwent Doppler US between August 1997 and November 1998 for measurement of the renal segmental arterial resistance index at least 3 months after transplantation. All of the patients were followed up for 3 or more years. The combined end point was a decrease of 50% or more in the creatinine clearance rate, allograft failure, or death.

Results.—A resistance index of 80 or higher was observed in 122 (20%) patients, of whom 84 (69%) had a decrease of 50% of more in creatinine clearance. In comparison, 56 of the 479 (12%) patients with a resistance index of less than 80 had a decrease of 50% or more in creatinine clearance. Fifty-seven patients with a higher resistance index (47%) required dialysis, as compared with 43 (9%) patients with a lower resistance index; 36 patients with a higher resistance index (30%) died, compared with 33 patients (7%) with a lower resistance index.

A total of 107 patients (88%) with a higher resistance index reached the combined end point, as compared with 83 (17%) patients with a lower resistance index. The multivariate relative risk of graft loss among patients with a higher resistance was 9.1. This risk was also increased by proteinuria, symptomatic cytomegalovirus infection, and a creatinine clearance rate of less than 30 mL/min/1.73 m^2 of body surface area.

Conclusion.—A renal arterial resistance index of 80 or higher measured at least 3 months after renal transplantation is associated with poor subsequent allograft performance and death.

▶ The majority of kidney transplants fail due to chronic allograft nephropathy. This study by Radermacher et al tested whether a renal arterial resistance index of less than 80 was predictive of the long-term survival of the transplanted kidney. The ethics committee of the University of Hannover approved the study and all patients gave written informed consent. Between August of 1997 and November of 1998, color Doppler was performed by a single investigator in 776 consecutive recipients of a kidney transplant and were followed up as outpatients in the clinic.

A total of 175 patients were excluded from the study because they had undergone transplantation less than 3 months previously. Follow-up data were available for all 601 patients. Patients with a resistance index value of 80 or higher were significantly older, had had their transplants for a longer time, had higher blood pressure, and were more likely to have coronary artery disease than patients with resistance index values below 80. A total of 122 patients (20%) had a resistance index of 80 or higher. Eighty-four of these patients (69%) had a decrease of 50% or more in the creatinine clearance rate, as compared with 56 of the 479 with a resistance index value of less than 80 (12%). Also, 57 patients with a higher resistance index required dialysis.

The authors found that a resistance index of 80 or higher in an allograft patient was a strong predictor of both allograft failure and death with a functioning graft. Various risk factors—older age, poor renal function at 1 year, the presence of proteinuria and hypertension, delayed graft function—have all been proposed as means for differentiating between patients with a good chance of long-term survival of the kidney allograft and those patients with a poor chance.

S. Klahr, MD

Chronic Renal Failure After Transplantation of a Nonrenal Organ
Ojo AO, Held PJ, Port FK, et al (Univ of Michigan, Ann Arbor)
N Engl J Med 349:931-940, 2003   36–2

Introduction.—The transplantation of nonrenal organs is frequently complicated by chronic renal disease associated with multifactorial causes. A population-based cohort analysis was performed to assess the occurrence of chronic renal failure, the risk factors for renal failure, and the associated hazard of death in recipients of nonrenal transplants.

Methods.—Pretransplantation and posttransplantation clinical variables and data from a registry of patients with end-stage renal disease (ESRD) were analyzed to estimate the cumulative incidence of chronic renal failure (glomerular filtration rate of 29 mL/min/1.73 m^2 of body surface area or less or the development of ESRD) and the associated risk of death among 61,321 patients who received nonrenal transplants in the United States between 1990 and 2000.

Results.—A total of 11,426 patients developed chronic renal failure at a mean follow-up of 36 months. Of these, 3297 (28.9%) needed maintenance dialysis or renal transplantation. The 5-year risk of chronic renal failure varied, according to the type of organ transplanted, from 6.9% for heart-lung transplant recipients to 21.3% for intestinal transplant recipients. Multivariate analysis revealed that an increased risk of chronic renal failure was linked with increasing age (relative risk (RR)/10-year increment, 1.36; $P <$ .001), female gender (RR among male patients vs female patients, 0.74; $P <$ .001), pretransplantation hepatitis C infection (RR, 1.15; $P <$ .001), hypertension (RR, 1.18; $P <$ .001), diabetes mellitus (RR, 1.42; $P <$ .001), and postoperative acute renal failure (RR, 2.3; $P <$ .001).

Chronic renal failure significantly increased the risk of death (RR, 4.55; $P <$ .001). Treatment of ESRD with kidney transplantation was linked with a 5-year risk of death that was significantly lower than that linked with dialysis (RR, 0.56; $P =$ .02).

Conclusion.—The 5-year risk of chronic renal failure after transplantation of a nonrenal organ ranges between 7% to 21%, depending on the type of organ transplanted. Chronic renal failure among patients with a nonrenal transplant is linked with an increase by a factor in excess of 4 for the risk of death.

▶ In this article, the authors report an analysis of kidney outcomes in almost 70,000 recipients of nonkidney organ transplants—such as heart, lung, both heart and lung, liver, and intestine—in the United States between 1990 and 2000. After a median follow-up of 36 months, severe chronic kidney disease (a glomerular filtration rate of less than 29 mL/min/1.73m² of body surface area) had developed in 16.5% of the patients, and almost one third of these patients had ESRD.

Ojo et al did not report the prevalence of chronic kidney impairment (a glomerular filtration rate of 30 to 59 mL/min/1.73m²) among recipients of nonrenal transplants, but a conservative estimate based on the general population suggests that its prevalence would be several times as high as the prevalence of severe chronic kidney disease in this population. This study indicates that severe chronic kidney disease is relatively common after the transplantation of a nonrenal organ and is associated with increased mortality.

The findings of Ojo et al should stimulate new studies in this area. The variability in risk among patients with different types of organ transplants in this study points to the existence of other important patient-specific and organ-specific susceptibility traits.

These data show that diabetes mellitus, hypertension, and hepatitic C infection are independent risk factors in the aggregate, although their prevalence and effect varied according to the type of organ transplanted. Recipients of liver transplants had a prevalence of hepatitis C of 21.4%, with an associated 22% excess risk of chronic kidney failure. In contrast, recipients of lung transplants had a prevalence of hepatitis C of about 1%. In conclusion, the 5-year risk of chronic kidney failure after transplantation of a nonrenal organ ranges from 7% to 21%, depending on the type of organ transplanted.

S. Klahr, MD

Graft Survival Following Living-Donor Renal Transplantation: A Comparison of Tacrolimus and Cyclosporine Microemulsion With Mycophenolate Mofetil and Steroids

Bunnapradist S, Daswani A, Takemoto SK (Cedars-Sinai Med Ctr, Los Angeles; Univ of California, Los Angeles)

Transplantation 76:10-15, 2003   36–3

Background.—Differences in graft survival rates may be more evident in analyses of data from registry databases than from randomized clinical trials, as the former have greater statistical power than the latter. Data on graft survival rates in patients using tacrolimus (tac) or cyclosporine (CsA) with mycophenolate mofetil (MMF) and steroids, and data on living-donor kidney transplant patients obtained from the United Network for Organ Sharing Renal Transplant Registry were analyzed.

Methods.—Data on 4686 patients receiving CsA-MMF and on 2393 receiving tac-MMF in 1998 and 1999 were analyzed (Table 2). The main endpoint was graft survival after adjusting for confounding factors.

Findings.—Unadjusted all-cause 2-year graft survival rates were 94.3% with CsA-MMF and 92.2% with tac-MMF, a significant difference (Fig 1). After adjusting for possible confounders, graft failure risk at 2 years was sig-

TABLE 2.—Demographics and Baseline Characteristics of Living-Donor Kidney Patients Transplanted 1998 To 1999 (Intent-to-Treat Population)

	tac-MMF (n=2,393)	Percent of Patients	CsA-MMF (n=4,686)
Recipient age			
0-20 years	9.6		9.9
21-55 years	72.8		71.1
>55 years	17.5		18.9
Unknown	0.1		0.0
P		NS	
Recipient sex			
Male	54.4		59.8
P		<0.001	
Recipient race			
White	63.8		71.3
Black	19.7		13.1
Hispanic	11.6		10.7
Asian	2.6		3.2
Other/unknown	2.2		2.0
P		<0.001	
Original disease			
Glomerulonephropathy	9.7		10.3
Diabetes mellitus	21.5		19.9
Hypertension	15.1		12.3
Unknown/other	53.8		57.5
P		<0.001	
Previous transplant			
0	87.3		93.9
1	10.5		5.7
>1	2.2		0.4
P		<0.001	
PRA status			
0-10	84.6		87.6
11-30	7.5		6.7
>30	7.9		5.6
P		<0.001	
Donor age			
<55 years	83.3		87.5
>55 years	7.3		8.2
Unknown	9.4		4.3
P		<0.001	
HLA compatibility			
0 haplotype mismatch	8.9		11.5
1 haplotype	55.9		54.2
2 haplotype	35.2		34.4
P		0.003	

Abbreviations: Tac, Tacrolimus; *MMF,* mycophenolate mofetil; *CsA,* cyclosporine; *NS,* not significant; *PRA,* panel reactive antibody; *HLA,* human leukocyte antigen.

(Courtesy of Bunnapradist S, Daswani A, Takemoto SK: Graft survival following living-donor renal transplantation: A comparison of tacrolimus and cyclosporine microemulsion with mycophenolate mofetil and steroids. *Transplantation* 76:10-15, 2003.)

nificantly greater for patients receiving tac-MMF than for those given CsA-MMF for all-cause graft failure and death-censored graft failure. The analysis also identified other independent risk factors for graft failure: recipient or donor age older than 55 years, female sex, pretransplant blood transfusions, 1 or 2 haplotype mismatches compared with zero haplotype mismatch, and panel reactive antibody (PRA) exceeding 30%.

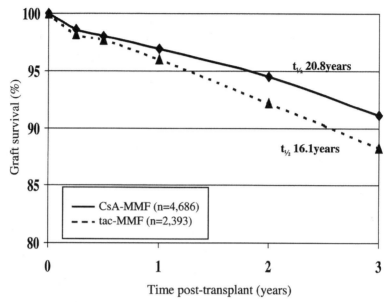

FIGURE 1.—Unadjusted graft survival rates for living donor patients receiving cyclosporine-myco-phenolate mofetil (CsA-MMF) (n=4,686) or tacrolimus (tac)-MMF (2,393) ($P = .0006$). The difference in graft half-life ($t_{1/2}$) was significant ($P < .001$). (Courtesy of Bunnapradist S, Daswani A, Takemoto SK: Graft survival following living-donor renal transplantation: A comparison of tacrolimus and cyclosporine microemulsion with mycophenolate mofetil and steroids. *Transplantation* 76:10-15, 2003.)

Conclusions.—In this analysis of large-scale registry data, 2-year renal allograft survival rates were significantly greater in living-donor recipients treated with CsA combined with MMF compared with those for tac combined with MMF as initial immunosuppression. Factors such as a decreased incidence of acute rejection may have changed the balance of determinants for graft survival after living-donor transplantation.

▶ The use of new immunosuppressive drugs during the last 10 to 15 years has provided transplant clinicians with a number of drug combinations and the opportunity to select regimens according to the risk profile and characteristics of individual patients.

This study by Bunnapradist et al in Los Angeles used analysis data from living-donor kidney transplant patients registered with the United Network for Organ Sharing (UNOS) Renal Transplant Registry to compare 2-year graft survival rates between the 2 commonly used immunosuppression regimens: tac or CsA in conjunction with MMF and steroids.

A total of 7079 living-donor kidney transplant patients who received their transplant during 1998 to 1999 were included in the analysis. Table 2 depicts the demographics and baseline characteristics of living-donor kidney patients transplanted during 1998 and 1999.

At 2 years posttransplant, the patient survival rate was 97.7% in the group in tac and 96.8% in the CsA, a difference that was not statistically significant.

There were 4686 patients that received CsA-MMF and 2393 that received tac-MMF.

The results of this study, based on more than 7000 patients receiving living-donor kidney transplants, showed significantly higher 2-year all-cause and death-censored graft survival rates in living-donor kidney transplant recipients managed with CsA-MMF compared with those managed by tac-MMF. This difference was sustained for a wide range of potentially confounding factors (see Fig 1).

S. Klahr, MD

Survival After Pancreas Transplantation in Patients With Diabetes and Preserved Kidney Function
Venstrom JM, McBride MA, Rother KI, et al (NIH, Bethesda, Md; Vanderbilt Univ, Nashville, Tenn; United Network for Organ Sharing, Richmond, Va; et al)
JAMA 290:2817-2823, 2003   36–4

Background.—Pancreatic transplantation is a therapeutic option for patients with complicated diabetes mellitus and is supported by the American Diabetes Association for patients with diabetes who have had, or need, a kidney transplant. In the absence of kidney failure, pancreas transplantation may be considered for patients with diabetes and severe and frequent metabolic instability. However, solitary pancreas transplantation remains a controversial issue because of procedure-associated morbidity and mortality, the toxicity of immunosuppression, the high costs, and unproved effects on the secondary complications of diabetes.

At present, it is unclear whether a survival advantage over conventional therapies is obtained from pancreas transplantation. The association between solitary pancreas transplantation and survival in patients with diabetes and preserved kidney function was investigated.

Methods.—This retrospective observational cohort study was conducted at 124 transplant centers in the United States and included 11,572 patients with diabetes mellitus on the waiting list for pancreas transplantation at the United Network for Organ Sharing/Organ Procurement and Transplantation Network from January 1, 1995, to December 31, 2000. Patients receiving a multiorgan transplant and those with a serum creatinine level greater than 2 mg/dL or who ultimately received a simultaneous pancreas-kidney transplant were excluded. The main outcome measure was all-cause mortality within 4 years after transplantation or within a comparable time on the waiting list for the group not undergoing transplantation.

Results.—The overall relative risk of all-cause mortality for transplant recipients over 4 years of follow-up was 1.57 (95% confidence interval [CI], 0.98-2.53) for pancreas transplant only, 1.42 (95% CI, 1.03-1.94) for pancreas-after-kidney transplant, and 0.43 (95% CI, 0.39-0.48) for simultaneous pancreas-kidney transplant. Survival rates for transplant patients at 1 and 4 years were 96.5% and 85.2% for pancreas transplant alone, respectively, and 95.3% and 84.5% for pancreas-after-kidney transplant. For patients on the waiting list, 1- and 4-year survival rates were 97.6% and 92.1%, respectively, for pancreas transplant alone and 97.1% and 88.1%, respectively, for pancreas-after-kidney transplant.

Conclusion.—In this analysis of outcomes in patients with diabetes and preserved kidney function who underwent pancreas transplantation from 1995 to 2000, survival was significantly worse compared with survival of patients on the waiting list who underwent conventional therapy.

▶ In this issue of *JAMA*, Venstrom et al examined the survival of patients who received simultaneous pancreas-kidney transplants and of patients with preserved kidney function who received pancreas transplants alone or pancreas-after- kidney transplants, compared with patients who remained on the waiting list for those procedures. The conclusions of the authors regarding the benefit of simultaneous pancreas-kidney transplantation differ markedly from the analyses of pancreas-after-kidney transplantation or pancreas transplantation alone, and yet the postsurgical survival for each procedure is quite similar. The reason appears to be that, while patients with diabetes and kidney failure awaiting a simultaneous pancreas-kidney transplant have a remarkably high annual death rate, patients awaiting a solitary pancreas transplant have a much better prognosis.

It is suggested that a randomized controlled trial would be the most appropriate way to evaluate the effects of pancreas transplantation on survival, but this design may not be feasible or ethical. At this point, clinicians and patients considering the pancreas transplant option must understand the risks and benefits, the expense, and the uncertainties associated with this surgery therapy.

Also mortality associated with long-term diabetes is markedly lower than that associated with other conditions similarly amenable to transplantation, such as end-stage renal disease and liver failure. The data of this group of investigators suggest that patients with complicated diabetes who are considering a solitary pancreas transplant must weigh the potential benefit of insulin independence against an apparent increase in mortality for at least the first 4 years post transplantation. The authors suggest that the solitary pancreas transplantation option for those with normal kidney function warrants a second look.

S. Klahr, MD

The Natural History of Chronic Allograft Nephropathy
Nankivell BJ, Borrows RJ, Fung CL-S, et al (Univ of Sydney, Australia)
N Engl J Med 349:2326-2333, 2003   36–5

Background.—Chronic allograft nephropathy is the primary cause of kidney transplant failure. Registry data can be used to define some risk factors for chronic allograft nephropathy, but the pathophysiology of this complication is poorly understood. Findings on biopsy of a chronically failing kidney transplant usually indicate nonspecific or end-stage changes, so the relative contributions of preexisting disease in the allograft and immunologic and nonimmunologic factors become difficult to distinguish. One significant problem has been the lack of prospective, longitudinal histologic data from studies of chronic graft dysfunction in humans. The natural history of chronic allograft nephropathy was described.

Methods.—A prospective study was conducted in 120 patients with type 1 diabetes; 119 of these patients received kidney-pancreas transplants. A total of 961 kidney transplant biopsy specimens were obtained from the time of transplantation to 10 years after transplantation.

Results.—There were 2 distinctive phases in the evolution of chronic allograft nephropathy. The initial phase involved early tubulointerstitial damage from ischemic injury, prior severe rejection, and subclinical rejection. This was predictive of mild disease by 1 year. This initial phase was present in 94.2% of patients. Early subclinical rejection was common and affected 45.7% of biopsy specimens at 3 months. The risk of rejection was increased by the occurrence of a prior episode of severe rejection, was reduced by tacrolimus and mycophenolate therapy, and gradually resolved after 1 year. Both subclinical rejection and chronic rejection were associated with increased tubulointerstitial damage.

After 1 year, a later phase of chronic allograft nephropathy was observed. This phase was characterized by microvascular and glomerular injury. Chronic rejection was not common (5.8%). Progressive high-grade arteriolar hyalinosis with luminal narrowing, increasing glomerulosclerosis, and additional tubulointerstitial damage was accompanied by the use of calcineurin inhibitors. Nephrotoxicity was nearly universal at 10 years, and severe chronic allograft nephropathy was found in 58.4% of patients, with sclerosis in 37.3% of glomeruli. Tubulointerstitial and glomerular damage was irreversible once established and resulted in a degradation of renal function and graft failure.

Conclusion.—Two distinctive phases of injury were identified in this study of the pathophysiology and natural history of chronic allograft nephropathy after transplantation. It is clear from these findings that chronic allograft nephropathy in kidney-pancreas transplantation recipients with diabetes is a sequential, multifactorial disease process that results from a series of time-dependent immunologic and nonimmunologic insults.

▶ This study from Australia evaluated the natural history of chronic allograft nephropathy of 120 recipients with type 1 diabetes, all but one of whom had received kidney-pancreas transplants. Chronic allograft nephropathy is the progressive kidney dysfunction with chronic interstitial fibrosis, tubular atrophy, vascular occlusive changes, and glomerulosclerosis. This entity is the major cause of kidney-transplant failure. Kidney biopsies were performed according to the protocol at the time of transplantation, at 1 and 2 weeks, at 1, 3, 5, and 12 months, and then yearly for 10 years.

Needle-core biopsy specimens were obtained. Renal histopathologic analysis was performed in a blinded fashion by 2 observers using the Banff working classification. Chronic allograft nephropathy was defined as chronic interstitial fibrosis and tubular atrophy, with or without fibrointimal vascular thickening, and was graded according to the proportion of cortical area affected.

The recipients were a mean of 38.2 ± 7 years old at the time of transplantation; 58.3 percent were male and all but 1 was white. Diabetes mellitus had been present for a mean of 24.9 ± 6.9 years before combined transplantation, and after transplantation the mean glycosylated hemoglobin level was 5.6% ± 1.3% and was accompanied by sustained euglycemia.

This study provides new insights into the pathophysiology and natural history of chronic allograft nephropathy. This nephropathy appears to consist of 2 distinctive phases of injury, occurring at different times after transplantation within different histologic compartments. Early tubulointerstitial damage correlates with immunologic factors, including severe acute rejection and persistent subclinical rejection with the addition of ischemia-reperfusion injury. Later damage is characterized by progressive arteriolar hyalinosis, ischemic glomerulosclerosis, and interstitial fibrosis associated with long-term calcineurin-inhibitor nephropathy.

Despite very good 1-year rates of graft survival achieved by the introduction of cyclosporine and then tacrolimus, reservations have been expressed about the long-term nephrotoxicity of these calcineurin inhibitors. The high prevalence of late nephrotoxicity, the irreversibility of progressive glomerulosclerosis, and its contribution to chronic allograft nephropathy suggest that calcineurin inhibitors are unsuitable as long-term immunosuppressive agents for kidney transplantation.

S. Klahr, MD

37 Dialysis

Introduction

It was reported by Knight et al (Abstract 37–1) that despite technological advances in hemodialysis over the last several years, the overall mortality rates for patients undergoing maintenance hemodialysis are high, especially in older individuals.

HIV-related renal diseases are the third leading cause of end-stage renal disease (ESRD) among African Americans aged 20 to 64 years. As reported by Szczech and colleagues (Abstract 37–2), based on the projected growth of the population of HIV-infected patients with ESRD, this study provides epidemiologic and clinical information that describes the clinical needs of this population.

In the study by Troyanov et al (Abstract 37–3), recent evidence suggests that dysregulation of apoptosis within the vessel wall is an important determinant for the development and progression of atherosclerosis in animal models and humans.

The risk of atherosclerotic cardiovascular disease (ASCVD) is 5 to 30 times greater in patients with ESRD compared with the general population. A study by Longenecker et al (Abstract 37–4) tested the hypothesis that small apolipoprotein(a) size, but not a lipoprotein(a) level, is associated with prevalent ASCVD in the United States in a cohort of patients in dialysis therapy.

Teng et al (Abstract 37–5) indicate that patients receiving paricalcitol while undergoing long-term hemodialysis appear to have a significant survival advantage when compared with those patients receiving calcitriol. The authors indicated that a prospective randomized study would be critical to confirm these findings.

Despite advances in renal replacement therapy, patients receiving hemodialysis continue to experience a high mortality rate due mainly to cardiovascular disease. In summary, a study by Danielski et al (Abstract 37–6) compared biomarkers of inflammation and oxidative stress in patients with severe hypoalbuminemia during hemodialysis.

In the study by Ota et al (Abstract 37–7), the use of argatroban, a synthetic antithrombin product that has been developed in Japan, is discussed. This agent selectively inhibits thrombin without affecting antithrombin III activity. It is expected that its use as an anticoagulant in hemodialysis patients with antithrombin III deficiency will be safe.

Saulo Klahr, MD

The Association Between Mental Health, Physical Function, and Hemodialysis Mortality
Knight EL, Ofsthun N, Teng M, et al (Harvard Med School, Boston; Harvard School of Public Health, Boston; Fresenius Med Care, Lexington, Mass)
Kidney Int 63:1843-1851, 2003   37–1

Background.—Individuals undergoing maintenance hemodialysis, especially those who are older, have especially high mortality rates; in 1999, elderly patients (75-79 years old) with end-stage renal disease (ESRD) survived an average of 2.3 years, and for those 85 years or older, the average decreased to 1.6 years. In the United States, in 1999, the average life expectancy for individuals was 10.1 years at age 77 years, 7.5 years at age 82 years, and 5.6 years at age 87 years or more. Poor outcomes may be improved if individuals with ESRD who are at highest risk for death can be identified and interventions can be implemented. Predictors of mortality have included self-reported mental health and physical function. These parameters were assessed at baseline and over time to determine whether their decline is linked to a higher risk of death.

Methods.—The study included 14,815 individuals 20 to 96 years old (mean age, 61 years) who had ESRD. The SF-36 Health Survey was completed 1 to 3 months after hemodialysis was initiated and again 6 months later to reveal any declines. Associations were sought between the initial SF-36 Health Survey mental component summary (MCS) and physical component summary (PCS) scores and the mortality during the follow-up, which lasted 2 years. Interactions between age plus MCS and PCS scores were also evaluated. The principal outcome measure was the mortality rate.

Results.—The mean MCS score was 46.0, and the mean PCS score was 31.6. The MCS scores of younger and older persons were similar, but older individuals had lower PCS scores than younger persons; in addition, they were less likely to be African Americans, weighed less, were more likely to have ESRD resulting from hypertension, and had lower levels of diastolic blood pressure and phosphorus than younger individuals. A negative correlation was found between age and PCS score, and a very weak positive correlation was noted between age and MCS score and between MCS and PCS scores. An independent association was noted between MCS and PCS scores and 1- and 2-year mortality rates. A graded association was seen between PCS score and mortality rates in younger individuals that was not found in the oldest age group. Of the 5773 individuals for whom information was available on both baseline and 6-month scores, the mean MCS score change was −1.6 and the mean PCS score change was −1.0. A 10-point decline in MCS or PCS score was linked to a significant additional increase in mortality rate. No significant interaction was found between age and 6-month MCS or PCS score changes.

Conclusions.—Lower self-reported mental health and physical function were significantly associated with increased mortality rates in this population of individuals undergoing hemodialysis for ESRD. This relationship was graded across a broad spectrum of mental health and physical function scores. A decline in these parameters during a period of 6 months signaled an increased risk of death. Thus, obtaining serial measurements of a patient's mental health and physical functioning may aid in assessing the risk of death for an individual undergoing hemodialysis.

▶ Despite technological advances in hemodialysis over the last several years, overall mortality rates for patients undergoing maintenance hemodialysis are high, especially in older individuals. The reported 1999 average life expectancy for patients with ESRD was 2.3 years for those 75 to 79 years old, 1.9 years for those 80 to 84 years old, and 1.6 years for those 85 years old and older. Individuals in this study had been undergoing hemodialysis for at least 3 months.

Low self-reported mental health and physical function were significantly associated with increased mortality rates in a graded fashion in a large hemodialysis population, and the magnitudes of the observed associations were comparable to the increased mortality rates associated with clinically significant decrements in serum albumin. A 6-month decline in self-reported mental health and physical function was also significantly associated with additional risk of mortality. These results suggest that serial measurements of mental health and physical function may complement other baseline measurements in assessing mortality risk in individuals undergoing hemodialysis. The authors found that the impact of self-reported physical function on mortality rates differed significantly by age group, so it is important to consider age when interpreting physical function data. One should note that depression, which is associated with a low MCS score, and poor physical functioning are both amenable to treatment. Future studies are needed to determine whether interventions targeted at improving physical function and mental health can reduce mortality rates for individuals undergoing hemodialysis.

S. Klahr, MD

The Clinical Characteristics and Antiretroviral Dosing Patterns of HIV-Infected Patients Receiving Dialysis
Szczech LA, for the Adult AIDS Clinical Trial Group Renal Complications Committee (Duke Univ, Durham, NC; et al)
Kidney Int 63:2295-2301, 2003   37–2

Background.—Among African Americans 24 to 60 years old, HIV-related renal disease constitutes the third leading cause of end-stage renal disease (ESRD). Antiretroviral medications have slowed the progression of these disorders, yet the number of HIV-infected patients who reach ESRD will increase exponentially in the next 10 years. The clinical characteristics and antiretroviral dosing patterns of HIV-infected patients who are undergoing dialysis were assessed retrospectively to determine the clinical requirements of these individuals.

Methods.—Data were collected from 5 medical centers from January 1, 1998, through January 1, 2001, and included both demographic and clinical information on all HIV-infected patients receiving dialysis. Hepatitis status, CD4 lymphocyte count, and use of antiretroviral medication were used to characterize various subgroups. Of the 89 patients whose data were included, 55 patients were alive when data were collected. Their ages ranged from 22.7 to 66.9 years (mean age, 44.6 years). Men accounted for 74.2% of the sample, and 83.2% of the patients were African American.

Results.—Only 45.9% of the patients who were having renal biopsies were diagnosed with HIV-associated nephropathy (HIVAN), but most of the patients who had not had a biopsy had this diagnosis. Testing revealed 19.7% of the patients were positive for hepatitis B surface antigen, and 67.1% were positive for hepatitis C. IV drug use and older age were more commonly found among patients diagnosed with hepatitis C. Of 89 patients, 54 (60.7%) were receiving antiretroviral therapy. The use of these medications was linked to an increase in the absolute CD4+ lymphocyte count among patients alive when data were collected. The absolute CD4+ count did not change for patients who were not receiving antiretroviral medications. HIV RNA levels decreased in those who were alive and receiving antiretroviral medications but did not change in those alive but not receiving these agents. Great variation was noted in the dosing regimens of individual medications. The most significant variations were found among the patterns of lamivudine use, there being 12-fold differences in dosing regimens.

Conclusions.—These patients with HIVAN who were undergoing hemodialysis often had coinfection with hepatitis C. In addition, the dosing regimens varied widely between individuals, suggesting that some patients may be inadequately treated and some may be experiencing unneeded drug toxicity. Because this population is growing, the epidemiologic and clinical information gleaned should prove useful in addressing the clinical requirements of these individuals.

▶ HIV-related renal diseases are the third leading cause of ESRD among African Americans 24 to 60 years old. Before the use of highly active antiretroviral therapy (HAART), HIV-infected ESRD patients had a high mortality rate with mean survival times of 3.0 months, 4.5 months, and 11.0 months, according to reports done in 1988, 1995, and 1996, respectively. Subsequently, an observational cohort study, reported in 2000, showed a longer mean survival time among patients treated with HAART as compared with 1 or 2 antiretroviral drugs (mean, 28 vs 13 months). In addition, an analysis of United States Renal Disease Study data, done in 2002, revealed an improved survival rate for patients beginning dialysis during and since 1997.

Although this study provides epidemiologic information on HIV-infected patients beginning dialysis in the post HAART era, these data have some limitations. Since the study is observational, associations described cannot be assumed to have a cause-effect relationship. Further, these data are unable to examine those factors that might result in a survival bias, selecting patients with a decreased mortality risk prior to or following the beginning of renal replacement therapy.

Additional questions in the care of the HIV-infected ESRD patient should be investigated. HIV-infected patients with renal disease who undergo kidney biopsy have differences in the distribution of histologic and clinical diagnoses as compared with patients not undergoing biopsy. At the patient level, more aggressive diagnostic evaluation using renal biopsy may result in better-directed treatment. The impact of this on outcomes is not known.

Finally, the wide variation in dosing of antiretroviral medications suggest that there are subgroups of patients who are not receiving the appropriate dose to maximally suppress viral replications or minimize drug toxicity. Based on the projected growth of the population of HIV-infected patients with ESRD, this study provides epidemiologic and clinical information that describes the clinical needs of this population.

S. Klahr, MD

Soluble Fas: A Novel Predictor of Atherosclerosis in Dialysis Patients
Troyanov S, Hébert M-J, Masse M, et al (Hôpital du Sacré-Coeur de Montréal; Université de Montréal; Université de Sherbrooke, Canada)
Am J Kidney Dis 41:1043-1051, 2003   37–3

Background.—The leading cause of death in patients with end-stage renal disease (ESRD) is cardiovascular disease (CVD), and atherosclerotic complications are extremely common. Atherosclerosis that occurs prematurely results from a multitude of factors; however a special role is accorded to the high prevalence of classic cardiovascular risk factors in patients with ESRD, specifically, diabetes, hypercholesterolemia, hypertension, and smoking. Apoptosis dysregulation has been noted to function as a determinant for the development and progression of atherosclerosis. The induction of apoptosis involves ligation of the cell-surface antigen Fas/CD95 by its natural ligand (Fas-L) and subsequent activation of initiator and effector caspases. The overexpression of Fas is involved in advanced atherosclerotic lesion development, most likely regulating the amount of tissue mass in diseased vessels. Soluble Fas (sFas) and its ligand (sFas-L) can be determined in human plasma and increased levels have been hypothesized to be linked with CVD, but whether these can serve as predicting factors for patients with ESRD was unknown. The ability of sFas and sFas-L to predict CVD or death or both was investigated.

Methods.—A prospective cohort study was designed to investigate the potential held by plasma sFas and sFas-L levels to independently predict the risk of CVD and death. The study included 107 patients (median age, 70 years) undergoing chronic hemodialysis who were evaluated and were followed up for a median of 27 months.

Results.—At least 1 CVD end point was experienced by 53 patients. Thirty-nine patients had coronary artery disease (CAD) end points, suffering 17 fatal or nonfatal myocardial infarctions, 23 episodes of unstable angina, and 16 sudden deaths. Twenty-eight patients had peripheral arterial occlusive disease (PAOD) end points, including 13 transient ischemic attacks or strokes and 15 peripheral vascular disease episodes in previously unaffected limbs. The sFas levels at baseline showed significant relationships with the occurrence of CVD end points, but the sFas-L levels did not. A significantly greater risk for CVD end points accompanied increased sFas levels independent of baseline CVD history, classic risk factors for atherosclerosis, and markers of inflammation. Increased levels of C-reactive protein (CRP) were also linked to cardiovascular end points. Patients in the highest sFas tertile had increased cardiovascular mortality when compared with that of patients in the lowest tertile.

Conclusions.—This study revealed sFas as a novel and independent marker of vascular disease in ESRD patients, being significantly and independently predictive of CVD end points.

▶ Recent evidence suggests that dysregulation of apoptosis within the vessel wall is an important determinant for the development and progression of atherosclerosis in animal models and humans. CVD is the leading cause of death in patients with ESRD. Compared with the general population, death rates from cardiovascular events are 10 to 40 times greater in dialysis patients. In the present study, more than 49% of patients presented with at least 1 cardiovascular event. Although very high, this rate is not unusual. The reported occurrence of CVD in patients with ESRD is 10 to 100 times that of the general population. Conventional risk factors for atherosclerosis do not completely account for this excess burden, and new insights are emerging regarding novel etiologic factors. Inflammation is now recognized as an important risk factor for cardiovascular events and mortality.

Apoptosis mediates the controlled deletion of unwanted cells. Apoptosis occurs when death is part of an organized tissue process, as in embryogenesis, metamorphosis, endocrine-dependent tissue atrophy, and the control of normalcy. The biological process involves a series of steps leading to the demise of cells by the activation of endogenous systems. Historically, apoptosis refers to a form of programmed cell death observed in animal tissues. A large number of factors can initiate apoptosis, such as hypoxia, ischemia, cytokines, growth factors, ANG II, tumor necrosis factor-α (TNF-α), reactive oxygen species, and mechanical stretch.

These factors act on a family of cell membrane receptors that include the tumor necrosis factor receptor and Fas (also known as CD95 or APO-7). Members of this family share a common intracytoplasmic domain called the death domain. Stimulation of these receptors leads to conformational changes in the death domain, which initiates the activation of a cascade of intracytoplasmic molecules that include TRAD, FADD/MORT1, RIP, and RAIDD/CRADD. This leads to activation of a number of cytoplasmic signaling cascades, the best known among which is probably the mitogen-activated protein kinase pathway.

This study was in patients with a high prevalence of vascular disease at baseline. The conclusion indicates that sFas is a novel marker of vascular disease in patients with ESRD.

S. Klahr, MD

Lipoprotein(a) and Prevalent Cardiovascular Disease in a Dialysis Population: The Choices for Health Outcomes in Caring for ESRD (CHOICE) Study
Longenecker JC, Coresh J, Marcovina SM, et al (Johns Hopkins Univ, Baltimore, Md; Univ of Washington, Seattle; New England Medical Center, Boston)
Am J Kidney Dis 42:108-116, 2003   37–4

Background.—Patients with end-stage renal disease (ESRD) have a risk for atherosclerotic cardiovascular disease (ASCVD) that is 5 to 30 times greater than the risk among the general population. However, traditional ASCVD risk factors do not completely explain the excess ASCVD risk in this population. Levels of lipoprotein(a) (Lp[a]) are elevated in patients with ESRD and are also inversely related to the size of apolipoprotein(a) [apo(a)], a glycoprotein that is bound to Lp(a). The association of Lp(a) level and apo (a) size with prevalent ASCVD in incident dialysis patients was investigated.

Methods.—The study group included 871 incident dialysis patients (261 blacks, 565 whites, 45 other). Lp(a) was measured with the use of apo(a) size-independent enzyme-linked immunoassay, and apo(a) size was determined by sodium dodecyl sulfate–agarose gel electrophoresis. Prevalent ASCVD was defined as coronary heart disease or cerebral or peripheral vascular disease and was determined from medical records. Analysis included the variables of age; sex; race; dialysis modality; diabetes; and serum creatinine, albumin, and low-density lipoprotein cholesterol levels.

Results.—Overall, the prevalence of ASCVD was 58%. Comparison of median Lp(a) levels of those with ASCVD versus those without showed 38 nmol/L versus 35 nmol/L for whites and 100 nmol/L versus 74 nmol/L for blacks, respectively. Lp(a) level was associated with ASCVD in patients younger than 60 years but not in patients aged 60 years and older. Odds ratios were 1.3 for all whites and 1.1 for all blacks. Odds ratios of ASCVD were 1.7 for whites younger than 60 years and 1.2 for blacks younger than 60 years. There was no association between apo(a) isoform size and ASCVD.

Conclusion.—This study found an association between Lp(a) level and prevalent ASCVD among whites younger than 60 years but not among blacks or patients older than 60 years. These findings suggest that baseline ASCVD is not likely to strongly confound the potential associations of Lp(a) level and prospectively identified ASCVD incident dialysis patients.

▶ The risk of ASCVD is 5 to 30 times greater in patients with ESRD compared with the general population. The levels of Lp(a) are elevated in dialysis patients, suggesting that Lp(a) may account for a portion of the increased atherosclerotic disease in the ESRD patients. In the United States, few studies of Lp(a), apo(a), and ASCVD in patients with ESRD have enrolled incident dialysis patients or a large population of blacks or used an apo(a) size-insensitive Lp(a) assay.

This study by Longenecker et al tested the hypothesis that small apo(a) size, but not an Lp(a) level, is associated with prevalent ASCVD in the United States in a cohort of patients in dialysis therapy. ESRD is a good setting in which to study the relationship between high Lp(a) levels and ASCVD, since both are highly prevalent in this setting. In addition, a large population of blacks was enrolled in this study. The authors found an association between Lp(a) level and ASCVD among whites younger than 60 years. No statistically significant associations were found among blacks.

The limitations of this study relate to its cross-sectional design. Such cross-sectional studies may fail to detect true associations of risk factors with such potentially fatal diseases as ASCVD. With this study design, it also is not possible to determine whether elevated Lp(a) level is causally related to prevalent ASCVD. This study found that high Lp(a) levels are common among patients with ESRD and are associated with prevalent cardiovascular disease among younger white patients. The association was weaker in older and black patients.

Apo(a) isoform size was not associated with prevalent ASCVD and did not modify the association of Lp(a) levels with ASCVD.

S. Klahr, MD

Survival of Patients Undergoing Hemodialysis With Paricalcitol or Calcitriol Therapy
Teng M, Wolf M, Lowrie E, et al (Fresenius Med Care North America, Lexington, Mass; Harvard Med School, Boston)
N Engl J Med 349:446-456, 2003   37–5

Background.—Parenteral vitamin D suppresses parathyroid secretion and is standard therapy for secondary hyperparathyroidism. Unfortunately, it also results in elevated calcium and phosphorus levels, which may accelerate vascular disease and mortality. In 1998, paricalcitol was approved for treatment of hyperparathyroidism caused by chronic renal failure. Paricalcitol is associated with less change in serum calcium and phosphorus than calcitriol. A historical cohort study was performed comparing mortality for a large group of patients undergoing long-term dialysis who were treated with either calcitriol or paricalcitol.

Study Design.—The study group consisted of 67,399 patients who were undergoing dialysis at more than 1000 dialysis care facilities in North America (Table 1). The primary study population consisted of all patients who began receiving treatment with either calcitriol (Calcijex) or paricalcitol (Zemplar) from 1999 to 2001. For those who switched formulations during the study, subgroup analyses were performed. Demographic

TABLE 1.—Baseline Characteristics According to Vitamin D Therapy*

Characteristic	Paricalcitol (N = 29,021)	Calcitriol (N = 38,378)	P Value
Mean age (yr)	60.7	61.3	<0.01
Male sex (% of patients)	52	53	<0.01
Race (% of patients)			<0.01
White	53	55	
Black	39	36	
Other	8	9	
Diabetes (% of patients)	48	49	<0.01
Glycosylated hemoglobin (%)†	6.8	6.8	0.23
Primary cause of renal failure (% of patients)			<0.01
Diabetes	36	37	
Hypertension	38	36	
Glomerulonephritis	11	11	
Other	15	16	
Duration of dialysis (days)	620	530	<0.01
Vascular access (% of patients)			<0.01
Fistula	21	19	
Graft	27	26	
Catheter	23	21	
Unknown	29	34	
Body-mass index‡	28.6	28.4	<0.01
Body-surface area (m²)	1.87	1.85	<0.01
Blood pressure (mm Hg)			
Systolic	149	149	0.92
Diastolic	79	78	<0.01
Albumin (g/dl)	3.7±1.0	3.6±0.5	<0.01
Calcium (mg/dl)	8.7±0.8	8.5±0.9	<0.01
Phosphorus (mg/dl)	5.6±1.6	5.3±1.5	<0.01
Calcium-phosphate product	49±15	45±14	<0.01
Parathyroid hormone (pg/ml)	496±364	413±336	<0.01
Alkaline phosphatase (U/liter)	128±92	129±100	0.06
Cholesterol (mg/dl)			
Total	169±45	170±47	0.09
Low-density lipoprotein§	93±35	93±36	0.80
Hemoglobin (g/dl)	10.8±1.5	10.7±1.6	<0.01
Ferritin (ng/ml)	382±424	364±437	<0.01
White-cell count (mm⁻³)	8±3	8±3	0.57
Bicarbonate (mmol/liter)	21±4	20±4	<0.01
Creatinine (mg/dl)	7.8±3.2	7.6±3.1	<0.01
Dialysate calcium (mEq/liter)	2.66	2.67	<0.01
Urea reduction ratio (%)¶	67±9	67±10	0.08

*Plus-minus values are means ± SD. Baseline laboratory values represent the mean value during the 3 months before initiation of treatment with injectable vitamin D. To convert the values for calcium to millimoles per liter, multiply by 0.250; to convert the values for phosphorus to millimoles per liter multiply by 0.3229; to convert the values for cholesterol to millimoles per liter multiply by 0.02586; to convert the values for creatinine to millimoles per liter multiply by 88.4; to convert the values for dialysate to millimoles per liter multiply by 0.5.
†Data on glycosylated hemoglobin were available for 7514 patients.
‡The body-mass index is the weight in kg divided by the square of the height in meters.
§Data on low-density lipoprotein cholesterol were available for 4134 patients.
¶The urea reduction ratio, a measure of the adequacy of dialysis, is calculated as 100 × [1 − (postdialysis blood urea nitrogen/predialysis blood urea nitrogen)].
(Reprinted with permission of *The New England Journal of Medicine* from Teng M, Wolf M, Lowrie E, et al: Survival of patients undergoing hemodialysis with paricalcitol or calcitriol therapy. *N Engl J Med* 349:446-456, 2003. Copyright 2003, Massachusetts Medical Society. All rights reserved.)

and laboratory data were collected prospectively. The 36-month survival rate was compared for these groups.

Findings.—The mortality rate among patients receiving calcitriol was 6,805/30,471 person-years or 0.223 per person-year, whereas the mortality rate among patients who received paricalcitol was 3,417/19,031 person-years or 0.180 per person-year (Fig 1). This difference was highly significant. The difference in mortality rate achieved significance at 1 year and increased over time. In the adjusted analysis, the mortality rate was 16% lower among paricalcitrol-treated patients. At 12 months, calcium levels increased 8.2% and phosphorus levels increased 13.9% in the calcitriol group, compared with 6.7% and 11.8% in the paricalcitol group. The 2-year survival rate was

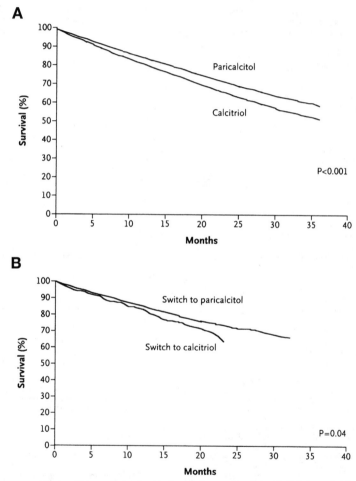

FIGURE 1.—Kaplan-Meier analysis of survival according to type of vitamin D therapy. Panel A shows the survival of patients treated with either paricalcitol or calcitriol who received the same therapy for the duration of the follow-up. Panel B shows the survival of patients who switched from calcitriol to paricalcitol or from paricalcitol to calcitriol during the follow-up period. The time of switching was approximately 900 days after initiation of dialysis for both groups. P values were calculated with the use of the log-rank test. (Reprinted with permission of *The New England Journal of Medicine* from Teng M, Wolf M, Lowrie E, et al: Survival of patients undergoing hemodialysis with paricalcitol or calcitriol therapy. *N Engl J Med* 349:446-456, 2003. Copyright 2003, Massachusetts Medical Society. All rights reserved.)

73% among those who switched from calcitriol to paricalcitol and 64% among those who switched from paricalcitol to calcitriol.

Conclusions.—This large historical cohort study of patients undergoing dialysis examined the effect on mortality rate of treatment with calcitriol versus paricalcitol. There was a significant survival advantage for patients who received paricalcitol. These conclusions need to be verified with a prospective, randomized clinical trial.

▶ Renal osteodystrophy is a disorder of bone and mineral metabolism, with elevated levels of parathyroid hormone and a high bone turnover. Parenteral vitamin D suppresses parathyroid hormone secretion and has been used as a therapy for secondary hyperparathyroidism.

Six years ago in 1998, paricalcitol (19-nor-1-25-diphydroxivitamin D_2) was approved for the treatment. It was noted that paricalcitol suppressed parathyroid hormone faster than calcitriol.

The primary study population consisted of patients on dialysis by Teng et al at Fresenius Medical Care North America. The primary study population consisted of all patients who started receiving treatment with zemplar or calcitriol. Between January 1, 1999, and December 31, 2001, treatment with injectable vitamin D was initiated in 69,492 patients undergoing treatment in Fresenius facilities. Of these, 67,399 (97%) were initially treated with paricalcitol or calcitriol and served as the primary study population (Table 1).

During the 3 years of follow-up, the mortality rate differed between the groups: among patients receiving paricalcitol, there were 3417 deaths during a total of 19,031 patient-years of observation compared with 6805 deaths during 30,471 patient-years, among those receiving calcitriol (Fig 1).

The authors indicated that patients receiving paricalcitol while undergoing long-term hemodialysis appear to have a significant survival advantage when compared with those patients receiving calcitriol. The authors indicated that a prospective randomized study would be critical to confirm these findings.

S. Klahr, MD

Linkage of Hypoalbuminemia, Inflammation, and Oxidative Stress in Patients Receiving Maintenance Hemodialysis Therapy
Danielski M, Ikizler TA, McMonagle E, et al (Maine Med Ctr, Portland; Maine Med Ctr Research Inst, Scarborough; Vanderbilt Univ, Nashville, Tenn)
Am J Kidney Dis 42:286-294, 2003   37–6

Background.—Patients on long-term maintenance hemodialysis have high cardiovascular mortality. Studies have linked the presence of hypoalbuminemia, inflammation and oxidative stress to cardiovascular morbidity and mortality, but the interrelationship among these prognostic factors is not clear. Biomarkers of inflammation and oxidation were examined in a hypoalbuminemic population on maintenance dialysis and compared with those in a normoalbuminemic maintenance dialysis population and to healthy controls.

Study Design.—The study group consisted of 18 patients on maintenance dialysis with serum albumin levels of no more than 3.2 g/dL, 18 age-, race-, sex-, and diabetes-matched hemodialysis patients and 18 matched healthy controls. Blood samples were drawn before dialysis for assessment of serum C-reactive protein (CRP), plasma interleukin-6 (IL-6), serum prealbumin, plasma protein-reduced thiol content, and plasma protein carbonyl content.

Findings.—Levels of serum CRP, IL-6, plasma protein thiol oxidation, and protein carbonyl formation were significantly higher in dialysis patients than in healthy controls. They were also significantly higher in hypoalbuminemic dialysis patients than in normoalbuminemic dialysis patients. Prealbumin levels were significantly lower in hypoalbuminemic dialysis patients than in the other 2 groups.

Conclusions.—This study compared biomarkers of inflammation and oxidative stress between hypoalbuminemic hemodialysis patients and matched normoalbuminemic dialysis patients and matched healthy controls. Biomarkers of inflammation and oxidative stress were increased in both dialysis populations, but they were further increased in the hypoalbuminemic population. This suggests that anti-inflammatory and antioxidative therapies may be useful in reducing cardiovascular morbidity and mortality in the maintenance dialysis population.

▶ Despite advances in renal replacement therapy, patients on hemodialysis continue to experience a high mortality caused mainly by cardiovascular disease.

The authors screened a dialysis population of more than 600 patients in 6 dialysis centers. Eighteen patients were identified with a serum albumin level of 3.2 g/dL or less. Both malnutrition and inflammation are prevalent in dialysis patients and contribute to cardiovascular morbidity and mortality.

Inflammation is common in patients with end-stage kidney disease. Cross-sectional studies indicate that 30% to 50% of hemodialysis patients have serologic evidence of an inflammatory response. An increase in oxidative stress has been implicated in the pathogenesis of cardiovascular complications in uremic patients.

Several cross-sectional studies also showed an inverse relationship between an elevation of CRP and IL-6 levels and serum albumin concentrations. CRP is an acute-phase response protein produced by the liver under the control of proinflammatory cytokines, including IL-6. High levels of IL-6 in plasma are associated with increased mortality, hypoalbuminemia, and erythropoietin resistance and greater in patients in hemodialysis compared with healthy individuals.

In summary, this study compared biomarkers of inflammation and oxidative stress in patients with severe hypoalbuminemia during hemodialysis. The authors found that levels of biomarkers of inflammation and oxidative stress are increased in both hemodialysis patient groups compared with healthy subjects. Therefore, anti-inflammatory and antioxidative drugs may be promising in attempting to reduce cardiovascular complications in this patient population.

S. Klahr, MD

Effects of Argatroban as an Anticoagulant for Haemodialysis in Patients With Antithrombin III Deficiency

Ota K, Akizawa T, Hirasawa Y, et al (Tokyo Women's Med Univ; Wakayama Med Univ, Japan; Shinrakuen Hosp, Niigata, Japan; et al)
Nephrol Dial Transplant 18:1623-1630, 2003   37–7

Background.—The use of an anticoagulant is an important component of hemodialysis. In patients with congenital or acquired antithrombin III deficiency undergoing hemodialysis, anticoagulation often results in coagulation or residual blood in the blood circuit and dialyser. Argatroban is a synthetic thrombin antagonist that directly inhibits the activity of thrombin in a manner that differs from that of heparin; thus, argatroban manifests an anticoagulating effect without the activation of antithrombin III. The anticoagulating effects of argatroban in patients with antithrombin III deficiency undergoing hemodialysis were investigated.

Methods.—This retrospective nationwide study was conducted among patients in Japan with congenital or acquired antithrombin III deficiency who had undergone hemodialysis with argatroban as an anticoagulant between1996 and April 2000. Patients were included in the study if they had antithrombin III activity less than 70% of normal or if blood coagulation or residual blood in the extracorporeal circuit could not be prevented by the use of heparin during hemodialysis.

Results.—Fifty-nine patients were included in the study. In comparison with data before the administration of argatroban, significant improvements of residual blood in the dialyser and arterial and venous drip chambers were observed at the last administration of argatroban. There was also a significant increase in antithrombin III activity. There were no adverse events reported in 66 of 80 (82.5%) safety analysis cases. One patient with severe adverse events demonstrated a bleeding tendency, and another had prolongation of prothrombin time.

Conclusion.—Argatroban is an effective and safe anticoagulant for use in patients undergoing hemodialysis for congenital or acquired antithrombin III deficiency.

▶ An important aspect of hemodialysis treatment is the use of an anticoagulant. Heparin has been used as an anticoagulant in hemodialysis, but heparin use is accompanied by several adverse reactions, including the development of hemorrhagic lesions, and osteoporosis, activation of platelets, and degradation of lipids. Argatroban is a synthetic antithrombin product that has been developed in Japan. This agent selectively inhibits thrombin without affecting antithrombin III activity. It is expected that its use as an anticoagulant in hemodialysis patients with antithrombin III deficiency will be safe.

A retrospective survey in Japan was conducted on congenital or acquired antithrombin III–deficient patients undergoing hemodialysis from April 1996 to April 2000. These patients, whose antithrombin III activity was less than 70 % of normal activity and in whom blood coagulation or residual in the blood in the extracorporeal circuit could not be prevented by the use of heparin, were studied. Of the 96 patients who received argatroban, 80 were eligible for the safety study analysis; 16 patients were not included due to refusal to participate in the study or because a complete study could not be done.

Argatroban was administered as an anticoagulant for hemodialysis to patients with antithrombin III deficiency in individuals with less than 70 % of normal activity in whom sufficient anticoagulation could not be achieved using heparin. A significant decrease in the appearance of residual blood in the extracorporeal circuit and an increase in antithrombin III activity were observed after the use of argatroban. No adverse reactions were observed in 82.5% of the patients. On the basis of these results, argatroban appears to be very effective as a safe anticoagulant for the treatment of patients on hemodialysis with reduced antithrombin III activity.

S. Klahr, MD

38 Calcium, Phosphorus, and Bone

Introduction

Hervás et al (Abstract 38–1) reported on a randomized study comparing sevelamer and calcium acetate to assess the efficacy of sevelamer in lowering serum phosphorus in hemodialysis patients.

The purposes of the study by Sawaya et al (Abstract 38–2) were: (1) to evaluate the relationship between intact parathyroid hormone (iPTH) levels and bone turnover in African American and white patients with end-stage renal disease on maintenance dialysis, and (2) to compare iPTH levels and bone histomorphometric parameters between the 2 races in patients with similar turnover rates.

Saulo Klahr, MD

Treatment of Hyperphosphatemia With Sevelamer Hydrochloride in Hemodialysis Patients: A Comparison With Calcium Acetate
Hervás JG, Prados D, Cerezo S (Univ of Granada, Spain)
Kidney Int 63, Supplement 85:S69-S72, 2003   38–1

Background.—Among the complications often seen with end-stage renal disease are secondary hyperparathyroidism and hyperphosphatemia, for which patients are restricted with regard to phosphorus intake and given carbonate or acetate salts of calcium plus vitamin D metabolites in some cases. Recently, sevelamer hydrochloride was approved as a calcium- and aluminum-free phosphate binder. The effectiveness of sevelamer hydrochloride in controlling hyperphosphatemia was compared with that of calcium acetate for patients undergoing hemodialysis.

Methods.—For a population of 61 patients, phosphate binder administration was suspended over a 2-week washout period, after which 51 patients were randomly given either sevelamer or calcium acetate; 40 patients

311

completed the study (Table 1). Monthly laboratory tests were carried out for 34 weeks to monitor the effect on patients' hyperphosphatemia.

Results.—The mean dose of sevelamer was 4.09 g/d; that of calcium acetate was 3.9 g/d. Patients tolerated sevelamer well, and side effects occurred at the same rate in the 2 groups. Thirty-eight percent of patients developed dyspepsia with sevelamer as did 36% of those with calcium acetate. Other side effects included diarrhea and constipation.

Both treatments produced statistically significant declines in the mean serum phosphorus levels; mean changes in the 2 groups from baseline to end of treatment were similar with the 2 therapies. Just over 7% of patients receiving sevelamer had at least 1 instance of hypercalcemia; this also occurred in about 9% of those receiving calcium acetate. Declines were noted in the intact parathyroid hormone levels with both treatments.

No significant change in serum alkaline phosphatase levels occurred with either therapy. The lipid profile for the sevelamer treatment group changed significantly from baseline (Fig 2), while that for the calcium acetate group did not. The mean changes with sevelamer treatment included total cholesterol, −30.5 mg/dL; low-density lipoprotein (LDL) cholesterol, −32.8 mg/dL; and high-density lipoprotein (HDL) cholesterol, 8.2 mg/dL.

Conclusion.—Sevelamer was able to effectively reduce the levels of serum phosphorus in patients undergoing hemodialysis. In addition, both total and LDL cholesterol levels were reduced with the use of sevelamer, with the degree of LDL cholesterol reduction similar to that obtained with cholesterol-

TABLE 1.—Baseline Patients' Characteristics

N	51
Age *years*	60.4 ± 15.1
Gender *% female*	40%
Primary renal disease	
Glomerulonephritis	17.5%
Interstitial	15%
Cystic	7.5%
Hypertension	15%
DM	15%
Unknown	25%
Others	5%
Length of dialysis *months*	56.9 ± 48.7
Previous phosphate binders	
Calcium acetate	79%
Calcium carbonate	21%
Dialysate calcium *mEq/L*	
2.5	79%
3.0	21%
Parathyroidectomy	10%
Vitamin D metabolites	70%
Kt/V	1.16 ± 0.15
Serum albumine	3.86 ± 0.41
Cholesterol-lowering agents	11.7%

(Courtesy of Hervás JG, Prados D, Cerezo S: Treatment of hyperphosphatemia with sevelamer hydrochloride in hemodialysis patients: A comparison with calcium acetate. *Kidney Int* 63 (suppl 85): S69-S72, 2003. Reprinted by permission of Blackwell Publishing.)

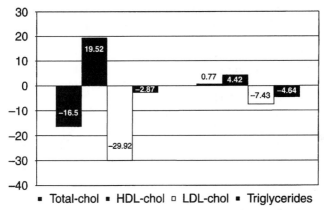

FIGURE 2.—Percentage change in total cholesterol, low-density lipoprotein (*LDL*) cholesterol, high-density lipoprotein (*HDL*) cholesterol, and triglyceride values. (Courtesy of Hervás JG, Prados D, Cerezo S: Treatment of hyperphosphatemia with sevelamer hydrochloride in hemodialysis patients: A comparison with calcium acetate. *Kidney Int* 63 (suppl 85): S69-S72, 2003. Reprinted by permission of Blackwell Publishing.)

lowering agents. HDL cholesterol levels were significantly increased or not affected by sevelamer. The advantages of modifying the lipid profile of hemodialysis patients are not currently known.

▶ Secondary hyperparathyroidism and hyperphosphatemia are common complications in end-stage renal disease. Treatment usually includes dietary restriction of phosphorus, use of carbonate or acetate salts of calcium, and often, the administration of vitamin D metabolites. Calcium salts have become the treatment choice for hyperphosphatemia, although the provision of calcium can lead to hypercalcemia and increase the risk of metastatic calcification, particularly in those patients on calcitriol therapy and patients with low bone turnover rates.

Sevelamer hydrochloride is a recently approved calcium- and aluminum-free phosphate binder. In previous studies, it effectively controlled serum phosphate in hemodialysis patients without their developing hypercalcemia. A randomized study comparing sevelamer and calcium acetate was performed to assess the efficacy of sevelamer in lowering serum phosphorus in hemodialysis patients. The study included male and female hemodialysis patients aged 18 years or older who were treated for at least 3 months with hemodialysis 3 times per week. Inclusion criteria required calcium-based phosphate binders and vitamin D therapy at stable doses for at least 1 month.

Patients were chosen and administration of calcium containing phosphate binder was discontinued during a 2-week washout period. Patients who developed a serum phosphorus level greater than 6 mg/dL during this washout were eligible for the study. After the 2-week washout phase, subjects were randomized to receive sevelamer hydrochloride or calcium acetate. Sevelamer was supplied in a capsule containing 403 mg (Renagel), while the calcium acetate was supplied as Royen, containing 500 mg calcium acetate (see Table 1).

Sevelamer treatment reduced both serum total cholesterol and LDL cholesterol. The 29% reduction in LDL cholesterol by sevelamer treatment is similar to the reduction obtained by cholesterol-lowering agents. Nevertheless, alternatives to HMG-CoA reductase inhibitors may be advisable, given the increased risk of drug-related side effects in patients with chronic renal failure (see Fig 2). In addition, sevelamer treatment significantly increases HDL cholesterol or has no effect at all.

The relative benefits of modifying the lipid profile in hemodialysis patients are also unknown. Changes in LDL cholesterol and HDL cholesterol induced by sevelamer in this study would be expected to reduce the rate of cardiovascular disease and potentially increase survival in these patients.

S. Klahr, MD

Differences in Bone Turnover and Intact PTH Levels Between African American and Caucasian Patients With End-Stage Renal Disease

Sawaya BP, Butros R, Naqvi S, et al (Univ of Kentucky, Lexington)
Kidney Int 64:737-742, 2003   38–2

Introduction.—Data derived from healthy research subjects indicate that African Americans have higher serum parathyroid hormone (PTH) levels and reduced bone responsiveness to PTH compared with whites. African American patients with end-stage renal disease (ESRD) also have higher serum PTH levels compared with whites. The association between intact PTH (iPTH) levels and bone turnover in African Americans and whites with ESRD on maintenance dialysis were examined. The iPTH levels and bone histomorphometric parameters between African Americans and whites were compared in patients with similar bone turnover rate.

Methods.—Serum iPTH and bone histomorphometric data were examined for racial differences in 76 patients with ESRD (48, white; 28, African American). Bone turnover was ascertained by means of histomorphometric determination of activation frequency in all patients.

Results.—Age, duration of dialysis, and calcium and phosphorus levels were similar in the 2 groups (Table 1). The mean iPHT levels were signifi-

---

TABLE 1.—Patients' Characteristics and Demographic Data

	Caucasians (C) (N = 48)	African Americans (AA) (N = 28)	P Value (C vs. AA)
Age *years*	47.7 ± 2.2	48 ± 2.6	NS
Male/female %	62/38	46/54	NS
Diabetics %	31	18	NS
Hemodialysis/peritoneal dialysis %	56/44	86/14	<0.01
Duration of dialysis *months*	20.1 ± 3.0	13.6 ± 2.9	NS
Vitamin D therapy %	20	23	NS

(Courtesy of Sawaya BP, Butros R, Naqvi S, et al: Differences in bone turnover and intact PTH levels between African American and Caucasian patients with end-stage renal disease. *Kidney Int* 64:737-742, 2003. Reprinted by permission of Blackwell Publishing.)

TABLE 2.—Intact Parathyroid Hormone and Biochemical Profile

	Caucasians (C) (N = 48)	African Americans (AA) (N = 28)	P Value (C vs. AA)
PTH (15-65 pg/mL)	270 ± 46	534 ± 79	<0.01
Calcium (8.4-10.2 mg/dL)	9.6 ± 0.2	9.1 ± 0.2	NS
Phosphorus (2.7-4.5 mg/dL)	6.4 ± 0.3	6.2 ± 0.4	NS
Alkaline phosphatase (20-70 U/L)	144 ± 43	162 ± 31	<0.01

Abbreviation: PTH, Parathyroid hormone.

(Courtesy of Sawaya BP, Butros R, Naqvi S, et al: Differences in bone turnover and intact PTH levels between African American and Caucasian patients with end-stage renal disease. *Kidney Int* 64:737-742, 2003. Reprinted by permission of Blackwell Publishing.)

cantly higher among African Americans than among whites (534 vs 270 pg/ mL; $P < .01$). The mean alkaline phosphatase levels (international units per liter) were significantly higher in African Americans than in whites (162 vs 144; $P < .01$). Correlations between PTH levels and activation frequency were $r = 0.60$ ($P < .01$) for whites and $r = 0.22$ ($P = NS$) for African Americans.

The mean PTH level in African American patients with histologic findings of low bone turnover was 460 versus 168 in white patients who had similar bone turnover ($P < .01$) (Table 2). Among patients with low bone turnover, African Americans had significantly higher osteoid volume and thickness, number of osteoblasts and osteoclasts, erosion surface, peritrabecular fibrosis, and single-label surface compared with whites. Erosion depth, bone formation rate per osteoblast, and mineralization apposition rate were similar between the 2 groups.

Conclusion.—No correlation was observed between iPTH and bone turnover in African Americans with ESRD. A marked number of African American patients with low bone turnover have very high serum PTH levels. Bone histomorphometric findings show differences in remodeling dynamics and responses to PTH between African American and white patients.

▶ The purposes of this study by Sawaya et al were: (1) to evaluate the relationship between iPTH levels and bone turnover in African American and white patients with ESRD on maintenance dialysis and (2) to compare iPTH levels and bone histomorphometric parameters between the 2 races in patients with similar turnover rates.

Patients who underwent bone biopsy between 1992 and 2000 were evaluated for this study. There was no difference in age, gender, diabetes status, duration of dialysis, or the use of vitamin D therapy between the African American and white groups (see Table 1). There were more white patients on peritoneal dialysis than African American patients. However, similar results were obtained when only hemodialysis patients were compared between the 2 racial groups. Therefore, the combined results of both hemodialysis and peritoneal patients were reported. African American patients had higher serum levels of iPTH despite similar serum phosphorus and calcium concentrations (Table 2). Alkaline phosphatase was also higher in the African American group (Table 2).

The results of this study confirm that African American patients with ESRD have higher serum PTH levels than whites. A significant positive correlation between PTH and bone turnover is seen only in white patients. The correlation coefficient for iPTH and bone turnover in this racial group is similar to that of other reports. However, there is no correlation between PTH and bone turnover in African American patients.

This study demonstrates that iPTH in African American patients with ESRD does not correlate with bone turnover as it does in white patients. Many African American patients with low bone turnover have substantially high iPTH levels. These findings have an impact on current clinical practice in defining the target iPTH level in ESRD patients.

S. Klahr, MD

Introduction

This section is organized by chapters. Articles selected for inclusion here reflect (in your editors' opinions) the clinical utility and novelty of the findings, not necessarily the prevalence or importance of the diseases in our practices. For example, the best and first descriptions of severe acute respiratory syndrome (SARS) are reviewed here. The disappointing failure of CT screening to provide a mortality benefit from lung cancer is also reported, as is evidence that continuous positive airway pressure (CPAP) reduces cardiovascular risk in patients with sleep apnea.

With regard to lung cancer, we report that cigar smokers are at increased risk just as cigarette smokers are, and that more vitamins are not necessarily better when it comes to reducing lung cancer risk in smokers.

Slow progress continues to be made in the treatment of chronic obstructive pulmonary diseases, the everyday challenge to the pulmonologist. We have new evidence that inhaled corticosteroids may confer benefit, as well as information about which patients are likely to require readmission or to benefit from noninvasive positive pressure ventilation (NIPPV) when they are admitted. In addition, the definitive report on the surgical treatment of emphysema is included here.

Treatment for asthma continues to advance. Montelukast and omalizumab appear to be useful additions to our pharmacologic armamentarium, and there is more evidence that obesity predisposes to wheezing.

In the ongoing battle with tuberculosis (TB), we have new information about the effects of bacille Calmette-Guérin (BCG) on skin testing, about even shorter-course treatment, and about the risk of drug-resistant TB in immigrants. The pneumococcal vaccination has turned out to be more valuable than we thought.

Spiral CT scanning may allow "one-stop" shopping for the evaluation of suspected pulmonary embolism. There are exciting new treatment options for pulmonary hypertension.

Evidence-based medicine begins to make headway in the critical care unit, and we learn more about physician staffing and outcomes, about the utility (or not!) of the pulmonary artery catheter, and about whether patients with advanced pulmonary fibrosis benefit from intubation.

Sleep apnea is more prevalent than we thought, and the "traditional" risk factors of obesity and male gender become less important after about age 50. Hormone replacement may reduce the increased risk of sleep apnea in postmenopausal women. Portable monitoring is reliable and reproducible.

Many useful and groundbreaking papers did not make the final cut into this volume. If you find this section interesting or helpful, you might also like to read the 2004 YEAR BOOK OF PULMONARY DISEASE. I hope you enjoy this section!

Barbara A. Phillips, MD, MSPH

39 Lung Cancer

Deposition of Cigar Smoke Particles in the Lung: Evaluation With Ventilation Scan Using ^{99m}Tc-Labeled Sulfur Colloid Particles
McDonald LJ, Bhatia RS, Hollett PD (Mem Univ of Newfoundland, St John's, Canada)
J Nucl Med 43:1591-1595, 2002   39–1

Introduction.—Recent years have seen an increase in cigar smoking, which at least partially reflects a belief that cigars are safer than cigarettes. A key question is whether cigar smokers inhale when they smoke, as cigarette smokers do. No studies of pulmonary particle deposition during cigar smoking have been performed. This issue was addressed in a study of cigar smokers that included a comparison of those with versus those without a history of cigarette smoking.

Methods.—The study included 24 men with some history of cigar smoking: 12 were current or past cigarette smokers, and 12 had never smoked cigarettes. All research subjects smoked a cigar using a holder that mixed the smoke with a radioaerosol of ^{99m}Tc-labeled sulfur colloid particles (total radioactivity dose, 100 MBq). After smoking, lung ventilation scanning was performed.

Results.—On a baseline questionnaire, 100% of the study participants without a history of cigarette smoking said they never or rarely inhaled when smoking cigars, as did 58% of those with a history of cigarette smoking. However, the lung uptake studies showed that all study participants inhaled cigar smoke to some degree. The mean total lung count was 6375.3 for the men with a history of cigarette smoking and 7737.4 for those without. However, counts varied widely, and the trend was not significant.

Conclusions.—This pulmonary particle deposition study strongly suggests that cigar smokers inhale when smoking cigars. This is so for cigar smokers with or without a history of cigarette smoking, regardless of whether they believe they inhale. The findings question the widespread belief that cigar smoking is safer than cigarette smoking.

▶ This article should be copied and given to all patients who report that they do not inhale cigar smoke! In this study, the authors directly examined particle deposition in the lungs during cigar smoking. Contrary to the belief by some that cigar smokers do not inhale, the results of this study show that all smokers inhaled cigar smoke to some degree and that they were generally unaware that they were doing so. This study is important because of the perception that cigars are safer than cigarettes and that individuals can regulate the degree to which they inhale. Cigar use is increasing in all ages, socioeconomic groups, and races. This is at a time when cigarette smoking is decreasing, largely due to social pressures. Thus, we must educate our patients that cigar smoking is not a benign habit that brings with it no risk.

N. E. Dunlap, MD, PhD

Fruits and Vegetables Are Associated With Lower Lung Cancer Risk Only in the Placebo Arm of the β-Carotene and Retinol Efficacy Trial (CARET)
Neuhouser ML, Patterson RE, Thornquist MD, et al (Fred Hutchinson Cancer Research Ctr, Seattle; Univ of Washington, Seattle; Univ of Michigan, Ann Arbor)
Cancer Epidemiol Biomarkers Prev 12:350-358, 2003   39–2

Introduction.—The β-Carotene and Retinol Efficacy Trial (CARET) and similar supplementation trials have indicated that supplementation with β-carotene increases rather than reduces the incidence of lung cancer. Yet, considerable interest remains in investigating how other compounds in fruits and vegetables can affect the risk of lung cancer. Data were used from 14,120 CARET participants who completed food frequency questionnaires to assess the relationship between diet and lung cancer risk.

Methods.—The CARET was a multicenter, randomized, double-blind, placebo-controlled chemoprevention trial to determine whether daily supplementation with 30 mg of β-carotene and 25,000 IU of retinyl palmitate would decrease the risk of lung cancer among 18,314 heavy smokers and asbestos-exposed workers. The intervention was ceased 21 months early in 1996 because of evidence that the supplements increased the risk of lung cancer and total mortality; however, active follow-up of all participants continued until September 2003. Dietary intake over the previous year was assessed at baseline and every 2 years thereafter with the use of a self-administered tool. Data were also collected concerning smoking, asbestos exposure, and demographics. The analyses were controlled for smoking, asbestos exposure, and other covariates.

Results.—Statistically significant correlations of fruit and vegetable intake with lower cancer risk were limited to the placebo arm. The risk ratio (RR) for highest versus lowest quintile of total fruit consumption in the placebo arm was 0.56 (95% confidence interval [CI], 0.39-0.81) with a two-sided P for trend = .003. Two specific botanical groups were linked with decreased risk of lung cancer. Compared with the lowest quintile of rosaceae fruit consumption, participants in the placebo group in the top quintile had a RR of 0.63 (95% CI, 0.42-0.94; P for trend = .02); for cruciferae vegetables, the RR was 0.68 (95% CI, 0.45-1.04; P for trend = .01).

Conclusion.—There were no statistically significant correlations between fruit and vegetable intake and lung cancer risk in participants randomly assigned to receive the CARET supplements (30 mg of β-carotene and 25,000

IU of retinyl palmitate). Plant foods have an important preventive effect in a population at high risk for lung cancer. Persons who use β-carotene supplements do not benefit from the protective compounds in plant foods.

▶ This report was interesting because the findings were somewhat unexpected. Although we all appreciate that fruits and vegetables have substances within them that protect against cancer, it was less obvious that adding additional vitamin supplements to a healthy diet would negate the positive effects. The authors suggested 3 possible reasons for the negating effects of the β-carotene and retinyl palmitate: (1) the β-carotene may upregulate the enzymes that result in accumulation of highly carcinogenic intermediate metabolites; (2) β-carotene may downregulate the RAR-β tumor suppressor gene and upregulate c-Fos, c-Jun, and cyclin D1, which induce cellular proliferation; and (3) the β-carotene supplements may inhibit the bioavailability of the dietary carotenoids. Results from this large randomized intervention trial will need to be confirmed by other studies, but thought should be given before substituting vitamin supplements for a diet rich in fruits and vegetables.

N. E. Dunlap, MD, PhD

Lung Cancer Screening With CT: Mayo Clinic Experience
Swensen SJ, Jett JR, Hartman TE, et al (Mayo Clinic, Rochester, Minn)
Radiology 226:756-761, 2003   39–3

Introduction.—Screening with spiral CT can identify lung cancers that are of a smaller size (<2 cm in diameter) and earlier stage (85%-93% at stage I) compared with those observed at chest radiography and in current clinical practice. It is not known whether detection of earlier-stage disease improves mortality rates. A large cohort of patients at high risk for lung cancer was assessed by using screening with low-dose spiral CT of the chest.

Methods.—A prospective cohort investigation was performed in 1520 persons aged 50 years or older who had smoked 20 pack-years or more. Three annual low-dose CT examinations of the chest and upper abdomen were performed. Data concerning characteristics of pulmonary nodules and additional findings were examined.

Results.—At 2 years after baseline CT scanning, 2832 uncalcified pulmonary nodules were detected in 1049 (69%) participants. Forty cases of lung cancer were diagnosed, of which 26 were diagnosed at baseline (prevalence) CT examinations, and 10 at subsequent annual (incidence) CT examinations. CT alone identified 36 cases, and sputum cytologic examination alone detected 2 cases. Two patients had interval cancers. Cell types were squamous cell tumor (n = 7), adenocarcinoma or bronchioloalveolar carcinoma (n = 24), large cell tumor (n = 2), non–small cell tumor (n = 3), and small cell tumors (n = 4). The mean size of the non–small cell cancers identified at CT was 15.0 mm. The stages of cancer were IA in 22 cases, IB in 3 cases, IIA in 4 cases, IIB in 1 case, IIIA in 5 cases, IV in 1 case, and limited small cell tumor in 4 cases. Twenty-one (60%) of 35 non–small cell cancers identified at CT were stage IA at diagnosis. Six hundred ninety-six additional findings of clinical importance were determined.

Conclusion.—CT can identify early stage lung cancers. The rate of benign nodule identification is high.

► In the 1970s, the National Cancer Institute sponsored a mass screening program with chest radiographs and sputum cytology at the Mayo Clinic to detect early lung cancer. The study found no difference in mortality between the screened and control groups. Thus, chest x-ray screening was discouraged. In this study, low-dose spiral CT scanning was used to screen 1520 patients aged 50 or older who were deemed to be at high risk for lung cancer. The findings show that many early stage lung cancers were detected. But as with the previous study, no mortality benefit was identified. Eight of 39 surgeries were performed on benign nodules. This raises the question as to whether CT screening should be promoted. With a mortality rate of 3.8% seen with wedge resection of a pulmonary nodule in community hospitals, it is hard to conclude that widespread CT screening should be endorsed. The National Cancer Institute has started another trial, The National Lung Screening Trial, which will evaluate the disease-specific mortality benefit of CT screening. This study may answer the question once and for all as to whether mass screening for lung cancer should be undertaken.

N. E. Dunlap, MD, PhD

Lung Cancer Risk Reduction After Smoking Cessation: Observations From a Prospective Cohort of Women
Ebbert JO, Yang P, Vachon CM, et al (Mayo Clinic, Rochester, Minn; Univ of Minnesota, Minneapolis)
J Clin Oncol 21:921-926, 2003   39–4

Introduction.—Lung cancer risk in female former smokers diminishes with increasing duration of smoking abstinence. The time that needs to pass before the risk of lung cancer among former smokers reaches that of never smokers is unknown. Lung cancer risk among former smokers was examined in a large prospective cohort of women to estimate the duration of excess lung cancer risk, to assess risk reduction by histologic cell type, and to determine the effect of smoking cessation.

Methods.—The Iowa Women's Health Study is a prospective cohort investigation of risk factors for cancer and chronic diseases in 41,836 women aged 55 to 69 years. In 1986, mailed questionnaires were used to obtain detailed smoking histories. Age-adjusted lung cancer incidence through 1999 was examined according to years of smoking abstinence.

Results.—A total of 37,078 females were included in the analytic cohort. Compared with never smokers, former smokers (any duration) had an elevated risk of lung cancer (relative risk, 6.6; 95% confidence interval, 5.0-8.7) up to 30 years after quitting smoking. The risk for adenocarcinoma remained elevated for as many as 30 years for both former heavy and former light smokers. A beneficial effect of smoking cessation was seen among recent and distant former smokers.

Conclusion.—The risk for lung cancer is increased for both current and former smokers compared with never smokers. The risk declines for former smokers with increasing duration of abstinence. The reduction in excess lung cancer risk among former smokers is prolonged compared with other trials, particularly for adenocarcinoma and for heavy smokers. This underscores the need to place more emphasis on smoking prevention and lung cancer chemoprevention.

▶ The results of this study are a sobering reminder that the effects of cigarette smoking are long-term. In this population-based cohort study from the Iowa Women's Health Study, the authors found that compared with never smokers, former smokers had an elevated risk of lung cancer for up to 30 years of follow-up. Lung cancer risk generally decreased with increasing time since smoking cessation. However, former light smokers (1-19 pack-years) still had a greater than 2-fold increased risk of cancer up to 30 years after smoking abstinence. This was primarily because of the persistent risk of adenocarcinoma among former smokers. On the brighter side, although the risk of cancer after smoking does not return to the nonsmoking baseline for decades, there was a significant decrease in the incidence of cancer in the first 10 years of abstinence. Although this questionnaire-based study has its limitations, these findings support the need to focus on prevention of smoking initiation, since former smokers have a prolonged elevated risk of lung cancer after smoking cessation.

N. E. Dunlap, MD, PhD

40 Emphysema/Chronic Obstructive Pulmonary Disease

Thirteen-Year Experience in Lung Transplantation for Emphysema
Cassivi SD, Meyers BF, Battafarano RJ, et al (Washington Univ, St Louis)
Ann Thorac Surg 74:1663-1670, 2002   40–1

Objective.—As the indications for lung transplantation continue to expand, emphysema continues to be the most common. A 13-year experience with lung transplantation for emphysema is reviewed, including a comparison of outcomes between patients with chronic obstructive pulmonary disease (COPD) and alpha-1 antitrypsin deficiency (AAD).

Patients.—The review included a total of 306 consecutive lung transplants performed for emphysema at 1 institution between 1988 and 2000. Two hundred twenty recipients had COPD and 86 had AAD; mean ages were 55 and 49 years, respectively. Follow-up data were available on all patients, and the average duration of follow-up was 3.7 years.

Outcomes.—In-hospital mortality was 6.2% and was similar for patients with COPD versus AAD and for recipients of single versus double lung transplants. From the first to the second half of the experience, hospital mortality decreased from 9.5% to 3.9%. The 5-year survival rate was 58.6%, and similar results were found for the COPD and AAD groups. However, recipients of bilateral lung transplants had a better 5-year survival rate than did recipients of single lung transplants: 66.7% versus 44.9%. Multivariate analysis identified 2 independent predictors of mortality: single lung transplantation (relative hazard, 1.98) and the use of cardiopulmonary bypass during the transplant procedure (relative hazard, 1.84).

Conclusions.—Among patients undergoing lung transplantation, outcomes are similar for those with COPD versus AAD, despite the younger age of patients with AAD. Survival is significantly better in recipients of double lung transplants. Experience and technical modifications appear to have produced gains in early and long-term survival rates in this 13-year single-center experience.

▶ The most common indication for lung transplantation is end-stage emphysema, a diagnosis that encompasses both COPD and AAD. In this article, the authors retrospectively review their institution's outcomes of 306 lung transplants for emphysema to identify differences in morbidity, mortality, and outcomes between COPD and AAD patients. The average 5-year survival rate for all patients was approximately 60%. There was no significant difference in longevity between groups, even though the AAD patients were, on average, 6 years younger at the time of transplant than their COPD counterparts. As previously reported elsewhere,[1,2] these authors also found a significant survival advantage for bilateral transplants over single lung transplants. Whether this is due to selection bias or increased lung reserve after transplantation is not clear. It is clear, however, that the long-term survival of lung transplant patients continues to improve as techniques evolve through experience.

N. E. Dunlap, MD, PhD

References

1. Sundaresan RS, Shiraishi Y, Trulock EP, et al: Single or bilateral lung transplantation for emphysema? *J Thorac Cardiovas Surg* 112:1485-1495, 1996.
2. Bavaria JE, Kotloff R, Palevsky H, et al: Bilateral versus single lung transplantation for chronic obstructive pulmonary disease. *J Thorac Cardiovasc Surg* 11:520-528, 1997.

Risk Factors of Readmission to Hospital for a COPD Exacerbation: A Prospective Study
Antó JM, for the EFRAM Investigators (Institut Municipal d'Investigació Mèdica (IMIM), Barcelona; et al)
Thorax 58:100-105, 2003   40–2

Introduction.—Exacerbations of chronic obstructive pulmonary disease (COPD) are a significant cause of hospital admission for men in many countries. Factors causing exacerbations are largely unknown. The correlation between readmission for COPD exacerbation and several modifiable potential risk factors were examined, after adjustment for sociodemographic and clinical factors.

Methods.—Three hundred forty patients with COPD from 4 tertiary hospitals were recruited between May 1, 1997, and April 30, 1998, by using a systematic sample of 1 out of every 2 patients admitted to the hospital or remaining in the emergency department for at least 18 hours for a COPD exacerbation. Patients were followed up for a mean of 1.1 years. Data were gathered regarding potential risk factors, including clinical and functional status, medical care and prescriptions, medication adherence, lifestyle, health status, and social support. The relative risk of readmission for COPD was calculated.

Results.—During the evaluation period, 63% of patients were readmitted at least once; 29% of patients died. The final multivariate analysis revealed these risk (or protective) factors: 3 or more admissions for COPD in the year before recruitment (hazard ratio, 1.66; 95% confidence interval [CI], 1.16-2.39), forced expiratory volume in 1 second percentage predicted (0.97; 95% CI, 0.96-0.99), oxygen tension (0.88; 95% CI, 0.79-0.98), higher levels of usual physical activity (0.54; 95% CI, 0.34-0.86), and taking anticholinergic drugs (1.81; 95% CI, 1.11-2.94). Exposure to passive smoking was also associated with increased risk of readmission with COPD after adjustment for clinical factors (1.63; 95% CI, 1.04-2.57); this did not remain in the final model.

Conclusion.—This is the first report to demonstrate a strong correlation between usual physical activity and decreased risk of readmission to the hospital with COPD, which is potentially important for rehabilitation and other therapeutic strategies.

▶ A number of factors have been identified that appear to be associated with an increase in or reductions in hospitalizations for COPD exacerbations. For example, obtaining influenza vaccination, respiratory rehabilitation, and inhaled corticosteroid use have been associated with a decrease in hospitalizations. However, these studies have often been small and the methodology has been less than robust so that most clinicians find these reports to be preliminary at best. The current report is larger (346 patients) and has a more robust methodology in that data were prospectively collected over a 1-year period and patients were monitored for at least a year from the day of discharge.

Using this methodology, some previously identified factors for increased exacerbations were identified. Three or more admissions in the previous year, lower forced expiratory volume in 1 second, and taking anticholinergic medications were all associated with an increased risk of admission. Interestingly, a high level of usual physical activity (more than 232 kcal/d) was associated with a 46% reduction in risk of admission. This parameter should be addressed as an outcome measure in future studies since it may further support the use of pulmonary rehabilitation in patients with advanced disease.

J. R. Maurer, MD

Inhaled Corticosteroids and Survival in Chronic Obstructive Pulmonary Disease: Does the Dose Matter?
Sin DD, Man SFP (Univ of Alberta, Edmonton, Canada)
Eur Respir J 21:260-266, 2003   40–3

Introduction.—Chronic obstructive pulmonary disease (COPD) is the only leading cause of mortality in the world whose incidence is rising. Inhaled corticosteroids (ICS) decrease the number of clinical exacerbations in COPD, but it is not known whether there is a dose-response relationship. The long-term influence of varying doses of ICS on COPD mortality was examined in a large population cohort of patients with moderate to severe COPD who were previously hospitalized.

Methods.—Hospital discharge data were used to identify 6740 patients aged 65 years and older who were hospitalized because of COPD between April 1, 1994, and March 31, 1998. The relative risk (RR) for all-cause mortality was compared across the various dose categories of ICS (none and low, medium, and high doses) after hospital discharge.

Results.—ICS therapy after discharge was correlated with a 25% relative reduction in risk for all-cause mortality (RR, 0.75; 95% confidence interval [CI], 0.68-0.82). Patients receiving medium- or high-dose therapy had lower risks for mortality compared with those receiving lower doses (RR 0.77, 95% CI, 0.69-0.86 for low dose; RR 0.48, 95% CI, 0.37-0.63 for medium dose; and RR 0.55, 95% CI, 0.44-0.69 for high dose).

Conclusion.—The use of ICS therapy after hospital discharge for COPD is associated with a significant decrease in the overall mortality rate. Low-dose therapy was inferior to both medium- and high-dose therapy in protecting against mortality in patients with COPD.

▶ Several recent large studies looking at the impact of inhaled corticosteroids in COPD have shown the somewhat unexpected finding that these drugs appear to reduce the number of disease exacerbations which, by extension, improves quality of life. Studies have not, however, shown an impact on the rate of fall of forced expiratory volume in 1 second (FEV_1).[1] Mixed data exist on reduction in mortality. The Global Initiative for Obstructive Lung Disease (GOLD) gives a qualified recommendation for use of inhaled steroids for patients with moderate and severe lung disease for these reasons. A 2002 systematic review of the literature concluded that the bulk of the existing literature did support reduced exacerbations in patients taking inhaled corticosteroids. However, it has also recently been documented that inhaled steroids, especially when given in higher doses, have some of the unwanted side effects that are well known with oral drug: osteoporosis and cataracts in particular.

The purpose of the current study was to determine whether the dose of inhaled steroids is important (presumably lower doses would have less of the negative side effects) in achieving the positive impact of inhaled corticosteroids. This large study did not measure numbers of exacerbations, but rather mortality, since it was an observational study using government hospital discharge and dispensed medication data. Over 3 years of follow-up, patients taking moderate and high doses of inhaled steroids (>500 µg/d) had a significant reduction in mortality. This finding presents a compelling reason to do large-scale prospective trials with different dosages of inhaled steroids, as none of the other medications used in COPD treatment, with the exception of oxygen, have been shown to impact mortality.

J. R. Maurer, MD

Reference

1. Highland KB, Strange C, Heffner JE:. Long-term effects of inhaled corticosteroids on FEV$_1$ in patients with chronic obstructive pulmonary disease: A meta-analysis. *Ann Intern Med* 138:969-973, 2003.

Which Patients With Acute Exacerbation of Chronic Obstructive Pulmonary Disease Benefit From Noninvasive Positive-Pressure Ventilation? A Systematic Review of the Literature

Keenan SP, Sinuff T, Cook DJ, et al (Royal Columbian Hosp, New Westminster, Canada; Univ of British Columbia, Vancouver, Canada; McMaster Faculty of Sciences, Hamilton, Ont, Canada; et al)
Ann Intern Med 138:861-870, 2003   40–4

Introduction.—During the past decade, noninvasive positive-pressure ventilation (NPPV) in patients with acute exacerbations of chronic obstructive pulmonary disease (COPD) has gained popularity. There are inconsistencies in reports that address the effectiveness of NPPV in these patients. A systematic literature review was conducted to evaluate the effects of NPPV on the incidence of endotracheal intubation, length of hospital stay, and in-hospital mortality in patients with an acute exacerbation of COPD and to ascertain the effect of exacerbation severity on these outcomes.

Methods.—Searches of MEDLINE (1966-2000) and EMBASE (1990-2002) were performed. Additional data sources were the Cochrane Library, personal files, abstract proceedings, reference lists of selected articles, and expert contact. All languages were accepted. Randomized controlled trials were chosen that (1) assessed patients with acute exacerbations of COPD; (2) compared NPPV and standard therapy with standard therapy alone; and (3) included requirement for endotracheal intubation, length of hospital stay, or hospital survival as an outcome.

Results.—The addition of NPPV to standard care in patients with acute exacerbation of COPD reduced the rate of endotracheal intubation (risk reduction, 28%; 95% confidence interval [CI], 15%-40%), length of hospital stay (absolute reduction, 4.57 days; CI, 2.30-6.83 days), and in-hospital mortality rate (risk reduction, 10%; CI, 5%-15%). Subgroup analysis revealed that these beneficial effects occurred only in patients with severe exacerbations and not in those with milder exacerbations.

Conclusion.—Patients with severe exacerbations of COPD benefit from the addition of NPPV to standard therapy, but those with mild COPD exacerbations do not appear to benefit from this therapeutic intervention.

▶ Keenan et al have presented a literature review of the current state of the art in the use of NPPV in patients with acute exacerbations of COPD. The studies selected had to be randomized controlled trials, and they had to examine patients with acute exacerbations and compare noninvasive ventilation and standard therapy with standard therapy alone. They had to report whether patients required intubation, the length of hospital stay, and hospital survival. The bottom line is that patients with severe disease seem to benefit from the use of noninvasive ventilation as an adjunct to therapy.

J. R. Maurer, MD

41 Asthma

Comparison of High-Dose Inhaled Flunisolide to Systemic Corticosteroids in Severe Adult Asthma
Lee-Wong M, Dayrit FM, Kohli AR, et al (Albert Einstein College of Medicine, New York)
Chest 122:1208-1213, 2002   41–1

Background.—Widely accepted guidelines indicate that systemic corticosteroids are standard treatment for patients with severe asthma exacerbations who require hospitalization. However, the role of inhaled corticosteroids in the treatment of asthma requiring hospitalization is unclear. Several investigations of its role in the treatment of asthma in the emergency department have reported beneficial effects. Whether, after 48 hours of IV treatment with corticosteroids, the use of high-dose inhaled flunisolide is as effective as systemic corticosteroids in adults hospitalized for a severe asthma exacerbation was investigated.

Methods.—Forty patients aged 18 to 55 years were enrolled in this randomized, double-blind, placebo-controlled study. All the patients experienced asthma exacerbations requiring hospitalization. The main intervention was the use of inhaled flunisolide by means of metered-dose inhaler (250 µg per activation), 8 puffs twice daily, compared with systemic corticosteroids alone after 8 doses of IV corticosteroids. The main outcome measurements were peak expiratory flow rate (PEFR), forced expiratory volume in 1 second (FEV_1), and symptom scores, which were recorded at presentation to the emergency department and on day 7 at an outpatient follow-up visit.

Results.—From day 1 to day 7, the mean PEFR increased from 190 to 379 L/min in the flunisolide group compared to 207 to 347 L/min in the systemic corticosteroids group. The mean FEV_1 increased from 1.6 to 2.3 L in the flunisolide group and from 1.4 to 2.1 L in the systemic corticosteroids group. Changes in symptom scores were −0.7 for the flunisolide group and −0.9 in the systemic corticosteroids group. Both groups had a hospital readmission rate of zero at day 7.

Conclusions.—High-dose inhaled corticosteroids are as effective as systemic corticosteroids in the 7 days after hospital admission for a severe exacerbation of asthma.

▶ Are escalated doses of anti-inflammatory therapy necessary after the first 48 hours in acute exacerbations of asthma? Can the traditional oral steroid taper be eliminated or replaced with inhaled corticosteroids (ICS)? If so, what is the best delivery method for ICS in acute asthma exacerbation?

The role of ICS in acute asthma exacerbations needs further examination. This small study showed no difference between high-dose ICS and oral steroid in the short-term treatment of asthma exacerbation. Clarification of the indications and appropriate dosing of ICS in asthma exacerbation may reduce oral steroid use, thus avoiding some of the adverse side effects. In addition, the introduction of ICS on hospital discharge may reinforce the importance of anti-inflammatory therapy in asthma treatment and improve compliance with care.

A. R. Blanchard, MD

Association of Body Mass Index With the Development of Methacholine Airway Hyperresponsiveness in Men: The Normative Aging Study
Litonjua AA, Sparrow D, Celedon JC, et al (Harvard Med School, Boston; Boston Univ; VA Med Ctr, Boston)
Thorax 57:581-585, 2002   41–2

Background.—The increase in prevalence of asthma in developed nations has coincided with the rising prevalence of obesity in these countries. Cross-sectional studies in children have found a higher prevalence of obesity in asthmatic subjects than in nonasthmatic controls. A Dutch study found that adult women with a body mass index (BMI) of 30 kg/m² or more had 1.8 times the risk of asthma as leaner women. However, a similar relationship was not observed among men. A prospective analysis of women participating in the Nurses' Health Study was the first to show a relationship between a high BMI and a subsequent doctor's diagnosis of asthma. The relationship between BMI and the development of an objective marker for asthma, methacholine airway hyperresponsiveness (AHR), in adult men was investigated.

Methods.—The study included 61 men with no AHR at initial methacholine challenge testing who developed AHR approximately 4 years later and 244 matched control participants. The effects of initial BMI and changes in BMI on the development of AHR were determined by means of conditional logistic regression models.

Results.—Initial BMI was found to have a nonlinear relationship with the development of AHR. Compared with men whose initial BMI was in the middle quintile, men whose BMI was in the lowest quintile (BMI 19.8 to 24.3 kg/m²) and those with BMI in the highest quintile (BMI greater than 29.4 kg/m²) were more likely to have AHR develop. These findings persisted after controlling for age, smoking, IgE level, and initial FEV_1. There was also a positive linear relationship between change in BMI over the period of observation and the subsequent development of AHR.

Conclusions.—This study found an association of both a low BMI and a high BMI with the development of airway hyperresponsiveness. However, the risk of AHR in men with low BMI appears to be partially mediated by weight gain. These findings may be indications of the mechanisms underlying the observed associations between obesity and asthma.

▶ Some epidemiologic surveys have shown that asthma is more prevalent in obese children and adults. Most of these were based on symptom reports rather than on pulmonary function testing/bronchial provocation. A number of studies have attempted to sort out the relationship, if any, between obesity and asthma. Chinn et al[1] reported the results of a large (n = 11,277) multicenter study showing that AHR increased with increasing BMI in men but showing a weak relationship in women. The present VA study found a U-shaped relationship between BMI and AHR, with both underweight and overweight men at risk of AHR. There was a positive linear relationship between weight gain and the development of AHR in this limited study. A few suggested mechanisms for an association between the 2—(a) weight gain produces reduced lung volumes/decreased airway caliber leading to AHR, (b) obesity is a risk factor for sedentary lifestyle and increased indoor allergen exposure, (c) obesity induces changes in T cell function,[2] and (d) there is increased systemic inflammation in the obese state.

This study emphasizes the need for further prospective research on the relationship between obesity and the development of objective findings of asthma.

A. R. Blanchard, MD

References

1. Chinn S, Jarvis D, Burney P: Relation of bronchial responsiveness to body mass index in the ECRHS. European Community Respiratory Health Survey. *Thorax* 57:1028-1033, 2002.
2. Mito N, Kitada C, Hosoda T, et al: Effect of diet-induced obesity on ovalbumin specific immune response in a murine asthma model. *Metabolism* 51:1241-1246, 2002.

National Trends in Asthma Visits and Asthma Pharmacotherapy, 1978-2002

Stafford RS, Ma J, Finkelstein SN, et al (Stanford Univ, Palo Alto, Calif; Massachusetts Inst of Technology, Cambridge; Massachusetts Gen Hosp, Boston; et al)
J Allergy Clin Immunol 111:729-735, 2003   41–3

Background.—Evidence-based asthma treatment guidelines have been published and recommend treatment to control asthma, with short-term medication used only for relief of acute symptoms. Data from the 1978 to 2002 National Disease and Therapeutic Index (NDTI) were used to document 25-year trends in asthma office visits and pharmacotherapy to determine whether asthma treatment has moved to be aligned with recommendations.

Study Design.—The NDTI is a continuing office-physician survey conducted by Integrated Medical Services (IMS) Health. The trends in asthma office visit frequency and patterns of asthma pharmacotherapy use were tracked from 1978 to 2002 in the United States.

Findings.—The NDTI database indicated that the annual number of asthma office visits increased continuously from 1978 through 1990 but then reached a plateau. The use of controller medications increased 8 times from 1978 to 2002, with the biggest increase in the use of corticosteroids. The use of medication for relief of acute asthma symptoms, especially β_2-agonists, decreased during this same time. The use of medication to control asthma exceeded that to relieve asthma symptoms for the first time in 2001. Xanthines, which dominated asthma therapy in 1978, were rarely used in 2002. More recent drugs have been rapidly adopted.

Conclusions.—Data from the 1978 to 2002 NDTI survey of physicians have documented changes in asthma office visits and pharmacotherapy that increasingly bring practice in line with published evidence-based treatment recommendations. The publication of these guidelines appears to have contributed to this shift in prescribing patterns for the treatment of asthma.

▶ Self-reported asthma prevalence, as well as morbidity and mortality rates, have increased over the last 20 years. Over the past 10 years, the roles of acute and chronic inflammation and airway remodeling in the pathogenesis of asthma have come into focus. With this recognition, national and international guidelines have been devised and revised to improve outcomes in asthma. The present study examined trends in asthma pharmacotherapy from 1978 to 2002 and found that pharmacotherapy has become more consistent with consensus guidelines emphasizing the use of controller medications. The challenge for the next decade is continued education of the patient population in order to encourage adherence.

A. R. Blanchard, MD

42 Pulmonary Infections

A Meta-analysis of the Effect of Bacille Calmette Guérin Vaccination on Tuberculin Skin Test Measurements
Wang L, Turner MO, Elwood RK, et al (Univ of British Columbia, Canada; Ctr for Clinical Epidemiology and Evaluation, Vancouver, BC, Canada)
Thorax 57:804-809, 2002   42–1

Background.—The accurate diagnosis of latent tuberculosis infection is essential to any program intended to control the spread of this significant global public health problem. Diagnosis is largely dependent on skin tuberculin skin testing, and the appropriate interpretation of skin test results requires an understanding of the factors that may affect these results, such as previous Bacille Calmette Guérin (BCG) vaccination. Another complicating factor is the variation in the strength with which recommendations are made to individual patients regarding the treatment of latent tuberculosis infection. The purpose of this meta-analysis was to address these issues by analysis of the available data regarding the effect of BCG vaccination on tuberculin skin testing in persons without active tuberculosis.

Methods.—The MEDLINE database was searched for relevant English language articles from 1966 to 1999. Bibliographies of relevant articles were reviewed for additional studies that may have been missed in the MEDLINE search. Articles were included in the meta-analysis if they had recorded tuberculin skin test results for subjects who had received the BCG vaccine more than 5 years previously and had a concurrent control group. Only prospective studies were included. Relevant data from these studies included the geographic location, the number of participants, the type of BCG vaccine used, the type of tuberculin skin test performed, and the results of the tuberculin skin test.

Results.—From 980 articles identified and 370 articles reviewed, 26 articles were included in the final analysis. Patients who had received BCG vaccination were more likely to have a positive skin test, but the effect of BCG vaccination on skin test results declined after 15 years. Positive skin tests with indurations of more than 15 mm are more likely to result from tuberculous infection than from BCG vaccination.

Conclusion.—In persons without active tuberculosis, immunization with BCG significantly increases the likelihood of a positive tuberculin skin test. These findings indicate the need to interpret the skin test in the individual clinical context and with an appreciation of other risk factors for infection.

The size of the induration should be an important consideration in any recommendation for treatment of latent infection.

▶ Every primary care physician and pulmonologist has wrestled with what to do in the case of a patient who has a "positive" tuberculin skin test (TST) and a past history of receiving a BCG vaccination. This article by Wang et al gives one a framework, based on a meta-analysis of data from 26 articles (117,507 subjects), of how to interpret skin test results after a BCG vaccination. They found that immunization with BCG does significantly increase the likelihood of having a TST reactivity of more than 10 mm. However, a TST of more than 15 mm is far less likely to be due to BCG vaccination. (This is a good reason to always record the size of tuberculin skin test induration in millimeters and not just report "positive" or "negative".) A BCG vaccination given in infancy is far less likely to cause a significant TST response later in life than is a BCG vaccination administered more than 15 years before the TST. This article provides many more important caveats for the clinician who wishes to counsel patients who have previously been immunized with BCG on their need to treat a possible latent tuberculosis infection as indicated by a "positive" TST.

N. E. Dunlap, MD, PhD

Short-Course Rifampin and Pyrazinamide Compared With Isoniazid for Latent Tuberculosis Infection: A Multicenter Clinical Trial

Jasmer RM, for the Short-Course Rifampin and Pyrazinamide for Tuberculosis Infection (SCRIPT) Study Investigators (Univ of California, San Francisco; et al)
Ann Intern Med 137:640-647, 2002   42–2

Background.—A regimen of rifampin and pyrazinamide is recommended for treating latent tuberculosis infection in adults without HIV infection. However, severe hepatotoxic effects have been reported in patients undergoing such treatment. The safety and tolerance of a 2-month rifampin and pyrazinamide regimen were compared with those of a 6-month regimen of isoniazid in patients with latent tuberculosis infection.

Methods.—Five hundred eighty-nine adults with latent tuberculosis infection were enrolled in the multicenter, prospective, open-label trial. Three hundred seven patients were assigned to rifampin and pyrazinamide daily for 2 months, and 282 were assigned to isoniazid daily for 6 months.

Findings.—Grade 3 or 4 hepatotoxic effects developed in 7.7% of patients receiving rifampin and pyrazinamide compared with 1% of those receiving isoniazid. The odds ratio of developing hepatotoxic effects with rifampin and pyrazinamide therapy was 8.46. In addition, this regimen was more likely to be discontinued because of hepatotoxic effects, the odds ratio of which was 5.19. The overall percentage of nonhepatotoxic adverse events in the rifampin–pyrazinamide and isoniazid groups were 20% and 16%, respectively. The percentages of patients completing the rifampin–pyrazinamide and isoniazid treatments were 61% and 57%, respectively.

Conclusions.—Compared with the 6-month regimen of isoniazid, the 2-month regimen of rifampin and pyrazinamide was associated with a greater risk of grade 3 or 4 hepatotoxic effects. During treatment, measures of liver enzymes need to be obtained regularly to assess possible liver injury and to prevent progression to severe toxic effects.

▶ The only way that we will ever be able to eliminate tuberculosis from our population is, in addition to finding and treating active cases, to identify and treat persons with latent tuberculosis infection. It is difficult to complete a treatment course in patients with latent infection because they have no symptoms from the infection, the treatment course with the traditional therapy, isoniazid, is relatively long (6-9 months), and often the medication makes them feel bad. Therefore, alternative drug regimens that can be given for a shorter period (2 months) would appear to be an attractive alternative. The authors of this study compared the traditional 6-month daily regimen of isoniazid with the 2-month daily regimen of rifampin and pyrazinamide in patients without HIV infection and noted toxic effects and rates of therapy completion. All medication was self-administered. They found that the 2-month regimen was associated with a significantly higher risk of hepatotoxic effects and that no significant difference occurred in the number of patients completing therapy. Their findings suggest that anyone who is undergoing the 2-month regimen of rifampin and pyrazinamide should be monitored closely for symptoms of hepatitis, and screening of liver enzymes, particularly after the first month of therapy, is advised.

N. E. Dunlap, MD, PhD

Short-Course Rifamycin and Pyrazinamide Treatment for Latent Tuberculosis Infection in Patients With HIV Infection: The 2-Year Experience of a Comprehensive Community-Based Program in Broward County, Florida

Narita M, Kellman M, Franchini DL, et al (Broward County Health Dept, Fort Lauderdale, Fla; A G Holley State Tuberculosis Hosp, Lantana, Fla; Florida Dept of Health, Tallahassee; et al)
Chest 122:1292-1298, 2002   42–3

Background.—Patients with HIV infection and positive tuberculin skin test results are much more likely to acquire tuberculosis (TB) than is the general population. Treatment for latent TB infection (LTBI) in HIV-infected patients is imperative in preventing acute TB. The completion rate and tolerability of short-course rifamycin and pyrazinamide in the treatment of LTBI in HIV-infected patients through a comprehensive community-based program were reported.

Methods.—A cohort of 3118 patients with HIV infection was screened for LTBI between February 1991 and March 2001. One hundred thirty-five of these patients were given rifamycin and pyrazinamide for 2 months and directly observed. This group was then compared with a historical control group that consisted of 93 HIV-infected patients taking self-administered isoniazid for 12 months between 1996 and 1998.

Findings.—Ninety-two percent of patients receiving rifamycin and pyrazinamide completed treatment. Five patients stopped treatment because of adverse effects, including allergic skin reactions in 4 and hepatitis in 1. By comparison, 61% of the control group completed treatment. None of the isoniazid recipients had significant adverse effects.

Conclusions.—This comprehensive community-based regimen of rifamycin and pyrazinamide for LTBI resulted in significantly better treatment compliance than did a traditional isoniazid regimen. The rifamycin–pyrazinamide regimen may, therefore, provide improved TB prevention in communities with a high number of HIV-infected individuals.

▶ After reading the previous article (Abstract 42–2), one may conclude that the 2-month regimen of rifampin and pyrazinamide for treatment of LTBI had no place in TB control. This article points out how this regimen, which has a higher rate of hepatotoxic effects, may not be the optimal regimen in an ideal world or controlled study but may have an important role in a practical, resource-limited TB control program.

In a world of resource constraints, these authors compared the completion rate and tolerability of the 2-month regimen of rifamycin and pyrazinamide given under direct observation with a self-administered daily regimen of isoniazid. They found that the completion rate with the 2-month regimen was significantly higher, probably due to the administration of the drug by public health workers with direct observation. The side effects from the medication were minimal in this group. This difference is likely due to the twice-weekly administration of medication compared with the previous article's daily administration of medication (Abstract 42–2). Although the effectiveness of the 2-month, twice-weekly dosing of rifamycin and pyrazinamide may not be as good as the 9-month regimen with isoniazid, in practice, this regimen may result in better long-term TB control. This is because the 2-month regimen required fewer public health resources to administer the medication by directly observed means compared with the 9-month regimen. In addition, because of the directly observed administration of medication, more patients completed the prescribed therapy. Sometimes the less effective therapy may be the best practical alternative for treating a disease more effectively!

N. E. Dunlap, MD, PhD

Global Drug-Resistance Patterns and the Management of Latent Tuberculosis Infection in Immigrants to the United States

Khan K, Muennig P, Behta M, et al (Cornell Univ, New York; Columbia Univ, New York; City Univ of New York)
N Engl J Med 347:1850-1859, 2002   42–4

Introduction.—Foreign-born individuals represent 10% of the population of the United States but account for half of all cases of tuberculosis. In many immigrants, the infection is resistant to isoniazid. Thus, both the Centers for Disease Control and Prevention and the Institute of Medicine have called for improvements in the detection and treatment of latent infection in new immigrants. A decision analysis model was constructed to examine the effectiveness and cost-effectiveness of 4 strategies to reduce the burden of tuberculosis in immigrants to the United States.

Methods.—The model used a hypothetical cohort of all adult documented immigrants entering the United States from developing nations during 2000. Region-specific drug-resistance profiles were derived from data on 30,388 cases of infection. The strategies examined were no intervention or tuberculin skin testing followed by treatment for those with a positive result, with the use of isoniazid, rifampin, or rifampin plus pyrazinamide. Among the costs included in the model were those related to medications, hospitalization, patients' time, and services of interpreters.

Results.—A strategy of detecting and treating latent tuberculosis infection among immigrants from developing nations would produce both health benefits and economic savings. Rifampin plus pyrazinamide was predicted to be more effective and less costly than rifampin alone, and the combination therapy was preferred for treatment of latent infection in immigrants from Vietnam, Haiti, and the Philippines.

Conclusion.—Screening of immigrants from developing nations for latent tuberculosis infection at the time of their entry into the United States could produce substantial health and economic benefits. As predicted by the model, implementation of such a strategy for a single year might avert approximately 9000 to 10,000 cases of active tuberculosis infection, and $60 million to $90 million could be saved over the expected lifetime of an immigrant cohort entering the country during a given year. The ultimate success at eliminating tuberculosis will require developed nations to reduce the burden of this disease in the rest of the world.

▶ As the number of tuberculosis cases in the United States declines, public health efforts are shifting to target individuals who are infected with *Mycobacterium tuberculosis* but are not yet diseased. These individuals with latent tuberculosis infection (LTBI) are often immigrants coming from countries in which drug-resistant tuberculosis is prevalent. The current guidelines from the Centers for Disease Control and Prevention (CDC) for treating patients with LTBI do not take into account global differences in drug-resistance patterns. The authors of this report developed a decision-analysis model using region-specific drug-resistance profiles and examined the efficacy and cost-effectiveness of different treatment strategies. The results provide some rational recommendations to clinicians for treating immigrants with LTBI based on their geographic region of origin. Although the economic analysis needs to be tested and confirmed, the mapping of drug-resistant tuberculosis throughout the world and the guidance that this analysis provides for clinicians working in conjunction with tuberculosis control programs is quite useful.

N. E. Dunlap, MD, PhD

43 Cough

Chronic Cough and Gastroesophageal Reflux Disease: Experience With Specific Therapy for Diagnosis and Treatment
Poe RH, Kallay MC (Highland Hosp, Rochester, NY; Univ of Rochester, NY)
Chest 123:679-684, 2003   43–1

Background.—One of the most common symptoms of gastroesophageal reflux disease (GERD) is cough, yet most patients with reflux-induced cough experience no other symptoms of GERD, which can make diagnosis challenging. Ambulatory esophageal pH monitoring can diagnose GERD-related cough, but it is relatively expensive and may be poorly tolerated. The utility of a therapeutic trial of proton-pump inhibitor therapy for diagnosing and treating GERD-related cough was investigated.

Methods.—The medical records of 183 patients (71 men and 112 women; mean age, approximately 55 years) referred over a 3.5-year period for cough of 3 or more weeks' duration were reviewed. All patients had normal chest x-ray findings, and none were taking an angiotensin-converting enzyme inhibitor. The diagnostic approach was initially based on symptoms. If symptoms were absent or noncontributory, patients were given a methacholine challenge test (to diagnose asthma) and an empirical trial of antihistamines or decongestants (to diagnose postnasal drip).

Patients who did not respond to these trials were treated with a once-daily proton-pump inhibitor (usually omeprazole or lansoprazole). If response to the proton-pump inhibitor was suboptimal or if esophageal dysfunction was suspected, a prokinetic agent (metoclopramide or cisapride) was added. If there was no response to this trial, patients underwent 24-hour ambulatory esophageal pH monitoring.

Results.—Of the 183 patients, 56 (31%) had GERD-related cough. These included 24 patients (43%) with GERD only, 29 patients (53%) with GERD and 1 other cause of cough, and 3 patients (5%) with GERD and 2 or more other causes of cough. In 24 patients (43%), the only symptom of GERD was cough. Proton-pump inhibitor therapy was successful in 44 patients (79%), of whom 24 responded to the inhibitor alone, 18 responded to the inhibitor plus a prokinetic agent, and 2 each responded to a histamine type-2 blocker or cisapride alone.

The trial of proton-pump inhibitor therapy markedly improved or eliminated cough in 38 patients after 4 weeks (86%) and in all patients by 12 weeks. Twelve patients with GERD-related cough (21%) did not respond to the trial of therapy and required 24-hour ambulatory esophageal pH monitoring. Six of these patients had aspiration as confirmed by bronchoscopy.

Of the 12 nonresponders, 4 responded to prolonged high-dose proton-pump inhibitor therapy combined with a prokinetic agent, 2 successfully underwent fundoplication, 2 refused fundoplication, 2 responded to alternative interventions (extended-release hyoscyamine sulfate, discontinuation of losartan), and 2 continued to cough despite maximal therapy.

Conclusion.—Once asthma and postnasal drip are ruled out or treated, a 4- to 6-week trial of therapy with a proton-pump inhibitor (with or without a prokinetic agent) can diagnose and treat about 80% of patients with GERD-induced cough. Ambulatory esophageal pH monitoring can thus be reserved for nonresponders. Nonresponders may be candidates for fundoplication and may be at higher risk of aspiration.

▶ Chronic cough is one of the most common causes for patients to seek medical attention. It is also one of the more common reasons for referral to a pulmonologist. This study nicely demonstrates a very reasonable approach to therapy in those thought to have cough due to GERD. Clearly, doing pH probes on every patient with a chronic cough is not cost effective. How does one reconcile the findings of this article with those of the American College of Chest Physicians Consensus Panel report?[1] I would split the patients into either a postnasal drip group or the GERD group to decide on initial therapy. (For postnasal drip, prescribe first generation antihistamines; for GERD, follow the approach outlined here.)

Unfortunately, we still have to also keep in mind that many patients will have more than one cause and, of course, that some will have cough due to angiotensin-converting enzyme inhibitor, asthma, chronic bronchitis, or recent infection. Finally, there has been recently described lymphocytic bronchitis, which would require bronchoscopy for diagnosis.

J. A. Barker, MD

Reference

1. Irwin RS, Boulet L-P, Cloutier MM, et al: Managing cough as a defense mechanism and as a symptom: A consensus panel report of the ACCP. *Chest* 114:133S-181S, 1998.

44 Thromboembolic Disease

Pulmonary Embolism: Comparison of Angiography With Spiral Computed Tomography, Magnetic Resonance Angiography, and Real-Time Magnetic Resonance Imaging

Haage P, Piroth W, Krombach G, et al (Univ of Technology, Aachen, Germany; Philips Research Labs, Hamburg, Germany)
Am J Respir Crit Care Med 167:729-734, 2003   44–1

Background.—The signs and symptoms of pulmonary embolism are nonspecific, so diagnosis requires imaging techniques. Clinically suspected pulmonary embolism may be evaluated by contrast-enhanced spiral CT, MR angiography (MRA), and real-time MRI with radial k-space scanning. The sensitivity of spiral CT is approximately 90% for central, lobar, or segmental pulmonary emboli. MRI uses even safer contrast agents than CT without radiation exposure and allows for the depiction of perfusion and ventilation, which might further aid the differential diagnosis of pulmonary embolism. However, patients with dyspnea often are not capable of holding their breath for a longer time, resulting in frequent image degradation. For these patients, real-time MRI with radial k-space scanning may be the most appropriate modality. This study is the first comparative analysis of all available modalities, including radial real-time MRI, for the diagnosis of suspected pulmonary embolism.

Methods.—Nine pigs with artificially induced pulmonary embolism were included in this study. Pulmonary angiography was used as the reference gold standard. All the images were independently evaluated for the presence of pulmonary emboli by 2 reviewers.

Results.—Forty-three filling defects were detected by conventional angiography on lobar and segmental levels. The sensitivity of CT images was 72.1% for reader 1 and 69.8% for reader 2. Sensitivity of MRA images was 79.1% for reader 1 and 81.4% for reader 2. However, with real-time MRI, the detection rate was 97.7% for both readers.

Conclusions.—In an animal model of pulmonary embolism, real-time MRI without the use of radiation or iodinated contrast material is comparable with angiography in the detection of pulmonary emboli.

▶ This study is highlighted since it introduces the modality of real-time MRI as a potential test in the diagnosis of pulmonary embolism. It has the advantages of no radiation, no iodinated contrast, and no needed breath hold. The interobserver agreement in this animal study was very high. The drawbacks of cost and claustrophobia will remain an issue for any MRI modality.

K. L. Lewis, MD

Heparin Plus Alteplase Compared With Heparin Alone in Patients With Submassive Pulmonary Embolism
Konstantinides S, for the Management Strategies and Prognosis of Pulmonary Embolism-3 Trial Investigators (Georg-August-Universität, Göttingen, Germany; et al)
N Engl J Med 347:1143-1150, 2002   44–2

Background.—Thrombolysis is an established treatment for patients with acute massive pulmonary embolism and hemodynamic instability or cardiogenic shock. In contrast, there has for several decades been an ongoing debate regarding the effect of thrombolytic agents on the outcome of hemodynamically stable patients who have submassive pulmonary embolism. Among the factors contributing to the ongoing controversy are the lack of a large, randomized study assessing clinical end points; the risk of serious hemorrhage associated with thrombolytic therapy; and the fact that patients' hemodynamic status may gradually improve with heparin therapy alone. The purpose of this randomized placebo-controlled study was to compare the effects of treatment with heparin plus placebo versus heparin plus alteplase on the outcome of patients with acute submassive pulmonary embolism.

Methods.—This study focused on 256 patients with acute pulmonary embolism and pulmonary hypertension or right ventricular dysfunction but without arterial hypotension or shock. Patients were assigned in double-blind fashion to either heparin plus 100 mg of alteplase (118 patients) or heparin plus placebo (138 patients). The primary end point was in-hospital death or clinical deterioration requiring an escalation of treatment, which was defined as catecholamine infusion, secondary thrombolysis, endotracheal intubation, cardiopulmonary resuscitation, or emergency surgical embolectomy or thrombus fragmentation by catheter.

Results.—The heparin-plus-placebo group had a significantly higher incidence of the primary end point than the heparin-plus-alteplase group, whereas the heparin-plus-alteplase group had a significantly higher probability of 30-day event-free survival. Mortality was low in both groups. However, treatment with heparin plus placebo was associated with nearly 3 times the risk of death or treatment escalation compared with heparin plus alteplase. There were no incidents of fatal bleeding or cerebral bleeding in patients receiving heparin plus alteplase.

Conclusions.—Alteplase administered in conjunction with heparin can improve the clinical course of stable patients who have acute submassive pulmonary embolism. Heparin plus alteplase also can prevent clinical deterioration requiring the escalation of treatment during the hospital stay.

Importance of Cardiac Troponins I and T in Risk Stratification of Patients With Acute Pulmonary Embolism

Konstantinides S, Geibel A, Olschewski M, et al (Georg-August-Universität Göttingen, Germany; Albert-Ludwigs-Universität Freiburg, Germany; St Josefs Hosp Wiesbaden, Germany)

Circulation 106:1263-1268, 2002   44–3

Background.—Risk stratification of patients with acute pulmonary embolism (PE) is difficult. Myocardial injury results in elevated serum levels of cardiac troponin I (cTnI) and cardiac troponin T (cTnT), and some data suggest that cTnI levels correlate with right ventricular dysfunction. The utility of serum cTnI and cTnT levels in risk stratification of patients with PE was examined.

Methods.—The subjects were 106 patients (40% men; mean age, 61 years) with confirmed acute PE. Blood samples for measuring cTnI and cTnT levels were drawn at admission and at 4, 8, and 24 hours thereafter. Cut-off points were set prospectively to define normal (less than 0.07 ng/mL), moderately elevated (0.07-1.5 ng/mL), and markedly elevated (more than 1.5 ng/mL) cTnI levels, and to define normal (less than 0.04 ng/mL), moderately elevated (0.04-0.1 ng/mL), and markedly elevated (more than 0.1 ng/mL) cTnT levels. All patients also underwent echocardiography to assess right ventricular function. cTnI and cTnT levels were correlated with echocardiographic findings and with in-hospital events. A complicated hospital course was defined as death or at least 1 of the following: need for thrombolytic therapy, catecholamine support of blood pressure (except for dopamine at the rate of 5 µg/kg/min or less), endotracheal intubation, and cardiopulmonary resuscitation.

Results.—cTnI levels were above normal in 43 (41%) patients, and cTnT levels were above normal in 39 (37%) patients. An elevated cTnI or cTnT level correlated significantly with electrocardiographic findings of right ventricular strain and with echocardiographic findings of right ventricular function, but not with arterial hypotension or other baseline clinical parameters. Seven patients (6.6%) died while hospitalized, and 19 patients (18%) had a complicated in-hospital course. Elevated cTnI and cTnT levels also correlated significantly with death and with a complicated in-hospital course.

The negative predictive values for an elevated cTnI or cTnT level in predicting a complicated clinical course were 92% and 93%, respectively, although the positive predictive values were lower (37% and 41%, respectively). Furthermore, the risk of poor outcome increased dramatically as the cTnI or cTnT level increased. Logistic regression analysis revealed that the risk of a poor outcome was significantly greater only in patients with markedly elevated cTnI or cTnT levels.

Conclusion.—Elevations in serum cTnI and cTnT levels correlated significantly with right ventricular function and with poorer outcomes in these patients with confirmed PE. Patients with markedly elevated cTnI or cTnT levels were 6.5 to 17 times more likely to die or to have a complicated in-hospital course than were patients with normal levels. Thus, measurements of serum cTnI and cTnT levels may be a useful marker for risk stratification among patients with PE. Further trials are warranted to determine whether measuring cTnI and/or cTnT levels can improve the management and outcomes of patients with PE.

Role of Helical CT in Detecting Right Ventricular Dysfunction Secondary to Acute Pulmonary Embolism

Contractor S, Maldjian PD, Sharma VK, et al (UMDNJ-NJ Med School, Newark)
J Comput Assist Tomogr 26:587-591, 2002   44–4

Background.—Pulmonary embolism (PE) has a high mortality rate. Pressure overload of the right ventricle results in right ventricular dysfunction (RVD), which may progress to ventricular failure and circulatory collapse. The role of helical CT in the early detection of RVD after acute PE was examined.

Study Design.—All 25 CT chest scans performed at 1 institution between July 1999 and December 2000 that had positive findings for acute PE were reviewed by a single reader for findings that suggested RVD. This reader was unaware of the results of echocardiography or angiography. The helical CT findings were then correlated with the results of echocardiography and pulmonary angiography to determine the sensitivity and specificity of CT in detecting RVD in patients with acute PE.

Findings.—Helical CT had a sensitivity of 78%, a specificity of 100%, and a positive predictive value of 100% for the detection of RVD in patients with acute PE.

Conclusions.—Helical CT seems to be useful in detecting RVD in patients with acute PE. The morphologic features of the ventricles and the position of the interventricular septum should be examined in all CT scans with positive findings for PE to assist in the early detection of RVD.

▶ The US Food and Drug Administration approved alteplase for use in patients with "massive" PE in 1990, despite the lack of large trials confirming a benefit in patient outcomes. The definition of *massive* is somewhat broad: it includes associated shock, refractory hypoxemia, a saddle embolus, more than 40% of the pulmonary vascular bed affected by emboli, and others. Few would argue against the use of a thrombolytic agent in PE with shock because this carries a mortality rate of approximately 35%.[1] However, systemic thrombolysis has been much more controversial in patients who were not in shock with documented PE since this group, when taken as a whole, has a much lower mortality rate. There has been a good deal of interest in trying to find ways to stratify patients who were not in shock but who might benefit from thrombolysis. This has led to the discovery that patients with evidence of acute pulmonary hypertension and right ventricular stress have poorer outcomes with an approximate mortality rate of 8%. The use of electrocardiographic, pulmonary artery catheter, or echocardiographic information can be used to identify such patients with submassive PE.

In a study sponsored by Boehringer Ingelheim Pharma, the Management Strategies and Prognosis of Pulmonary Embolism-3 (MAPPET-3) investigators (Abstract 44–2) performed the largest study of thrombolytic use in patients with PE ever done and focused on this important group of patients with submassive embolism and evidence of right ventricular strain. For this reason, it is highlighted in this edition of the Year Book, and the authors are to be commended. Unfortunately, that is where the commendations end. The authors concluded that the use of heparin plus alteplase was associated with a reduced risk of death or escalation of treatment when compared with the use of heparin plus placebo. They suggest that the role of alteplase in PE should definitely be extended to include the group of patients studied, a view supported in an accompanying editorial in *The New England Journal of Medicine*.[2] These conclusions are misleading and require further examination.

First, the use of alteplase in this study did not reduce the mortality rate at 30 days. In fact, there was a trend toward an increased mortality rate. The study was not powered to assess a mortality difference because the actual mortality rates were much lower than the estimated 8% going into the study. Second, the majority of patients who initially received heparin alone and required an escalation of treatment received rescue alteplase. Almost all patients who received "rescue" alteplase did not have shock develop but were said to have worsening symptoms and respiratory failure. However, only 3 of 24 patients in that subgroup required mechanical ventilation, which suggests a very liberal application of "rescue" alteplase and an inherent study bias toward the use of thrombolysis. Interestingly, 3 patients who were initially randomized to receive alteplase required mechanical ventilation, a number equal to the heparin alone group. Third, recurrent PE rates were not different between the 2 groups. Fortunately, the rates of significant bleeding events in this study were low and not significantly different. Therefore, this study leaves more questions than it does answers, and recommending alteplase for PE in the absence of shock is risky at best at this time.

Perhaps alternative methods of patient stratification in pulmonary embolism could help better guide clinical decisions, including thrombolysis. One potential method was described by the same authors in the MAPPET-2 study published in *Circulation* (Abstract 44–3). The finding that cardiac troponins in documented PE correlate well with mortality rates should prove to be very useful in clinical practice and in guiding future research.

Another interesting approach was evaluated by Contractor et al (Abstract 44–4) using the helical CT findings of right ventricular dilation or interventricular septal deviation as evidence of RVD in acute PE. Although further validation is required, the stage is being set for helical CT to become "one stop shopping" for venous thromboembolic diseases. Currently, helical CT can be used to assess for PE, deep vein thrombosis, and RVD with a single study in those patients who can handle the contrast.

K. L. Lewis, MD

References

1. Dalen J: Pulmonary embolism: What have we learned since Virchow? *Chest* 122:1801-1817, 2002.
2. Goldhaber S: Thrombolysis for pulmonary embolism. *N Engl J Med* 347:1131-1132, 2002.

45 Pulmonary Hypertension

Sildenafil for Long-term Treatment of Nonoperable Chronic Thromboembolic Pulmonary Hypertension
Ghofrani HA, Schermuly RT, Rose F, et al (Justus-Liebig-Univ Giessen, Germany)
Am J Respir Crit Care Med 167:1139-1141, 2003   45–1

Background.—Recently it was reported that oral sildenafil is a more potent acute pulmonary vasodilator than inhaled nitric oxide in patients with pulmonary hypertension. Sildenafil is an inhibitor of phosphodiesterase type 5 that is approved for the treatment of erectile dysfunction. Phosphodiesterase type 5 is abundantly expressed in lung tissue and thus stabilizes the second messenger cGMP. The long-term effects of oral sildenafil in patients with nonoperable severe chronic thrombembolic pulmonary hypertension (CTEPH) were investigated.

Methods.—The effects of oral sildenafil on hemodynamics and exercise capacity were examined in 12 patients with nonoperable CTEPH. All the patients had progressive disease despite long-term treatment with adequate anticoagulation and the best supportive care. They had severe pulmonary hypertension, as determined by a pulmonary vascular resistance index of 1935 ± 228 dynes/sec/cm^5 per m^2, a cardiac index of 2.0 L/min/m^2, and a 6-minute walking distance of 312 ± 30 m.

Results.—After approximately 6 months of treatment with oral sildenafil, pulmonary hemodynamics and exercise capacity were significantly improved, with a pulmonary vascular resistance index of 1361 ± 177 L/min/m^2, a cardiac index of 2.4 ± 0.2 L/min/m^2, and 6-minute walking distance of 366 ± 28 m. There were no serious adverse effects related to the medication.

Conclusions.—These findings indicate that oral sildenafil may be a new alternative for the medical treatment of patients with nonoperable chronic thromboembolic pulmonary hypertension.

▶ The use of oral sildenafil is something to get *excited* about (please refrain from the Viagra jokes!). Ghofrani et al published encouraging data last year on the combined use of sildenafil and inhaled iloprost in patients with pulmonary hypertension.[1] Now they present the use of oral sildenafil in a subgroup of patients that is often refractory to medical therapy. The 6-minute walk distance improvements were similar to those seen with bosentan, and the hemodynamic improvements were substantial.[2] It is important to point out that a fair number of patients with pulmonary hypertension will be on nitrates, a consideration that must be taken into account when contemplating sildenafil use.

K. L. Lewis, MD

References

1. Ghofrani HA, Wiedemann R, Rose F, et al: Combination therapy with oral sildenafil and inhaled iloprost for severe pulmonary hypertension. *Ann Intern Med* 136:515-522, 2002.
2. Rubin LJ, Badesch DB, Barst RJ, et al: Bosentan therapy for pulmonary arterial hypertension. *N Engl J Med* 346:896-903, 2002.

Intravenous Iloprost for Treatment Failure of Aerosolised Iloprost in Pulmonary Arterial Hypertension

Hoeper MM, Spiekerkoetter E, Westerkamp V, et al (Hannover Med School, Germany)

Eur Respir J 20:339-343, 2002   45–2

Background.—Pulmonary arterial hypertension (PAH) is characterized by progressive obliteration of the pulmonary vascular bed that, in nearly all cases, results in progressive failure of the right side of the heart and death. Treatment with continuous IV prostacyclin (epoprostenol) has been shown to improve exercise capacity, hemodynamics, and survival duration in patients with pulmonary hypertension. In some countries, continuous IV iloprost, a stable prostacyclin analogue, has been found to be as efficient as epoprostenol in these patients. The requirement of a permanent central venous access is a major drawback of continuous IV prostaglandin treatment, as this access site is prone to infection. Inhaled iloprost, oral beraprost, and subcutaneous treprostinil have recently been introduced as alternatives to IV prostaglandin treatment. However, it is not known whether the inhaled form of iloprost is as safe and efficacious as IV iloprost therapy. Whether patients whose clinical condition deteriorates under treatment with aerosolized iloprost would benefit from switching to continuous IV iloprost was determined.

Methods.—The study group included 16 patients with severe PAH who received continuous IV iloprost after primary or secondary failure of treatment with aerosolized iloprost. The main outcome measures were survival, New York Heart Association (NYHA) class, and walking distance in the 6-minute walk test. These 16 patients were part of a group of 93 patients with PAH being treated with aerosolized iloprost.

Results.—These 16 patients had severe failure of the right side of the heart. Five of the 16 patients showed no improvement and eventually died. Three patients had further deterioration in NYHA class and exercise capacity, and 2 of these patients underwent lung transplantation. The third patient was still living at publication. Eight patients showed significant improvement with continuous IV iloprost: 1 underwent transplantation, and the remaining 7 patients were alive and stable at publication. Among these 8 patients, the walking distance in the 6-minute walk test increased from 205 ± 94 m to 329 ± 59 m. This study was unable to identify any clinical or hemodynamic variables that would predict whether switching from inhaled to IV iloprost would have a beneficial effect.

Conclusions.—Among patients with PAH whose conditions deteriorated while being treated with inhaled iloprost, 50% experienced a significant improvement in exercise capacity after switching to continuous IV iloprost. It was not possible to predict the individual effects of this approach, so IV prostaglandin treatment should be considered in patients with PAH who deteriorate while receiving aerosolized iloprost.

▶ Prostacyclin (epoprostenol, PGI_2) has significant vasodilatory properties and has been one of the mainstays of the treatment of patients with primary pulmonary hypertension, together with antithrombotic agents and calcium channel blockers. Unfortunately, this IV medication requires a continuous infusion because it is somewhat unstable and has a short half-life. The need for central venous access, the development of tachyphylaxis, and rebound pulmonary hypertension are just a few of the challenges that patients and clinicians face during prostacyclin use. A prostacyclin analogue, iloprost, is longer acting, more stable, and available in the IV and inhaled forms in a few countries (not in the United States). Enthusiasm about its use, particularly in the inhaled form, has grown due to the obvious need for alternatives to high-risk prostacyclin therapy. Inhaled iloprost is a noninvasive medicine that has less systemic vasodilation and offers potential improvements in ventilation perfusion relationships over IV infusions.[1] Its major drawback is its short duration of hemodynamic efficacy, leading to nonsustained pulmonary vasodilation and a need for 6 to 9 inhalations daily. Nonetheless, it represents a significant advance in the therapeutic options for patients with pulmonary hypertension. Also, the discovery that the oral dual endothelin receptor blocker, bosentan, causes significant hemodynamic and clinical improvements in pulmonary hypertension gives hope that the era of invasive infusion therapy for pulmonary hypertension is drawing to a close.[2]

However, what does one do when noninvasive approaches are failing? Hoeper et al sought to determine whether continuous infusion therapy with iloprost offered a benefit to the patient worsening while being treated with inhaled therapy. Eight of 16 patients did improve, as seen by dramatic increases in their 6-minute walk distances, but there was no ability to predict who would respond. It would seem that a reasonable approach to patients with pulmonary hypertension would be initial therapy with an inhaled or oral agent (or perhaps both, if available) and a move to infusion therapy with a prostanoid in patients not responding to noninvasive therapy.

K. L. Lewis, MD

References

1. Olschewski H, Ardeschir G, Walmrath D, et al: Inhaled prostacyclin and iloprost in severe pulmonary hypertension secondary to lung fibrosis. *Am J Respir Crit Care Med* 160:600-607, 1999.
2. Rubin L, Badesch D, Barst R, et al: Bosentan therapy for pulmonary arterial hypertension. *N Engl J Med* 346:896-903, 2002.

Survival in Primary Pulmonary Hypertension: The Impact of Epoprostenol Therapy
McLaughlin VV, Shillington A, Rich S (Rush-Presbyterian-St Luke's Med Ctr, Chicago; EPI-Q Inc, Oakbrook Terrace, Ill)
Circulation 106:1477-1482, 2002   45-3

Background.—Primary pulmonary hypertension (PPH) is a severe and progressive disease that, if untreated, has a median survival of 2.8 years and survival rates of 68%, 48%, and 34% at 1, 3, and 5 years, respectively. In 1980 the National Institutes of Health (NIH) established a registry on PPH that described the clinical characteristics of the disease and its natural history over a 5-year period. In 1990, IV epoprostenol was the first drug to win Food and Drug Administration approval for the treatment of PPH. Since then, epoprostenol has become the standard of care for the treatment of patients with advanced PPH. The long-term effects of epoprostenol on PPH have not been defined.

Methods.—The study included 162 consecutive patients with a diagnosis of PPH who were treated with epoprostenol were followed up for a median of 31 months. A customized database was used to gather data, including functional class, exercise tolerance, and hemodynamics. Each patient's vital status was verified.

Results.—The observed rate of survival of patients treated with epoprostenol was 87.8% at 1 year, 76.3% at 2 years, and 62.8% at 3 years, all significantly greater than the expected survival rates of 58.9%, 46.3%, and 35.4%, respectively—figures based on historical data. At baseline, predictors of survival were exercise tolerance, functional class, right atrial pressure, and vasodilator response to adenosine. After the first year of therapy, predictors of survival included functional class and improvement in exercise tolerance, cardiac index, and mean pulmonary artery pressure.

Conclusions.—These findings indicate that IV epoprostenol is effective in improving the long-term survival of patients with primary pulmonary hypertension.

Outcome in 91 Consecutive Patients With Pulmonary Arterial Hypertension Receiving Epoprostenol

Kuhn KP, Byrne DW, Arbogast PG, et al (Vanderbilt Univ, Nashville, Tenn)
Am J Respir Crit Care Med 167:580-586, 2003   45–4

Background.—Pulmonary artery hypertension (PAH) is characterized by sustained elevation of the pulmonary vascular resistance (PVR). In untreated patients, right heart failure and death eventually occur. PAH occurs in an idiopathic form known as primary pulmonary hypertension (PPH) and in association with other disorders, including connective tissue disease and congenital heart disease. The introduction of epoprostenol has significantly improved the treatment of PAH; however, the survival benefit from epoprostenol therapy has not been well defined. An effort was made to determine the long-term effects of epoprostenol on mortality rate and to identify factors associated with outcome in patients with different forms of PAH.

Methods.—From June 1995 to August 2001, 91 patients with PAH were treated with epoprostenol at a single institution. All of the patients were treated with IV epoprostenol after either failure to improve clinically with calcium channel blocker therapy or failure to demonstrate a significant decrease in mean pulmonary arterial pressure. The effects of long-term epoprostenol therapy were analyzed to identify features associated with outcome.

Results.—Predictors of worse outcome in these patients included older age at onset of disease; World Health Organization functional class IV, either at baseline or at follow-up; and scleroderma spectrum of disease. No baseline or follow-up hemodynamic factors were found to be predictive of outcome.

Conclusions.—These findings indicate that treatment with epoprostenol improves the survival of patients with PPH compared with survival predicted by the National Institutes of Health Primary Pulmonary Hypertension Registry's survival equation. It also appears from these findings that epoprostenol provides significantly better survival in PPH patients than in patients with the scleroderma spectrum of PAH. However, survival is significantly shorter in older patients treated with epoprostenol, regardless of the cause of their PAH.

▶ The use of epoprostenol therapy in PPH is intensive, costly, and risky. However, because the survival rates for the disease, when untreated, are so low, such measures may be necessary. To this point, the evidence supporting epoprostenol's use has been short term only, with no clear indication of how long-term therapy impacted disease progression and outcome. The information from the Rush-Presbyterian registry published by McGlaughlin et al (Abstract 45–3) showed a dramatic survival advantage from epoprostenol therapy at least to 3 years when compared with the expected survival of untreated patients. Meticulous attention to anticoagulation, calcium channel blockade, and overall care in a pulmonary hypertension specialty center probably impacted the survival benefit, but this in no way detracts from the importance of the result as it pertains to infused epoprostenol. During the observational period, a total of 119 local line infections, 70 sepsis episodes, 10 tunnel infections, and 72 catheter replacements were identified. Also, it appeared that 4 deaths were attributed to line sepsis, and 1 death was due to epoprostenol infusion interruption. Thus, the potential harm of therapy should always be discussed with patients. Fortunately, this information will help provide better education for patients about the chance for a good long-term outcome with epoprostenol infusion therapy. Finally, data presented in this article should prove useful in guiding transplantation decisions, since NYHA functional classification at each evaluation while the patient was undergoing therapy was a good indicator of what the survival would be over a period of months to years.

Data from Vanderbilt by Kuhn et al (Abstract 45–4) on 91 consecutive patients showed 1-, 2-, and 3-year survival rates remarkably similar to the Rush registry in patients with PPH who were treated with continuous epoprostenol. Patients who had scleroderma associated pulmonary hypertension fared much more poorly during infusion therapy. A third study published in 2002 by Sitbon et al[1] showed epoprostenol-treated PPH survival rates almost identical to the 2 studies reviewed here, leaving little doubt about the expected outcomes in this patient group.

K. L. Lewis, MD

Reference

1. Sitbon O, Humbert M, Nunes H, et al: Long-term intravenous epoprostenol infusion in primary pulmonary hypertension: Prognostic factors and survival. *Am Coll Cardiol* 40:780-788, 2002.

46 Critical Care

A Randomised, Controlled Trial of the Pulmonary Artery Catheter in Critically Ill Patients
Rhodes A, Cusack RJ, Newman PJ, et al (St George's Hosp, London)
Intensive Care Med 28:256-264, 2002   46–1

Introduction.—The pulmonary artery catheter (PAC) is commonly used by critical care practitioners worldwide. Some observational trials have suggested that use of the PAC increases mortality rates. The survival and clinical outcomes of critically ill patients treated with the use of a PAC were compared with those treated without a PAC in a prospective, randomized, controlled clinical investigation.

Methods.—Between October 1997 and February 1999, 201 critically ill adults in the ICU were randomly assigned to either a PAC group or a control, non-PAC group (95 and 106 patients, respectively). One patient in the control group was withdrawn, and 5 in the PAC group did not receive a PAC. All remaining participants were available for follow-up. Survival to 28 days, intensive care and hospital length of stay, and organ dysfunction were compared on an intention-to-treat basis and on a subgroup basis for participants who successfully received a PAC.

Results.—There were no significant between-group differences in mortality rates between the PAC group and the controls (47.9% vs 47.6%; $P > .99$). The mortality rate for patients who had management decisions based on information derived from a PAC was 45% ($P = .77$). The PAC group had significantly more fluids administered in the initial 24 hours than the controls (4953 vs 4292 mL), as well as an increased incidence of renal failure at day 3 postrandomization (35% vs 20%; $P < .05$) and thrombocytopenia ($P < .03$).

Conclusion.—There was no evidence of an increased mortality rate in the PAC group as compared with the non-PAC group.

▶ I admire this well-done, prospective, randomized, controlled trial. It clearly shows no difference in mortality rates in this group of very ill patients with septic shock, whether a PAC was used or not. Therapy was different in the groups, however: the PAC group received significantly more fluid. Still, is the intervention worthwhile? Mortality rates and outcomes did not differ in the 2 groups. Perhaps the catheter allows us to make more logical decisions, but the difference in therapy is really insignificant in the overall scheme of the patient.

J. A. Barker, MD

Outcome of Patients With Idiopathic Pulmonary Fibrosis Admitted to the Intensive Care Unit

Saydain G, Islam A, Afessa B, et al (Mayo Clinic, Rochester, Minn)
Am J Respir Crit Care Med 166:839-842, 2002   46–2

Background.—Idiopathic pulmonary fibrosis (IPF) carries a poor prognosis, and the risk of mortality may be even higher when patients with IPF have life-threatening comorbid conditions develop. The effectiveness of standard ICU treatments for patients with IPF who have life-threatening complications was examined.

Methods.—The medical records of 38 patients with IPF (25 men and 13 women; mean age, 68.3 years) admitted to the ICU with a life-threatening complication were reviewed.

Results.—The reasons for ICU admission were respiratory failure in 32 patients (84%), gastrointestinal bleeding in 2, hypotension in 2, and acute abdomen in 2. At hospital admission, 20 patients (52.6%) were taking corticosteroids and 24 (63.2%) had been using home oxygen therapy. During hospitalization, 19 patients (50%) required mechanical ventilation. According to the Acute Physiologic and Chronic Health Evaluation III score, the predicted ICU mortality rate was 12% and the predicted in-hospital mortality rate was 26%. However, actual rates were markedly higher, at 45% and 61%, respectively.

Survivors and nonsurvivors did not differ significantly in pulmonary function, echocardiographic findings, the use or duration of mechanical ventilation, or the development of sepsis or multiple organ failure. Of the 13 patients who survived to hospital discharge and for whom follow-up information was available, all but 1 (92%) died at a median of 2 months after hospital discharge.

Conclusion.—Patients with IPF admitted to the ICU have poorer outcomes than predicted on the basis of common risk factors. Patients with IPF and their families should be aware of these poor outcomes so that they can make informed decisions about life support and ICU care.

▶ These results confirm my own experience with IPF patients admitted to the ICU. They do poorly. Even if they do survive the experience, the majority (92%) are dead within 2 months. Why would this be so? Their lung compliance (lung stiffness) is so poor that many do not improve upon going from noninvasive to mechanical ventilation. The long-standing high minute ventilation requirements have reduced both their exercise tolerance and their nutritional status to below normal. Finally, it is tempting to surmise that IPF is a disease of diffuse inflammation, which might explain the high rate of multiorgan failure found in this study. Patients and physicians alike should think twice about entering the ICU for this disorder at its end stage.

J. A. Barker, MD

Short-term Noninvasive Pressure Support Ventilation Prevents ICU Admittance in Patients With Acute Cardiogenic Pulmonary Edema

Giacomini M, Iapichino G, Cigada M, et al (Polo Universitario Ospedale San Paolo, Milan, Italy; "Aldo e Cele Daccò," Ranica, Bergamo, Italy)
Chest 123:2057-2061, 2003   46–3

Introduction.—Most patients with acute cardiogenic pulmonary edema (ACPE) are initially managed in the emergency department (ED). When patients do not respond to conventional medical treatment, ventilatory assistance is required. If the duration of treatment was short enough, noninvasive pressure support ventilation (NIPSV) could be used in the ED, thus avoiding admission to the ICU. There are no predictive criteria for lack of response to NIPSV for ACPE, making it difficult to ascertain how long NIPSV has to be continued before determining whether it is successful. Patients in the ED with ACPE were evaluated to determine whether a short attempt at NIPSV could avoid ICU admittance and to identify lack of response prediction variables. Fifty-eight consecutive patients with ACPE who were unresponsive to medical treatment and admitted between January 1999 and December 2000 were evaluated in an uncontrolled, prospective, inception cohort investigation.

Methods.—Pressure support ventilation was begun with a full-face mask until resolution of respiratory failure. A 15-minute "weaning test" was performed to assess clinical stability. Patients who responded were moved to a medical ward, and those who were nonresponders were intubated and admitted to the ICU. Patients were followed up for optimal length of intervention, avoidance of ICU admittance, incidence of myocardial infarction, and predictive lack of response criteria.

Results.—The mean time for the NIPSV trial was 96 minutes. None of the 43 responders (74%) were subsequently ventilated or admitted to the ICU. Two patients had a myocardial infarction, and 13 died. A mean arterial pressure of less than 95 mm Hg (odds ratio [OR], 10.6; 95% confidence interval [CI], 1.8-60.8; $P < .01$) and chronic obstructive pulmonary disease (COPD) (OR, 9.4; 95% CI, 1.6-54.0; $P < .05$) at baseline were predictive of lack of response to noninvasive ventilation.

Conclusion.—A short attempt at noninvasive ventilation is effective in averting mechanical ventilation. A 15-minute weaning test can identify patients who will not require further invasive ventilatory support. Both COPD and hypotension at baseline are negative predictive criteria.

▶ Noninvasive ventilation is now commonly used for episodes of acute pulmonary edema. This ingenious prospective study outlined a relatively rapid method of determining which patients would benefit from it. In addition, the authors tested a 15-minute rapid wean test that likewise split patients into those who needed only medical therapy from then on versus those who needed continued partial ventilatory assistance. It is no surprise to me that hypotensive patients and patients with underlying COPD required invasive ventilation more often. Still, these are very useful data for stratifying patients for this common problem.

J. A. Barker, MD

Physician Staffing Patterns and Clinical Outcomes in Critically Ill Patients: A Systematic Review
Pronovost PJ, Angus DC, Dorman T, et al (Johns Hopkins Univ, Baltimore, Md; Univ of Pittsburgh, Pa)
JAMA 288:2151-2162, 2002   46–4

Introduction.—ICUs that are staffed with critical care physicians (intensivists) may have improved clinical outcomes and a reduced use of resources. Because studies reporting the benefits of staffing ICUs with intensivists have been observational in nature, a systemic review was designed to examine the effect of ICU physician staffing on hospital and ICU mortality rates and length of stay (LOS).

Methods.—Studies eligible for review were randomly selected for observational controlled trials of critically ill adults or children, ICU physician staffing strategies, hospital and ICU mortality rates, and LOS. MEDLINE was searched for the period from January 1, 1965, through September 30, 2001. Additional sources of data included EMBASE, the related articles feature of PubMed, and a hand search of abstracts from selected scientific meetings. Data were abstracted independently by the 2 primary reviewers and verified for accuracy by the third reviewer.

Results.—A review of 2590 abstracts led to the identification of 26 observational studies, 1 of which included 2 comparisons, for a total of 27 comparisons of alternative staffing strategies. Twenty studies focused on a single ICU. Staffing of ICUs was classified as low intensity (no intensivist or elective intensivist consultation) or high intensity (mandatory intensivist consultation or direction of all care by an intensivist). In 16 of 17 studies, high-intensity staffing was associated with a lower hospital mortality rate. High-intensity staffing was associated with a lower ICU mortality rate in 14 of 15 studies, reduced hospital LOS in 10 of 13 studies, and reduced ICU LOS in 14 of 18 studies without case-mix adjustment. The few studies that adjusted for case mix generally favored high-intensity physician staffing.

Conclusion.—Hospital and ICU mortality rate and hospital and ICU LOS were reduced by the strategy of high-intensity ICU physician staffing. These findings were consistent across a variety of populations and hospital settings. In contrast to the United States, the closed ICU approach by intensivists is common in Europe and Australia.

▶ This systematic review carefully and in terrific detail outlines the mounting evidence that closed ICUs or open ICUs with intensivist staffing lead to improved hospital mortality rates as well as lower LOS. Some articles showed both lower hospital LOS and ICU LOS. Intensivists were also shown to reduce inappropriate ICU admissions. (Presumably, this means patients who were either not sick enough for intensive care or patients who were clearly terminal.) Not mentioned in this particular review are changes in ventilator days and the consequent decreases in ventilator-associated pneumonia (VAP) rates. VAP rates correlate directly with hospital mortality rates as well. Likewise not included were other potential advantages, such as reduction in pharmacy costs by use of sedation and ventilator protocols, by increased use of noninvasive ventilation, and by antibiotic streamlining.

Public interest in improved hospital care and safety is at an all-time high. The Leapfrog Group and others are now using the results summarized in this article to foment change in ICU staffing in the United States.[1] Intensivists must understand these data and issues.

J. A. Barker, MD

Reference

1. Birkmeyer JD, et al: Leapfrog safety standards: Potential benefits of universal adoption. The Leapfrog Group, Washington, DC, 2000 (www.leapfroggroup.org).

Morbidity, Mortality, and Quality-of-Life Outcomes of Patients Requiring ≥14 Days of Mechanical Ventilation
Combes A, Costa M-A, Trouillet J-L, et al (Groupe Hospitalier Pitié-Salpêtrière, Paris)
Crit Care Med 31:1373-1381, 2003   46–5

Background.—Fewer than 10% of all ICU admissions are for patients who require long-term mechanical ventilation (MV), yet these patients are high consumers of health care resources, often being chronically ill and having multiple organ failure. Thus, the ICU mortality among these patients is high for a variety of reasons, including age, severity of underlying medical status on admission, and MV duration, and their mortality and cost of care remain high after discharge. Health-related quality of life (HRQL) is an important component in evaluating outcome and can have an impact on choosing management strategies. Patients who had MV for a minimum of 14 days in the ICU were evaluated to determine their outcome and HRQL status.

Methods.—Enrollees included 347 consecutive patients who received MV for at least 14 days. Preadmission health status was measured by using the New York Heart Association (NYHA) functional class score. Outcomes and factors affecting those outcomes were determined along with the HRQL after a median follow-up of 3 years by using the Nottingham Health Profile and St. George's Respiratory questionnaires.

Results.—Forty-three percent of the patients died, which was a significantly higher percentage than among patients ventilated for less than 14 days (33%). Factors found to be independent predictors of ICU death were 65 years or older, preadmission NYHA functional class of 3 or greater, preadmission immunocompromised status, septic shock on admission to the ICU, renal replacement therapy while in the ICU, and nosocomial septicemia. Of the 197 patients discharged alive from the ICU, 157 completed long-term follow-up, with overall cumulative probabilities of death of 20% at 6 months, 25% at 12 months, and 33% at 36 months. Fifty-eight patients died 1 to 57 months after discharge. Actuarial survival curves showed significantly better long-term survival for patients who had undergone cardiac surgery than for other patient groups. Age of 65 or older, immunocompromised status, and use of MV for more than 35 days were independent predictors of death after ICU discharge. HRQL questionnaires were completed by 87 patients an average of 3 years after discharge from the ICU, when all but one patient lived at home. Compared with a matched general French population, the scores for these patients were significantly worse in all areas except social isolation, indicating more difficulties were experienced. Pain, sleep, energy, emotional reaction, mobility, and pulmonary function were particularly affected, with survivors of acute respiratory distress syndrome having significantly more pulmonary-specific problems.

Conclusions.—The HRQL of patients who underwent MV for at least 14 days was poorer than that of a matched general population. However, 99% of those responding after 3 years remained independent and living at home despite their impairments. Patients having had cardiac surgery had a higher probability of long-term survival than other patient groups.

▶ There are several interesting findings in this study. First, patients receiving MV for 14 days or more do poorly. There were only 99 of 347 patients who were clearly alive (50 lost to follow-up) 1 to 5 years later. Second, those with prolonged ventilation after heart surgery clearly have better survival curves. Finally, quality of life remains below that of peer groups, yet survivors are largely still living independently. Certainly these data may be very helpful for patients and families struggling with ethical dilemmas related to ICU care. The authors' suggestions to evaluate rehabilitation issues further are prescient—although there are no data on those issues in this study.

J. A. Barker, MD

47 Pleural Effusions

Is It Meaningful to Use Biochemical Parameters to Discriminate Between Transudative and Exudative Pleural Effusions?
Romero-Candeira S, Hernández L, Romero-Brufao S, et al (Hosp Gen Universitario de Alicante, Spain)
Chest 122:1524-1529, 2002

47–1

Background.—The general consensus is that definition of a pleural effusion as a transudate limits the differential diagnosis to a small number of disorders and terminates the need for further diagnostic workup of the pleural effusion. The consequences of this course are dramatic reductions in cost and morbidity. Less than 5% of neoplastic effusions may be transudative, but in these patients the classification remains useful. The use of Light's criteria to discriminate transudates from exudates has been considered the first step in the study of a pleural effusion of unknown cause. However, there is increasing concern about the usefulness of this technique, particularly regarding the limitations of Light's criteria in patients receiving diuretic therapy. The added value of biochemical criteria to clinical judgment for separating transudates from exudates was evaluated.

Methods.—This prospective randomized study included 249 consecutive patients referred for diagnostic thoracentesis. Two physicians classified the pleural effusion as transudate or exudate on the basis of all available information just before the thoracentesis was performed. The sensitivity, specificity, and accuracy of the clinical presumption were compared with the sensitivity, specificity, and accuracy of Light's criteria, serum-pleural fluid albumin, and protein gradients. The combined accuracy of biochemical and clinical criteria was also assessed.

Results.—The accuracy of Light's criteria was 93%, which was significantly higher than the accuracy of clinical presumption (84%), serum-pleural fluid albumin gradient (87%), and serum-pleural fluid protein gradient (86%). In patients receiving diuretic therapy, the accuracy of Light's criteria (83%) was not significantly different from that of the albumin gradient (88%) or the protein gradient (86%).

Conclusions.—Light's criteria are significantly more accurate than the clinical presumption for separating pleural transudates from exudates. However, Light's criteria lose accuracy in patients receiving diuretics, and in these patients the accuracy of Light's criteria was similar to that obtained from alternative biochemical criteria alone or a combination of biochemical criteria and clinical judgment.

Exudative Effusions in Congestive Heart Failure

Eid AA, Keddissi JI, Samaha M, et al (Univ of Oklahoma, Oklahoma City)
Chest 122:1518-1523, 2002   47–2

Background.—Congestive heart failure (CHF) is the most frequent cause of pleural effusions. Typically, pleural effusion associated with heart failure has the characteristics of a transudate. It resolves when the underlying cardiac problem is treated. Because CHF is a common clinical presentation, it is not unusual for a patient with heart failure to have an exudative pleural effusion as a result of a coexisting condition such as pneumonia. Occasionally, however, a patient with CHF will have an exudative effusion in the absence of an apparent cause other than heart failure. The incidence and clinical significance of these exudative effusions were determined.

Methods.—The study group was composed of all patients at 1 institution who had CHF and effusion during a 7-year period from January 1994 through December 2000. These patients were identified from their hospital discharge diagnoses and radiographs; those who had undergone thoracentesis were identified through a review of library logs. The presenting symptoms and clinical course were determined from a review of the medical records. The effect of red blood cell (RBC) contamination on pleural fluid lactate dehydrogenase levels was determined by measuring the lactate dehydrogenase activity of mock pleural fluid containing known amounts of RBC.

Results.—A total of 770 patients were identified, but only 175 patients underwent a thoracentesis. Of these 175 patients, 86 patients had transudates and 89 had exudates. A noncardiac cause for the exudate was readily identified in 59 patients by hospital discharge, and 7 additional patients had a cause discovered during follow-up. Of the remaining 23 patients, 11 had undergone coronary artery bypass graft (CABG) surgery 1 year or more before presentation, and 50% of effusions in patients who had undergone CABG surgery were exudates. Thus, only 12 patients had CHF-related exudates, and in 4 of these patients the exudates could be explained by RBC contamination of the pleural fluid. The clinical presentation of patients with CHF-associated exudates was similar to the presentation of CHF in patients with transudates.

Conclusions.—The results of this study suggest that exudative effusions caused only by CHF are rare. There is a noncardiac cause for pleural effusion in most patients who have congestive heart failure and an exudative effusion. The high frequency of exudates in patients with a history of CABG is indicative of a persistent impairment in lymphatic clearance from the pleural cavity.

▶ It has been presumed that testing offered superiority to clinical assessment only, but data supporting this are surprisingly sparse. The authors did show that biochemical testing was superior, but their clinical suspicions were right almost 85% of the time, which was unexpectedly high. For some time, Light's criteria for separating transudates from exudates has been the standard (namely, pleural fluid/serum protein ratio, pleural fluid/serum LDH ratio, and pleural fluid LDH concentration).[1] In this investigation, Light's criteria continued to be superior to other approaches. However, the accuracy of Light's criteria is reduced in patients taking diuretics. In the setting of diuretic use, the assessment of pleural fluid cholesterol using a cutoff of 45 mg/dL can be particularly helpful in separating transudates from exudates. In fact, the combination of pleural fluid cholesterol and pleural fluid LDH concentrations has been shown to be as reliable as Light's criteria without the need for serum specimens.[2] Pleural fluid cholesterol was not studied by Romero-Candeira et al (Abstract 47–1).

Many patients taking diuretics are doing so for the diagnosis of congestive heart failure (CHF). Despite the reduced accuracy of Light's criteria in the setting of diuretic use, Eid and colleagues (Abstract 47–2) found that most exudates (using Light's criteria) in the setting of CHF were in fact not due to the CHF, despite the universal use of diuretics. Therefore, an exudate in a patient with CHF taking diuretics should not be presumed to be a "pseudoexudate" but should instigate a search for a cause other than CHF. The use of pleural fluid cholesterol was also not studied by Eid et al.

K. L. Lewis, MD

Reference

1. Light RW, Macgregor MI, Luchsinger PC, et al: Pleural effusions: The diagnostic separation of transudates and exudates. *Ann Intern Med* 77:507-513, 1972.
2. Costa M, Quiroga T, Cruz E: Measurement of pleural fluid cholesterol and lactate dehydrogenase. A simple and accurate set of indicators for separating exudates from transudates. *Chest* 108:1260-1263, 1995.

48 Sleep Apnea

Incidence of Sleep-Disordered Breathing in an Urban Adult Population: The Relative Importance of Risk Factors in the Development of Sleep-Disordered Breathing
Tishler PV, Larkin EK, Schluchter MD, et al (Harvard Med School, Boston; Case Western Reserve Univ, Cleveland, Ohio)
JAMA 289:2230-2237, 2003   48–1

Background.—Sleep-disordered breathing (SDB) is a prevalent condition associated with serious chronic disease. The 5-year incidence of SDB and the risk factors influencing it were investigated.

Methods.—The study included 286 participants in the Cleveland Family Study who were eligible, according to the study inclusion criteria, by being 18 years or older and having had 2 in-home sleep studies 5 years apart, with the first study yielding normal results. Information on medical and family history and SDB symptoms was obtained. Height, body weight, blood pressure, waist and hip circumference were measured, serum cholesterol concentrations determined, and overnight sleep monitored.

Findings.—Sixteen percent of the eligible group had a second-study apnea hypopnea index (AHI) of at least 10, and 10% had a second-study AHI result of at least 15. For the AHI findings of at least 15, an estimated 2.5% may have represented test variability. In an ordinal logistic regression analysis, AHI correlated significantly with age, body mass index (BMI), male sex, waist-to-hip ratio, and serum cholesterol concentration. Age interacted with sex and BMI. The odds ratio (OR) for increased AHI per 10-year increase in age was 1.15 in men and 2.41 in women. The OR for men versus women declined from 5.04 at 30 years of age to 0.54 at 60 years of age. The OR for increased AHI per 1-unit increase in BMI declined from 1.21 to 1.05 between 20 and 60 years of age.

Conclusions.—The 5-year incidences for moderately severe and mild to moderately severe SDB are 7.5% and 16%, respectively. Age, sex, BMI, waist-to-hip ratio, and serum cholesterol concentration independently influence the incidence of SDB. The predominance of SDB seen in men decreases with advancing age. By 50 years of age, men and women have similar incidence rates. In addition, the influence of BMI declines with age and may be negligible at 60 years of age.

▶ A 5-year incidence of 37% for an AHI that many would consider to be diagnostic of obstructive sleep apnea is alarming. To put this in context, CMS (Centers for Medicare and Medicaid Services, formerly known as HCFA or Health Care Financing Administration) will pay for continuous positive airway treatment (CPAP) for patients who have an AHI of 5 or more with just about any symptom,[1] and for symptomatic patients who have an AHI of 15 or more (which developed in 10% of this study population over the course of 5 years). The authors refer to "sleep-disordered breathing," or to absolute AHIs rather than claiming that a certain percentage of study participants had obstructive sleep apnea syndrome (OSAS). This is smart, given that they used a nonstandard definition of oxygen desaturation for identifying apneas and hypopneas (this study used an oxygen desaturation of 2.5 %, instead of the more standard 4%),[2] and that AHIs must be correlated with symptoms to make a diagnosis. However, they report a 5-year incidence of 10% (2% per year) for an AHI of 15 events per hour of sleep, which most sleep medicine clinicians would consider to be unequivocal OSA. Given that the risk of cardiovascular disease is correlated with AHI and is certainly significant at AHIs of 15 events per hour of sleep or more,[3] quibbling about what constitutes OSA becomes somewhat irrelevant.

The bread and butter sleep clinic patient is a 48 year-old, obese, hypertensive man. This study clearly documents that sex and obesity become negligible risk factors for SDB after the ages of 50 and 60 years, respectively. This has been reported before.[4] Since older patients with OSA do not match the classic stereotype, they may be overlooked; this is unfortunate, since we know that sleep apnea causes many of the afflictions of older age, such as hypertension,[5] cardiovascular disease,[3,6] and cognitive decline,[7] and that CPAP can reverse these changes.[8-10]

Take home messages: Sleep apnea is common, and becoming more so. Because the "typical" risk factors (obesity, male sex) become much less important in the older patient, we probably are seriously underdiagnosing SDB in geriatric patients, and may be missing opportunities to preserve function and quality of life in this age group.

B. A. Phillips, MD, MSPH

References

1. www.hcfa.gov (go to http://www.hcfa.gov/coverage/8b3%2Dbbb1.htm)
2. Meoli AL, Casey KR, Clark RW, et al: Hypopnea in sleep-disordered breathing in adults. *Sleep* 24:469-470, 2001.
3. Shahar E, Whitney CW, Redline S, et al: Sleep-disordered breathing and cardiovascular disease. Cross-sectional results of the Sleep Heart Health Study. *Am J Respir Crit Care Med* 163:19-25, 2001.
4. Young T, Shahar E, Nieto FJ, et al: Predictors of sleep-disordered breathing in community-dwelling adults: The Sleep Heart Health Study. *Arch Intern Med* 162:893-900, 2002.
5. Peppard PE, Young T, Palta M, et al: Prospective study of the association between sleep-disordered breathing and hypertension. *N Engl J Med* 342:1378-1384, 2000.

6. Peker Y, Hedner J, Norum J, et al: Increased incidence of cardiovascular disease in middle-aged men with obstructive sleep apnea. A 7-year follow-up. *Am J Respir Crit Care Med* 166:159-165, 2002.
7. Kim H, Young T, Matthews G, et al: Sleep-disordered breathing and neuropsychological deficits. *Am J Respir Crit Care Med* 156:1813-1819, 1997.
8. Pepperell JCT, Ramdassingh-Dow S, Crosthwaite N, et al: Ambulatory blood pressure after therapeutic and subtherapeutic nasal continuous positive airway pressure for obstructive sleep apnoea: A randomised parallel trial. *Lancet* 359:204-214, 2002.
9. Engelman HM, Kingshott RN, Wraith PK et al: Randomized placebo-controlled crossover trial of continuous positive airway pressure for mild sleep apnea/hypopnea syndrome. *Am J Respir Crit Care Med* 159:461-467, 1999.
10. Kanedo Y, Floras JS, Usui K, et al: Cardiovascular effects of continuous positive airway pressure in patients with heart failure and obstructive sleep apnea. *N Engl J Med* 348:1233-1241, 2003.

Hormone Replacement Therapy and Sleep-Disordered Breathing

Shahar E, for the Sleep Heart Health Study Research Group (Univ of Minnesota, Minneapolis; Case Western Reserve Univ, Cleveland, Ohio; Univ of Wisconsin, Madison; et al)
Am J Respir Crit Care Med 167:1186-1192, 2003   48–2

Background.—Disordered breathing during sleep occurs more commonly among postmenopausal than premenopausal women. This may be because of diminishing concentrations of estrogen and progesterone. The association between the use of replacement hormones and sleep-disordered breathing (SDB) among women, 50 years or older, was investigated.

Methods.—The sample of 2852 non-institutionalized women were participants in the Sleep Heart Health Study. Unattended, single-night polysomnography was done at the participant's home to determine the frequency of apneas and hypopneas per hour of sleep.

Findings.—The prevalence of SDB, defined as an apnea-hypopnea index of 15 or greater, was about half as high in hormone users as in nonusers. This association was only moderately attenuated by multivariable adjustment for known determinants of the disorder, such as age, body mass index, and neck circumference. The inverse correlation between hormone use and SDB was apparent in various subgroups, being especially strong in 50- to 59-year-old individuals.

Conclusions.—Increasing evidence suggests that replacement hormone therapy may help prevent or alleviate SDB among postmenopausal women. Additional research is warranted.

Menopausal Status and Sleep-Disordered Breathing in the Wisconsin Sleep Cohort Study

Young T, Finn L, Austin D, et al (Univ of Wisconsin-Madison)
Am J Respir Crit Care Med 167:1181-1185, 2003   48–3

Background.—Menopause is considered a risk factor for sleep-disordered breathing (SDB). However, this hypothesis has not been tested sufficiently. The association between menopausal status and SDB was determined in a population-based sample.

Methods.—The study included 589 women enrolled in the Wisconsin Sleep Cohort Study. Menopausal status was based on menstrual history, gynecologic surgery, hormone replacement therapy (HRT), follicle-stimulating hormone, and vasomotor symptoms. In-laboratory polysomnography established the frequency of SDB.

Findings.—The odds ratios (ORs) for 5 or more apnea and hypopnea events per hour were 1.2 in perimenopausal women and 2.6 in postmenopausal women, after adjustment for age, body habitus, smoking, and other potential confounding variables. The ORs for 15 or more apnea and hypopnea events per hour were 1.1 in perimenopausal women and 3.5 in postmenopausal women.

Conclusions.—Menopausal transition correlates significantly with an increased likelihood of having SDB, independent of known confounding variables. Menopausal women who report snoring, daytime sleepiness, or unsatisfactory sleep should be evaluated for SDB.

▶ Nearly simultaneously, the Sleep Heart Health Study (Abstract 48–2) and the Wisconsin Sleep Cohort Study (Abstract 48–3) deliver a "good news, bad news" message for aging women. The bad news: menopause is an independent risk factor for Obstructive Sleep Apnea. The good news: hormone replacement therapy (HRT) may have a role in preventing or reducing SDB in menopausal women. These studies are much more powerful than previous work on this topic. The cohorts are large, important confounders (body mass index, age, smoking) that are identified and controlled for, and the statistics are carefully done. Amidst all the confusion about the risks and benefits of HRT, these findings may not be particularly welcome. But for those of us who see *beaucoup* middle-aged women with mild sleep apnea who are not particularly keen on continuous positive airway pressure, HRT may be another treatment option worth considering.

B. A. Phillips, MD, MSPH

Short-term Variability of Respiration and Sleep During Unattended Nonlaboratory Polysomnogaphy—The Sleep Heart Health Study

Quan SF, for the Sleep Heart Health Study (SHHS) Research Group (Univ of Arizona, Tucson; et al)

Sleep 25:843-849, 2002   48–4

Background.—The Sleep Heart Health Study (SHHS) is a large multicenter cohort study that explores the link between sleep-disordered breathing and cardiovascular and cerebrovascular mortality and morbidity in the general population. This report presents findings from a substudy conducted among a sample of participants in the SHHS. The goal was to determine the short-term variability of 2 nights of unattended nonlaboratory nocturnal polysomnography conducted several months apart.

Methods.—This study group was composed of a subset of 99 participants in the SHHS who agreed to undergo a repeat polysomnography within 4 months of their original study. Acceptable repeat polysomnograms were obtained from 91 participants. The respiratory disturbance index ($RDI_{3\%}$; apnea or hypopnea events associated with $\geq 3\%$ oxygen desaturation) and sleep data from initial and repeated polysomnography were compared.

Results.—There was no significant bias in RDI between study nights with the use of several different RDI definitions, including $RDI_{3\%}$ and apnea or hypopnea events associated with oxygen desaturation of 4% or more ($RDI_{4\%}$). Variability between studies estimated with intraclass correlations (ICC) ranged from 0.77 to 0.81. For study participants with and $RDI_{3\%}$ of less than 15, the variability between studies increased as a function of increasing RDI. However, for participants with an $RDI_{3\%}$ of 15 or greater, variability was constant. Body mass index, sleep efficiency, gender, and age were not directly predictive of RDI variability. At $RDI_{4\%}$, cutpoints of 5 or less, 10 or less, or 15 or less events per hour, 79.1%, 85.7%, and 87.9% of patients, respectively had the same classification of sleep disordered breathing status on both nights of study. There was no significant bias in sleep staging, sleep efficiency, or arousal index between studies. However, variability between studies was greater with ICC values ranging from 0.37 (percentage of time in rapid eye movement) to 0.76 (arousal index).

Conclusions.—The SHHS provided accurate estimates of the severity of sleep-disordered breathing and the quality of sleep with 1 night of unattended nonlaboratory polysomnography. These findings may be applicable to other large epidemiologic studies that use similar recording techniques and quality-assurance procedures.

▶ This study confirms and elaborates what many other studies of home monitoring have demonstrated. As the authors of this study say ". . . our results provide evidence to support the utility of NPSG [nocturnal polysomnography] data obtained in a single night [of home testing] to yield reliable indices of the RDI [respiratory disturbance index] . . ." Fig 1 (see original article) shows reproducibility data for the unattended (aka home monitoring) system used in the Sleep Heart Health Study.

Home monitoring is no longer coming. It's here. Too bad. While I think home monitoring is as good as polysomnography at diagnosing sleep apnea, I doubt either one is as good as a skilled clinician who takes a directed history and physical. And while I think that errors of both underdiagnosis and overdiagnosis are made with any system, the risks of "unnecessary" CPAP are far outweighed by the risks of failure to diagnose or delay in diagnosis of sleep apnea. Our overreliance on technology and diagnostic testing is costing lives. Because untreated sleep apnea is a driving risk,[1-5] some of the lives cost by the unnecessary and nonstandardized testing we do are not even those of the patients affected!

B. A. Phillips, MD, MSPH

References

1. Wright J, Johns R, Watt I, et al: The health effects of obstructive sleep apnoea and the effectiveness of treatment with continuous positive airway pressure: A systematic review of the research evidence. *BMJ* 314:851-860, 1997.
2. Zhang J, Fraser S, Lindsay J, et al: Age-specific patterns of factors related to fatal motor vehicle traffic crashes: Focus on young and elderly drivers. *Public Health* 112:289-295, 1998.
3. Findley LJ, Unverzagt ME, Suratt PM: Automobile accidents involving patients with obstructive sleep apnea. *Am Rev Respir Dis* 138:337-340, 1988.
4. Barbe F, Pericas J, Munoz A, et al: Automobile accidents in patients with sleep apnea syndrome: An epidemiological and mechanistic study. *Am J Respir Crit Care Med* 158:18-22, 1998.
5. Findley LJ, Weiss JW, Jabour ER: Drivers with untreated sleep apnea: A cause of death and serious injury. *Arch Intern Med* 151:1451-1452, 1991.

Increased Incidence of Cardiovascular Disease in Middle-Aged Men With Obstructive Sleep Apnea: A 7-Year Follow-up
Peker Y, Hedner J, Norum J, et al (Sahlgrenska Univ, Gothenburg, Sweden)
Am J Respir Crit Care Med 166:159-165, 2002   48–5

Background.—Obstructive sleep apnea (OSA) occurs in 24% of middle-aged men and in 9% of women in the United States, but the treatment criterion for OSA, daytime sleepiness, is reported by 17% of middle-aged men and by 22% of women. There is increasing evidence of an independent association between OSA and cardiovascular disease, mainly hypertension and coronary artery disease. However, no convincing evidence of a causal link has been found. Previous studies of OSA and cardiovascular disease have been limited by poor documentation, significant loss of study participants to follow-up, inadequate control of confounding factors, and pre-existing cardiovascular disease in more than half of the study population at baseline. The potential link between OSA and cardiovascular disease was further explored.

Methods.—The incidence of cardiovascular disease was explored in a consecutive sleep clinic cohort of 182 middle-aged men with or without OSA. All study participants were free of hypertension or other cardiovascular disease, pulmonary disease, diabetes mellitus, psychiatric disorders, alcohol dependency, and malignancy at baseline. Data were obtained from the Swedish Hospital Discharge Register for a 7-year period ending on December 31, 1998, and from questionnaires. The effectiveness of OSA treatment, age, body mass index (BMI), systolic blood pressure, diastolic blood pressure at baseline, and smoking habits were controlled for.

Results.—The incidence of at least 1 cardiovascular disease was observed in 22 of 60 research subjects with OSA (36.7%) compared with 8 of 122 research subjects without OSA (6.6%). Multiple logistic regression showed that significant predictors of the incidence of cardiovascular disease were OSA at baseline and age after adjustment for BMI, systolic blood pressure, and diastolic blood pressure. Efficient treatment was associated with a significant risk reduction for cardiovascular disease incidence after adjustment for age and systolic blood pressure at baseline in the research subjects with OSA.

Conclusions.—It would seem that the risk of having cardiovascular disease is increased in middle-aged individuals with OSA independently of age, BMI, blood pressure, and smoking status. Effective treatment of OSA reduces the excess risk of cardiovascular disease, and treatment may also be considered for relatively mild cases of OSA without regard to daytime sleepiness.

▶ Sleep apnea has been implicated as a cause of cardiovascular disease[1] and is well-established as a cause of hypertension.[2-7] The article by Peker et al is important because it is a longitudinal study controlling for the important risk factors of BMI, age, blood pressure, and smoking. The study is notable because it shows that effective treatment of sleep-disordered breathing reduces the risk of cardiovascular disease.

What surprised me about this study was that uvulopalatopharyngoplasty was ultimately as effective as continuous positive airway pressure in reducing cardiovascular risk in this cohort. The "success" rate for uvulopalatopharyngoplasty was about what it usually is (50%), but the compliance rate for continuous positive airway pressure was even worse! Ultimately, about two thirds of the patients with sleep-disordered breathing in this study were not effectively treated. This jibes with my clinical impression and experience. We have a long way to go to improve outcomes for this largely lifestyle-induced disease.

B. A. Phillips, MD, MSPH

References

1. Shahar E, Whitney CW, Redline S, et al: Sleep-disordered breathing and cardiovascular disease. Cross-sectional results of the Sleep Heart Health Study. *Am J Respir Crit Care Med* 163:19-25, 2001.
2. Pepperell JCT, Ramdassingh-Dow S, Crosthwaite N, et al: Ambulatory blood pressure after therapeutic and subtherapeutic nasal continuous positive airway pressure for obstructive sleep apnoea: A randomised parallel trial *Lancet* 359:204-214, 2002.
3. Lavie P, Herer P, Hoffstein V: Obstructive sleep apnoea syndrome as a risk factor for hypertension: Population study. *BMJ* 320:479-482, 2000.

4. Nieto FJ, Young TB, Lind BK, et al: Association of sleep-disordered breathing, sleep apnea, and hypertension in a large community-based study. *JAMA* 283:1829-1836, 2000.

5. Grote L, Ploch T, Heitmann J, et al: Sleep-related breathing disorder is an independent risk factor for systemic hypertension. *Am J Respir Crit Care Med* 160:1875-1882, 1999.

6. Peppard PE, Young T, Palta M, et al: Prospective study of the association between sleep-disordered breathing and hypertension. *N Engl J Med* 342:1378-1384, 2000.

7. Leung RS, Bradley TD: Sleep apnea and cardiovascular disease. *Am J Respir Crit Care Med* 164:2147-2165, 2001.

Elevated Levels of C-Reactive Protein and Interleukin-6 in Patients With Obstructive Sleep Apnea Syndrome Are Decreased by Nasal Continuous Positive Airway Pressure

Yokoe T, Minoguchi K, Matsuo H, et al (Showa Univ, Tokyo; Toho Univ, Tokyo)
Circulation 107:1129-1134, 2003   48–6

Background.—Obstructive sleep apnea syndrome (OSAS) is associated with increased cardiovascular morbidity and mortality. Patients with OSAS have increased levels of C-reactive protein (CRP) and interleukin (IL)-6, which are important risk factors for atherosclerosis and coronary heart disease. Because treatment with nasal continuous positive airway pressure (nCPAP) decreases the risk of cardiovascular mortality in patients with severe OSAS, it may also inhibit atherosclerosis in these patients. The serum levels of CRP and IL-6 and the production of IL-6 by monocytes were examined in patients with OSAS and the effects of nCPAP on these levels were investigated.

Methods.—In the first part of the study, a group of 30 patients with OSAS and 14 obese control subjects underwent polysomnography, after which venous blood was collected at 5 AM. Serum levels of CRP and IL-6 and spontaneous production of IL-6 by monocytes were assayed. In the second part of the study, the effects of 1 month of nCPAP were studied in patients with moderate to severe OSAS. After 1 month of nCPAP therapy, polysomnography was repeated while the patient received nCPAP, and samples of venous blood were obtained. These samples were evaluated for levels of CRP and IL-6 and production of IL-6 by monocytes.

Results.—CRP and IL-6 levels were significantly higher in patients with OSAS than in obese control subjects. In the patients with OSAS, the primary factors affecting levels of CRP were the severity of OSAS and body mass index, while the primary factors influencing IL-6 levels were body mass index and nocturnal hypoxia. Treatment with nCPAP significantly decreased levels of both CRP and IL-6 as well as IL-6 production by monocytes.

Conclusion.—The levels of CRP and IL-6 and the spontaneous production of IL-6 by monocytes are elevated in patients with OSAS, but treatment with nCPAP lowers these levels. Because IL-6 and CRP are important risk factors for atherosclerosis and coronary artery disease, the use of nCPAP in patients with OSAS may reduce their risk for cardiovascular morbidity and mortality.

▶ This article presents more evidence that CPAP can reduce the cardiovascular risk of OSA. As more and more data demonstrate that OSA causes significant cardiovascular morbidity and mortality, and that treatment with CPAP can reduce this health burden, it is becoming increasingly difficult to justify the delays and cost of our current approach to OSA diagnosis. This is especially true since many of those with OSA can be diagnosed with simple clinical tools such as a history, physical examination, and/or questionnaires![1-8] As awareness grows, it is likely that careful clinical evaluation, home monitoring, and auto-titrating (or "smart") CPAP will improve access and patient convenience.

B. A. Phillips, MD, MSPH

References

1. Maislin G, Pack AI, Kribbs NB, et al: A survey screen for prediction of apnea. *Sleep* 18:158-166, 1995.
2. Crocker BD, Olson LG, Saunders NA, et al: Estimation of the probability of disturbed breathing during sleep before a sleep study. *Am Rev Respir Dis* 142:14-18, 1990.
3. Flemons WW, Whitelaw WA, Brant R, et al: Likelihood ratios for a sleep apnea clinical prediction rule. *Am J Respir Crit Care Med* 150:1279-1285, 1994.
4. Viner S, Szalai JP, Hoffstein V: Are history and physical examination a good screening test for sleep apnea? *Ann Intern Med* 115:356-359, 1991.
5. Rowley JA, Aboussouan LS, Badr S: The use of clinical prediction formulae in the evaluation of obstructive sleep apnea. *Sleep* 23:929-938, 2000.
6. Kushida CA, Efron B, Guilleminault C: A predictive morphometric model for the obstructive sleep apnea syndrome. *Ann Intern Med* 127:581-587, 1997.
7. Netzer NC, Stoohs RA, Netzer CM, et al: Using the Berlin Questionnaire to identify patients at risk for the sleep apnea syndrome. *Ann Intern Med* 131:485-491, 1999.
8. Mallampati SR, Gatt SP, Gugino LD, et al: A clinical sign to predict difficult tracheal intubation: A prospective study. *Can Anaesth Soc J* 32:429-434, 1985.

Effect of Nasal Continuous Positive Airway Pressure Treatment on Blood Pressure in Patients With Obstructive Sleep Apnea

Becker HF, Jerrentrup A, Ploch T, et al (Philipps-Univ, Marburg, Germany; Univ of Sydney, Australia)
Circulation 107:68-73, 2003   48–7

Background.—Increasing evidence suggests that obstructive sleep apnea (OSA) is an independent risk factor for arterial hypertension. However, no controlled studies have been done showing a marked effect of nasal continuous positive airway pressure (nCPAP) treatment on hypertension in OSA. Thus, the effects of treatment on cardiovascular sequelae have been questioned. The effect of nCPAP on arterial hypertension in patients with OSA was determined.

Methods.—The study included 60 consecutive patients with moderate to severe OSA. By random assignment, patients were given therapeutic or sub-therapeutic nCPAP for a mean of 9 weeks. Nocturnal polysomnography and continuous noninvasive blood pressure recording was performed for 19 hours before treatment and during treatment. Sixteen patients in each group completed treatment.

Findings.—In the therapeutic group, apneas and hypopneas were decreased by about 95%. In the subtherapeutic group, they were reduced by 50%. Effective nCPAP reduced mean arterial blood pressure by a mean of 9.9 mm Hg. Subtherapeutic nCPAP produced no relevant change. Mean blood pressure and diastolic and systolic blood pressures declined significantly by about 10 mm Hg during the day and night.

Conclusions.—Effective nCPAP therapy in patients with moderate to severe OSA results in a marked decrease in day and night arterial blood pressure. The 10-mm Hg decline in mean blood pressure is predicted to decrease risk of coronary heart disease events by 37% and risk of stroke by 56%.

▶ This study emphasizes that subtherapeutic CPAP does not lower blood pressure. It is also notable for the fact that only half the cohort actually completed the study and that blood pressure changes were seen within 9 weeks. Others[1,2] have reported falls in blood pressure with CPAP treatment, but the 10-mm Hg fall reported here is huge.

B. A. Phillips, MD, MSPH

References

1. Pepperell JCT, Ramdassingh-Dow S, Crosthwaite N, et al: Ambulatory blood pressure after therapeutic and subtherapeutic nasal continuous positive airway pressure for obstructive sleep apnoea: A randomised parallel trial. *Lancet* 359:204-214, 2002.
2. Kanedo Y, Floras JS, Usui K, et al: Cardiovascular effects of continuous positive airway pressure in patients with heart failure and obstructive sleep apnea. *N Engl J Med* 348:1233-1241, 2003.

Comparison Between Automatic and Fixed Positive Airway Pressure Therapy in the Home

Massie CA, McArdle N, Hart RW, et al (Suburban Lung Associates, Elk Grove Village, Ill; Univ of Western Australia, Perth; Sleep Medicine Associates of Texas, Dallas; et al)

Am J Respir Crit Care Med 167:20-23, 2003   48–8

Background.—Obstructive sleep apnea-hypopnea syndrome (OSAHS) can be effectively treated with continuous positive airway pressure (CPAP), which has been shown to reduce excessive daytime sleepiness and may also decrease the hypertension and vascular risk associated with OSAHS. However, the rates of CPAP use are suboptimal in both short- and long-term studies, averaging 3 to 5 hours per night. The use of CPAP may be limited by side effects such as pressure intolerance, difficulty in exhaling, mask dislodgment, mask leak, and air leak through the mouth. Changes in weight, body position, alcohol use, and nasal patency can alter patients' acute and chronic CPAP requirements. Whether objective CPAP use, quality of life, and daytime sleepiness can be improved by the use of an autotitrating CPAP device was assessed in patients with OSAHS who required higher CPAP (10 cm H_2O or greater).

Methods.—The multisite, randomized, single-blind crossover study included 44 patients with a mean age of 49 ± 10 years. The patients were randomly assigned to 6 weeks at laboratory-determined fixed pressure and 6 weeks on autotitrating CPAP.

Results.—The average nightly use of CPAP was greater in the automatic mode than in the fixed-pressure mode (306 vs 271 minutes), and the median and 95th centile pressures were lower in automatic mode. Automatic CPAP also provided better SF-36 Vitality scores (80 ± 14 vs 75 ± 18) and mental health scores. However, there was no significant difference in Epworth scores between the 2 groups. During automatic therapy, patients reported more restful sleep, better quality sleep, less discomfort from pressure, and less trouble getting to sleep in both the first week of therapy and in the averaged scores for weeks 2 through 6.

Conclusion.—This comparison between automatic and fixed CPAP in home-based treatment of OSAHS showed that patients with high fixed CPAP requirements utilize autotitrating CPAP more often and report greater benefit from this therapy.

▶ We will see more and more of these kinds of articles, both because of growing awareness of OSAHS and its consequences, and also because of an actual increase in the prevalence of sleep-disordered breathing. We simply cannot afford either the fiscal cost or the public health risk of requiring in-lab CPAP titrations for those who cannot be titrated during a "split night" (single night used both for diagnosis and treatment). In my experience and opinion, the "in lab CPAP titration" is a sacred cow, venerated and exalted by those who stand to gain from perpetuating it, eg, those with vested interest in sleep laboratories.

When you think about it, isn't it a little far fetched to think that a technician, even if he/she is a respiratory therapist (which most are not), can determine, in 4 to 8 hours, the magical CPAP pressure that will work for a given patient, in all situations, including drinking too much, supine sleeping, rapid eye movement rebound, having a cold, gaining or losing weight, or any combination of the above? Autotitrating CPAP, if the algorithm is good, can adjust for all these conditions. Based on this report, a "real life" in-home study, the algorithm of this device is good.

The most vexing issue confronting sleep clinicians is CPAP compliance.[1,2] At this point, only humidity and education have been shown to increase compliance. This article adds to the growing body of evidence that autotitrating CPAP is associated with lower overall pressures and increased compliance.[3-6] The authors also report better outcomes for some subjective measures that are commonly disregarded by physicians but of no small importance to patients, such as more restful sleep, less discomfort from pressure, and improved vitality.

B. A. Phillips, MD, MSPH

References

1. Janson C, Noges E, Svedberg-Brandt S, et al: What characterizes patients who are unable to tolerate continuous positive airway pressure (CPAP) treatment? *Respir Med* 94:145-149, 2000.
2. McArdle N, Devereux G, Heidarnejad H, et al: Long-term use of CPAP therapy for sleep apnea/hypopnea syndrome. *Am J Respir Crit Care Med* 159:1108-1114, 1999.
3. Fleury B, Rakotonanahary D, Hausser-Hauw C, et al: A laboratory validation study of the diagnostic mode of the Autoset system for sleep-related respiratory disorders. *Sleep* 19:497-501, 1996.
4. Sharma S, Wali S, Pouliot Z, et al: Treatment of obstructive sleep apnea with a self-titrating continuous positive airway pressure (CPAP) system. *Sleep* 19:497-501, 1996.
5. Stradling JR, Barbour C, Pitson DJ, et al: Automatic nasal continuous positive airway pressure in the laboratory: Patient outcomes. *Thorax* 52:72-75, 1997.
6. Randerath W, Schraeder O, Galetke W, et al: Autoadjusting CPAP therapy based on impedance efficacy, compliance and acceptance. *Am J Crit Care Med* 163:652-657, 2001.

PART SIX

HEART AND CARDIOVASCULAR DISEASE
WILLIAM H. FRISHMAN, MD

Introduction

The results of many outstanding basic science and clinical research studies were reported on last year that relate to the prevention, diagnosis, and treatment of cardiovascular disease. The articles selected for abstracting in this section of the 2004 YEAR BOOK OF MEDICINE were chosen from among the more than 5000 articles that were reviewed. Each selected abstract is followed by my editorial comments, and when appropriate, additional references are cited. Abstracted articles are provided that are relevant to the pathophysiology of cardiovascular disease and associated clinical situations.

The first chapter includes 6 selections related to cardiovascular disease risk factors and markers. The level of physical activity in the elderly is associated inversely with the risk of clinical cardiovascular disease, reinforcing similar observations made in middle-aged individuals. An elevated C-reactive protein level, a marker of possible vascular inflammation, is reduced by alcohol intake, explaining some of the benefit of mild to moderate alcohol intake in reducing the risk of coronary artery disease (CAD). Stress and depression are considered to be risk factors for CAD. Marital stress, but not work stress, predicts a worse prognosis for CAD in women. Cognitive behavior therapy to treat depression was not shown to affect morbidity or mortality in patients with CAD; however, patients did have relief of depressive symptoms with treatment. Cigarette smoking remains an important risk factor for CAD and appears to be associated with a higher prevalence of other risk factors and markers of active inflammation. Treatments to cause cessation of cigarette smoking are probably the best interventions for reducing cardiac disease risk. An elevation in low-density lipoprotein (LDL)-cholesterol is considered to be a risk factor for CAD, and the presence of smaller shaped LDL particles adds considerable additional risk. Pharmacologic approaches to reduce LDL-cholesterol while augmenting LDL particle size could be of great clinical benefit.

Acute coronary syndromes are discussed in the next chapter. Echocardiography is often done as part of an assessment during an acute myocardial infarction, and the presence of an enlarged left atrium implies a poor clinical prognosis. In patients with acute coronary syndromes, where there may also be "aspirin resistance," short- and long-term treatment with both aspirin and clopidogrel appears to provide greater benefit than aspirin use alone. In contrast, the use of antibiotic therapy has not shown benefit in reducing subsequent cardiovascular risk in survivors of a myocardial infarction, suggesting that active coronary disease may not relate to an infectious process. Aggressive reduction of LDL-cholesterol is associated with a reduced risk of morbidity and mortality in patients with CAD. Statin drugs appear to reduce LDL-cholesterol and associated serum markers of inflammation such as C-reactive protein. New markers of increased mortality risk for patients with unstable CAD include increased serum levels of soluble CD40 ligand, an elevated C-reactive protein, and an elevated white blood cell count. In patients with chest pain syndromes, an elevated troponin appears to be a superior marker of ischemic injury than isoenzyme of creatine phosphokinase (CPK-MB) values.

The next chapter discusses 4 articles related to chronic CAD. Again, elevations in C-reactive protein are associated with inducible ischemia in patients with chronic CAD, especially in those not receiving statins and beta blockers. Another disease marker for an increased risk of cardiovascular events in chronic CAD is a low level of red-cell glutathione peroxidase-1, which may be another therapeutic target similar to C-reactive protein. There is still an ongoing debate regarding the optimal treatment for stable symptomatic CAD: invasive versus optimal medical therapy. More studies are suggesting the greater benefits of optimal medical therapy, especially in older subjects.

Specific endothelial growth factors are being evaluated in patients with CAD and peripheral vascular disease as a means to augment angiogenesis. Most of the reported studies have shown equivocal clinical benefit with those interventions compared with placebo.

Highlighted in the next chapter are the major advances in the interventional management of CAD. Vascular brachytherapy (endoluminal radiotherapy) at the time of coronary restenting reduces the risk of recurrent restenosis and appears to improve subsequent clinical outcomes. However, with drug-eluting stents containing either sirolimus or paclitaxel, the rate of restenosis may be significantly reduced from the time of the initial intervention. Elevations in C-reactive protein in patients undergoing stenting are associated with a less favorable prognosis after coronary stenting. Perhaps with aggressive risk factor control this increased risk can be attenuated.

There have always been questions concerning a gender bias, a racial bias, or a socioeconomic bias regarding the access to appropriate cardiovascular care. Race and socioeconomic factors appear to unfavorably affect the likelihood of revascularization after myocardial infarction in New York City and may pose a problem nationwide.

An innovative experimental approach under evaluation for treating myocardial ischemia is the intramyocardial transplantation of autologous endothelial cells to achieve neovascularization. A possible application of this technology is the use of intramyocardial cell therapy with coronary bypass surgery in cardiac regions where surgical revascularization is not possible.

There have been many advances in the therapy of acute and chronic congestive heart failure. Hemodilution is common in patients with advanced heart failure, highlighting the need to have diuretics as a cornerstone of therapy. Eplerenone, a selective aldosterone inhibitor, was shown to be of benefit in patients with left ventricular dysfunction. Aldosterone inhibition, as well as loop diuretics, angiotensin-converting enzyme inhibitors, and beta blockers, has become the standard treatment for symptomatic systolic ventricular failure. Eplerenone was recently approved for clinical use in hypertension and heart failure.

Other innovative treatments for symptomatic heart failure include the use of biventricular cardiac pacing in patients having a wide ECG QRS interval.

In addition, continuous positive pressure therapy has been shown to be of benefit in patients with heart failure and obstructive sleep apnea.

Heart transplantation and permanent left ventricular assist devices are available for only a small percentage of patients with advanced heart failure. Of growing interest is the use of cell therapy by means of injections of autologous bone marrow cells or cardiac stem cells to regenerate the heart. Clinical studies are now in place that use this innovative approach.

Valvular heart disease and its clinical complications remain major problems in cardiovascular medicine. In patients with complicated native valve left-sided valvular endocarditis, a risk stratification scheme can be used to determine prognostic severity. There is more evidence to show that percutaneous balloon angioplasty can be a viable alternative to open mitral valve commissurotomy in patients having mitral stenosis with pliable valves. The results of repeat percutaneous valvuloplasty to treat postcommissurotomy restenosis also appear to be favorable. In symptomatic patients with significant valvular aortic stenosis, an intraoperative approach was considered to be the only treatment for improving outcomes. However, IV nitroprusside has been shown to bring about a rapid improvement in symptoms in some patients with aortic stenosis, raising the possibility of long-term oral vasodilator therapy as an alternative to surgery.

The next chapter presents 4 articles that describe advances in nonoperative cardiac diagnosis. Intravascular ultrasound (IVUS) appears to be a useful technology for qualitatively evaluating atherosclerotic plaques in patients with CAD, which a routine coronary angiogram cannot do. The data derived from IVUS may help in therapeutic decision-making. MRI is a noninvasive technique for quantitatively evaluating the presence and extent of CAD and can differentiate between ischemic and nonischemic cardiomyopathy.

Electron beam tomography is a technique for establishing the presence of CAD and may be of use in predicting future cardiovascular events, in addition to standard cardiovascular risk factors.

In addition to echocardiography, tissue Doppler imaging can help to identify asymptomatic individuals at risk of clinically significant hypertrophic cardiomyopathy. There is preliminary evidence that early treatment with angiotensin II receptor blockers and/or calcium channel blockers may reverse the disease process in asymptomatic individuals.

There have been many advances in the diagnosis and treatment of various cardiac arrhythmias. Frequent ventricular ectopy during recovery after exercise was found to be a better predictor of an increased risk of sudden death than ectopy occurring during exercise. The finding of postexercise ventricular ectopy should lead to additional diagnostic testing and treatment interventions.

Pacemakers were thought to be of use in patients having frequent vasovagal syncope (common faint) episodes. However, a clinical trial revealed little to no benefit from this intervention. Survivors of out-of-hospital cardiac arrest and defibrillation have excellent long-term prognoses, similar to that of disease-matched patients who have not had a cardiac arrest. Patients with heart failure who have atrial fibrillation have a worse prognosis than those patients without the arrhythmia. These atrial fibrillation patients should undergo anticoagulation if it can be tolerated.

Patients with long QT interval syndrome have varying clinical courses depending on their genetic type, which could influence subsequent treatment approaches.

In the last chapter, studies on various topics are presented. Cilostazol, a selective type III phosphodiesterase inhibitor, has been shown to be the most effective agent for improving exercise tolerance in patients with intermittent claudication.

The course of carcinoid heart disease is influenced by whether patients with metastatic disease receive cancer chemotherapy or not. There appears to be no treatment for preventing cardiac involvement related to metastatic carcinoid tumors of the liver.

Early repolarization detected on the ECG is a benign condition, often seen in young black subjects; however, it is commonly confused with the ECG abnormalities seen with pericarditis, hyperkalemia, hypothermia, and myocardial ischemia.

Patients with cocaine-induced chest pain may or may not have myocardial ischemia as the cause. Patients with no recurrent symptoms nor evidence of myocardial ischemia can be safely discharged after 4-12 hours of observation.

An association has been observed between atherosclerotic disease and peripheral venous thrombosis. Atherosclerosis may be a cause of venous thrombosis.

William H. Frishman, MD

49 Risk Factors

Relative Intensity of Physical Activity and Risk of Coronary Heart Disease
Lee I-M, Sesso HD, Oguma Y, et al (Harvard School of Public Health, Boston;
Harvard Med School, Boston; Keio Univ, Yokohama, Japan; et al)
Circulation 107:1110-1116, 2003   49–1

Introduction.—Physical activity is linked to a reduced risk of chronic disease. There is controversy concerning the intensity of activity needed for reduced risk. A limitation when determining activity intensity on an absolute scale is that a particular activity may require different relative efforts among persons depending on their fitness levels. It may be that when one is prescribing physical activity, a relative scale to gauge intensity is more appropriate than an absolute scale. There are no published data that examine the relationship between relative intensity of physical activity and the risk of development of chronic diseases. This question was investigated for coronary heart disease (CHD) in the ongoing Harvard Alumni Health Study.

Methods.—The study evaluated 7337 men (mean age, 66 years) who completed a questionnaire in 1988. Participants reported actual activities and used the Borg Scale to note their perceived level of exertion when exercising (relative intensity).

Results.—During a mean follow-up of 5.3 years, 551 participants developed CHD. After multivariate adjustments, the relative risks of CHD among men who perceived their exercise exertion as "moderate," "somewhat strong," and "strong" or more intense were 0.86 (95% confidence interval, 0.66-1.13), 0.69 (0.51-0.94), and 0.72 (0.52-1.00), respectively (P_{trend} = .02), compared with those who rated their exertion as "weak" or less intense. This inverse relationship extended to men not fulfilling current recommendations (expending less than 4.2 MJ/wk in physical activity or not engaging in activities of 3 metabolic equivalents or more [P_{trend} = .03 and .007, respectively]).

Conclusion.—There is an inverse correlation between relative intensity of physical activity (an individual's perceived level of exertion) and risk of CHD, even among men who are not satisfying current activity recommendations. Recommendations for "moderate" intensity physical activity may need to consider individual fitness levels rather than globally prescribing activities at fixed metabolic equivalent intensities.

▶ Physical activity is associated with a decreased risk of CHD and its complications.[1] In older individuals, there is an inverse relationship between the relative intensity of physical activity and the risk of developing CHD, even among those not satisfying current recommendations for physical activity. Other lifestyle measures showing benefit in the elderly include an increased consumption of dietary cereal fiber.[2]

W. H. Frishman, MD

References

1. NIH Consensus Development Panel on Physical Activity and Cardiovascular Health: Physical activity and cardiovascular health. *JAMA* 276:241-246, 1996.
2. Mozaffarian D, Kumanyika SK, Lemaitre RN, et al: Cereal, fruit, and vegetable fiber intake and the risk of cardiovascular disease in elderly individuals. *JAMA* 289:1659-1666, 2003.

Alcohol Consumption and Plasma Concentration of C-Reactive Protein
Albert MA, Glynn RJ, Ridker PM (Harvard Med School, Boston)
Circulation 107:443-447, 2003   49–2

Background.—Moderate alcohol consumption has been correlated with a lower mortality rate from cardiovascular causes. However, the relationship between C-reactive protein (CRP), which predicts cardiovascular risk, and alcohol intake is not clear. This association was assessed in a cross-sectional survey and over time.

Methods.—Data were obtained from 1732 men and 1101 women participating in the Pravastatin Inflammation/CRP Evaluation Study. Participants were placed into 5 categories on the basis of levels of alcohol intake: no alcohol or less than 1 drink per month, 1 to 3 drinks per month, 1 to 4 drinks weekly, 5 to 7 drinks weekly, and 2 or more drinks daily.

Findings.—The median CRP levels in the 5 categories, from lowest to highest alcohol intake, were 2.6, 2.2, 1.7, 1.6, and 1.8 mg/L, respectively. This association was observed among men, women not receiving hormone replacement therapy, nonsmokers, and persons with and without a history of cardiovascular disease. The association between alcohol intake and CRP remained significant even after adjustment for traditional cardiovascular risk factors in a multivariate analysis. Alcohol intake had no significant effect on the changes in CRP or lipid concentrations related to statin use.

Conclusions.—Moderate alcohol intake correlated with decreased CRP levels compared with no or occasional alcohol consumption. This effect was independent of alcohol-related effects on lipids. Drinking alcohol may attenuate cardiovascular mortality partly through an anti-inflammatory mechanism.

▶ Alcohol consumption in moderation has shown benefit both in men and women for reducing the risk of coronary artery disease (CAD).[1] The mechanism of this benefit has not been explained; however, there is now evidence of an anti-inflammatory action with reduced CRP levels.

It has also been suggested that statins may have an anti-inflammatory action as part of its benefit. High-risk patients suitable for statin therapy can be identified by increased CRP levels even when cholesterol values are normal.[2,3] In addition to CRP, a high erythrocyte sedimentation rate can identify high-risk CAD.[4]

W. H. Frishman, MD

References

1. Frishman WH, Del Vecchio A, Sanal S, et al: Cardiovascular manifestations of substance abuse: II. Alcohol, amphetamines, heroin, cannabis, and caffeine. *Heart Dis* 5:253-271, 2003.
2. Blake GJ, Ridker PM, Kuntz SM: Potential cost-effectiveness of C-reactive protein screening followed by targeted statin therapy for the primary prevention of cardiovascular disease among patients without overt hyperlipidemia. *Am J Med* 114:485-494, 2003.
3. Takano M, Mizuno K, Yokoyama S, et al: Changes in coronary plaque color and morphology by lipid-lowering therapy with atorvastatin: Serial evaluation by coronary angioscopy. *J Am Coll Cardiol* 42:680-686, 2003.
4. Natali A, L'Abbate A, Ferrannini E: Erythrocyte sedimentation rate, coronary atherosclerosis, and cardiac mortality. *Eur Heart J* 24:639-648, 2003.

Effects of Treating Depression and Low Perceived Social Support on Clinical Events After Myocardial Infarction: The Enhancing Recovery in Coronary Heart Disease Patients (ENRICHD) Randomized Trial
Berkman LF, for the ENRICHD Investigators (Harvard Univ, Boston; et al)
JAMA 289:3106-3116, 2003   49–3

Background.—The prevalence of major depression among patients with coronary heart disease is almost 20%, and the prevalence of minor depression is about 27%. In patients who experience a myocardial infarction (MI), depression is a risk factor for mortality independent of the severity of the cardiac disease. There is some evidence that the antidepressant sertraline hydrochloride may be effective in treating recurrent depression in patients with either an acute MI or an episode of unstable angina. However, no clinical trial has determined whether treatment of depression with counseling or antidepressants after an acute MI improves survival or reduces cardiac risk.

Another risk factor for cardiac morbidity and mortality in patients with coronary heart disease is the absence of social support. Whether mortality and recurrent infarction are reduced by treatment of depression and low perceived social support (LPSS) with cognitive behavior therapy (CBT), supplemented by a selective serotonin reuptake inhibitor antidepressant when indicated, was determined.

Methods.—This randomized clinical trial enrolled 2481 MI patients from 8 centers; all the patients were enrolled within 28 days of their MI. The presence of major or minor depression was diagnosed by modified criteria from the *Diagnostic and Statistical Manual of Mental Disorders*, 4th Edition, and the severity by the 17-item Hamilton Rating Scale for Depression (HRSD).

LPSS was determined by the Enhancing Recovery in Coronary Heart Disease Patients (ENRICHD) Social Support Instrument (ESSI). The patients were randomly assigned to either usual medical care or CBT-based psychosocial intervention. CBT was initiated at a median of 17 days after the index MI, for a median of 11 individual sessions throughout 6 months, along with group therapy when feasible, with administration of selective serotonin reuptake inhibitors to patients scoring higher than 24 on the HRSD or having a less than 50% reduction in Beck Depression Inventory scores after 5 weeks. The main outcome measures were the composite primary end point of death or recurrent MI; secondary outcomes included a change in HRSD (for depression) or ESSI scores (for LPSS) at 6 months.

Results.—Treatment with CBT-based psychosocial intervention was associated with greater improvement in psychosocial outcomes at 6 months. At an average of 29 months of follow-up, there was no significant difference in event-free survival between usual care (75.9%) and psychosocial intervention (75.8%). Nor were there differences in survival between the psychosocial intervention and usual-care arms in any of the 3 psychosocial risk groups—depression, LPSS, and depression and LPSS patients.

Conclusion.—This intervention for depression after MI did not increase event-free survival. The CBT intervention improved depression and social isolation in these patients, but the relative improvement in the psychosocial intervention group versus the usual-care group was not as great as expected because of substantial improvement in the patients who received usual care.

▶ There is mounting evidence that psychiatric depression is an independent risk factor for morbidity and mortality[1-7] in patients with coronary artery disease. Different mechanisms have been proposed for this increased risk, including an increased level of platelet aggregation and a pro-inflammatory state.[8,9]

CBT does not appear to affect the event-free survival rate. Anti-depressant medications do appear safe to use in patients who have survived an MI, but there is no definitive evidence as yet that they affect the rate of subsequent cardiovascular events. However, the antidepressant drugs and/or psychotherapy favorably affect mood and should not be avoided in depressed patients who have survived an MI or in those individuals at risk for a first cardiovascular event.

W. H. Frishman, MD

References

1. Feinstein RE: Cardiovascular effects of novel antipsychotic medications. *Heart Dis* 4:184-190, 2002.
2. Glassman AH, O'Connor CM, Califf RM, et al: Sertraline treatment of major depression in patients with acute MI or unstable angina. *JAMA* 288:701-709, 2002.
3. Ruo B, Rumsfeld JS, Hlatky MA, et al: Depressive symptoms and health-related quality of life. *JAMA* 290:215-221, 2003.
4. Frasure-Smith N, Lesperance F: Depression and other psychological risks following myocardial infarction. *Arch Gen Psych* 60:627-636, 2003.

5. Blumenthal JA, for the NORG Investigators: Depression as a risk factor for mortality after coronary artery bypass surgery. *Lancet* 362:604-609, 2003.
6. Frasure-Smith N, Lesperance F: Depression—A cardiac risk factor in search of a treatment (editorial). *JAMA* 289:3171-3172, 2003.
7. Jiang W, Babyak MA, Rozanski A, et al: Depression and increased myocardial ischemic activity in patients with ischemic heart disease. *Am Heart J* 146:55-61, 2003.
8. Laghrissi-Thode F, Wagner WR, Pollock BG, et al: Elevated platelet factor 4 and beta-thromboglobulin plasma levels in depressed patients with ischemic heart disease. *Biol Psychiatry* 42:290-295, 1997.
9. Miller GE, Stetler CA, Carney RM, et al: Clinical depression and inflammatory risk markers for coronary heart disease. *Am J Cardiol* 90:1279-1283, 2002.

Relationship Between Cigarette Smoking and Novel Risk Factors for Cardiovascular Disease in the United States

Bazzano LA, He J, Muntner P, et al (Tulane Univ, New Orleans, La; Natl Inst of Environmental Health Sciences, Research Triangle Park, NC)

Ann Intern Med 138:891-897, 2003   49–4

Background.—The relationship between cigarette smoking and novel risk factors for cardiovascular disease in a general population has not been well studied. Few studies have included a biochemical marker of current smoking. The association between smoking and serum C-reactive protein (CRP), fibrinogen, and homocysteine concentrations was investigated.

Methods.—A cross-sectional study was done that included 4187 current smokers, 4791 former smokers, and 8375 "never smokers," 18 years and older. All had been participants in the Third National Health and Nutrition Examination Survey performed between 1988 and 1994.

Findings.—Smoking was associated with increased concentrations of CRP, fibrinogen, and homocysteine, after adjustment for traditional cardiovascular disease. Current smoking, compared with never smoking, correlated with CRP levels in the detectable or clinically increased ranges. Increased fibrinogen and homocysteine levels were also associated with current smoking. Positive, significant dose-response relationships were documented between measures of cigarette smoking and increased levels of novel risk factors.

Conclusions.—Cigarette smoking is strongly, positively, and independently associated with increased CRP levels in a dose-response relationship. Smoking is also strongly associated with increased fibrinogen and homocysteine concentrations. Therefore, inflammation and hyperhomocysteinemia may be important mechanisms by which smoking promotes atherosclerotic disease.

▶ Novel risk factors associated with the development of cardiovascular disease continue to be identified.[1] These factors include hyperhomocysteinemia,[2] inflammation,[3] increased levels of various clotting factors[4] and adhesion molecules,[5] increased levels of osteoprotegerin[6] and various matrix metalloproteinases,[7,8] and deficiencies in matrix metalloproteinase inhibitors[9] and thyroid functioning.[10] There also appear to be significant interactions between traditional risk factors for coronary artery disease, such as cigarette smoking, and the newly described factors, such as hyperhomocysteinemia and inflammation.[11,12] These interactions may explain how traditional risk factors accelerate the atherosclerotic process.

W. H. Frishman, MD

References

1. Hackam DG: Emerging risk factors for atherosclerotic vascular disease. A critical review of the evidence. *JAMA* 290:932-940, 2003.
2. Frishman WH, Retter A, Misailidis J, et al: Innovative pharmacologic approaches to the treatment of myocardial ischemia, in Frishman WH, Sonnenblick EH, Sica DA (eds): *Cardiovascular Pharmacotherapeutics*, ed 2. New York, McGraw Hill, 2003, pp 655-690.
3. Kaplan RC, Frishman WH: Systemic inflammation as a cardiovascular disease risk factor and as a potential target for drug therapy. *Heart Dis* 3:326, 2001.
4. Wu KK, Aleksic N, Ballantyne CM, et al: Interaction between soluble thrombomodulin and intercellular adhesion molecule-1 in predicting risk of coronary heart disease. *Circulation* 107:1729-1732, 2003.
5. Frishman WH, Retter A, Mobati D, et al: Innovative drug targets for treating cardiovascular disease: Adhesion molecules, cytokines, neuropeptide Y, calcineurin, bradykinin, urotensin, and heat shock protein, in Frishman WH, Sonnenblick EH, Sica DA (eds): *Cardiovascular Pharmacotherapeutics*, ed 2. New York, McGraw Hill, 2003, pp 705-739.
6. Schoppet M, Sattler AM, Schaefer JR, et al: Increased osteoprotegerin serum levels in men with coronary artery disease. *J Clin Endocrinol Metab* 88:1024-1028, 2003.
7. Blankenberg S, Rupprecht HJ, Poirier O, et al: Plasma concentrations and genetic variation of matrix metalloproteinase 9 and prognosis of patients with cardiovascular disease. *Circulation* 107:1579-1585, 2003.
8. Smeglin A, Frishman WH: Elastinolytic matrix metalloproteinases and their inhibitors as therapeutic targets in atherosclerotic plaque instability. *Cardiol Rev* 12:141-150, 2004.
9. Frishman WH, Ahangar BA, Sinha S: Matrix metalloproteinases and their inhibitors in cardiovascular disease, in Frishman WH, Sonnenblick EH, Sica DA (eds): *Cardiovascular Pharmacotherapeutics*, ed 2. New York, McGraw Hill, 2003, pp 797-811.
10. Iervasi G, Pingitore A, Landi P, et al: Low-T3 syndrome. A strong prognostic predictor of death in patients with heart disease. *Circulation* 107:708-713, 2003.
11. Sano T, Tanaka A, Namba M, et al: C-reactive protein and lesion morphology in patients with acute myocardial infarction. *Circulation* 108: 282-285, 2003.
12. Dibra A, Mehilli J, Braun S, et al: Association between C-reactive protein levels and subsequent cardiac events among patients with stable angina treated with coronary artery stenting. *Am J Med* 114:715-722, 2003.

Marital Stress Worsens Prognosis in Women With Coronary Heart Disease: The Stockholm Female Coronary Risk Study

Orth-Gomér K, Wamala SP, Horsten M, et al (Karolinska Institutet, Stockholm; Univ of Miami, Fla; Harvard School of Public Health, Boston)
JAMA 284:3008-3014, 2000   49–5

Introduction.—Psychosocial stress has been linked with coronary heart disease (CHD) in men. The prognostic impact of psychosocial stress has rarely been examined in women. The prognostic impact of psychosocial work stress and marital stress was examined in a population-based, prospective follow-up investigation.

Methods.—Two hundred seventy-nine of 292 consecutive women who were working or cohabitating with a male partner and who were hospitalized for acute myocardial infarction or unstable angina pectoris between February 1991 and February 1993 were evaluated. All women between the ages of 30 and 65 years were enrolled. Patients were followed up from the date of clinical examination to August 1997 (median, 4.8 years). Patients were followed up for recurrent coronary events, including cardiac death, acute myocardial infarction, and revascularization procedures. They were categorized by marital status with use of the Stockholm Marital Stress Scale and by work stress with use of the ratio of work demand to work control.

Results.—In 187 women who were married or cohabitating with a male partner, marital stress was correlated with a 2.9-fold increased risk (95% confidence interval, 1.3-6.5) of recurrent events after adjusting for age, estrogen status, educational level, smoking, diagnosis at the index event, diabetes mellitus, systolic blood pressure, triglyceride level, high-density lipoprotein cholesterol level, and left ventricular ejection dysfunction. Work stress among 200 women who worked did not significantly predict recurrent coronary events (hazard ratio, 1.6; 95% confidence interval, 0.8-3.3).

Conclusion.—Marital stress, not work stress, predicted a poor prognosis in women aged 30 to 65 years with CHD. These findings differ from those in male populations and indicate that specific preventive measures need to be tailored to the needs of women with CHD.

▶ Women appear to be at the same risk for developing clinical CHD, albeit at a later time. Marital stress, the stress of child rearing and pregnancy,[1] peripheral adiposity,[2] the presence of polycystic ovary syndrome,[3] and the effects of premenopausal oopherectomy[4] provide additional factors contributing to the risk of CHD in women. Work stress does not appear to be a risk factor in women. Women benefit from interventions that address traditional risk factors for CHD, such as cigarette smoking and hypercholesterolemia. Studies need to be done to demonstrate a benefit from addressing these newly identified factors.

W. H. Frishman, MD

References

1. Lawlor DA, Emberson JR, Ebrahim S, et al: Is the association between parity and coronary heart disease due to biological effects of pregnancy or adverse lifestyle risk factors associated with child-rearing? Findings from the British Women's Heart and Health Study and the British Regional Heart Study. *Circulation* 107:1260-1264, 2003.
2. Tankó LB, Bagger YZ, Alexandersen P, et al: Peripheral adiposity exhibits an independent dominant antiatherogenic effect in elderly women. *Circulation* 107:1626-1631, 2003.
3. Christian RC, Dumesic DA, Behrenbeck T, et al: Prevalence and predictors of coronary artery calcification in women with polycystic ovary syndrome. *J Clin Endocrinol Metab* 88:2562-2568, 2003.
4. Hsia J, Barad D, Margolis K, et al: Usefulness of prior hysterectomy as an independent predictor of Framingham Risk Score (The Women's Health Initiative). *Am J Cardiol* 92:264-269, 2003.

Relationships Between Low-Density Lipoprotein Particle Size, Plasma Lipoproteins, and Progression of Coronary Artery Disease: The Diabetes Atherosclerosis Intervention Study (DAIS)

Vakkilainen J, for the DAIS Group (Helsinki Univ; et al)
Circulation 107:1733-1737, 2003   49–6

Introduction.—The risk of cardiovascular morbidity and mortality is significantly higher in persons with diabetes, compared with those who do not have that disease. The Diabetes Atherosclerosis Intervention Study (DAIS) reported that fenofibrate treatment is linked with significantly less progression of focal coronary artery disease (CAD) (40% less progression of minimal lumen diameter vs placebo, $P = .029$; 42% less progression in percentage diameter stenosis vs placebo, $P = .02$) and an improved plasma lipid profile in persons with type 2 diabetes.

Fenofibrate produces a shift toward larger, more buoyant low-density lipoprotein (LDL) particles, which is a potentially antiatherogenic change. A total of 418 patients with type 2 diabetes were evaluated to determine whether changes in LDL particle size may contribute to the favorable effect of fenofibrate on CAD progression in DAIS participants.

Methods.—Participants were randomly assigned to treatment with either 200 mg micronized fenofibrate daily or placebo. The mean follow-up was 39.6 months. The LDL peak particle diameter (LDL size) was ascertained by means of polyacrylamide gradient gel electrophoresis in 405 participants at baseline and at trial completion. The progression of CAD was determined by quantitative coronary angiography. The LDL size increased significantly more in the fenofibrate versus the placebo group (0.98 nm vs 0.32 nm; $P < .0010$).

In the combined group, small LDL size was significantly correlated with progression of CAD measured as the increase in percentage diameter stenosis ($r = -0.16$; $P = .002$) and reductions in minimum ($r = -0.11$; $P = .030$) and mean ($r = -0.10$; $P = .045$) lumen diameter. High on-treatment LDL cholesterol, apolipoprotein B, and triglyceride concentrations were also linked with progression of CAD. In regression analyses, small LDL size added to the effect of LDL cholesterol and apolipoprotein B added to the progression of CAD. Similar correlations were seen in the fenofibrate group. In the placebo group, lipoprotein variables were not significantly associated with the progression of CAD.

Conclusion.—Changes in LDL size and plasma lipid level are responsible for part of the antiatherogenic effect of fenofibrate in patients with type 2 diabetes.

▶ Interventions that reduce total cholesterol and LDL cholesterol have been shown to reduce the risk of cardiovascular disease and stroke.[1,2] The presence of smaller shaped LDL particles has also been shown to be a risk factor, even when the total LDL concentration is normal. Interventions that can reduce the numbers of small LDL particles may be contributing to an anti-atherosclerotic benefit.

The newest cholesterol-lowering drug to become available is ezetimibe, which is best used with the statins in a combination regimen.[3] A niacin-statin combination is also available.[1] Statins remain the drugs of choice for the treatment of hypercholesterolemia, and multiple mechanisms have now been elucidated to explain their benefit in causing atherosclerotic plaque stabilization,[4] including favorable effects on nitrotyrosine levels[5] and inflammation.[1] Raising high-density lipoprotein cholesterol and reducing triglyceride levels also have important risk reducing effects.[6,7]

W. H. Frishman, MD

References

1. Shachter NS, Zimetbaum P, Frishman WH: Lipid-lowering drugs, in Frishman WH, Sonnenblick EH, Sica DA (eds): *Cardiovascular Pharmacotherapeutics*, ed 2. New York, McGraw Hill, 2003, pp 317-353.
2. Chien PC, Frishman WH: Lipid disorders, in Crawford MH (ed): *Current Diagnosis & Treatment in Cardiology*, ed 2. New York, Lange Medical Books/McGraw Hill, 2002, pp15-30.
3. Kerzner B, Corbelli J, Sharp S, et al: Efficacy and safety of ezetimibe coadministered with lovastatin in primary hypercholesterolemia. *Am J Cardiol* 91:418-424, 2003.
4. Libby P, Aikawa M: Mechanisms of plaque stabilization with statins. *Am J Cardiol* 91(suppl): 4B-8B, 2003.
5. Shishehbor MH, Aviles RJ, Brennan M-L, et al: Association of nitrotyrosine levels with cardiovascular disease and modulation by statin therapy. *JAMA* 289:1675-1680, 2003.
6. Sowers JR: Effects of statins on the vasculature: Implications for aggressive lipid management in the cardiovascular metabolic syndrome. *Am J Cardiol* 91(suppl):14B-22B, 2003.
7. Sprecher DL, Wakins TR, Behar S, et al: Importance of high-density lipoprotein cholesterol and triglyceride levels in coronary heart disease. *Am J Cardiol* 91:575-580, 2003.

50 Acute Coronary Syndromes

Left Atrial Volume: A Powerful Predictor of Survival After Acute Myocardial Infarction

Møller JE, Hillis GS, Oh JK, et al (Mayo Clinic, Rochester, Minn)

Circulation 107:2207-2212, 2003

50–1

Introduction.—Several Doppler echocardiographic variables may be used to evaluate left ventricular (LV) diastolic function. During ventricular diastole, the left atrium is directly exposed to LV pressures via the open mitral valve. The left atrium size is thus largely determined by the same factors that impact diastolic LV filling. Left atrial (LA) filling is a more stable indicator and reflects the duration and severity of diastolic function. Patients who had a comprehensive evaluation of LV systolic and diastolic function, including assessment of LA volume early after acute myocardial infarction (AMI), were evaluated retrospectively to determine if LA volume would predict long-term outcome after AMI.

Methods.—Between October 1999 and July 2001, 314 unselected patients with AMI who had a transthoracic echocardiogram with assessment of LV systolic and diastolic function and measurement of LA volume during admission were identified. The LA volume was corrected for body surface area and the cohort was divided according to a LA volume index of 32 mL/m^2 (2 standard deviations above normal). The main end point was all-cause mortality.

Results.—The median patient age was 70 years (range, 32-94 years). The LA volume index was higher than 32 mL/m^2 in 142 patients (45%). Compared with patients with a LA volume index of 32 mL^2 or below, these patients were older; had a greater prevalence of hypertension, diabetes, and previous revascularization; initially had more frequent non-ST elevation AMI; and were less likely to undergo percutaneous coronary intervention. Forty-six patients (15%) died during a median follow-up of 15 months (range, 0-33 months). The LA volume index was a powerful predictor of mortality (Fig 1) and continued to be an independent predictor (hazard ratio, 1.05 per 1-mL/m^2 change; 95% confidence interval, 1.03-1.06; $P < .001$) after adjustment for clinical characteristics, LV systolic function, and Doppler-derived parameters of diastolic function.

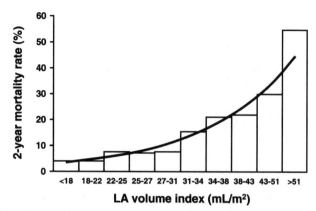

FIGURE 1.—Unadjusted 2-year mortality rates in 10 equal groups of patients according to left atrial (*LA*) volume index. Increase in mortality with increasing LA volume appeared exponential (*solid line*). (Courtesy of Møller JE, Hillis GS, Oh JK, et al: Left atrial volume: A powerful predictor of survival after acute myocardial infarction. *Circulation* 107:2207-2212, 2003.)

Conclusion.—LA enlargement indicates a poor prognosis in patients with AMI. Measurement of LA volume may become a simple and important tool for risk stratification and be useful for future surveillance and therapy in patients with AMI.

▶ LA enlargement assessed by Doppler echocardiography implies a poor clinical prognosis in patients with AMI. An increase in LA volume index appears to provide prognostic information incremental to other indexes of risk, which include while blood cell counts, B-type natriuretic peptide levels,[1] plasminogen activator inhibitor–1 studies,[2] cardiac enzyme studies, ECG indexes,[3] and measurements of LV systolic function.

W. H. Frishman, MD

References

1. Richards AM, Nicholls G, Espiner EA, et al: B-type natriuretic peptides and ejection fraction for prognosis after myocardial infarction. *Circulation* 107:2786-2792, 2003.
2. Collet JP, Montalescot G, Vicaut E, et al: Acute release of plasminogen activator inhibitor-1 in ST-segment elevation myocardial infarction predicts mortality. *Circulation* 108:391-394, 2003.
3. Rathore SS, Weinfurt KP, Gross CP, et al: Validity of a simple ST-elevation acute myocardial risk index. Are randomized trial prognostic estimates generalizable to elderly patients? *Circulation* 107:811-816, 2003.

Early and Late Effects of Clopidogrel in Patients With Acute Coronary Syndromes

Yusuf S, for the CURE (Clopidogrel in Unstable angina to prevent Recurrent Events) Trial Investigators (McMaster Univ, Hamilton, Ont, Canada; et al)
Circulation 107:966-972, 2003   50–2

Introduction.—Unstable angina and non–ST-elevation myocardial infarction are usually considered acute coronary syndromes (ACSs). These conditions place patients at high risk of death, myocardial infarction, or stroke both early in the hospital phase and also late during the subsequent months and years. Strategies to prevent these early and late events are needed.

The Clopidogrel in Unstable angina to prevent Recurrent Events (CURE) Trial reported the benefits of clopidogrel when added to standard therapy that includes aspirin for patients with an ACS. Treatment was started within 24 hours of symptom onset and was continued for up to 1 year. The rapidity with which treatment was effective and its sustainability over 1 year was examined, along with the rates of bleeding over the same periods.

Findings.—A total of 12,562 patients with ACS were randomly assigned to receive clopidogrel (300 mg initially followed by 75 mg/d) or placebo for 3 to 12 months. The proportion of patients who experienced cardiovascular death, myocardial infarction, or stroke (primary outcome) at 30 days was 5.4% for placebo and 4.3% for the active group (relative risk, 0.79; 95% confidence interval, 0.67-0.92) (Fig 1). There was no significant excess in life-threatening bleeds in each period (0.75% vs 1.28%; relative risk, 1.09; 95% confidence interval, 0.75-1.59 for 31 days to 12 months). Further subdivision of the early data suggests benefits within 24 hours with consistently lower rates of the primary outcome in combination with refractory or severe ischemia.

Conclusion.—Clopidogrel diminishes the risk of ischemic vascular events; benefits emerge within 24 hours of initiation of treatment and continue throughout the 12 months (mean, 9 months) of the trial.

▶ Innovative anticoagulation strategies have been developed for managing patients with unstable coronary syndromes which include various antiplatelet agents, low molecular weight heparins, and direct thrombin inhibitors.[1-4] There is growing evidence that at least 2 antiplatelet drugs are needed to maximize cardioprotection, both during and up to 1 year after an ACS. Part of this approach may relate to the well-documented occurrence of "aspirin resistance" in a significant number of individuals at risk.

W. H. Frishman, MD

References

1. Frishman WH, Lerner RG, Klein MD, et al: Antiplatelet and antithrombotic drugs, in Frishman WH, Sonnenblick EH, Sica DA (eds): *Cardiovascular Pharmacotherapeutics*, ed 2. New York: McGraw Hill 2003, pp 259-298.

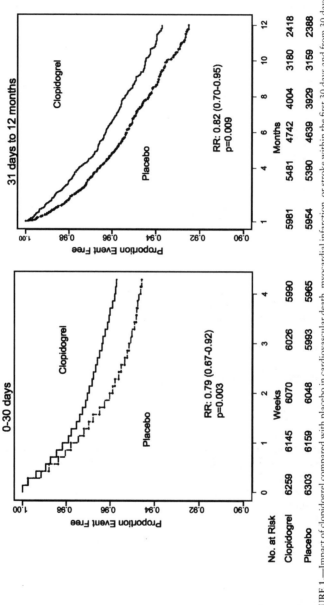

FIGURE 1.—Impact of clopidogrel compared with placebo in cardiovascular death, myocardial infarction, or stroke within the first 30 days and from 30 days to 12 months. *Abbreviation: RR*, Relative risk. (Courtesy of Yusuf S, for the CURE [Clopidogrel in Unstable angina to prevent Recurrent Events] Trial Investigators: Early and late effects of clopidogrel in patients with acute coronary syndromes. *Circulation* 107:966-972, 2003.)

2. Goodman SG, Fitchett D, Armstrong PW, et al: Randomized evaluation of the safety and efficacy of enoxaparin versus unfractionated heparin in high-risk patients with non–ST-segment elevation acute coronary syndromes receiving the glycoprotein IIb/IIIa inhibitor eptifibatide. *Circulation* 107:238-244, 2003.
3. Wallentin L, Bergstrand L, Dellborg M, et al, for the ASSENT Plus Investigators: Low molecular weight heparin (dalteparin) compared to unfractionated heparin as an adjunct to rt-PA (alteplase) for improvement of coronary artery patency in acute myocardial infarction—The ASSENT Plus study. *Eur Heart J* 24:897-908, 2003.
4. Gurbel PA, Bliden KP, Hiatt BL, et al: Clopidogrel for coronary stenting. Response variability, drug resistance, and the effect of pretreatment platelet reactivity. *Circulation* 107:2908-2913, 2003.

Antibiotic Therapy After Acute Myocardial Infarction: A Prospective Randomized Study

Zahn R, for the Arbeitsgemeinschaft Leitender Kardiologischer Krankenhausärzte (Working Group of Leading Hospital Cardiologists; ALKK); et al (Herzzentrum Ludwigshafen, Germany; et al)
Circulation 107:1253-1259, 2003

50–3

Introduction.—Inflammation has an important role in the pathogenesis of arteriosclerosis, particularly in acute coronary syndromes. Seroepidemiologic trials have questioned whether bacterial infections, particularly with *Chlamydia pneumoniae*, contribute to this inflammatory process. A higher prevalence of *C pneumoniae* has been observed in diseased versus normal coronary arteries. Treatment with the macrolide antibiotic roxithromycin was assessed to determine whether it would decrease mortality or morbidity in patients with acute myocardial infarction (AMI).

Methods.—The Antibiotic Therapy After an Acute Myocardial Infarction Study was a prospective, randomized, placebo-controlled, double-blind investigation that examined the effect of treatment with roxithromycin for patients with AMI. A total of 872 patients with AMI were randomly assigned to receive either double-blind treatment with 300 mg roxithromycin or placebo daily for 6 weeks (433 patients, roxithromycin; 439, placebo). The major end point was total mortality during 12 months of follow-up.

Results.—Baseline characteristics, reperfusion therapy, and medical therapy were similar in the 2 groups. A higher proportion of patients in the active treatment group had an anterior wall AMI (48.1% vs 40.2%; $P = .027$) and a lower prevalence of chronic obstructive pulmonary disease (3.5% vs 6.9%; $P = .028$). More participants in the roxithromycin group interrupted their study medication before 4 weeks of treatment (78 of 433 [18%] vs 48 of 439 [11%]; $P = .003$; odds ratio, 1.8; 95% confidence interval, 1.2-2.6).

Evaluation at 12-month follow-up was possible in 868 of 872 (99.5%) patients. The total mortality rate at 12 months was 6.5% (28/431) for the roxithromycin group versus 6.0% (26/437) for the placebo group (odds ratio, 1.1; 95% confidence interval, 0.6-1.9; $P = .739$) (Fig 2). There were no significant between-group differences in the secondary combined end points at 12 months.

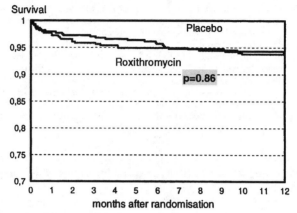

FIGURE 2.—Kaplan-Meier survival curve. (Courtesy of Zahn R, for the Arbeitsgemeinschaft Leitender Kardiologischer Krankenhausärzte [Working Group of Leading Hospital Cardiologists; ALKK]: Antibiotic therapy after acute myocardial infarction: A prospective randomized study. *Circulation* 107:1253-1259, 2003.)

Conclusion.—Treatment of AMI with roxithromycin did not decrease event rates during the initial 12 months of follow-up after AMI. These findings do no support the routine use of antibiotic therapy with a macrolide in patients with AMI.

▶ Inflammation appears to play an important role in the pathogenesis of coronary atherosclerosis and its complications. It was thought that this inflammatory process was triggered by various infectious agents.[1] However, this hypothesis has been challenged by multiple antibiotic trials, revealing no benefit on outcomes in patients with AMI.[2,3]

There is evidence of heightened pro-inflammatory cytokine activity and complement activation in patients with acute coronary syndromes and a lessening of anti-inflammatory cytokine activity.[4,5] It is still not known what triggers inflammation in acute coronary syndromes; however, various therapies, such as statins, may inhibit the inflammatory process.[6]

W. H. Frishman, MD

References

1. Kaplan RC, Frishman WH: Systemic inflammation as a cardiovascular disease risk factor and as a potential target for drug therapy. *Heart Dis* 3:326-332, 2001.
2. Anderson JL, Muhlestein JB, Carlquist J, et al: Randomized secondary prevention trial of azithromycin in patients with coronary artery disease and serological evidence of *Chlamydia pneumoniae* infection. The Azithromycin in Coronary Artery Disease: Elimination of Myocardial Infection with Chlamydia (ACADEMIC) study. *Circulation* 99:1540-1547, 1999.
3. O'Connor CM, Dunne MW, Pfeffer MA, et al, for the Investigators in the WIZARD Study: Azithromycin for the secondary prevention of coronary heart disease events: The WIZARD Study: A randomized controlled trial. *JAMA* 290:1459-1466, 2003.

4. Heeschen C, Dimmeler S, Hamm CW, et al: Serum levels of the anti-inflammatory cytokine interleukin-10 is an important prognostic determinant in patients with acute coronary syndromes. *Circulation* 107:2109-2114, 2003.
5. Damas JK, Waehre T, Yndestad A, et al: Interleukin-7–mediated inflammation in unstable angina: Possible role of chemokines and platelets. *Circulation* 107:2670-2676, 2003.
6. Granger CB, for the COMMA Investigators: Pexelizumab, an anti-C5 complement antibody, as adjunctive therapy to primary percutaneous coronary intervention in acute myocardial infarction. The COMplement inhibition in Myocardial infarction treated with Angioplasty (COMMA) Trial. *Circulation* 108:1184-1190, 2003.

Soluble CD40 Ligand in Acute Coronary Syndromes

Heeschen C, for the CAPTURE Study Investigators (Univ of Frankfurt, Germany; et al)
N Engl J Med 348:1104-1111, 2003   50–4

Introduction.—The CD40 ligand is expressed on platelets and is released from them upon activation. Increasing evidence indicates that the CD40 ligand has an important role in disease progression and plaque destabilization. The predictive value of soluble CD40 ligand as a marker for clinical outcome and the therapeutic effect of glycoprotein IIb/IIIa receptor inhibition were examined in patients with acute coronary syndromes (ACSs).

Methods.—Serum levels of soluble CD40 ligand were determined in 1088 patients with ACSs previously enrolled in a randomized trial comparing abciximab with placebo before coronary angioplasty and in 626 patients with acute chest pain. Soluble CD40 ligand, soluble P-selectin, high-sensitivity tumor necrosis factor α, and soluble intracellular adhesion molecule 1 were determined via enzyme-linked immunosorbent assay. Also measured were troponin T and C-reactive protein. In a subgroup of 161 patients with chest pain, platelet activation was evaluated.

Results.—The levels of soluble CD40 ligand were elevated in excess of 5.0 µg/L in 221 patients with ACSs (40.6%). In the placebo group, elevated soluble CD40 ligand levels indicated a significantly increased risk for death or nonfatal myocardial infarction during 6 months of follow-up (adjusted hazard ratio as compared with patients with low levels of the ligand [5.0 µg/L or less], 2.71; 95% confidence interval [CI], 1.51-5.35; $P = .001$) (Fig 1).

The prognostic value of this marker was validated in patients with chest pain, for whom elevated soluble CD40 ligand levels identified those with ACSs at high risk for death or nonfatal myocardial infarction (adjusted hazard ratio as compared with those with low levels of the ligand, 6.65; 95% CI, 3.18-13.89; $P < .001$). The increased risk in patients with elevated soluble CD40 ligand levels was significantly diminished by treatment with abciximab (adjusted hazard ratio as compared with those receiving placebo, 0.37; 95% CI, 0.20-0.68; $P = .01$). There was no significant treatment effect of abciximab in patients with low levels of soluble CD40 ligand.

Conclusion.—In patients with unstable coronary artery disease, elevation of soluble CD40 ligand levels signifies increased risk of cardiovascular

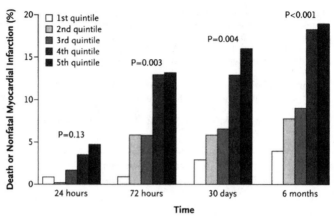

FIGURE 1.—Association between soluble CD40 ligand levels and the rate of cardiac events (death or nonfatal myocardial infarction) at 24 hours, 72 hours, 30 days, and 6 months among 544 patients receiving placebo. The patients were divided into quintiles according to the serum level of soluble CD40 ligand, as follows: first quintile, below 1.93 µg/L; second quintile, 1.93 to 3.50 µg/L; third quintile, 3.51 to 5.00 µg/L; fourth quintile, 5.01 to 6.30 µg/L; and fifth quintile, above 6.30 µg/L. *P values* are for trend at each time point. (Reprinted by permission of *The New England Journal of Medicine* from Heeschen C, for the CAPTURE Study Investigators: Soluble CD40 ligand in acute coronary syndromes. *N Engl J Med* 348:1104-1111, 2003. Copyright 2003, Massachusetts Medical Society. All rights reserved.)

events. Elevation of soluble CD40 ligand identifies a subgroup of patients at risk who will probably benefit from antiplatelet treatment with abciximab.

▶ Increasing evidence suggests that soluble CD40 ligand plays an important role in coronary artery disease progression and plaque instability. It also appears to be a prognostic marker that provides information beyond that provided by elevations in troponins, C-reactive protein,[1,2] tumor necrosis factor α, and soluble intracellular adhesion molecules. Choline appears to be another prognostic marker that may aid in prognostication in ACSs.[3]

W. H. Frishman, MD

References

1. Kinjo K, Sato H, Ohnishi Y, et al: Impact of high-sensitivity C-reactive protein on predicting long-term mortality in acute myocardial infarction. *Am J Cardiol* 91:931-935, 2003.
2. Varo N, de Lemos JA, Libby P, et al: Soluble CD40L: Risk prediction after acute coronary syndromes. *Circulation* 108:1049-1052, 2003.
3. Danne O, Möckel M, Lueders C, et al: Prognostic implications of elevated whole blood choline levels in acute coronary syndromes. *Am J Cardiol* 91:1060-1067, 2003.

Prognostic Value of Isolated Troponin Elevation Across the Spectrum of Chest Pain Syndromes

Rao SV, Ohman EM, Granger CB, et al (Duke Clinical Research Inst, Durham, NC; Univ of North Carolina, Chapel Hill; Univ of Alberta, Edmonton, Canada; et al)

Am J Cardiol 91:936-940, 2003   50–5

Introduction.—Patients with chest pain who have baseline isolated troponin elevation without ST-segment deviation, creatine kinase (CK)-MB elevation, or other high-risk clinical characteristics are clinically challenging since their risk of death or recurrent myocardial infarction (MI) is not clear. The importance of baseline isolated troponin elevation was examined across a spectrum of cardiac risk to ascertain the early and short-term risk of death or MI.

Methods.—Baseline CK-MB and troponin data from the Platelet IIb/IIIa Antagonism for the Reduction of Acute Coronary Syndrome Events in a Global Organization Network (PARAGON) B troponin substudy, the Global Utilization of Strategies to Open Occluded Coronary Arteries (GUSTO) IIa troponin substudy, and the Chest Pain Evaluation by Creatine Kinase-MB, Myoglobin, and Troponin I (CHECKMATE) study were examined. Patients were placed in 1 of 4 categories, based on marker status (troponin-positive/CK-MB–positive, troponin-positive/CK-MB–negative, troponin-negative/CK-MB–positive, or troponin-negative/CK-MB–negative).

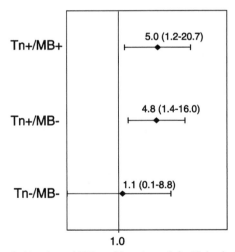

FIGURE 2.—Adjusted odds ratios and 95% confidence intervals for 30-day death or myocardial infarction by marker status in the CHECKMATE population (patients with negative results for CK-MB and troponin [*Tn-/MB-*] are the reference group). *Abbreviations:* +, Positive; −, negative. (Reprinted from *American Journal of Cardiology* courtesy of Rao SV, Ohman EM, Granger CB, et al: Prognostic value of isolated troponin elevation across the spectrum of chest pain syndromes. *Am J Cardiol* 91:936-940, 2003. Copyright 2003 with permission from Excerpta Medica Inc.)

The adjusted odds of death or MI occurring at 24 hours and 30 days was evaluated by baseline marker status using multivariable logistic regression. The group negative for both markers was used as the reference.

Results.—Patients positive for both markers had the highest odds of the 24-hour and 30-day end point. The adjusted odds of the 30-day end point for participants with isolated troponin elevation were 1.3 (95% confidence interval, 0.7-2.3) and 4.8 (95% confidence interval, 1.4-16.0) for high- and low-risk patients, respectively (Fig 2). The risk for 24-hour and 30-day death or MI with isolated positive CK-MB results was lower, compared to isolated positive troponin results; it was not significantly higher than if the 2 markers were negative.

Conclusion.—In patients with high- and low-risk chest pain, baseline troponin elevation without CK-MB elevation was linked to increased risk for early and short-term adverse outcomes. It is recommended that these patients be admitted to the hospital and monitored in either an ICU or a stepdown unit.

▶ Chest pain units are being formed in many EDs across the country to aid in patient triage and decision making regarding hospital admission.[1] These units utilize multiple laboratory measures including CK-MB, myoglobin, and troponin. It appears that troponin elevation in the absence of CK-MB evaluation is predictive of early and late adverse events across the spectrum of patients with chest pain. Troponin appears to be a superior marker, and measurements of CK-MB may be redundant in the assessment of patients with chest pain disorders.

W. H. Frishman, MD

Reference

1. Kogan A, Shapira R, Silman-Stoler Z, et al: Evaluation of chest pain in the ED: Factors affecting triage decisions. *Am J Emerg Med* 21:68-70, 2003.

51 Chronic Coronary Artery Disease

C-Reactive Protein and Ischemia in Users and Nonusers of β-Blockers and Statins: Data From the Heart and Soul Study

Beattie MS, Shlipak MG, Liu H, et al (Univ of California, San Francisco; VA Med Ctr, San Francisco; California Pacific Med Ctr, San Francisco)

Circulation 107:245-250, 2003   51–1

Background.—Increased C-reactive protein (CRP) levels have been associated with an increased risk of coronary events. However, it is unclear whether inflammation correlates with inducible ischemia in patients with stable coronary disease.

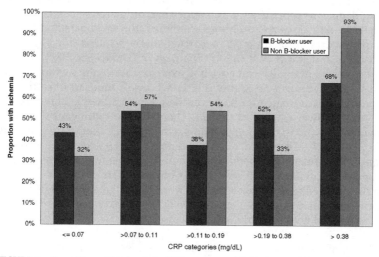

FIGURE 1.—Proportion with ischemia by CRP category and β-blocker use. (Courtesy of Beattie MS, Shlipak MG, Liu H, et al: C-reactive protein and ischemia in users and nonusers of β-blockers and statins: Data from the Heart and Soul Study. *Circulation* 107:245-250, 2003.)

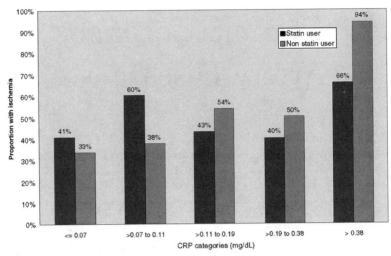

FIGURE 2.—Proportion with ischemia by CRP category and statin use. (Courtesy of Beattie MS, Shlipak MG, Liu H, et al: C-reactive protein and ischemia in users and nonusers of β-blockers and statins: Data from the Heart and Soul Study. *Circulation* 107:245-250, 2003.)

Methods.—One hundred eighteen persons with exercise-induced ischemia and 111 without inducible ischemia, as determined by stress echocardiography, were studied. CRP concentrations were measured.

Findings.—Seventy-five percent of the participants in the highest CRP category, defined as more than 0.38 mg/dL, had inducible ischemia compared with 45% in the lower 4 categories combined, for an adjusted odds ratio of 4.2. This correlation differed in participants who used and did not use β-blockers and statins. Of the 89 nonusers of β-blockers, 93% of the patients in the highest CRP category had exercise-induced ischemia compared with 42% in the lower categories (Fig 1). Of the 67 nonusers of statins, 94% in the highest CRP category had exercise-induced ischemia compared with 44% in the lower categories (Fig 2). There was no significant relationship between CRP and ischemia in patients treated with either of these agents.

Conclusions.—Increased CRP concentrations appear to be associated strongly and independently with inducible ischemia in patients with stable coronary disease, especially in nonusers of β-blockers or statins. Further research is needed to explore the mechanisms underlying the relationship between inflammation and ischemia, as well as possible ways to prevent ischemia associated with inflammatory processes.

▶ High CRP levels have been observed in patients with chronic ischemic heart disease.[1] β-Blockers and statins appear to have favorable effects on CRP levels, perhaps because of an anti-inflammatory effect of these treatments.[2,3] Statins also appear to reduce plaque instability and thrombogenicity,[3] and β-blockers have been thought to do likewise.[4]

Patients with symptomatic coronary artery disease who receive aggressive lipid lowering therapy have also been shown to have improved symptom status and ischemia that appears to reflect improved vascular function and not reduced atheroma burden.[4]

Selective COX-2 inhibitors have been shown to improve vascular function in patients with symptomatic coronary artery disease.[5]

W. H. Frishman, MD

References

1. Yamashita H, Shimada K, Seki E, et al: Concentrations of interleukins, interferon, and C-reactive protein in stable and unstable angina pectoris. *Am J Cardiol* 91:133-136, 2003.
2. Son JW, Koh KK, Ahn JY, et al: Effects of statin on plaque stability and thrombogenicity in hypercholesterolemic patients with coronary artery disease. *Int J Cardiol* 88:77-82, 2003.
3. Horne BD, for the Intermountain Heart Collaborative (IHC) Study Group: Statin therapy interacts with cytomegalovirus seropositivity and high C-reactive protein in reducing mortality among patients with angiographically significant coronary disease. *Circulation* 107:258-263, 2003.
4. Fathi R, Haluska B, Short L, et al: A randomized trial of aggressive lipid reduction for improvement of myocardial ischemia, symptom status, and vascular function in patients with coronary artery disease not amenable to intervention. *Am J Med* 114:445-453, 2003.
5. Chenevard R, Hürlimann D, Béchir M, et al: Selective COX-2 inhibition improves endothelial function in coronary artery disease. *Circulation* 107:405-409, 2003.

The VIVA Trial: Vascular Endothelial Growth Factor in Ischemia for Vascular Angiogenesis
Henry TD, for the VIVA Investigators (Minneapolis Heart Inst Foundation, Minn; et al)
Circulation 107:1359-1365, 2003   51–2

Background.—In animal models, recombinant human vascular endothelial growth factor protein (rhVEGF) has been shown to stimulate angiogenesis. In addition, rhVEGF has been reported to be well tolerated in phase I clinical trials. This double-blind placebo-controlled study was designed to assess the safety and efficacy of intracoronary and IV infusions of rhVEGF in patients with stable exertional angina not suitable for standard revascularization.

Methods.—One hundred seventy-eight patients were randomly assigned to placebo, low-dose rhVEGF ($17\ ng\cdot kg^{-1}\cdot min^{-1}$), or high-dose rhVEGF ($50\ ng\cdot kg^{-1}\cdot min^{-1}$) by coronary infusion at baseline and IV infusion on days 3, 6, and 9. Patients underwent exercise treadmill testing, angina class determination, and quality of life assessment at baseline and on days 60 and 120. Also at baseline and on day 60, myocardial perfusion imaging was performed.

Findings.—Change in exercise treadmill test (ETT) time between day 60 and baseline did not differ between groups. Angina class and quality of life were improved significantly in each group, with no significant differences among the groups. On day 120, placebo recipients showed decreased benefit on all 3 measures, but did not differ significantly from patients in the low-dose rhVEGF group (Fig 1). High-dose rhVEGF recipients, however, had

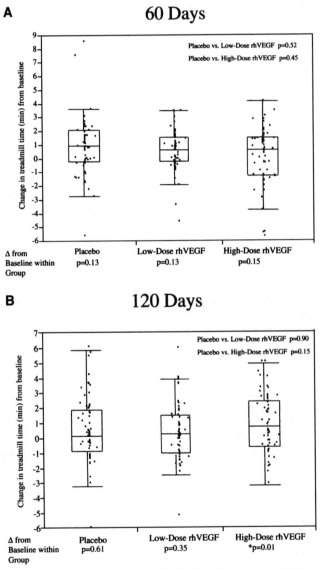

FIGURE 1.—Change in ETT time (minutes) from baseline for all 3 groups at day 60 (**A**) and day 120 (**B**). Box plots represent 25th to 75th percentiles with median and individual data. Missing values were assigned least rank for statistical analysis but not imputed in the figure. (Courtesy of Henry TD, for the VIVA Investigators: The VIVA trial: Vascular endothelial growth factor in ischemia for vascular angiogenesis. *Circulation* 107:1359-1365, 2003.)

significant improvement in angina class, with nonsignificant trends in ETT time and angina frequency compared with the placebo group.

Conclusions.—In this trial, rhVEGF was not more effective than placebo on any measure by day 60. By day 120, high-dose rhVEGF was associated with significant improvement in angina, with a favorable trend in ETT time and angina frequency. This agent appears to be safe and well tolerated.

▶ Various strategies have been developed to treat inoperable patients with refractory angina pectoris, including external counterpulsation, spinal stimulation, and angiogenesis. Various angiogenesis growth factors have been used in treating angina, with mixed results being reported.[1,2] These growth factors also need to be given with a catheter-based approach.

Other treatments being evaluated for stable angina treatment include ranolazine (free fatty-acid enhancer),[3] ivabradine (a sinus node inhibitor),[4] nicorandil (a coronary vasodilator),[3] magnesium,[5] and arginine.[6]

W. H. Frishman, MD

References

1. Frishman WH, Ganem A, Nelson MA, et al: Therapeutic angiogenesis: a new treatment modality for ischemic heart disease, in Frishman WH, Sonnenblick EH, Sica DA (eds): *Cardiovascular Pharmacotherapeutics*, ed 2. New York, McGraw Hill, 2003, pp 691-704.
2. Nelson MA, Passeri J, Frishman WH: Therapeutic angiogenesis: A new treatment modality for ischemic heart disease. *Heart Dis* 2:314-325, 2000.
3. Frishman WH, Retter A, Misailidis J, et al: Innovative pharmacologic approaches to the treatment of myocardial ischemia, in Frishman WH, Sonnenblick EH, Sica DA (eds): *Cardiovascular Pharmacotherapeutics*, ed 2. New York, McGraw Hill, 2003, pp 655-690.
4. Borer JS, Fox K, Jaillon P, et al: Antianginal and antiischemic effects of ivabradine, an I$_f$ inhibitor, in stable angina: A randomized, double-blind, multicentered, placebo-controlled trial. *Circulation* 107:817-823, 2003.
5. Shechter M, Merz CNB, Stuehlinger H-G, et al: Effects of oral magnesium therapy on exercise tolerance, exercise-induced chest pain, and quality of life in patients with coronary artery disease. *Am J Cardiol* 91:517-521, 2003.
6. Piatti PM, Fragasso G, Monti LD, et al: Acute intravenous L-arginine infusion decreases endothelin-1 levels and improves endothelial function in patients with angina pectoris and normal coronary arteriograms: Correlation with asymmetric dimethylarginine levels. *Circulation* 107:429-436, 2003.

Outcome of Elderly Patients With Chronic Symptomatic Coronary Artery Disease With an Invasive vs Optimized Medical Treatment Strategy: One-year Results of the Randomized TIME Trial

Pfisterer M, for the Trial of Invasive Versus Medical Therapy in Elderly Patients (TIME) Investigators (Univ Hosp, Basel, Switzerland; et al)
JAMA 289:1117-1123, 2003　　　　　　　　　　　　51–3

Background.—In younger adult patients with coronary artery disease (CAD), revascularization procedures are of demonstrated benefit in improving symptoms and quality of life. However, the risks and benefits of invasive treatment for elderly patients with CAD remain unclear. The recent Trial of Invasive Versus Medical Therapy in Elderly patients (TIME) study found significant improvement in quality of life with invasive therapy over short-term follow-up, with some associated increase in mortality rate. The 1-year follow-up outcomes of elderly patients in the TIME study are reported.

Methods.—The planned analysis included 282 patients aged 75 or older with symptomatic, chronic CAD. All had class 2 or higher angina, based on Canadian Cardiac Society criteria, despite treatment that included at least 2 antianginal medications. The 1-year follow-up study included only patients who survived at least 6 months after random assignment to revascularization or optimized medical therapy. The mean patient age was 80 years; 42% of the patients were women. Quality of life was evaluated by standardized assessments, including the Short Form 36. Death and other major adverse cardiac events were also assessed.

Results.—Both revascularization and medical management were associated with significant improvements in angina and quality of life, compared with baseline. However, the earlier advantage of revascularization was no longer present at 1-year follow-up. Patients undergoing invasive therapy had a significantly lower rate of subsequent hospitalization with revascularization and a hazard ratio (HR) of 0.19. However, the 1-year mortality rate was significantly higher, HR 1.51. The rate of other major adverse events (ie, death or nonfatal myocardial infarction) was not significantly different between groups. The overall rate of major adverse cardiac events was higher for patients receiving medical therapy (49.3% vs 19.0% at 6 months and 64.2% vs 25.5% at 12 months).

Conclusions.—For patients over the age of 75 with chronic, symptomatic CAD, the early quality-of-life advantages of revascularization over optimized medical therapy are not preserved through 1-year follow-up. These 2 approaches also offer similar outcomes in terms of symptom status and risk of death or nonfatal myocardial infarction. Medical treatment is associated with a substantially higher risk of subsequent hospitalization and revascularization, for a higher overall rate of major adverse cardiac events.

▶ Elderly patients with stable angina pectoris appear to have similar clinical outcomes when optimal medical therapy is compared with revascularization. Older patients should be kept on maximal medical therapy until unstable disease develops, which may then warrant an invasive treatment strategy.

Elderly patients also benefit from cardiac rehabilitation programs in a similar fashion as do younger patients.[1]

W. H. Frishman, MD

Reference

1. Marchionni N, Fattirolli F, Fumagalli S, et al: Improved exercise tolerance and quality of life with cardiac rehabilitation of older patients after myocardial infarction: Results of a randomized, controlled trial. *Circulation* 107:2201-2206, 2003.

Glutathione Peroxidase 1 Activity and Cardiovascular Events in Patients With Coronary Artery Disease

Blankenberg S, for the AtheroGene Investigators (Johannes Gutenberg Univ Mainz, Germany; et al)
N Engl J Med 349:1605-1613, 2003   51–4

Introduction.—Cellular antioxidant enzymes, including glutathione peroxidase and superoxide dismutase, have an important role in the control of reactive oxygen species. In vitro data and trials that use animal models indicate that these enzymes may protect against atherosclerosis. Little is understood concerning their relevance in human disease. The risk of cardiovascular (CV) events linked with baseline erythrocyte glutathione peroxidase 1 and superoxide dismutase activity was prospectively examined.

Methods.—A total of 636 patients seen between November 1996 and December 1997 with suspected coronary artery disease were included. Blood was drawn to determine glutathione peroxidase 1 and superoxide dismutase activity. The mean levels and proportions of baseline CV risk factors were determined for participants in whom a CV event did and did not occur subsequently. In all survival analyses, the end point was death from CV causes or

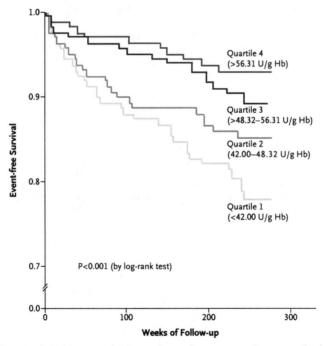

FIGURE 1.—Kaplan-Meier curves showing cardiovascular events according to quartile of glutathione peroxidase 1 activity. The numbers of cardiovascular events were 33, 23, 16, and 11 in quartiles 1, 2, 3, and 4, respectively. Glutathione peroxidase 1 activity is shown in units per gram of hemoglobin. (Reprinted by permission of *The New England Journal of Medicine* from Blankenberg S, for the AtheroGene Investigators: Glutathione peroxidase 1 activity and cardiovascular events in patients with coronary artery disease. *N Engl J Med* 349:1605-1613, 2003. Copyright 2003, Massachusetts Medical Society. All rights reserved.)

nonfatal myocardial infarction. The median and maximum follow-ups were 4.7 years and 5.4 years, respectively.

Results.—Glutathione peroxidase 1 activity was among the strongest univariate predictors of the risk of CV events; superoxide dismutase activity was not linked with risk. The risk of CV events was inversely correlated with increasing quartiles of glutathione peroxidase 1 activity (P for trend $< .001$); patients in the highest quartile of glutathione peroxidase 1 activity had a hazard ratio of 0.29 (95% CI, 0.15-0.58; $P < .001$) versus those in the lowest quartile (Fig 1). Glutathione peroxidase 1 activity was impacted by gender and smoking status; it retained its predictive power in these subgroups. The inverse relationship between glutathione peroxidase 1 activity and CV events remained almost unchanged.

Conclusion.—In patients with coronary artery disease, a low level of activity of red-cell glutathione peroxidase 1 is independently correlated with increased risk of CV events. Glutathione peroxidase 1 activity may be prognostically useful in addition to the traditional risk factors. It is possible that increasing glutathione peroxidase 1 activity lowers the risk of CV events.

▶ Clinicians have been searching for markers of occult coronary disease that would help identify those individuals requiring aggressive preventative treatment. Diagnostic screening modalities include exercise electrocardiography, exercise scintigraphy,[1] C-reactive protein levels, erythrocyte, glutathione peroxidase-1 activity, and plasma myeloperoxidase.[2] The complaint of penile erectile dysfunction has also been identified as a clinical marker of underlying coronary disease.[3]

W. H. Frishman, MD

References

1. Blumenthal RS, Becker DM, Yanek LR, et al: Detecting occult coronary disease in a high-risk asymptomatic population. *Circulation* 107:702-707, 2003.
2. Brennan M-L, Penn MS, Van Lente F, et al: Prognostic value of myeloperoxidase in patients with chest pain. *N Engl J Med* 349:1595-1604, 2003.
3. Solomon H, Man JW, Wierzbicki AS, et al: Relation of erectile dysfunction to angiographic coronary artery disease. *Am J Cardiol* 91:230-231, 2003.

52 Coronary Intervention Procedures

Intracoronary Radiation Therapy Improves the Clinical and Angiographic Outcomes of Diffuse In-Stent Restenotic Lesions: Results of the Washington Radiation for In-Stent Restenosis Trial for Long Lesions (Long WRIST) Studies
Waksman R, Cheneau E, Ajani AE, et al (Washington Hosp Ctr, DC; Scripps Clinic, La Jolla, Calif)
Circulation 107:1744-1749, 2003   52–1

Introduction.—Long and diffuse in-stent restenosis (ISR) continues to be challenging in percutaneous coronary interventions. The length and pattern of ISR is associated with the treatment failure of ISR with conventional treatment. Vascular brachytherapy (VBT) has potential for decreasing the recurrence of ISR, compared with conventional therapy, for short and intermediate ISR lesions with the use of both γ and β emitters. The Washington Radiation for In-Stent Restenosis Trial for long lesions (Long WRIST) was designed to ascertain the safety and efficacy of VBT in the treatment of diffuse ISR. The 6-month angiographic and 12-month clinical outcomes of the Long WRIST and the Long WRIST High Dose investigations are discussed.

Methods.—The efficacy of γ-radiation was compared with placebo therapy in the treatment of long and diffuse ISR. All patients had previously undergone intracoronary stent implantation in a native coronary artery with angina symptoms and evidence of diffuse ISR. Inclusion criteria were angiographic lesion length ranging between 36 and 80 mm, artery diameter between 3.0 and 5.0 mm, patient age 30 to 80 years, and long angiographically normal segments proximal and distal to the lesion. Patients were randomly assigned to radiation treatment with either ^{192}Ir with 15 Gy at 2 mm from the source axis or placebo. After enrollment, an additional 120 patients (using the same inclusion criteria) were treated with ^{192}Ir with 18 Gy. They were included in the Long WRIST High Dose registry. Antiplatelet therapy was initially prescribed for 1 month initially; it was extended to 6 months in the last 60 patients in the Long WRIST High Dose registry. At 6 months, the binary radiographic restenosis rate was 73%, 45%, and 38% for the placebo group and the 15 Gy and 18 Gy radiated groups, respectively ($P < .05$). At the 1-year follow-up, the primary clinical end point of major cardiac events was

63% and 42%, respectively, in the placebo group and the radiated group with 15 Gy ($P < .05$). Late thrombosis was 12%, 15%, and 9% for controls, the 15 Gy group with 1-month antiplatelet therapy, and the 18 Gy group with 6-month antiplatelet therapy, respectively.

Conclusion.—Vascular brachytherapy with ^{192}Ir is safe and decreases the incidence of recurrent restenosis in patients with diffuse ISR. Efficacy of VBT on angiographic and clinical outcomes is enhanced with a radiation dose of 18 Gy and prolonged antiplatelet therapy.

▶ Intravascular brachytherapy has been shown to be a useful treatment modality for treating ISR after percutaneous coronary interventions.[1] Even more diffuse restenotic lesions can be treated with brachytherapy. However, brachytherapy has been hampered by edge restenosis, late thrombosis, and adverse vascular remodeling.[2] With the advent of the new drug-eluting coronary stents, the problem of ISR may be eliminated.[3] However, longer-term follow-up of patients who have received these new stents is needed to document their efficacy.

W. H. Frishman, MD

References

1. Urban P, et al for the RENO investigators: A multicentre European registry of intraluminal coronary beta brachytherapy. *Eur Heart J* 24:604-612, 2003.
2. Frishman WH, Landzberg BR, Weiss M: Pharmacologic therapies for the prevention of restenosis following percutaneous coronary artery interventions, in Frishman WH, Sonnenblick EH, Sica DA (eds): *Cardiovascular Pharmacotherapeutics*, ed 2. New York, McGraw Hill, 2003, pp 741-776.
3. Moses JW, for the SIRIUS Investigators: Sirolimus-eluting stents versus standard stents in patients with stenosis in a native coronary artery. *N Engl J Med* 349:1315-1323, 2003.

A Paclitaxel-Eluting Stent for the Prevention of Coronary Restenosis
Park S, Shim WH, Ho DS, et al (Asan Med Ctr, Seoul, South Korea; Univ of Hong Kong; Cardiovascular Angiography Analysis Lab, Houston; et al)
N Engl J Med 348:1537-1545, 2003   52–2

Introduction.—Intimal hyperplasia after stent placement and its resulting restenosis restricts the efficacy of coronary stenting. The antiproliferative agent paclitaxel inhibits cell processes that are dependent on microtubular turnover, including mitosis, cell proliferation, and cell migration, while cells stay viable and in a cytostatic state. Paclitaxel has been considered for intracoronary delivery to arrest the process for neointimal hyperplasia after angioplasty and stenting. A coronary stent coated with paclitaxel as a means of preventing restenosis was examined in a multicenter (3 centers), prospective, randomized, triple-blind controlled investigation.

Methods.—One hundred seventy-seven patients with discrete coronary lesions (<15 mm in length, 2.25-3.5 mm in diameter) underwent implantation with either paclitaxel-eluting stents (low dose, 1.3 µg/mL² or high dose,

3.1 µg/mL^2) or control stents. Antiplatelet therapies included aspirin with ticlopidine, clopidogrel, or cilostazol in 120, 18, and 37 patients, respectively. Patients were clinically evaluated at 1 month and 4 to 6 months. Angiographic follow-up was at 4 to 6 months.

Results.—Technical success was observed in 99% of patients (176/177 patients). The high-dose group versus controls had significantly better outcome for the degree of stenosis (mean, 14% vs 39%; $P < .001$), late loss of luminal diameter (0.29 mm vs 1.04 mm; $P < .001$), and restenosis of over 50% (4% vs 27%; $P < .001$). Intravascular US analysis revealed a dose-dependent decrease in the volume of intimal hyperplasia (31, 18, and 13 mm^3, in the high-dose, low-dose, and control groups, respectively). There was a higher incidence of major cardiac events in patients who received cilostazol versus those who received ticlopidine or clopidogrel. In patients who received ticlopidine or clopidogrel, the event-free survival was 98% in the high-dose and 100% in the control group at 1 month; it was 96% in both groups, respectively, at 4 to 6 months.

Conclusion.—Paclitaxel-eluting stents used with conventional antiplatelet therapy for prevention of coronary restenosis effectively inhibits restenosis and neointimal hyperplasia and has a safety profile similar to that of standard stents.

▶ Restenosis after angioplasty with or without stenting has been a common problem.[1] Drug-eluting stents appear to reduce the risk of postcoronary angioplasty restenosis. Drug-eluting stents that use the antiproliferative agents sirolimus (rapamycin) and paclitaxel can reduce neointimal hyperplasia but long-term results regarding late restenosis need to be obtained.[1-7]

Early thrombotic complications have been observed with the sirolimus stent that is commercially available, but this may relate to the "learning curve," as more operators deploy these stents in a growing number of patients. In-stent restenosis has been described in some patients who received these stents.[7]

Other drug-eluting stents under investigation include those that use corticosteroids, and the matrix metalloproteinase inhibitor batimastat.[1] Heparin-coated stents have been used successfully in the treatment of stenoses in small coronary arteries.[8]

W. H. Frishman, MD

References

1. Frishman WH, Landzberg BR, Weiss M: Pharmacologic therapies for the prevention of restenosis following percutaneous coronary artery interventions, in Frishman WH, Sonnenblick EH, Sica DA (eds): *Cardiovascular Pharmacotherapeutics*, ed 2. New York, McGraw Hill, 2003, pp 741-776.
2. Moses JW, for the SIRIUS Investigators: Sirolimus-eluting stents versus standard stents in patients with stenosis in a native coronary artery. *N Engl J Med* 349:1315-1323, 2003.
3. Morice MC, Serruys PW, Sousa JE, et al: A randomized comparison of a sirolimus-eluting stent with a standard stent for coronary revascularization. *N Engl J Med* 346:1773-1780, 2002.

4. Tanabe K, Serruys PW, Grube E, et al: TAXUS III Trial. In-stent restenosis treated with stent-based delivery of paclitaxel incorporated in a slow-release polymer formulation. *Circulation* 107:559-564, 2003.

5. Hong M-K, Mintz GS, Lee CW, et al: Paclitaxel coating reduces in-stent intimal hyperplasia in human coronary arteries: A serial volumetric intravascular ultrasound analysis from the ASian Paclitaxel-Eluting Stent Clinical Trial (ASPECT). *Circulation* 107:517-520, 2003.

6. Ferreira AC, Peter AA, Salerno TA, et al: Clinical impact of drug-eluting stents in changing referral practices for coronary surgical revascularization in a tertiary care center. *Ann Thorac Surg* 75:485-489, 2003.

7. Colombo A, Orlic D, Stankovic G, et al: Preliminary observations regarding angiographic pattern of restenosis after rapamycin-eluting stent implantation. *Circulation* 107:2178-2180, 2003.

8. Haude M, for the COAST Trial Investigators: Heparin-coated stent placement for the treatment of stenoses in small coronary arteries of symptomatic patients. *Circulation* 107:1265-1270, 2003.

Association Between C-Reactive Protein Levels and Subsequent Cardiac Events Among Patients With Stable Angina Treated With Coronary Artery Stenting

Dibra A, Mehilli J, Braun S, et al (Deutsches Herzzentrum and Medizinische Klinik Rechts der Isar, Munich; Institut für Laboratoriumsmedizin, Deutsches Herzzentrum, Munich; Institut für Klinische Chemie und Pathochemie, Munich; et al)

Am J Med 114:715-722, 2003   52–3

Introduction.—Several trials have reported a link between elevated serum C-reactive protein (CRP) levels and increased risk of subsequent cardiovascular events in patients with or without evidence of coronary artery disease. The prognostic value of CRP levels was examined in patients with stable angina who underwent coronary stenting.

Methods.—A consecutive series of 1152 patients with stable angina who had undergone coronary stenting between May 1999 and April 2000 were monitored. Baseline CRP levels were determined with the use of a high-sensitivity assay. Of these, 651 (57%) had elevated CRP levels (>5 mg/L). The major end point was either death or myocardial infarction within 1 year after coronary artery stenting. Angiographic restenosis was considered to be 50% or greater diameter stenosis at follow-up angiography.

Results.—During the 1-year follow-up period, 62 (9.5%) of the 651 patients with an elevated CRP level and 24 (4.8%) of 501 patients with normal levels either died or had a myocardial infarction ($P = .002$). Multivariate analysis showed that elevated baseline CRP levels were linked with nearly a 2-fold increase in the rate of death or myocardial infarction after coronary restenting (hazard ratio = 1.8; 95% CI, 1.1-2.9). Most of the difference in the event rates occurred within the first 30 days (Fig 2). Baseline CRP levels were not associated with restenosis.

Conclusion.—Elevated preprocedural CRP levels are linked with a less favorable prognosis in patients with stable angina who undergo coronary stenting. Determination of CRP levels in these patients may help to identify

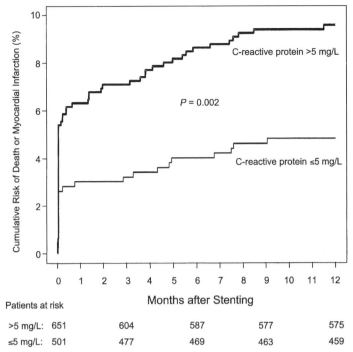

FIGURE 2.—Combined risk of death or myocardial infarction during 1-year follow-up, by baseline C-reactive protein level. Most of the difference between the 2 groups occurred early after stenting. (Reprinted from Dibra A, Mehilli J, Braun J, et al: Association between C-reactive protein levels and subsequent cardiac events among patients with stable angina treated with coronary artery stenting. *Am J Med* 114:715-722, 2003. Copyright 2003, with permission from Excerpta Medica, Inc.)

those who may benefit from a treatment strategy focused on attenuation of inflammation.

▶ Elevated serum CRP levels have been shown to be associated with a less favorable prognosis in patients undergoing coronary stenting. It has been suggested that CRP levels be obtained before angiography to identify high-risk patients who might benefit the most from preventative interventions.

Various therapies have been evaluated as treatments for reducing the short- and long-term complication rates and the morbidity and mortality rates after angioplasty and stenting. These treatments include the use of antiplatelet agents (aspirin, clopidogrel, and IIb/IIIa glycoprotein receptor antagonists) and heparin.[1,2] Statins appear to reduce mortality among patients with high CRP levels.[3] Beta-adrenergic blockers have been shown to reduce the incidence of myocardial infarction during angioplasty, and in addition, may reduce short-term complications.[4] The lipid-lowering drug probucol has been suggested as a treatment to reduce long-term complications after angioplasty.[5] The patient undergoing angioplasty and/or stenting needs to be treated with a wide variety of agents to maximize the short- and long-term benefits of these interventions (antiplatelet drugs, statins, beta blockers, and probably angiotensin-converting enzyme inhibitors). Percutaneous left ventricular assistance has also been used to support patients undergoing high-risk percutaneous coronary interventions.[6]

W. H. Frishman, MD

References

1. Frishman WH, Lerner RG, Klein MD, et al: Antiplatelet and antithrombotic drugs, in Frishman WH, Sonnenblick EH, Sica DA (eds): *Cardiovascular Pharmacotherapeutics*, ed 2. New York, McGraw Hill, 2003, pp 259-300.
2. Gurbel PA, Bliden KP, Hiatt BL, et al: Clopidogrel for coronary stenting: Response variability, drug resistance, and the effect of pretreatment platelet reactivity. *Circulation* 107:2908-2913, 2003.
3. Chang AW, Bhatt DL, Chew DP, et al: Relation of inflammation and benefit of statins after percutaneous coronary interventions. *Circulation* 107:1750-1756, 2003.
4. Wang FW, Osman A, Otero J, et al: Distal myocardial protection during percutaneous coronary intervention with an intracoronary β blocker. *Circulation* 107:2914-2919, 2003.
5. Tardif J-C, for the Canadian Antioxidant Restenosis Trial (CART-1) investigators: Effects of AGI-1067 and probucol after percutaneous coronary interventions. *Circulation* 107:552-558, 2003.
6. Lemos PA, Cummins P, Lee C-H, et al: Usefulness of percutaneous left ventricular assistance to support high-risk percutaneous coronary interventions. *Am J Cardiol* 91:479-481, 2003.

Is Geography Destiny for Patients in New York With Myocardial Infarction?

Fang J, Alderman MH (Albert Einstein College of Medicine, Bronx, NY)
Am J Med 115:448-453, 2003   52–4

Introduction.—White patients receive more cardiac services than African American patients in the United States. This disparity remains after accounting for insurance and socioeconomic status. Revascularization rates in patients hospitalized for myocardial infarction (MI) were assessed to ascertain the influence of race and socioeconomic factors on the likelihood of revascularization after MI in various parts of New York City.

Methods.—Statewide Planning and Research Cooperative System data from 1998 through 1999 from the New York State Department of Health was used to determine revascularization rates among patients hospitalized with MI in 2 socioeconomically disadvantaged communities in New York City (the South Bronx, which has no hospitals with revascularization facilities, and Harlem, which has 3 revascularization facilities). The remainder of New York City acted as reference. Demographic, clinical characteristics and revascularization rates were determined for each community.

Results.—Among patients hospitalized with MI, the age-adjusted revascularization rates were 29.2% for white patients, 12.5% for African American patients, and 19.9% for Hispanic patients ($P < .01$). In Harlem, mid-Manhattan, and the remainder of New York City, the revascularization rates were 12.0%, 23.0%, and 38.4%, respectively (*P* < .05). Logistic regression analysis, adjusted for age, gender, race, insurance status, comorbidity, clinical complications, and year of admission, showed that South Bronx patients were about 20% less likely to be revascularized versus the remainder of New York City; patients living in Harlem were twice as likely to undergo revascularization than residents living in the rest of New York City. Among patients admitted to hospitals with cardiac revascularization facilities, lower use among South Bronx residents remained; after adjusting for patient characteristics, Harlem residents were significantly less likely to undergo revascularization versus those from the remainder of New York City.

Conclusion.—Race and socioeconomic factors affect the likelihood of revascularization after MI among New York City residents. In addition, the lack of availability of revascularization further diminishes its use by residents of disadvantaged neighborhoods.

▶ The number of coronary artery revascularization procedures appears to be related to the ability to access hospitals that can provide this treatment. Because timely angioplasty with stenting is now considered the treatment of choice in managing most patients with acute MI,[1] it is imperative that all patients have equal access to clinical facilities that can provide these procedures. Free-standing cardiac catheterization laboratories (without onsite cardiothoracic surgery) that can perform angioplasty and stenting should soon become the "norm" to ensure that all patients with MI receive this state-of-the-art treatment close to home.[2]

Race and socioeconomic factors continue to influence the types of treatment patients with MI receive.

W. H. Frishman, MD

References

1. Grines CL: Should thrombolysis or primary angioplasty be the treatment of choice for acute myocardial infarction? Primary angioplasty: The strategy of choice. *N Engl J Med* 335:1313-1317, 1996.
2. Alter DA, Naylor CD, Austin PC, et al: Long-term MI outcomes at hospitals with or without on-site revascularization. *JAMA* 285:2101-2108, 2001.

Intramyocardial Transplantation of Autologous Endothelial Progenitor Cells for Therapeutic Neovascularization of Myocardial Ischemia

Kawamoto A, Tkebuchava T, Yamaguchi J, et al (Tufts Univ, Boston; Tokai Univ, Japan)

Circulation 107:461-468, 2003

52–5

Introduction.—Endothelial progenitor cells (EPCs) have a potential therapeutic role in ischemic disease. There are 2 important obstacles that must be overcome before considering actual clinical applications for EPCs: dosage and immunologic rejection. In vivo investigations were performed to address these limitations. Catheter-based transplantation of freshly isolated, autologous EPC-enriched fraction was evaluated in a swine chronic myocardial ischemia model. To confirm the therapeutic usefulness of the freshly isolated, human EPC-enriched fraction, intramyocardial transplantation was also performed in immunodeficient rats with myocardial ischemia using freshly isolated human CD34+ mononuclear cells (MNCs).

Methods.—Myocardial ischemia was caused by placing an ameroid constrictor around the swine's left circumflex artery. At 4 weeks after placement of the constrictor, CD31+ MNCs were freshly isolated from the peripheral blood of each pig. The CD31+ MNCs were incubated overnight in noncoated plates and nonadhesive cells (NA/CD31+ MNCs) were harvested as the EPC-enriched fraction. Nonadhesive CD31− cells (NA/CD31− MNCs) were also processed. Autologous transplantation of 10^7 NA/CD31+ MNCs, 10^7 NA/CD31− MNCs or phosphate-buffered saline solution (PBS) was achieved with the use of a NOGA mapping injection catheter to target ischemic myocardium. In a parallel investigation, 10^5 human CD34+ MNCs, 10^5 human CD34− MNCs or PBS was transplanted into ischemic myocardium of nude rats 10 minutes after the left anterior descending coronary artery was ligated.

Results.—In the swine trial, ischemic area by NOGA mapping, Rentrop grade angiographic collateral development, and echocardiographic left ventricular fraction improved significantly at 4 weeks after transplantation of NA/CD31− MNCs and not after injection of NA/CD31− MNCs or PBS. Capillary density in ischemic myocardium 4 weeks after transplantation was significantly higher in the NA/CD31− group versus controls. In the rat trial, echocardiographic left ventricular systolic function and capillary density were significantly better preserved in the CD34+ MNC group versus controls at 4 weeks after myocardial ischemia.

Conclusion.—Percutaneous delivery of autologous, freshly isolated EPCs targeted to sites of ischemia may be a practical strategy for revascularization of patients with chronic myocardial ischemia.

▶ There is increasing experimental evidence that the percutaneous delivery of autologous endothelial progenitor cells can provide neovascularization of the ischemic myocardium.[1,2] The percutaneous delivery of progenitor bone marrow cells and cardiac stem cells may 1 day provide an alternative way of treating acute myocardial injury and chronic congestive heart failure.[3-5]

W. H. Frishman, MD

References

1. Yamaguchi J-I, Kusano KF, Masuo O, et al: Stromal cell-derived factor-1 effects on ex vivo expanded endothelial progenitor cell recruitment for ischemic neovascularization. *Circulation* 107:1322-1328, 2003.
2. Frishman WH, Ganem A, Nelson MA, et al: Therapeutic angiogenesis: a new treatment modality for ischemic heart disease, in Frishman WH, Sonnenblick EH, Sica DA (eds): *Cardiovascular Pharmacotherapeutics*, ed 2. New York, McGraw Hill, 2003, pp 691-704.
3. Frishman WH, Anversa P: Stem cell therapy for myocardial regeneration: The future is now (editorial). *Heart Dis* 4:205, 2002.

4. Beltrami AP, Barlucci L, Torella D, et al: Adult cardiac stem cells are multipotent and support myocardial regeneration. *Cell* 114:763-776, 2003.
5. Frishman WH, Retter A, Misailidis J, et al: Innovative pharmacologic approaches to the treatment of myocardial ischemia, in Frishman WH, Sonnenblick EH, Sica DA (eds): *Cardiovascular Pharmacotherapeutics*, ed 2. New York, McGraw Hill, 2003, pp 655-690.

53 Congestive Cardiomyopathy

Hemodilution Is Common in Patients With Advanced Heart Failure
Androne A, Katz SD, Lund L, et al (Columbia Univ, New York)
Circulation 107:226-229, 2003   53–1

Background.—Because of chronic disease, bone marrow depression resulting from excessive cytokine production, malnutrition, accompanying renal disease, and/or drug therapy, patients with chronic heart failure (CHF) often have anemia, a condition that has a poor prognosis. Patients with edema, hypervolemia, and even those appearing clinically euvolemic may suffer hemodilution; plasma and red blood cell (RBC) volume estimates that use I[131]-tagged albumin may identify patients with CHF who have hemodilution, a condition that also has clinical implications. Specifically, patients with hemodilution require no further evaluation, but those with true anemia do. The prevalence of hemodilution and prognosis of CHF plus hemodilution were assessed.

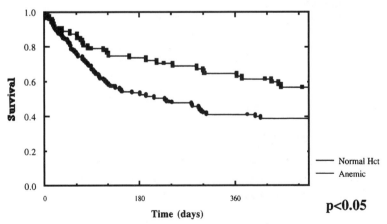

FIGURE 1.—Survival curves of patients with and without anemia. Hct indicates hematocrit. (Courtesy of Androne A, Katz SD, Lund L, et al: Hemodilution is common in patients with advanced heart failure. *Circulation* 107:226-229, 2003.)

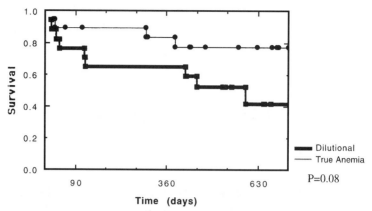

FIGURE 2.—Survival curves of the patients with true anemia versus hemodilution. (Courtesy of Androne A, Katz SD, Lund L, et al: Hemodilution is common in patients with advanced heart failure. *Circulation* 107:226-229, 2003.)

Methods.—The study included 196 patients with CHF who were evaluated for the presence of anemia. The prevalence of hemodilution was assessed in 37 ambulatory anemic patients with I^{131}-tagged albumin to measure RBC and plasma volume. Clinical outcomes were noted.

Results.—Anemia was found in 61% of the patients. Of the 37 anemic patients who had blood volume analysis, 46% had normal RBC volume with excess plasma volume; this was noted in 39% of men and only 16% of women. The hematocrit of patients with hemodilution was higher than that in patients with anemia; the mean plasma volume excess in hemodilution patients was 1460 mL, or 149% of predicted. The hemodilution group had significantly higher pulmonary capillary wedge pressure, but other parameters were similar in the anemia and hemodilution groups. Fifty-six percent of hemodilution patients appeared euvolemic. At 1 year, the survival rate of anemic patients was 41%, whereas that of patients with normal hematocrit levels was 63% (Fig 1). During a mean follow-up of 417 days, 4 anemia and 9 hemodilution patients died or required urgent transplantation. Survival rate curves did not differ significantly between the 2 groups, but patients with hemodilution tended to have worse outcomes than those with anemia only. However, the difference in adverse events between the 2 groups was significant (Fig 2).

Conclusions.—The clinical outcome for patients with CHF who also have anemia and hemodilution is poorer than that noted for patients with true anemia alone. Active correction is required to avoid adverse events, such as death or need for urgent transplantation. The volume overload may serve as an important mechanism contributing to the worse outcome.

▶ Hemodilution and true anemia are commonly observed in patients with advanced heart failure and appear to be risk factors for adverse patient outcomes.[1,2] When found in patients with CHF, both conditions should be actively corrected.[3] Improved nutrition and vitamin supplementation with or without erythropoietin[4] should be used to treat true anemia and aggressive CHF therapy used to address hypervolemia and hemodilution.

W. H. Frishman, MD

References

1. McClellan W, Flanders W, Langston R, et al: Anemia and renal insufficiency are independent risk factors for death among patients with congestive heart failure admitted to community hospitals: A population based study. *J Am Soc Nephrol* 13:1928-1936, 2002.
2. Horwich T, Fonarow G, Hamilton M, et al: Anemia is associated with worse symptoms, greater impairment in functional capacity and a significant increase in mortality in patients with advanced heart failure. *J Am Coll Cardiol* 39:2780-2786, 2002.
3. LeJemtel TH, Sonnenblick EH, Frishman WH: Diagnosis and medical management of heart failure, in Fuster V, Alexander RW, O'Rourke RA, et al (eds): *Hurst's The Heart*, ed 11. New York, McGraw Hill, 2004.
4. Silverberg D, Wexler D, Sheps D, et al: The use of subcutaneous erythropoietin and intravenous iron for the treatment of anemia of severe, resistant, congestive heart failure improves cardiac and renal function and functional cardiac class and markedly reduces hospitalization. *J Am Coll Cardiol* 35:1737-1744, 2000.

Eplerenone, a Selective Aldosterone Blocker, in Patients With Left Ventricular Dysfunction After Myocardial Infarction
Pitt B, for the Eplerenone Post-Acute Myocardial Infarction Heart Failure Efficacy and Survival Study Investigators (Univ of Michigan, Ann Arbor; et al)
N Engl J Med 348:1309-1321, 2003   53–2

Background.—Aldosterone blockade decreases mortality and morbidity rates for patients with severe heart failure. It also prevents ventricular remodeling and collagen formation in patients with left ventricular (LV) dysfunction after acute myocardial infarction (AMI); its role in decreasing hospitalization rate and mortality rate in these patients is unknown. The Eplerenone Post-Acute Myocardial Infarction Heart Failure Efficacy and Survival Study (EPHESUS) is a multicenter, international, randomized, double-blind, placebo-controlled investigation. Whether eplerenone, a selective aldosterone blocker, has an influence on morbidity and mortality rates for patients with AMI complicated by LV dysfunction and heart failure was investigated.

Methods.—The study included patients from 674 centers in 37 countries who were evaluated between December 27, 1999 and December 31, 2001. Patients were selected randomly to treatment with either eplerenone (25 mg/day initially, titrated to a maximum of 50 mg/day; n = 3313) or placebo (n = 3319) in addition to optimal medical treatment. The primary end points were time to death from any cause, time to death from cardiovascular cause, and first hospitalization for a cardiovascular event (heart failure, AMI, stroke, or ventricular arrhythmia).

Results.—At a mean follow-up of 16 months, 478 deaths occurred in the eplerenone group and 554 deaths in the placebo group (relative risk [RR],

0.85; 95% confidence interval [CI], 0.75-0.96; P = .008). In the eplerenone and placebo groups, cardiovascular causes resulted in 407 and 483 deaths, respectively, (RR, 0.83; 95% CI, 0.72-0.94; P = .005). The death rate from cardiovascular cause or hospitalization for cardiovascular events was significantly decreased in the eplerenone group (RR, 0.87; 95% CI, 0.79-0.95; P = .002), as was death from any cause or any hospitalization (RR, 0.92; 95% CI, 0.86-0.98; P = .02) (Fig 1). In addition, the rate of sudden death from cardiac causes was also significantly decreased (RR, 0.79; 95% CI, 0.64-0.97; P = .03). The incidence of serious hyperkalemia was 5.5% and

FIGURE 1

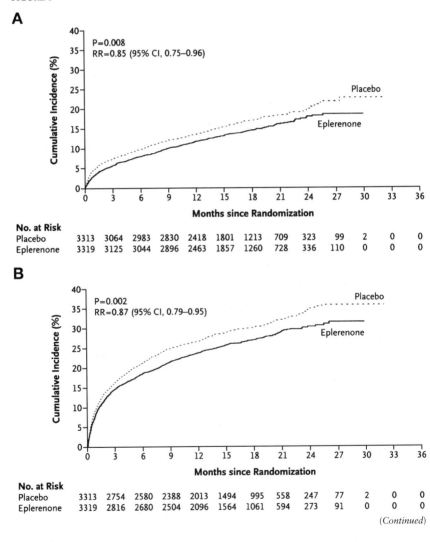

(*Continued*)

FIGURE 1 (cont.)

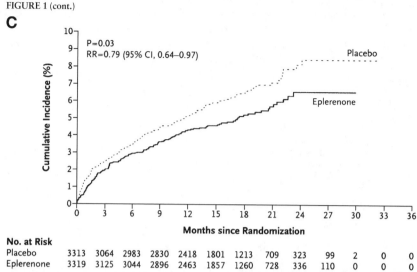

C

FIGURE 1.—Kaplan-Meier estimates of the rate of death from any cause. *Abbreviations: RR*, Relative risk; CI, confidence interval.(Reprinted by permission of *The New England Journal of Medicine* from Pitt, B for the Eplerenone Post-Acute Myocardial Infarction Heart Failure Efficacy And Survival Study investigators: Eplerenone, a selective aldosterone blocker, in patients with left ventricular dysfunction after myocardial infarction. *N Engl J Med* 248:1309-1321, 2003. Copyright 2003, Massachusetts Medical Society. All rights reserved.)

3.9% in the eplerenone and placebo groups, respectively, ($P = .002$), and the rate of hypokalemia was 8.4% and 13.1%, respectively ($P < .001$).

Conclusion.—The addition of eplerenone to optimal medical therapy decreases morbidity and mortality rates for patients with AMI complicated by LV dysfunction and heart failure.

▶ Inhibition of aldosterone with spironolactone[1] or eplerenone in addition to standard medical therapy appears to reduce morbidity and mortality in patients with LV dysfunction and heart failure. Eplerenone is a more specific aldosterone blocker and is associated with less gynecomastia than spironolactone.[2] Eplerenone was recently approved for clinical use in patients with congestive heart failure and in patients with hypertension. Angiotensin-converting enzyme (ACE) inhibition and angiotensin receptor blockade (ARB) do not completely suppress aldosterone production and activity, which may explain why aldosterone antagonism provides additional benefit in heart failure patients. Aldosterone inhibition also provides other pharmacologic benefits related to the prevention of myocardial fibrosis, an action unrelated to its effects on the kidney.[2] Standard therapy for symptoms of heart failure and LV dysfunction now includes an ACE inhibitor with or without an ARB, a loop diuretic and an aldosterone antagonist, and a β-adrenergic blocker with or without digoxin. Clinicians should be aware of the risk of hyperkalemia with this combination regimen, especially in patients with concomitant renal disease.

Other pharmacologic therapies under investigation for the treatment of congestive heart failure include vasopressin antagonists[3,4] and drugs that block both angiotensin and natriuretic peptide activity.[5,6] Treatment with the monoclonal antibody infliximab in patients with moderate to severe heart failure was shown to have no benefit on clinical outcomes.[7]

W. H. Frishman, MD

References

1. Pitt B, Zannad F, Remme WJ, et al: The effect of spironolactone on morbidity and mortality in patients with severe heart failure. *N Engl J Med* 341:709-717, 1999.
2. Stier CT Jr, Koenig S, Lee DY, et al: Aldosterone and aldosterone antagonism in cardiovascular disease: Focus on eplerenone (Inspra). *Heart Dis* 5:102-118, 2003.
3. Gheorghiade M, for the Tolvaptan Investigators: Vasopressin V$_2$-receptor blockade with tolvaptan in patients with chronic heart failure: Results from a double-blind, randomized trial. *Circulation* 107:2690-2696, 2003.
4. Frishman WH, Klapholz M, Acharya N, et al: Vasopressin and vasopressin-receptor antagonists in the treatment of cardiovascular disease, in Frishman WH, Sonnenblick EH, Sica DA (eds): *Cardiovascular Pharmacotherapeutics*, ed 2. New York, McGraw Hill, 2003; pp 601-616.
5. Frishman WH, Nawarskas J, Rajan V, et al: Vasopeptidase inhibitors: Neutral endopeptidase inhibitors and dual inhibitors of angiotensin-converting enzyme and neutral endopeptidase, in Frishman WH, Sonnenblick EH, Sica DA (eds): *Cardiovascular Pharmacotherapeutics*, ed 2. New York, McGraw Hill, 2003, pp 813-820.
6. LeJemtel TH, Sonnenblick EH, Frishman WH: Diagnosis and medical management of heart failure, in Fuster V, Alexander RW, O'Rourke RA, et al (eds): *Hurst's The Heart*, ed 11. New York, McGraw Hill, 2004.
7. Chung ES, for the ATTACH Investigators: Randomized, double-blind, placebo-controlled, pilot trial of infliximab, a chimeric monoclonal antibody to tumor necrosis factor-α, in patients with moderate-to-severe heart failure: Results of the Anti-TNF Therapy Against Congestive Heart Failure (ATTACH) Trial. *Circulation* 107:3133-3140, 2003.

Plasma Homocysteine and Risk for Congestive Heart Failure in Adults Without Prior Myocardial Infarction
Vasan RS, Beiser A, D'Agostino RB, et al (Framingham Heart Study, Mass; Boston Univ; Beth Israel Beaconess Med Ctr, Boston; et al)
JAMA 289:1251-1257, 2003   53-3

Background.—Among the risk factors already identified for congestive heart failure (CHF) are advancing age, myocardial infarction (MI), hypertension, valvular disease, diabetes mellitus, and obesity. A major vascular disease risk factor recently identified is plasma homocysteine, with increased levels linked to a greater risk of atherosclerotic sequelae, such as cardiovascular mortality, coronary heart disease, and stroke. It was hypothesized that the risk of CHF would be greater for patients with increased plasma homocysteine levels. This hypothesis was tested in a community-based sample of adults who had no previous MI.

Methods.—The study included 2491 adults with a mean age of 72 years. All had participated in the Framingham Heart Study during the examinations held in 1979-1982 and 1986-1990; none had CHF or previous MI at baseline. The incidence of experiencing a first episode of CHF was the main outcome measure; the follow-up was 8 years.

Results.—Hyperhomocysteinemia was found in 23% of women and 28% of men at baseline. CHF developed in 156 subjects. A dramatically higher crude cumulative incidence of CHF was noted in patients in the top 2 homocysteine quartiles than in patients in the lower 2 quartiles. Twenty-eight of the 88 women and 23 of the 68 men with incident cases of CHF experienced MI before CHF developed. The risk of CHF increased about 25% among men and 49% among women per quartile increment in the plasma homocysteine level. For women, the CHF risk increased at the second plasma homocysteine quartile, with an additional increase at the top quartile. For men, CHF risk increased only beyond the second quartile of plasma homocysteine. For both men and women, increased plasma homocysteine levels were predictive of CHF.

Conclusions.—Increased plasma homocysteine level was an independent predictor of risk for developing CHF in adults who had no previous MI.

▶ Elevated homocysteine levels appear to be an important risk factor for developing CHF, even in the absence of clinical coronary artery disease. The mechanism for homocysteine causing heart failure is not known.[1] At this juncture, awaiting results of future clinical trials, it is best to recommend vitamin therapy with folic acid alone, or in combination with pyridoxine and vitamin B12 for patients with symptomatic CHF or in those at risk of its development.[2,3]

W. H. Frishman, MD

References

1. Kruger NA, Frishman WH, Hussain J: Fish oils, the B vitamins, and folic acid as cardiovascular protective agents, in Frishman WH, Sonnenblick EH, Sica DA (eds): *Cardiovascular Pharmacotherapeutics* ed 2. New York, McGraw Hill, 2003, pp 381-405.
2. LeJemtel TH, Sonnenblick EH, Frishman WH: Diagnosis and management of heart failure, in Fuster V, Alexander RW, O'Rourke RA, et al (eds): *Hurst's The Heart* ed 11. New York, McGraw Hill, in press.
3. Jacques PF, Selhub J, Bostom AG, et al: The effect of folic acid fortification on plasma folate and total homocysteine concentrations. *N Engl J Med* 340:1449-1454, 1999.

Combined Cardiac Resynchronization and Implantable Cardioversion Defibrillation in Advanced Chronic Heart Failure: The MIRACLE ICD Trial
Young JB, for the Multicenter InSync ICD Randomized Clinical Evaluation (MIRACLE ICD) Trial Investigators (Cleveland Clinic Found, Ohio; et al)
JAMA 289:2685-2694, 2003

53–4

Background.—Cardiac resynchronization therapy (CRT) by means of biventricular pacing is an effective approach for treatment of heart failure in patients with a wide QRS interval. However, few data are available regarding outcomes for patients requiring CRT and implantable cardioverter defibrillator (ICD) therapy. The hypotheses that patients with moderate to severe symptoms of heart failure, a wide QRS interval, and an established indication for an ICD would benefit from CRT, and that the use of CRT would not be proarrhythmic nor compromise ICD therapy were investigated.

Methods.—The efficacy and safety of combined CRT and ICD therapy were determined in 369 patients with New York Heart Association (NYHA) class III or IV congestive heart failure, despite appropriate medical management. About one half of the group (n = 182) served as control patients (ICD activated, CRT off). The remaining 187 patients comprised the CRT group (ICD on, CRT on). The main outcome measures were changes between baseline and 6 months in quality of life (QOL), functional class, and distance covered during a 6-minute walk. Additional outcome measures included changes in exercise capacity, plasma neurohormones, left ventricular function, and overall heart failure status. In addition, survival rates, incidence of ventricular arrhythmias, and rates of hospitalization were compared between the 2 groups.

Results.—Patients in the CRT group demonstrated a greater improvement at 6 months in median QOL score and functional class than control patients but were no different from the control group in the change in distance walked in 6 minutes. The peak oxygen consumption was increased by 1.1 mL/kg per minute in the CRT group versus 0.1 mL/kg per minute in the control patients. However, the duration of treadmill exercise increased by a median 56 seconds in the CRT group and decreased by 11 seconds in the control group. No significant differences between the groups were noted in changes in left ventricular size or function, overall heart failure status, and hospitalization and survival rates. No proarrhythmia was observed, and arrhythmia termination capabilities were not compromised.

Conclusions.—Cardiac resynchronization for patients with appropriate pre-existing and continuing vigorous medical management improved the QOL, functional status, and exercise capacity for patients with moderate to severe heart failure, a wide QRS interval, and life-threatening arrhythmias, without interfering with ICD function.

▶ In addition to standard medical therapy, CRT using biventricular pacing in patients with congestive heart failure and a wide ECG QRS interval (a cause of cardiac dyssynchrony) improves quality of life, functional capacity, and exercise performance.[1,2] It was recently shown that CRT leads to improved systolic and diastolic function, and decreased mitral regurgitation.[3] Improved left ventricular remodeling also appears to contribute to the symptomatic benefits of CRT.[3]

Pacing has also been used to treat children having right bundle branch block and right ventricular failure.[4] Right-sided atrioventricular pacing was shown to augment right ventricular and systemic performance.

W. H. Frishman, MD

References

1. LeJemtel TH, Sonnenblick EH, Frishman WH: Diagnosis and medical management of heart failure, in Fuster V, Alexander RW, O'Rourke RA, et al (eds): *Hurst's The Heart*, ed 11. New York, McGraw Hill, 2004.
2. Abraham WT, Hayes DL: Cardiac resynchronization therapy for heart failure. *Circulation* 108:2596-2603, 2003.
3. St. John Sutton MG, Plappert T, Abraham WT, et al for the MIRACLE Study Group: Effect of cardiac resynchronization therapy on left ventricular size and function in chronic heart failure. *Circulation* 107:1985-1990, 2003.
4. Dubin AM, Feinstein JA, Reddy M, et al: Electrical resynchronization: A novel therapy for the failing right ventricle. *Circulation* 107:2287-2289, 2003.

Cardiovascular Effects of Continuous Positive Airway Pressure in Patients With Heart Failure and Obstructive Sleep Apnea

Kaneko Y, Floras JS, Usui K, et al (Toronto Rehabilitation Inst; Toronto Gen Hosp; Univ of Toronto)

N Engl J Med 348:1233-1241, 2003   53–5

Introduction.—Obstructive sleep apnea (OSA) is correlated with significantly increased odds of having heart failure. Recurrent OSA disrupts sleep and subjects the heart to periods of hypoxia, exaggerated negative intrathoracic pressure, and bursts of sympathetic activity provoking surges in blood pressure and heart rate. Twenty-four patients with depressed left ventricular ejection fraction (LVEF) (45% or less) and OSA who were receiving optimal medical treatment for heart failure were evaluated in a randomized controlled trial.

Methods.—All patients underwent polysomnography. On the next morning, their blood pressure (BP) and heart rate were determined by means of digital photoplethysmography, and left ventricular dimensions and LVEF were determined by means of echocardiography. Patients were randomly assigned to medical therapy either alone (controls) or with the addition of continuous positive airway pressure (CPAP) for 1 month. The assessment protocol was repeated after therapy.

Results.—In control subjects, there were no significant changes in the severity of OSA, daytime BP, heart rate, left ventricular end-systolic dimension, or LVEF during the evaluation period. In the CPAP group, markedly decreased OSA decreased the daytime systolic blood pressure (SBP) from a mean of 126 mm Hg to 116 mm Hg ($P = .02$), decreased the heart rate (HR) from 68 to 64 beats per minute ($P = .007$), decreased the left ventricular end-systolic dimension from 54.5 to 51.7 mm ($P = .009$), and improved the LVEF from 25.0 to 33.8% ($P < .001$) (Figs 1 and 2).

Conclusion.—In medically treated patients with heart failure, the treatment of coexisting obstructive sleep apnea with CPAP decreases SBP and improves left ventricular systolic function. Physicians need to be aware that OSA may have an adverse pathophysiologic role in heart failure that can be addressed via targeted therapy. Routine screening for sleep apnea may be important in patients with heart failure.

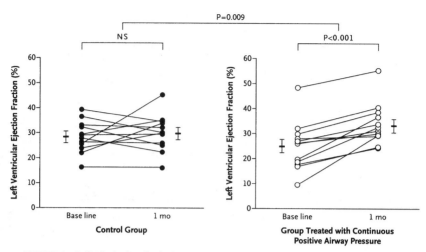

FIGURE 1.—Individual values for the lVEF in all patients. In the control group, there was no significant change in the LVEF from baseline to 1 month (from a mean [±SE] of 28.5% ± 1.8% to 30.0% ± 2.1%). In contrast, the LVEF increased in all 12 subjects treated with CPAP, and the mean increase was significant (from 25.0% ± 2.8% to 33.8% ± 2.4%, P < .001). The change in the LVEF from baseline to 1 month was significantly greater in the group treated with CPAP than in the control group (8.8% ± 1.6% vs 1.5% ± 2.3%, P = .009). The 1 patient in the group that received CPAP who had a baseline LVEF of 48% met the pretrial screening eligibility criterion (the LVEF was 39%). *Short horizontal lines and I bars are means ± SE. Abbreviations: LVEF,* Left ventricular ejection fraction; *CPAP,* continuous positive airway pressure; *NS,* not significant. (Reprinted by permission of *The New England Journal of Medicine* from Kaneko Y, Floras JS, Usui K, et al: Cardiovascular effects of continuous positive airway pressure in patients with heart failure and obstructive sleep apnea. *N Engl J Med* 348:1233-1241, 2003. Copyright 2003, Massachusetts Medical Society. All rights reserved.)

▶ CPAP therapy has been used for advanced heart failure with improvements shown in both ventricular performance and neurohormonal activation.[1] The patients who get the most benefit appear to be those having OSA.[2] Sleep apnea has been reported to occur in up to one third of patients with heart failure.[3] It is suggested that routine screening for sleep apnea in heart failure patients might identify patients who would benefit from CPAP. However, a less involved methodology than polysomnography in a sleep laboratory will need to be used as a cost-effective screening tool.

W. H. Frishman, MD

References

1. Midelton GT, Frishman WH, Passo SS: Congestive heart failure and continuous positive airway pressure therapy: Support of a new modality for improving the prognosis and survival of patients with advanced congestive heart failure. *Heart Dis* 4:102-109, 2002.
2. Sin DD, Logan AG, Fitzgerald FS, et al: Effects of continuous positive airway pressure on cardiovascular outcomes in heart failure patients with and without Cheyne-Stokes respiration. *Circulation* 102:61-66, 2000.
3. Sin DD, Fitzgerald F, Parker JD, et al: Risk factors for central and obstructive sleep apnea in 450 men and women with congestive heart failure. *Am J Respir Crit Care Med* 160:1101-1106, 1999.

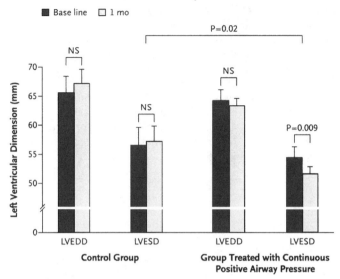

FIGURE 2.—Mean (±SE) changes in left ventricular dimensions. There were no significant changes in LVEDD or LVESD during the study period in the control group (LVEDD changed from 65.6 ± 2.8 mm to 67.2 ± 2.4 mm, and LVESD from 56.6 ± 3.0 mm to 57.3 ± 2.5 mm). In the group treated with CPAP, there was no significant change in LVEDD during the study period (LVEDD changed from 64.3 ± 1.8 mm to 63.4 ± 1.8 mm). However, there was a significant reduction in LVESD (from 54.5 ± 1.8 mm to 51.7 ± 1.2 mm, P = .009). The change in LVESD from baseline to 1 month was significantly greater in the group that received CPAP than in the control group (−2.8 ± 1.1 mm vs 0.7 ± 0.8 mm, P = .02). *Abbreviations: LVEDD,* Left ventricular end-diastolic dimension; *LVESD,* left ventricular end-systolic dimension; *CPAP,* continuous positive airway pressure; *NS,* not significant. (Reprinted by permission of *The New England Journal of Medicine* from Kaneko Y, Floras JS, Usui K, et al: Cardiovascular effects of continuous positive airway pressure in patients with heart failure and obstructive sleep apnea. N Engl J Med 348:1233-1241, 2003. Copyright 2003, Massachusetts Medical Society. All rights reserved.)

▶ Just think: a nonpharmacologic treatment for congestive heart failure that is cheap and has minimal side effects! Heart failure is a prevalent and expensive condition with high morbidity and mortality. Patients with heart failure have high rates of both OSA and central sleep apnea; it is likely that OSA is the cause of the heart failure, and central sleep apnea is the result.[1,2] No matter; CPAP is highly effective treatment for both![3,4]

This is the first controlled study to demonstrate that nocturnal CPAP significantly improves the daytime cardiac function of optimally treated heart failure patients. It also demonstrates a dramatic (10 mm Hg) fall in daytime SBP and HR, suggesting that reduced afterload is 1 likely mechanism of its beneficial effect.

It is notable that these patients were not very sleepy; no one had an Epworth Sleepiness Score of over 10, which is thought to be the cut-off range for normal. Yet they wore CPAP anyway and benefited significantly. In addition to improving cardiac function and reducing sleepiness, CPAP can lower blood pressure,[5] improve daytime cognition,[6] reduce car wrecks,[7] improve quality of life,[8] and reduce health care costs.[9] Yet the vast majority of patients with OSA are probably not being treated.[10] There are many barriers to treatment of sleep apnea, including limited access to sleep testing, the requirement to spend 1 or 2 nights in the sleep laboratory, third-party payers, and lack of awareness both by patients and by physicians.

With the growing body of evidence that sleep apnea causes significant cardiovascular morbidity and mortality and that treatment with CPAP can reduce this health burden, it is becoming increasingly difficult to justify the delays and cost of our current approach to sleep apnea diagnosis. This is especially true since many cases of sleep apnea can be diagnosed with simple clinical tools such as a history, physical examination, and questionnaires![11-18] As awareness grows, it is likely that careful clinical evaluation, home monitoring, and autotitrating (or "smart") CPAP will improve access and patient convenience. In the meantime, we owe it to our patients to look for this very treatable condition.

B. A. Phillips, MD, MSPH

References

1. Sin DD, Fitzgerald F, Parker JD, et al: Risk factors for central and obstructive sleep apnea in 450 men and women with congestive heart failure. *Am J Respir Crit Care Med* 160:1101-1106, 1999.
2. Javaheri S, Parker TJ, Liming JD, et al: Sleep apnea in 81 ambulatory male patients with stable heart failure: Types and their prevalences, consequences, and presentations. *Circulation* 97:2154-2159, 1998.
3. Malone S, Liu PP, Holloway R, et al: Obstructive sleep apnoea in patients with dilated cardiomyopathy: Effects of continuous positive airway pressure. *Lancet* 338:1480-1484, 1991.
4. Naughton MT, Liu PP, Bernard DC, et al: Treatment of congestive heart failure and Cheyne-Stokes respiration during sleep by continuous positive airway pressure. *Am J Respir Crit Care Med* 151:92-97, 1995.
5. Pepperell JCT, Ramdassingh-Dow S, Crosthwaite N, et al: Ambulatory blood pressure after therapeutic and subtherapeutic nasal continuous positive airway pressure for obstructive sleep apnoea: A randomised parallel trial. *Lancet* 359:204-214, 2002.
6. Bardwell WA, Ancoli-Israel S, Berry CC, et al: Neuropsychological effects of one-week continuous positive airway pressure treatment in patients with obstructive sleep apnea: A placebo-controlled study. *Psychosom Med* 63:579-584, 2001.
7. Findley L, Smith C, Hooper J, et al: Treatment with nasal CPAP decreases automobile accidents in patients with sleep apnea. *Am J Respir Crit Care Med* 161:857-859, 2000.
8. Sanner BM, Klewer J, Trumm A, et al: Long-term treatment with continuous positive airway pressure improves quality of life in obstructive sleep apnoea syndrome. *Eur Respir J* 16:118-122, 2000.
9. Bahammam A, Delaive K, Ronald J, et al: Health care utilization in males with obstructive sleep apnea syndrome two years after diagnosis and treatment. *Sleep* 22:740-747, 1999.
10. Kapur V, Strohl KP, Redline S, et al: Underdiagnosis of sleep apnea syndrome in U.S. communities. *Sleep Breath* 6:49-54, 2002.
11. Maislin G, Pack AI, Kribbs NB, et al: A survey screen for prediction of apnea. *Sleep* 18:158-166, 1995.
12. Crocker BD, Olson LG, Saunders NA, et al: Estimation of the probability of disturbed breathing during sleep before a sleep study. *Am Rev Respir Dis* 142:14-18, 1990.
13. Flemons WW, Whitelaw WA, Brant R, et al: Likelihood ratios for a sleep apnea clinical prediction rule. *Am J Respir Crit Care Med* 150:1279-1285, 1994.
14. Viner S, Szalai JP, Hoffstein V: Are history and physical examination a good screening test for sleep apnea? *Ann Intern Med* 115:356-359, 1991.

15. Rowley JA, Aboussouan LS, Badr S: The use of clinical prediction formulae in the evaluation of obstructive sleep apnea. *Sleep* 23:929-938, 2000.
16. Kushida CA, Efron B, Guilleminault C: A predictive morphometric model for the obstructive sleep apnea syndrome. *Ann Intern Med* 127:581-587, 1997.
17. Netzer NC, Stoohs RA, Netzer CM, et al: Using the Berlin Questionnaire to identify patients at risk for the sleep apnea syndrome. *Ann Intern Med* 131:485-491, 1999.
18. Mallampati SR, Gatt SP, Gugino LD, et al: A clinical sign to predict difficult tracheal intubation: A prospective study. *Can Anaesth Soc J* 32:429-434, 1985.

Transendocardial, Autologous Bone Marrow Cell Transplantation for Severe, Chronic Ischemic Heart Failure

Perin EC, Dohmann HF, Borojevic R, et al (Texas Heart Inst, Houston; Hosp Procardiaco, Rio de Janeiro, Brazil; Federal Univ, Rio de Janeiro, Brazil; et al)
Circulation 107:2294-2302, 2003   53–6

Background.—Because native angiogenesis cannot prevent remodeling after a significant injury to the heart, infarct-related heart failure is a major contributor to morbidity and mortality rates. In stem cell therapy investigation, pluripotential cells have exhibited the potential to differentiate into cardiomyocytes and endothelial cells, and pluripotential cells from bone marrow have improved myocardial function and perfusion in ischemic heart disease in animal models. The safety of endocardial bone marrow mononuclear cell (BMMNC) injections was determined, and the ability of endocardial injections of autologous BMMNCs (ABMMNCs) to promote neovascularization and overcome failure of the natural myocardial healing processes was assessed.

Methods.—The study included 14 patients who served as the treatment group and 7 as a control group in a prospective nonrandomized open-label study. At baseline, complete clinical and laboratory evaluations were done, and patients underwent exercise stress, 2-dimensional (2D) Doppler echocardiograms, single-photo emission CT (SPECT) perfusion scan, and 24-hour Holter monitoring. Mononuclear cells were harvested from the bone marrow, isolated, washed, and resuspended in saline solution for injection; 15 injections of 0.2 mL each were given (Fig 2). Viable myocardium was identified using electromechanical mapping (EMM). Follow-up evaluations were noninvasive at 2 months, and treatment patients had a 4-month invasive follow-up evaluation, with the same procedures used as at baseline.

Results.—The mapping and injection required a total mean time of 81 minutes. No major periprocedural complications developed, and all patients were discharged the third hospital day. At 2 months, serum creatinine levels were significantly increased in the control group in comparison to those in the treatment group, and the brain natriuretic peptide (BNP) levels trended toward increased differences between the 2 groups, with an increase in levels in the control group. Less heart failure and fewer anginal symptoms were reported by the treatment group. Significant differences were found in the end-systolic volume (ESV), end-diastolic volume (EDV), and left ventricular ejection fraction (LVEF) measures between the 2 groups at 2 months, with

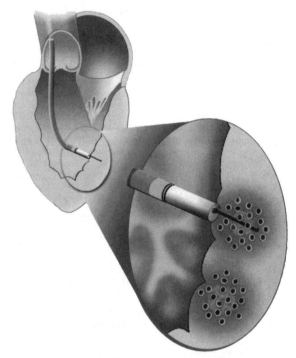

FIGURE 2.—Injection catheter advanced into the left ventricle through the aortic valve. The catheter tip is placed against the endocardial surface (*insert*) with the needle extended into the myocardium delivering ABMMNCs. *Abbreviation: ABMMNC,* Autologous bone marrow mononuclear cell. (Courtesy of Perin EC, Dohmann HF, Borojevic R, et al: Transendocardial, autologous bone marrow cell transplantation for severe, chronic ischemic heart failure. *Circulation* 107:2294-2302, 2003.)

the control group having smaller LV volumes and trending toward higher baseline ejection fractions. Cardiac function increased 6% in the treatment group, and it decreased in the control group. A significant reduction in ESV values was noted among treatment patients. A 73% reduction in the total reversible defect was also found in the treatment group, but no change was noted in the control patients. At 4 months, LVEF showed a sustained improvement from baseline, increasing from 20% to 29% in the treatment group. ESV was reduced, and EDV remained unchanged. The injected segments showed significant improvement in mechanical function, as illustrated by EMM.

Conclusions.—The use of intramyocardial injections of bone marrow-derived stem cells was found to be relatively safe for humans with severe heart failure. Myocardial blood flow may be improved and regional and global LV function enhanced.

▶ There is now a growing body of data to suggest that the heart has the ability to regenerate itself in response to tissue injury.[1] Recently, a pluripotent cardiac stem cell has been identified with the capacity to regenerate myocardial cells, connective tissue, and vascular tissue in the heart. Other innovative strategies include the injection of pluripotent bone marrow cells[2-7] and skeletal myoblasts[8] to achieve cardiac repair in acute myocardial injury and in chronic heart failure. These approaches may also have value in reversing the effects of cardiac aging and lengthening the natural life span of the human myocardium.

W. H. Frishman, MD

References

1. Beltrami AP, Barlucci L, Torella D, et al: Adult cardiac stem cells are multipotent and support myocardial regeneration. *Cell* 114:763-776, 2003.
2. Orlic D, Kajstura J, Chimenti S, et al: Bone marrow cells regenerate infarcted myocardium. *Nature* 410:701-705, 2001.
3. Saito T, Kuang J-Q, Lin CCH, et al: Transcoronary implantation of bone marrow stromal cells ameliorates cardiac function after myocardial infarction. *J Thorac Cardiovasc Surg* 126:114-123, 2003.
4. Kocher AA, Schuster MD, Szabolcs MJ, et al: Neovascularization of ischemic myocardium by human bone marrow-derived angioblasts prevents cardiomyocyte apoptosis, reduces remodeling and improves cardiac function. *Nat Med* 7:430-436, 2001.
5. Strauer BE, Brehm M, Zeus T, et al: Repair of infarcted myocardium by autologous intracoronary mononuclear bone marrow cell transplantation in humans. *Circulation* 106:1913-1918, 2002.
6. Assmus B, Schächinger V, Teupe C, et al: Transplantation of progenitor cells and regeneration enhancement in acute myocardial infarction (TOPCARE-AMI). *Circulation* 106:3009-3017, 2002.
7. Frishman WH, Anversa P: Stem cell therapy for myocardial regeneration: The future is now. *Heart Dis* 4:205, 2002.
8. Borenstein N, Bruneval P, Hekmati M, et al: Noncultured, autologous, skeletal muscle cells can successfully engraft into ovine myocardium. *Circulation* 107:3088-3092, 2003.

54 Valvular Heart Disease

Complicated Left-Sided Native Valve Endocarditis in Adults: Risk Classification for Mortality
Hasbun R, Vikram HR, Barakat LA, et al (Tulane Univ, New Orleans, La; Hosp of St Raphael, New Haven, Conn; Griffin Hosp, Derby, Conn)
JAMA 289:1933-1940, 2003   54–1

Introduction.—Patients with native valve endocarditis associated with complications that are likely to have an adverse effect on their prognosis may benefit from valve surgery. Management decisions in such cases are difficult, however, because of a lack of valid data. To facilitate individual treatment decisions, a retrospective observational cohort study sought to classify patients according to mortality risk.

Methods.—Research patients were identified through a review of medical records at 7 Connecticut hospitals. Patients with complicated left-sided native valve endocarditis were divided into derivation and validation cohorts. The derivation cohort consisted of 259 patients older than 16 who were diagnosed at 1 of 5 hospitals serving New Haven, West Haven, and Bridgeport, Conn, from January 1990 to January 2000. Included in the validation cohort were 254 patients diagnosed at 2 hospitals serving Hartford, Conn, during the same period. Items analyzed were baseline clinical information, comorbid conditions, laboratory and imaging studies, and type and duration of therapy. The primary outcome was all-cause mortality at 6 months after baseline.

Results.—The 6-month mortality rates were similar in the 2 cohorts: 25% in the derivation cohort and 24% in the validation cohort. Five baseline features were independently associated with 6-month mortality: comorbidity, abnormal mental status, moderate to severe congestive heart failure, bacterial cause other than viridans streptococci, and medical therapy without valve surgery. With the use of these features, a prognostic classification system was developed. Point scores were assigned to each feature, and quartiles of risk for 6-month mortality determined for the derivation cohort (≤6 points, 7-11 points, 12-15 points, and >15 points). Six-month mortality risks for these quartiles were, respectively, 5%, 15%, 31%, and 59%. Risks were similar in the validation cohort: 7%, 19%, 32%, and 69%, respectively.

Conclusion.—In patients with complicated left-sided native valve endocarditis, baseline clinical data can be used to provide an accurate prognostic classification of 6-month mortality risk. Such a system might aid in management decisions.

▶ Left-sided native valve endocarditis still remains a major problem, despite the availability of both antibiotics and open heart surgery.[1] Surgery is becoming a more important treatment modality and the identification of these patients who would benefit the most from an operative procedure is a clinical challenge. Echocardiography has provided a major advance in diagnosis, prognostication, and therapeutic decision making, with the ability to assess valvular and ventricular function and both the presence and size of valvular vegetations.

W. H. Frishman, MD

Reference

1. Frishman WH, Shazer RL, Naseer N, et al: Infective endocarditis and rheumatic fever, in Frishman WH, Sonnenblick EH, Sica DA (eds): *Cardiovascular Pharmacotherapeutics Manual*, ed 5. New York, McGraw Hill, 2004, pp 554-585.

Nitroprusside in Critically Ill Patients With Left Ventricular Dysfunction and Aortic Stenosis
Khot UN, Novaro GM, Popović ZB, et al (Indiana Heart Physicians, Indianapolis; Cleveland Clinic Florida, Weston; Cleveland Clinic Foundation, Ohio)
N Engl J Med 348:1756-1763, 2003   54–2

Introduction.—Vasodilator therapy is used increasingly in the management of left ventricular dysfunction, but it has been viewed as contraindicated, despite a lack of supporting data, in patients with severe aortic stenosis. The Use of Nitroprusside in Left Ventricular Dysfunction and Obstructive Aortic Valve Disease (UNLOAD) Study prospectively investigated the use of this potent IV vasodilator in critically ill patients with congestive heart failure and severe aortic stenosis.

Methods.—Eligible patients were undergoing invasive hemodynamic monitoring of heart failure in the ICU. All had depressed left ventricular function, a depressed cardiac index, and severe aortic stenosis. Hypotension was an exclusion criterion, but coexisting valve disease and coronary artery disease were not. IV nitroprusside was administered to 25 patients in a dose titrated to produce a mean arterial pressure between 60 and 70 mm Hg. After approximately 6 and 24 hours of nitroprusside infusion, the patients' heart rate, blood pressure, and hemodynamic variables were recorded and compared with baseline values.

Results.—The mean baseline values were 0.21 for ejection fraction, 0.6 cm² for aortic valve area (with peak and mean gradients of 65 mm Hg and 39 mm Hg, respectively), and 1.60 L/min per square meter for the cardiac index. Six hours after the initiation of nitroprusside therapy (when the mean dose had increased to 103 µg/min), the mean cardiac index had increased to 2.22 L/min per square meter. A further increase to a mean of 2.52 L/min per square meter was recorded after 24 hours (when the mean dose was 128 µg/min). The cardiac index did not decrease in any patients during nitroprusside therapy (Fig 1), and the infusion was well tolerated. Nitroprusside was continued until surgery, conversion to medical maintenance therapy, or death. The overall 30-day survival rate in this critically ill patient group was 76%.

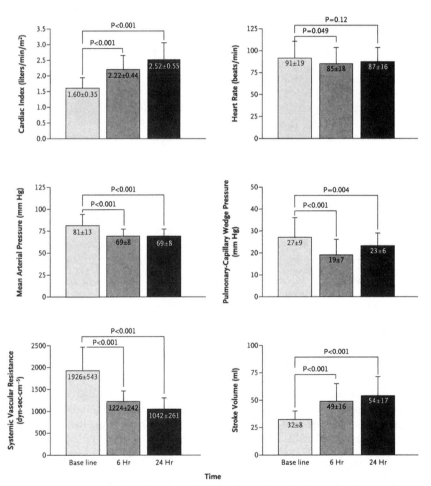

FIGURE 1.—Mean (±SD) Hemodynamic values at baseline and 6 and 24 hours after the start of nitroprusside infusion. (Reprinted by permission of *The New England Journal of Medicine* from Khot UN, Novaro GM, Popović ZB, et al: Nitroprusside in critically ill patients with left ventricular dysfunction and aortic stenosis. *N Engl J Med* 348:1756-1763, 2003. Copyright 2003, Massachusetts Medical Society. All rights reserved.)

Conclusion.—Nitroprusside therapy brought about a marked and rapid improvement in patients with severe aortic stenosis and left ventricular systolic dysfunction. The infusion provided a safe and effective bridge until patients could undergo aortic-valve replacement or receive effective oral vasodilator therapy.

▶ Patients with severe aortic stenosis and left ventricular dysfunction appear to benefit from the use of nitroprusside and/or IV inotropes such as dobutamine and milrinone. This approach can be used as a bridge to stabilize patients for aortic valve replacement.

In patients undergoing aortic valve replacement, there is often increased bleeding in the perioperative period. Recently it was shown that many patients with severe aortic stenosis have an acquired type IIA von Willebrand syndrome.[1] Proteolysis of von Willebrand factor as it passes through the stenotic valve is 1 of the proposed causes of the bleeding.[2] The bleeding dyscrasia is reversed by valve replacement[3] unless there is a mismatch between the patient and the valvular prosthesis.

Elevations in plasma natriuretic peptide are observed in patients with symptomatic aortic stenosis.[4] Measurement of natriuretic peptide has been found useful in assessing other cardiac conditions,[5] and in patients with aortic stenosis, can compliment the information gained from clinical assessment and echocardiography.

W. H. Frishman, MD

References

1. Vincentelli A, Susen S, Le Tourneau T, et al: Acquire von Willebrand syndrome in aortic stenosis. *N Engl J Med* 349:343-349, 2003.
2. Pareti FI, Lattuada A, Bressi C, et al: Proteolysis of von Willebrand factor and shear stress-induced platelet aggregation in patients with aortic valve stenosis. *Circulation* 102:1290-1295, 2000.
3. Anderson RP, McGrath K, Street A: Reversal of aortic stenosis, bleeding gastrointestinal angiodysplasia, and von Willebrand syndrome by aortic valve replacement. *Lancet* 347:689-690, 1996.
4. Gerber IL, Stewart RAH, Legget ME, et al: Increased plasma natriuretic peptide levels reflect symptom onset in aortic stenosis. *Circulation* 107:1884-1890, 2003.
5. Frishman WH, Sica DA, Cheng JWM, et al: Natriuretic and other vasoactive peptides, in Frishman WH, Sonnenblick EH, Sica DA (eds): *Cardiovascular Pharmacotherapeutics*, ed 2. New York, McGraw Hill, 2003, pp 451-477.

Effectiveness of Percutaneous Mechanical Mitral Commissurotomy Using the Metallic Commissurotome in Patients With Restenosis After Balloon or Previous Surgical Commissurotomy

Eltchaninoff H, Tron C, Cribier A (Univ of Rouen, France)

Am J Cardiol 91:425-428, 2003   54–3

Background.—The outcomes of balloon mitral valvuloplasty appear to be as or less effective after previous commissurotomy than after a first procedure. Percutaneous mechanical mitral commissurotomy (PMMC) is a new method untested in this patient subgroup. The safety and immediate outcomes of PMMC in a selected group of patients who had had previous commissurotomy were reported.

Methods.—One hundred seventy-three of 1175 patients (14.7%) had had previous commissurotomy. This group was older than those who had not had previous commissurotomy, mean ages being 40 and 35 years, respectively. The percentage of atrial fibrillation was higher in the former group, at 34%, than in the latter group, at 21%. In addition, the baseline transmitral gradient was lower and the echocardiographic Wilkins score higher in patients who had previous commissurotomy. The 2 groups were comparable in the baseline mitral valve area.

Findings.—Initial outcomes were judged to be satisfactory. Results were slightly less favorable after previous commissurotomy, the final mitral valve area being 2.01 cm² compared with 2.12 cm² in persons who had not had previous commissurotomy. Also, the residual transvalvular gradients in the 2 groups were 5 and 4.2 mm Hg, respectively. Procedural success and severe complication rates, at 93% and 4.7%, respectively, were similar in the 2 groups.

Conclusions.—PMMC appears to be safe and effective in patients with mitral restenosis after previous commissurotomy. The success rate in the current series was very high at 93%, the same as in patients who did not have previous commissurotomy. Outcomes were slightly but significantly less favorable in patients who had had the procedure previously.

▶ Balloon mitral valvuloplasty has become an important treatment modality for select patients having mitral stenosis, with results comparable to those observed with surgery.[1,2] In the past, the results with repeat valvuloplasty for restenosis were not as favorable as the initial procedure. However, with improved techniques, the repeat procedures are showing better results.

W. H. Frishman, MD

References

1. Iung B, Garbarz E, Michaud P, et al: Late results of percutaneous mitral commissurotomy in a series of 1024 patients. Analysis of late clinical deterioration: frequency, anatomic findings, and predictive factors. *Circulation* 99:3272-3278, 1999.
2. Farhat MB, Ayari M, Maatouk F, et al: Percutaneous balloon versus surgical closed and open mitral commissurotomy: Seven-year follow-up results of a randomized trial. *Circulation* 97:245-250, 1998.

55 Noninvasive Testing

Intravascular Ultrasound Analysis of Infarct-Related and Non–Infarct-Related Arteries in Patients Who Presented With an Acute Myocardial Infarction
Kotani J, Mintz GS, Castagna MT, et al (Washington Hosp Ctr, DC; Cardiovascular Research Foundation, New York)
Circulation 107:2889-2893, 2003   55–1

Introduction.—Earlier trials have reported diffuse destabilization of atherosclerotic plaques in patients with acute myocardial infarction (AMI). Intravascular ultrasound (IVUS) can examine vessel wall architecture and remodeling in a manner not feasible with angiography or angioscopy. The characteristics of the "culprit plaque" were compared with those of nonculprit plaques of both infarct-related artery (IRA) and non-IRA in patients with AMI.

Methods.—Between April 1997 and May 2000, IVUS was conducted in 2 or more native arteries in 38 patients (78 coronary arteries) within 1 week of onset of AMI. The IVUS analysis included qualitative and quantitative measurements of reference and lesion external elastic membrane (EEM), lumen, and plaque plus media (P&M) area. Positive remodeling was considered a lesion per mean reference EEM of more than 1.0. Culprit lesions were detected by a combination of ECG, wall motion abnormalities (ventriculogram or echogram), scintigraphic perfusion defects, and coronary angiogram.

Results.—Culprit lesions had more thrombus in culprit plaques than that in nonculprit plaques and non-IRA plaques (23.7% vs 3.4% and 3.1%; P = .0011). Culprit lesions were generally more hypoechoic (63.2% vs 37.9% and 28.1%, respectively; P = .0022). Culprit lesions were longer (17.5, vs 9.8, and 10.3 mm respectively; P < .0001), had a larger EEM area (15.0 vs 11.5, and 12.6 mm², respectively; P = .0353); a larger P&M area (13.0 mm² vs 7.5, and 9.3 mm², respectively; P < .0001), had smaller lumens (2.0 vs 4.1, and 3.4 mm², respectively; P = .0009) and more positive remodeling (79.4% vs 59.0% and 50.8%, respectively; P = .0155). The rate of plaque rupture/ dissection on multivessel imaging was greater in culprit, nonculprit IRA, and non-IRA plaques in patients with AMI, compared with that in a control group of patients with chronic stable angina.

Conclusion.—Culprit plaques have more markers of instability that are not typically seen elsewhere. This indicates that vascular events in patients with AMI are determined by local pre-event lesion morphologies.

▶ AMI is caused by a presumptive rupture of an atherosclerotic plaque with subsequent thrombosis. IVUS is a modality that can help to differentiate between vulnerable atherosclerotic plaques and stable plaques, which a routine coronary angiogram cannot do. IVUS has been used to analyze the progression of atherosclerotic plaque in clinical trials with various treatment modalities. As an invasive procedure, however, it cannot be used as a routine diagnostic tool.

There are preliminary results with a noninvasive modality for assessing atherosclerotic plaques that might have future application in identifying high-risk patients with coronary artery disease.[1]

W. H. Frishman, MD

Reference

1. Kanai H, Hasegawa H, Ichiki M, et al: Elasticity imaging of atheroma with transcutaneous ultrasound. Preliminary study. *Circulation* 107:3018-3021, 2003.

Value of Magnetic Resonance Imaging for the Noninvasive Detection of Stenosis in Coronary Artery Bypass Grafts and Recipient Coronary Arteries
Langerak SE, Vliegen HW, Jukema JW, et al (Leiden Univ Med Ctr, The Netherlands; Interuniversity Cardiology Inst of the Netherlands, Utrecht)
Circulation 107:1502-1508, 2003   55–2

Introduction.—Extensive work has been performed in native coronary arteries with MRI to demonstrate its ability to discern patent from occluded coronary arteries, identify stenosis in proximal coronary arteries, and to quantify flow. No trials have used MRI to identify stenotic vein grafts and recipient vessels. The value of MRI with baseline and stress flow measurements in identifying grafts, including recipient vessels with flow-limiting stenosis, was assessed in 173 patients with recurrent chest pain after coronary artery bypass surgery.

Findings.—The study included 69 eligible patients with 166 grafts (81 single vein, 44 sequential vein, and 41 arterial) who underwent MRI with baseline and stress flow mapping. Both evaluations were successful in 80% of grafts. The grafts and recipient vessels were separated into groups of stenosis: 50% or greater or 70% or greater (72 and 48, respectively). The probability for the presence of stenosis for each graft type was predicted by means of multiple MRI variables. The sensitivity and specificity of identifying single vein grafts with stenosis of 50% or greater or 70% or greater were 94% (95% confidence interval [CI], 48-79) and 96% (95% CI, 87-100), respectively.

Conclusion.—MRI with flow mapping is helpful in identifying grafts and recipient vessels with flow-limiting stenosis. Flow scans were possible in

80% of grafts. This proof-of-concept investigation indicates that noninvasive MRI detection of stenotic grafts in patients with recurrent chest pain after coronary artery bypass surgery may be helpful in identifying patients in need of an invasive procedure.

▶ The applications of MRI for the noninvasive assessment of cardiac function and diagnosis are increasing. MRI can help identify stenoses in coronary bypass grafts and recipient coronary arteries. The technology can be used to detect in-stent stenosis,[1] and myocardial ischemia,[2] and can help to differentiate patients with heart failure who have idiopathic dilated cardiomyopathy and ischemic cardiomyopathy.[3]

W. H. Frishman, MD

References

1. Nagel E, Thouet T, Klein C, et al: Noninvasive determination of coronary blood flow velocity with cardiovascular magnetic resonance in patients with stent deployment. *Circulation* 107:1738-1743, 2003.
2. Kuijpers D, Ho KYJAM, van Dijkman PRM, et al: Dobutamine cardiovascular magnetic resonance for the detection of myocardial ischemia with the use of myocardial tagging. *Circulation* 107:1592-1597, 2003.
3. McCrohon JA, Moon JC, Prasad SK, et al: Differentiation of heart failure related to dilated cardiomyopathy and coronary artery disease using gadolinium-enhanced cardiovascular magnetic resonance. *Circulation* 108:54-59, 2003.

Electron-Beam Tomography Coronary Artery Calcium and Cardiac Events: A 37-Month Follow-up of 5635 Initially Asymptomatic Low- to Intermediate-Risk Adults
Kondos GT, Hoff JA, Sevrukov A, et al (Univ of Illinois, Chicago; Northwestern Univ, Chicago)
Circulation 107:2571-2576, 2003   55–3

Introduction.—Conventional coronary artery disease (CAD) risk factors are unable to explain almost 50% of CAD events. The relationship between electron-beam tomography (EBT) coronary artery calcium (CAC), and cardiac events in initially asymptomatic, low- to intermediate-risk persons was determined, with adjustment for the presence of hypercholesterolemia, hypertension, diabetes, and history of cigarette smoking.

Methods.—Between January 1993 and December 1995, 10,132 asymptomatic persons (ages 30-76 years) self-referred for EBT CAC screening were evaluated. Those who met inclusion criteria (n = 8855) completed a questionnaire that addressed conventional CAD risk factors. At a mean of 37 months, data regarding the occurrence of cardiac events were obtained and verified with the use of medical records and death certificates.

Results.—In men, 192 events were linked with the presence of CAC (relative risk [RR], 10.5; $P < .001$), diabetes (RR, 1.98; $P = .008$), and smoking (RR, 1.4; $P = .025$). In women, 32 events were related to the presence of CAC (RR, 2.6; $P = .037$); no risk factors were related to cardiac events. The presence of CAC provided incremental prognostic data in addition to age and other risk factors.

Conclusion.—The correlation between EBT CAC and cardiac events in this cohort of initially asymptomatic middle-aged, low- to intermediate-risk persons undergoing screening indicates that knowledge of EBT CAC provides incremental data in addition to that defined by conventional CAD risk assessment. Population-based trials evaluating the usefulness of EBT CAC screening as an adjunct to office-based CAD risk assessment are recommended.

▶ Electron beam tomography (EBT) coronary artery calcification has been used as a means to identify individuals at risk of developing symptomatic heart disease.[1] However, using the finding of coronary calcification from screening to motivate patients to make changes in risk factors was not found to influence modifiable cardiovascular risk in asymptomatic patients.[2] Coronary calcium scores obtained by EBT can help identify those patients with symptomatic disease who are at greater risk.[3]

W. H. Frishman, MD

References

1. Greenland P, Gaziano JM: Selecting asymptomatic patients for coronary computer tomography or electrocardiographic exercise testing. *N Engl J Med* 349:465-473, 2003.
2. O'Malley PG, Feuerstein IM, Taylor AJ: Impact of electron beam tomography with or without case management, on motivation, behavioral change, and cardiovascular risk profile. A randomized controlled trial. *JAMA* 289: 2215-2223, 2003.
3. Möhlenkamp S, Lehmann N, Schmermund A, et al: Prognostic value of extensive coronary calcium quantities in symptomatic males—A 5-year follow-up study. *Eur Heart J* 24:845-854, 2003.

Tissue Doppler Imaging Predicts the Development of Hypertrophic Cardiomyopathy in Subjects With Subclinical Disease

Nagueh SF, McFalls J, Meyer D, et al (Baylor College of Medicine, Houston; Mayo Clinic, Scottsdale, Ariz)
Circulation 108:395-398, 2003   55-4

Introduction.—The elucidation of the molecular genetic basis of hypertrophic cardiomyopathy (HCM) has underscored the need for early identification of mutation carriers. Recent observations in both a transgenic rabbit model of HCM and in humans have revealed decreased myocardial Doppler velocities in research subjects with HCM mutations without cardiac hypertrophy. These findings have raised the possibility of the use of tissue Doppler (TD) imaging (TDI) for the early detection of persons with such mutations. The ability of TDI to identify persons with HCM-causing mutations who later develop left ventricular (LV) hypertrophy was assessed in 2 age- and sex-matched adult HCM families.

Methods.—Serial 2-dimensional and Doppler echocardiography were conducted in 12 patients, 17 to 51 years old, with HCM-causing mutations on 2 occasions: before development of LV hypertrophy and 2 years later. Twelve age- and sex-matched family members without mutations acted as control subjects.

Results.—In participants with mutations, the mean septal thickness and LV mass were 1.07 cm and 103.0 g at baseline, respectively. These values increased significantly to 1.30 cm and 193.0 g at 2-year follow-up ($P < .01$); 6 participants satisfied HCM diagnostic criteria. The mean systolic (Sa) and diastolic (Ea) myocardial velocities in participants with mutations were less, compared with those of control subjects at baseline and follow-up (lateral Sa, 15 vs 8.2 cm/s; lateral Ea, 16.5 vs 8.1 cm/s; $P < .01$). At 2-year follow-up, left atrial volume and pulmonary venous flow indices of LV filling pressures significantly increased ($P < .05$) and TD early and late diastolic velocities significantly decreased ($P < .05$) in participants with mutations. Control subjects showed no significant interval changes of any measured parameters.

Conclusion.—The subsequent development of HCM in persons with initially decreased TD velocities established TDI as a reliable technique for the early detection of HCM mutation carriers.

▶ Early diagnosis of HCM could allow interventions to prevent development of the clinical phenotype. Echocardiography in asymptomatic individuals can identify asymptomatic disease when asymmetric hypertrophy of the left ventricle is present. Tissue Doppler imaging provides another modality for identifying subclinical disease. There is a suggestion from animal studies that early treatment with angiotensin II receptor blockers and calcium blockers could reverse HCM in the early subclinical stage of the disease.[1,2] If this is true in humans, it would make preclinical screening imperative.

W. H. Frishman, MD

References

1. Lim DS, Lutucuta S, Bachireddy P, et al: Angiotensin II blockade reverses myocardial fibrosis in a transgenic mouse model of human hypertrophic cardiomyopathy. *Circulation* 103:789-791, 2001.
2. Semsarian C, Ahmad I, Giewat M, et al: The L-type calcium channel inhibitor diltiazem prevents cardiomyopathy in a mouse model. *J Clin Invest* 109:1013-1020, 2002.

56 Arrhythmias

Frequent Ventricular Ectopy After Exercise as a Predictor of Death
Frolkis JP, Pothier CE, Blackstone EH, et al (Cleveland Clinic Found, Ohio)
N Engl J Med 348:781-790, 2003   56–1

Introduction.—Ventricular ectopy is sometimes observed during exercise stress testing, but its relation with coronary artery disease or cardiovascular risk is unclear. A delay in vagal reactivation during recovery from exercise might reflect the presence of ventricular ectopy that is not suppressed. The effects of timing of ventricular ectopy—during recovery compared with during exercise—on the associated risk of death were assessed.

Methods.—The prospective study included 29,244 patients undergoing clinically indicated symptom-limited treadmill testing. The patients were 70% men (mean age, 56 years), none with a history of heart failure, valve disease, or arrhythmia. The occurrence and timing of ventricular ectopy were noted and correlated with risk of death over a mean 5.3 years of follow-up. Frequent ventricular ectopy was defined as 7 or more ventricular premature beats per minute, ventricular bigeminy, ventricular trigeminy, or ventricular couplets; or, in more severe cases, ventricular triplets, ventricular tachycardia, torsades de pointes, or ventricular fibrillation.

Results.—Rates of frequent ventricular ectopy were 3% during exercise only, 2% during recovery only, and 2% during both exercise and recovery. A total of 1862 deaths occurred during follow-up. The 5-year mortality rate was 9% for patients with frequent ventricular ectopy during exercise compared with 5% for patients without this finding (hazard ratio, 1.8). Risk was even higher for patients with frequent ventricular ectopy during recovery: 11% compared with 5% (hazard ratio, 2.4). With propensity matching for confounding variables, frequent ventricular ectopy during recovery was associated with an adjusted hazard ratio of 1.5 (Fig 2). In contrast, frequent ventricular ectopy during exercise was no longer significantly associated with death.

Conclusions.—In patients undergoing exercise stress testing, frequent ventricular ectopy during the recovery phase is strongly associated with an increased risk of death during 5-year follow-up. In contrast, frequent ventricular ectopy during exercise alone does not predict an increased risk of death. The findings highlight the role of vagal mediation in cardiac function, as well as showing that the exercise stress test is an important tool for assessing cardiac prognosis and risk.

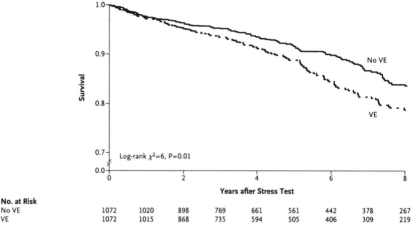

No. at Risk

No VE	1072	1020	898	769	661	561	442	378	267
VE	1072	1015	868	735	594	505	406	309	219

FIGURE 2.—Kaplan-Meier analysis of association of frequent ventricular ectopy (*VE*) during recovery from exercise with survival in the propensity-matched cohort. The cohort was derived by using propensity scores to match patients with VE during recovery to patients who did not have VE during recovery. Of 1080 patients who had VE during recovery, 1072 were matched. The characteristics of the cohort are shown in Table 2. (Reprinted by permission of *The New England Journal of Medicine* from Frolkis JP, Pothier CE, Blackstone EH, et al: Frequent ventricular ectopy after exercise as a predictor of death. *N Engl J Med* 348:781-790, 2003. Copyright 2003, Massachusetts Medical Society. All rights reserved.)

▶ Frequent ventricular ectopy occurring during recovery from exercise is an important independent predictor of death. Ventricular ectopy occurring only during exercise is not predictive. A relationship also exists between an attenuated recovery of the heart rate after exercise and an elevated risk of death.[1,2] Individuals having abnormal exercise tests with ventricular ectopy after exercise should undergo further diagnostic testing, including echocardiography, to assess for ventricular dysfunction. In addition, aggressive risk factor assessment and management of identified risk factors are justified.

W. H. Frishman, MD

References

1. Cole CR, Blackstone EH, Pashkow FJ, et al: Heart rate recovery immediately after exercise as a predictor of mortality. *N Engl J Med* 341:1351-1357, 1999.
2. Nishime EO, Cole CR, Blackstone EH, et al: Heart rate recovery and treadmill exercise score as predictors of mortality in patients referred for exercise ECG. *JAMA* 284:1392-1398, 2000.

Pacemaker Therapy for Prevention of Syncope in Patients With Recurrent Severe Vasovagal Syncope: Second Vasovagal Pacemaker Study (VPS II): A Randomized Trial

Connolly SJ, for the VPS II Investigators (McMaster Univ, Hamilton, Ont, Canada; et al)

JAMA 289:2224-2229, 2003

56–2

Background.—Vasovagal syncope is a common problem with no highly effective pharmacologic treatment. Episodes of vasovagal syncope are often associated with bradycardia, so pacemakers have been proposed as a potential treatment. The results of 3 small randomized trials have supported this proposal for patients with severe recurrent vasovagal syncope. However, these trials were not double-blind designs; thus, they may have been biased in their assessment of outcomes. In addition, a placebo effect from surgery may have been present. Whether pacing therapy reduces the risk of syncope for patients with vasovagal syncope was determined.

Methods.—The study included 100 patients who underwent implantation of a dual-chamber pacemaker and were then randomly assigned to either dual-chamber pacing (DDD) with rate drop response or sensing only without pacing (ODO). The main outcome measure was the time to first recurrence of syncope.

Results.—Of the 52 patients randomized to ODO, 22 (42%) had recurrent syncope within 6 months compared with 16 (33%) of 48 patients in the DDD group. The cumulative risk of syncope at 6 months was 40% for patients in the ODO group and 31% for patients in the DDD group. The relative risk reduction in time to syncope with DDD pacing was 30%. Seven patients experienced lead dislodgement or repositioning. One patient experienced vein thrombosis, 1 patient had pericardial tamponade resulting in removal of the pacemaker system, and an infection involving the pacemaker generator developed in 1 patient.

Conclusions.—Pacemaker therapy did not reduce the risk of recurrent syncope in patients with vasovagal syncope. In light of the weak evidence of efficacy of pacemaker therapy, and the risk of complications, pacemaker therapy should not be recommended as a first-line therapy for patients with recurrent vasovagal syncope.

▶ Vasovagal syncope ("common faint") is a common problem in medical practice, and there appears to be no effective pharmacologic treatment.[1] Pacemaker therapy was suggested as a possible therapy for vasovagal syncope; however, there is little evidence of benefit.

W. H. Frishman, MD

Reference

1. Frishman WH, Azer V, Sica D: Drug treatment of orthostatic hypotension and vasovagal syncope. *Heart Dis* 5:49-64, 2003.

Long-term Outcomes of Out-of-Hospital Cardiac Arrest After Successful Early Defibrillation

Bunch TJ, White RD, Gersh BJ, et al (Mayo Clinic, Rochester, Minn)
N Engl J Med 348:2626-2633, 2003   56–3

Introduction.—Rapid defibrillation is the single most important determinant of outcome after an out-of-hospital cardiac arrest with ventricular fibrillation. Rates of survival to hospital discharge are significantly increased when emergency personnel can provide treatment with automated external defibrillators. The long-term outcome of patients who underwent successful early defibrillation was examined in a population-based study.

Methods.—Included in the analysis were all patients who had an out-of-hospital cardiac arrest between November 1990 and January 2001 and received defibrillation from emergency personnel in Olmsted County, Minnesota. Advanced life support was provided by paramedics, and all patients were transported to the Mayo Clinic. Quality of life of survivors was assessed by the Medical Outcomes Study 36-Item Short-Form General Health Survey (SF-36). The survival rate of the study group was compared with that of an age-, sex- and disease-matched control population of county residents who had not had an out-of-hospital cardiac arrest and with that of age- and sex-matched control subjects from the general population of the United States (Fig 2).

Results.—Two hundred of 330 patients who had an out-of-hospital cardiac arrest during the study period had ventricular fibrillation; 145 (72%) of these patients maintained spontaneous circulation after defibrillation and were admitted to hospital. Demographic results were available for 142 patients, 79 of whom survived to hospital discharge. The mean time from the

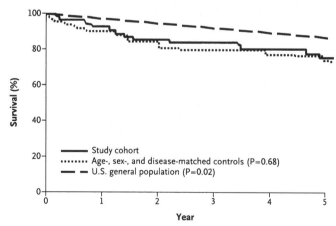

FIGURE 2.—Overall survival among the 79 survivors, as compared with age- and sex-matched controls from the general US population and an age-, sex-, and disease-matched population of patients from Olmsted County, Minn, who did not have out-of-hospital cardiac arrest. (Reprinted by permission of *The New England Journal of Medicine* from Bunch TJ, White RD, Gersh BJ, et al: Long-term outcomes of out-of-hospital cardiac arrest after successful early defibrillation. *N Engl J Med* 348:2626-2633, 2003. Copyright 2003, Massachusetts Medical Society. All rights reserved.)

911 call to administration of the first shock was 5.7 minutes among survivors and 6.6 minutes among nonsurvivors. During a mean follow-up of 4.8 years, 19 of 79 patients who survived to hospital discharge died. The expected 5-year survival rate for the out-of-hospital cardiac arrest survivors was identical to that of age-, sex-, and disease-matched control subjects (79%) but lower than that of the general population control subjects (86%). The SF-36 scores of 50 long-term survivors indicated a near normal quality of life and a return to work for the majority. Only the vitality score, a measure of fatigue, was reduced in survivors compared with the general population.

Conclusion.—Previous studies have reported a reduced quality of life among survivors of out-of-hospital cardiac arrest. But with the early administration of defibrillation by emergency personnel, a high rate of survival to hospital discharge and long-term survival with a near normal quality of life can be achieved.

▶ Patients who survive out-of-hospital cardiac arrest with ventricular fibrillation appear to have an excellent long-term prognosis.[1,2] Implantable defibrillators can prevent sudden cardiac death in patients at risk[3]; however, not all survivors of a ventricular fibrillation cardiac arrest may need the device. Electrophysiologic studies might be helpful to identify high-risk individuals, especially those with ventricular dysfunction and a history of coronary artery disease.

W. H. Frishman, MD

References

1. Rea TD, Crouthamel M, Eisenberg MS, et al: Temporal patterns in long-term survival after resuscitation from out-of-hospital cardiac arrest. *Circulation* 108:1196-1201, 2003.
2. Stiell I, for the OPALS Study Group: Health-related quality of life is better for cardiac arrest survivors who received citizen cardiopulmonary resuscitation. *Circulation* 108:1939-1944, 2003.
3. Ezekowitz JA, Armstrong PW, McAlister FA: Implantable cardioverter defibrillators in primary and secondary prevention: A systematic review of randomized, controlled trials. *Ann Intern Med* 138:445-452, 2003.

Temporal Relations of Atrial Fibrillation and Congestive Heart Failure and Their Joint Influence on Mortality: The Framingham Heart Study
Wang TJ, Larson MG, Levy D, et al (Harvard Med School, Boston; Boston Univ; Natl Heart, Lung and Blood Inst, Bethesda, Md)
Circulation 107:2920-2925, 2003   56–4

Introduction.—It is widely perceived that the combination of atrial fibrillation (AF) and congestive heart failure (CHF) carries a worse prognosis than either of these conditions alone. The joint epidemiology of AF and CHF in the large, community-based cohort of the Framingham Heart Study was analyzed.

Methods.—Participants in the Framingham Heart Study with new-onset AF or CHF between 1948 through 1995 underwent routine assessments of medical history, physical examination, and ECG at regularly scheduled evaluation points. Records were obtained for all medical encounters associated with cardiovascular disease and examined by a committee of 3 investigators. Multivariable Cox proportional hazards models with time-dependent variables were used to assess whether mortality after AF or CHF was impacted by the occurrence and timing of other conditions. Hazards ratios (HRs) were adjusted for both time period and cardiovascular risk factors.

Results.—During the evaluation period, 1470 participants had AF, CHF or both develop. Among 382 participants with both AF and CHF, 38% had AF first, 41% had CHF first, and 21% were diagnosed with both on the same day. The incidence of CHF among participants with AF was 33 per 1000 person-year; the incidence of AF among those with CHF was 54 per 1000 person-year. In participants with AF, the subsequent development of CHF was correlated with increased mortality (males: HR 2.7; 95% CI, 1.9-3,7; females: HR 3.1; 95% CI, 2.2-4.2). Similarly, in persons with CHF, later development of AF was linked with increased mortality (males: HR 1.6; 95% CI, 1.2-2.1; females: HR 2.7; 95% CI, 2.0-3.6). Preexisting CHF adversely impacted survival in persons with AF; preexisting AF was not linked with adverse survival in persons with CHF.

Conclusion.—Persons with AF or CHF who subsequently had the other condition develop also have a poor prognosis. It may be that prophylactic therapies to decrease the incidence of the second condition in high-risk persons with AF or CHF may be therapeutically beneficial.

▶ Atrial fibrillation remains a common problem in clinical practice. Patients with heart failure who subsequently have AF develop have a worse prognosis. Elderly patients with AF may also be in a prothrombotic state, making them susceptible for having thrombotic strokes as well as embolic strokes.[1-3] It is not known whether conversion of AF to normal sinus rhythm will directly reduce this prothrombotic state.

W. H. Frishman, MD

References

1. Conway DSG, Heeringa J, Van Der Kuip DAM, et al: Atrial fibrillation and the prothrombotic state in the elderly. The Rotterdam Study. *Stroke* 34:413-417, 2003.
2. Penado S, Cano M, Acha O, et al: Atrial fibrillation as a risk factor for stroke recurrence. *Am J Med* 114:206-210, 2003.
3. Page RL, for the Azimilide Supraventricular Arrhythmia Program (ASAP) Investigators: Asymptomatic or "silent" atrial fibrillation: Frequency in untreated patients and patients receiving azimilide. *Circulation* 107:1141-1145, 2003.

Risk Stratification in the Long-QT Syndrome

Priori SG, Schwartz PJ, Napolitano C, et al (Istituto di Ricovero e Cura a Carattere Scientifico Fondazione S Maugeri, Pavia, Italy; Istituto di Ricovero e Cura a Carattere Policlinico San Matteo, Pavia, Italy; Univ of Pavia, Italy)
N Engl J Med 348:1866-1874, 2003   56–5

Background.—The natural history of the long-QT syndrome (LQTS) remains incompletely characterized more than 40 years after its initial description, caused, primarily, by the fact that the LQTS is uncommon, cardiac events may be separated by long periods without symptoms, and the initial manifestation of the syndrome may occur late in life. Consequently, approaches to risk stratification are not well defined. Five genes have been linked to the LQTS, and mutations in the potassium-channel genes *KCNQ1* (*LQT1* locus) and *KCNH2* (*LQT2* locus) and the sodium-channel gene *SCN5A* (*LQT3* locus) are the most common causes of the LQTS. The risk of LQTS was stratified on the basis of genotype, in conjunction with other clinical variables, such as sex and the length of the QT interval.

Methods.—The study assessed 647 patients from 193 consecutively genotyped families with the LQTS. The cumulative probability of a first cardiac event (defined as the occurrence of syncope, cardiac arrest, or sudden death before the age of 40 years and before the initiation of therapy) was determined according to genotype, sex and the QT interval corrected for heart rate (QTc). Risk in the 4 categories derived from a combination of sex and QTc (<500 ms) or (500 msec) were assessed within each genotype.

Results.—The incidence of a first cardiac event before age 40 years and before the initiation of therapy was less among patients with a mutation at the *LQT1* locus (30%) than among those with a mutation at the *LQT2* locus (46%) or those with mutation at the *LQT3* locus (42%). Multivariate analysis showed that genetic locus and the QTc, but not sex, were independent predictors of risk. The QTc was an independent predictor of risk among patients with a mutation at the *LQT1* or *LQT2* locus but not among patients with a mutation at the *LQT3* locus. However, sex was independently predictive of events only among patients with a mutation at the *LQT3* locus.

Conclusion.—The clinical course of the LQTS is affected by the locus of the causative mutation, which also modulates the effects of the QTc and sex on clinical variables.

▶ Beta blockers have been shown to be effective in reducing mortality in patients with the L-QTS.[1] Implantable defibrillators should probably be used in those patients identified by genetic studies to be at high risk.[2]

W. H. Frishman, MD

References

1. Frishman WH: Alpha- and beta–adrenergic blocking drugs, in Frishman WH, Sonnenblick EH, Sica DA (eds): *Cardiovascular Pharmacotherapeutics*, ed 2. New York, McGraw Hill, 2003, pp 67-98.
2. Zareba W, Moss AJ, Daubert JP, et al: Implantable cardioverter defibrillator in high-risk long QT syndrome patients. *J Cardiovasc Electrophysiol* 14:337-341, 2003.

57 Other Topics

Meta-analysis of Results From Eight Randomized, Placebo-controlled Trials on the Effect of Cilostazol on Patients With Intermittent Claudication

Thompson PD, Zimet R, Forbes WP, et al (Hartford Hosp, Conn; Otsuka America Pharmaceutical, Inc., Rockville, Md)

Am J Cardiol 90:1314-1319, 2002   57–1

Background.—As treatment for intermittent claudication, cilostazol, a selective type III phosphodiesterase inhibitor, promotes vasodilation, which improves blood flow through narrowed arteries. Platelet aggregation can be reduced by a factor 10 to 30 times greater than that of aspirin. Eight studies have assessed the effect of cilostazol on symptomatic improvement and walking ability in patients with intermittent claudication, and a meta-analysis was done.

Methods.—The effects experienced by 2702 patients who had stable moderate to severe claudication were noted in 8 randomized, double-blind, placebo-controlled trials. Cilostazol therapy was administered for 12 to 24 weeks. Pain-free and maximal walking distance (MWD) and quality of life measures were reported.

Results.—MWD was improved by cilostazol in 6 of the trials, with increases of 44% to 50% over baseline measurements at twice-daily doses of 50 and 100 mg, respectively. Similar improvement was noted in pain-free walking distance, with increases of 60% and 67% with twice-daily doses of 50 and 100 mg, respectively (Fig 2). Men, women, older patients ($\geq$65 years), younger patients, and patients with and without diabetes had similar results with cilostazol. High-density lipoprotein cholesterol levels were increased by 12.8% and triglycerides decreased by 15.8% with 100-mg doses of cilostazol twice daily. No changes in hematologic parameters, liver function, electrolytes, or renal function developed with cilostazol use. Physical function subscale results showed greater improvement with the twice-daily 100-mg cilostazol than with placebo. With cilostazol, patients were able to walk at faster speeds and over greater distances with less severe claudication than with placebo in 6 trials where the Walking Impairment Questionnaire (WIQ) was given. Those taking the 100-mg twice-daily dose had greater improvement in walking speed and walking distance than placebo, with average increases of 6.1 and 6.6 points, respectively.

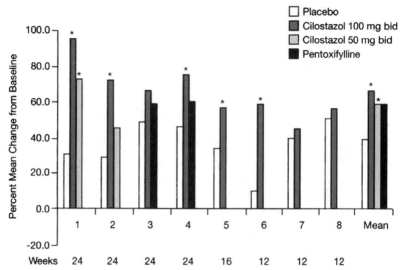

FIGURE 2.—Percent mean change in pain-free walking distance from baseline to end of treatment. *Cilostazol, 50 or 100 mg twice daily (bid), versus placebo ($P < .05$). (Reprinted from Thompson PD, Zimet R, Forbes WP, et al: Meta-analysis of results from eight randomized, placebo-controlled trials on the effect of cilostazol on patients with intermittent claudication. *Am J Cardiol* 90:1314-1319, 2002. Copyright 2002 with permission from Excerpta Medica Inc.)

Conclusions.—Cilostazol produced significant increases over placebo in walking distance and quality of life measures in patients who had intermittent claudication. No major adverse effects resulted from its use.

▶ Cilostazol, a selective type III phosphodiesterase inhibitor, appears to be the drug of choice for relieving symptomatic peripheral vascular disease.[1] Adjunctive therapy with antiplatelet agents, lipid-lowering drugs, and angiotensin-converting enzyme inhibitors appear to affect clinical outcomes.[1] High dose, short-term treatment with statins may also improve exercise tolerance, ankle-brachial pressure indices, and symptoms of claudication in hypercholesterolemic patients with peripheral vascular disease.[2]

W. H. Frishman, MD

References

1. Eberhardt RT, Coffman JD: Drug treatment of peripheral vascular disease, in Frishman WH, Sonnenblick EH, Sica DA (eds): *Cardiovascular Pharmacotherapeutics* ed 2. New York, McGraw Hill, 2003, pp 919-934.
2. Mondillo S, Ballo P, Barbati R, et al: Effects of simvastatin on walking performance and symptoms of intermittent claudication in hypercholesterolemic patients with peripheral vascular disease. *Am J Med* 114:359-364, 2003.

Factors Associated With Progression of Carcinoid Heart Disease

Møller JE, Connolly HM, Rubin J, et al (Mayo Clinic, Rochester, Minn)
N Engl J Med 348:1005-1015, 2003   57–2

Introduction.—Carcinoid tumors release serotonin and other vasoactive substances into the circulation that can cause right-sided valvular heart disease. Knowledge concerning the mechanisms involved in the progression of the cardiac lesions may lead to the development of treatments that attenuate the process. The factors associated with the progression of valvular dysfunctions in patients with metastatic carcinoid disease were reviewed retrospectively.

Methods.—The study included 71 patients with carcinoid syndrome who underwent serial echocardiographic evaluations performed more than 1 year apart, and 32 patients who were referred directly for surgical intervention after an initial echocardiographic examination. A score for carcinoid heart disease was assigned on the basis of an assessment of valvular anatomy and function and the function of the right ventricle. An increase of more than 25% in the score between studies was regarded as suggestive of disease progression. Tumor progression was based on abdominal CT scans and changes in the level of urinary 5-hydroxyindoleacetic acid (5-HIAA), a metabolite of serotonin.

Results.—Among patients who underwent serial echocardiographic evaluations, 25 (35%) had an increase of more than 25% in the cardiac score. Compared with patients whose score changed by 25% or less, these patients had higher urinary peak 5-HIAA levels (median, 265 mg/24 h [interquartile range, 209-593] vs 189/24 h [interquartile range, 75-286]; $P = .004$) and were more likely to have biochemical progression (10/25 patients vs 9/46; $P = .05$) and to have received chemotherapy (13/25 vs 10/46; $P = .009$). Logistic regression analysis revealed that a higher peak urinary 5-HIAA level and previous chemotherapy were predictive of an increase in the cardiac score that exceeded 25% (odds ratio [OR] for each increase in 5-HIAA of 25 mg/24 h, 1.08 [95% confidence interval [CI], 1.03-1.13]; $P = .009$). The OR linked with chemotherapy was 3.65 (95% CI, 1.74-7.48; $P = .001$).

Conclusion.—Serotonin is associated with progression of carcinoid heart disease. The risk of progressive heart disease is higher among patients who undergo chemotherapy compared with those who do not undergo this regimen.

▶ Carcinoid heart disease is caused by the release of serotonin from metastatic carcinoid tumors of the liver. The right heart is exposed to high levels of a serotonin metabolite 5-HIAA, which causes endocardial damage, leading to valvular dysfunction and right-sided heart failure.[1-3] Cytoxic chemotherapy is associated with a higher risk of developing heart disease. Treatment with somatostatin, hepatic dearterialization, or both, does not prevent the development of cardiac disease.

W. H. Frishman, MD

References

1. Pellikka PA, Tajik AJ, Khandheria BK, et al: Carcinoid heart disease: Clinical and echo-cardiographic spectrum in 74 patients. *Circulation* 87:1188-1196, 1993.
2. Denney WD, Kemp WE Jr, Anthony LB, et al: Echocardiographic and biochemical evaluation of the development and progression of carcinoid heart disease. *J Am Coll Cardiol* 32:1017-1022, 1998.
3. Robiolio PA, Rigolin VH, Wilson JS, et al: Carcinoid heart disease: Correlation of high serotonin levels with valvular abnormalities detected by cardiac catheterization and echocardiography. *Circulation* 92:790-795, 1995.

▶ Carcinoid tumors are rare, with about 20% to 30% presenting with advanced disease. The carcinoid syndrome is well known (diarrhea, cutaneous vasomotor flushing, bronchospasm), but less well described are the cardiac abnormalities associated with chronic exposure to serotonin and other vasoactive substances. This is an excellent article and review on the topic.

P. J. Loehrer, Sr, MD

The Early Repolarization Normal Variant Electrocardiogram: Correlates and Consequences
Klatsky AL, Oehm R, Cooper RA, et al (Kaiser Permanente Med Care Program, Oakland, Calif)
Am J Med 115:171-177, 2003   57–3

Introduction.—Early repolarization is not considered a marker of cardiovascular disease. Yet, it is an important finding because it may mimic the ECG of acute myocardial infarction, pericarditis, ventricular aneurysm, hyperkalemia, or hypothermia. The characteristics and outcomes of persons with early repolarization ECGs were compared with those of individuals with normal ECGs.

Methods.—Between 1983 and 1985, photocopies were obtained of 2234 selected ECGs from 73,008 persons undergoing health examinations. One hundred fifty-three ECGs with missing data or that were considered either abnormal by demonstrating early repolarization, borderline characteristics, or normal (670, 330, and 1081 ECGs, respectively) were extracted and re-interpreted in 2000 by cardiologists. Characteristics and outcomes of individuals with early repolarization ECGs were compared with persons with normal ECGs. Data concerning exercise were available for 325 participants.

Results.—Persons with early repolarization were more likely to be male (81% vs 33%), younger than 40 years old (60% vs 37%), African American (48% vs 26%) and more athletically inclined (10.4 vs 6.4 h/wk of activity), compared with the same variables of persons with normal ECGs. Those with early repolarization were not more likely to be hospitalized (hazard ratio [HR], 1.0; 95% confidence interval [CI], 0.9-1.2) or to die (HR, 0.8; 95% CI, 0.6-1.2) during follow-up, than the likelihood for individuals with normal ECGs. Outpatient diagnoses were not more frequent in those with early repolarization, and arrhythmias were actually less common ($P < .01$).

Conclusion.—Early repolarization is particularly more prevalent in young, athletic, African American men. Yet it is not rare in other individuals. The long-term prognosis of early repolarization may be considered benign.

▶ The early repolarization variant ECG pattern is commonly confused with the ECG patterns of acute myocardial infarction, pericarditis, ventricular aneurysm, hyperkalemia and hypothermia.[1] The repolarization variant is a benign condition. However, when associated with atypical chest pain, its presence may be confused with ischemia, leading to unnecessary diagnostic studies and treatment.

This ECG pattern is more prevalent in young, athletic, black men; however, it has also been seen in women, elderly patients, and inactive individuals. Individuals who have this pattern as part of their normal ECG should always keep a copy of their tracing with them, so comparisons can be made with subsequent ECGs obtained in other clinical settings.

W. H. Frishman, MD

Reference

1. Wang K, Asinger RW, Marriott HJL: ST-segment elevation in conditions other than acute myocardial infarction. *N Engl J Med* 349:2128-2135, 2003.

Validation of a Brief Observation Period for Patients With Cocaine-Associated Chest Pain

Weber JE, Shofer FS, Larkin GL, et al (Univ of Michigan, Ann Arbor; Hurley Med Ctr, Flint, Mich; Univ of Texas, Dallas; et al)
N Engl J Med 348:510-517, 2003   57–4

Background.—Retrospective studies of patients with cocaine-related chest pain treated by a strategy of discharge from the ED after 12 hours of observation and no evidence of ischemia have been reported. The complication rate in these reports appears to be very low. The safety of a 9- to 12-hour observation period for patients with cocaine-related chest pain at low to intermediate risk for cardiovascular events was assessed prospectively.

Methods.—Three hundred forty-four patients with cocaine-related chest pain receiving protocol-driven care in a chest-pain observation unit were included. These were consecutive patients who had reported or tested positive for cocaine use. Patients with normal troponin I levels, with no new ischemic changes on ECG, and who had no cardiovascular complications during 9 to 12 hours of observation were discharged. Death from cardiovascular causes at 30 days was the main outcome measure.

Findings.—Twelve percent of the patients were admitted directly to the hospital. Thus, 302 patients remained in the study cohort. None of the patients died of cardiovascular causes within 30 days of discharge. Of 256 patients with detailed follow-up data, only 4 (1.6%) subsequently had a nonfatal myocardial infarction. All 4 of these patients had continued to use cocaine.

Conclusions.—For patients with cocaine-related chest pain, a policy of 9 to 12 hours of observation followed by discharge appears to be safe. However, such patients should still be examined for potential acute coronary syndromes. Those who do not have recurrent symptoms, increased levels of markers of myocardial necrosis, or dysrhythmias may be safely released after 9 to 12 hours of observation. Strategies for substance abuse treatment are needed for such patients, as their likelihood of nonfatal myocardial infarction is increased if they continue to use cocaine.

▶ Cocaine use has increased in recent years, and the number of cardiovascular events related to its use have increased significantly.[1,2] Most patients with cocaine-associated chest pain need to be observed in an emergency department setting, but those individuals having no recurrent symptoms or evidence of myocardial ischemia or arrhythmia can safely be released after a 9- to 12-hour observation period.

Chest pain observation units in emergency departments are a cost-effective way of managing individuals with various chest pain syndromes that do not warrant hospital admission.

W. H. Frishman, MD

References

1. Lange RA, Hillis RD: Cardiovascualr complications of cocaine use. *N Engl J Med* 345:351-358, 2001 (Erratum, *N Engl J Med* 345:1432, 2001).
2. Frishman WH, DelVecchio A, Sanal S, et al: Cardiovascular manifestations of substance abuse. Part 1: Cocaine. *Heart Dis* 5:187-201, 2003.

An Association Between Atherosclerosis and Venous Thrombosis
Prandoni P, Bilora F, Marchiori A, et al (Univ of Padua, Italy; Univ of Amsterdam; Univ of Maastricht, The Netherlands)
N Engl J Med 348:1435-1441, 2003   57–5

Background.—The pathogenesis of venous thromboembolism has not been fully elucidated. Classic risk factors include cancer, surgery, immobilization, fractures, paralysis, pregnancy, childbirth, and use of estrogens. However, the cause of venous thromboembolism remains unexplained in about one third of patients. Atherosclerosis is associated with activation of both platelets and blood coagulation and an increase in fibrin turnover, all of which may predispose to blood coagulation. Whether atherosclerosis is associated with an increased risk of venous thrombosis was determined.

Methods.—US of the carotid arteries was performed in 299 unselected patients with deep venous thrombosis of the legs without symptomatic atherosclerosis and in 150 control subjects. The patient group included those with spontaneous thrombosis and those with secondary thrombosis from acquired risk factors. Both patients and controls were assessed for the presence of plaques.

Results.—At least one carotid plaque was identified in 72 of 153 patients with spontaneous thrombosis (47.1%), in 40 of 146 patients with secondary thrombosis (27.4%), and 48 of 150 control subjects (32%). The odds ratios for carotid plaques in patients with spontaneous thrombosis, compared with patients with secondary thrombosis and controls, were 2.3 and 1.8, respectively. The strength of this association did not change on multivariate analysis that adjusted for risk factors for atherosclerosis.

Conclusions.—An association was found between atherosclerotic disease and spontaneous venous thrombosis. Atherosclerosis may induce venous thrombosis, or the 2 conditions may have common risk factors.

▶ Spontaneous venous thrombi and pulmonary emboli are commonly associated with atherosclerotic disease. Detecting patients at risk for pulmonary emboli and venous thrombosis remains a clinical challenge. Various clinical models and diagnostic modalities have been suggested to increase the recognition of pulmonary emboli.[1,2] Various coagulation abnormalities have been identified in patients at risk of venoembolic disease.[3,4] It has been shown that patients with a spontaneous venous thromboembolism and D-dimer levels under 250 ng/mL have a lower risk of venous thromboembolic recurrence.[5]

W. H. Frishman, MD

References

1. van Strijen MJL, de Monyé W, Schiereck J, et al: Single-detector helical computed tomography as the primary diagnostic test in suspected pulmonary embolism: A multicenter clinical management study of 510 patients. *Ann Intern Med* 138:307-314, 2003.
2. Minati M, Monti S, Bottai M: A structured clinical model for predicting the probability of pulmonary embolism. *Am J Med* 114:173-179, 2003.
3. Kyrle PA, Minar E, Hirschl M, et al: High plasma levels of factor VIII and the risk of recurrent venous thromboembolism. *N Engl J Med* 343:457-462, 2000.
4. Martinelli I: Risk factors in venous thromboembolism. *Thromb Haemost* 86:395-403, 2001.
5. Eichinger S, Minar E, Bialonczyk C, et al: D-dimer levels and risk of recurrent venous thromboembolism. *JAMA* 290:1071-1074, 2003.

PART SEVEN

THE DIGESTIVE SYSTEM
JAMIE S. BARKIN, MD

Introduction

This section features the most important advances in gastroenterology and hepatology over the past year. The article abstracts and commentaries cover the entire spectrum of maladies of the esophagus, including obesity as a risk factor for gastroesophageal reflux disease (GERD) and screening and surveillance in patients with Barrett's esophagus. The stomach chapter includes which patients who use nonsteroidal anti-inflammatory drugs should have a gastroprotective regime and the approach to patients with dyspepsia.

In the small bowel chapter, the focus is on celiac disease, which is the most common gastrointestinal inherited disease and must be considered in all patients with presumed diarrhea-predominant irritable bowel syndrome (IBS). The therapy of patients with constipation predominant IBS is reviewed.

The colon chapter covers the appropriate screening of patients for colorectal cancer, including the significance of a single Hemoccult stool exam and the role of virtual colonoscopy.

The liver chapter encompasses screening for the hemochromatosis, the most frequent genetic liver disease, approach to the patient with elevated liver function tests, and review of nonalcoholic fatty liver disease.

The information imparted in this section will allow a ready source of up-to-date data, which I hope you will find useful, informative, and of benefit to you in caring for your patients.

Jamie S. Barkin, MD

58 Esophagus

Obesity and Estrogen as Risk Factors for Gastroesophageal Reflux Symptoms
Nilsson M, Johnsen R, Ye W, et al (Karolinska Institutet, Stockholm; Norwegian Univ, Trondheim, Norway; Levanger Hosp, Norway; et al)
JAMA 290:66-72, 2003   58–1

Background.—The prevalences of obesity and gastroesophageal reflux are increasing. The relation between body mass and gastroesophageal reflux symptoms and the influence of female sex hormones were investigated in a population-based, cross-sectional, case-control study.

Methods.—Data were obtained from 2 consecutive public health surveys in 1 county in Norway from 1984 to 1986 and from 1995 to 1997. Of the 65,363 participants in the second survey, 3113 reported severe heartburn or regurgitation in the last 12 months and were considered cases; 39,872 participants reporting no reflux symptoms were considered control subjects.

Findings.—A dose-response relation was observed between increasing body mass index (BMI) and reflux symptoms in men and women. This association was significantly stronger in women. The risk of reflux increased significantly among severely obese men and women compared with those with a BMI of less than 25. The relation between BMI and reflux symptoms was stronger in premenopausal women than in postmenopausal women. The use of hormone treatment after menopause increased the strength of this association. A decrease in BMI correlated with a reduced risk of reflux symptoms.

Conclusions.—Body mass is significantly related to gastroesophageal reflux symptoms. This association is stronger in women than men, especially before menopause. The use of hormone treatment after menopause strengthens the correlation. Thus, estrogens appear to play an important role in the cause of reflux disease.

► Gastroesophageal reflux disease (GERD) is one of the most common patients complaints. The factors that contribute to GERD are hiatal hernia, low lower esophageal pressure, occurrence of transient lower esophageal relaxations, decreased esophageal clearance, and possibly decreased gastric emptying.

The prevalence of obesity is increasing in frequency in the United States, as is that of GERD. Nilsson et al, in a cross-sectional, case-controlled study in

Sweden, evaluated whether obesity and estrogen intake are risk factors for GERD symptoms. They demonstrated a strong dose-dependent association between increasing BMI and symptomatic reflux in women and a moderate association among men. The association between hormone therapy and reflux was stronger. This finding supports a role of female sex in the etiology of reflux disease. Interestingly, this study showed that weight loss is associated with reduced risk of reflux symptoms.

This study reinforces our clinical impression that our patients have fewer GERD symptoms with weight loss; whether this is due to a decrease in the volume of meals, alteration of their contents (eg, less fat or carbohydrates), or the effects of decreased BMI per se is unclear. Discontinuing the use of estrogen medication in women with reflux symptoms may improve their symptoms, especially in those with increased BMI.

J. S. Barkin, MD

Colonic Fermentation Influences Lower Esophageal Sphincter Function in Gastroesophageal Reflux Disease
Piche T, Bruley des Varannes S, Sacher-Huvelin S, et al (U 539-Centre Hospitalier Universitaire-Hôtel Dieu, Nantes, France; Univ of Copenhagen; Hôpital Edouard Herriot, Lyon, France)
Gastroenterology 124:894-902, 2003   58–2

Background.—In healthy persons, colonic fermentation of carbohydrates influences gastric and esophageal motility. The effects of colonic fermentation induced by oral administration of fructooligosaccharides (FOS) was investigated in patients with gastroesophageal reflux disease (GERD).

Methods.—Nine patients with symptomatic GERD were included in the crossover study. The patients ate a low-residue diet of 10 g fiber/day during 2 7-day periods, separated by a washout period of at least 3 weeks. After each of their 3 meals a day, the patients were given FOS, 6.6 g, or placebo. On day 7, esophageal motility and pH were documented in fasting conditions and after a test meal.

Findings.—Compared with placebo, FOS significantly increased the number of transient lower esophageal sphincter relaxations and reflux episodes, esophageal acid exposure, and the GERD symptom score. The integrated glucagonlike peptide-1 plasma response was significantly greater after FOS than after placebo.

Conclusions.—In these patients with symptomatic GERD, colonic fermentation of indigestible carbohydrates increased transient lower esophageal sphincter relaxations rates, the number of acid reflux episodes, and GERD symptoms. Excess release of glucagonlike peptide-1 may partly account for these effects, although different mechanisms are probably involved.

▶ The lifestyle changes that we suggest to our patients to are to eat smaller meals with a decrease in fat and to resist from lying down within 3 hours of eating. Ropert et al[1] have previously shown in normal subjects that short-chain fatty acids in the colon, which result normally from unabsorbed carbohydrates, result in a dose-dependent relaxation of the proximal stomach, which is then followed by transient lower esophageal relaxations that could facilitate GERD.[1] Piche et al confirmed this hypothesis in patients with GERD who had sustained activation of colonic fermentation. This resulted in an increased rate of transient lower esophageal relaxations that was associated with a significant increase of acid reflux episodes, esophageal acid exposure, and GERD symptoms.

The colonic fermentation used in this study resulted from ingestion of FOS. These FOS are found in onions, garlic, asparagus root, pastry, and confectionery and dairy products. Thus, we need to counsel our GERD patients regarding reduced intake of foods that contain FOS. This study confirms our clinical impression that intake of these foods results in symptomatic GERD.

J. S. Barkin, MD

Reference

1. Ropert A, Cherbut C, Roze C, e al: Colonic fermentation and proximal gastric tone in humans. *Gastroenterology* 111:289-296, 1996.

Screening and Surveillance for Barrett Esophagus in High-Risk Groups: A Cost-Utility Analysis
Inadomi JM, Sampliner R, Lagergren J, et al (Univ of Michigan, Ann Arbor; Univ of Arizona, Tucson; Karolinksa Inst, Stockholm; et al)
Ann Intern Med 138:176-186, 2003   58–3

Background.—One-time screening for Barrett's esophagus has been suggested for patients with gastroesophageal reflux disease (GERD). The cost-effectiveness of this strategy is unknown. The cost-effectiveness of screening high-risk groups for Barrett's esophagus and providing surveillance to patients with Barrett's esophagus and dysplasia or to all patients with Barrett's esophagus was investigated.

Methods.—A decision analytic model was used. The target population was 50-year-old white men with GERD symptoms. The cost of screening or surveillance and screening and surveillance for Barrett's esophagus with dysplasia only or Barrett's esophagus without dysplasia every 2 to 5 years was determined. Surveillance was every 6 months for low-grade dysplasia and every 3 months for high-grade dysplasia. The target population was followed up until 80 years of age or death.

Findings.—When compared with no screening or surveillance, screening with surveillance only of patients with Barrett's esophagus with dysplasia cost $10,440 for quality-adjusted life-year (QALY) saved. Compared with surveillance of patients with Barrett's esophagus with dysplasia, the incremental cost-effectiveness ratio of surveillance every 5 years in patients with Barrett's esophagus but no dysplasia was $596,000 for QALY saved. Sensitivity analysis indicated that the annual incidence of adenocarcinoma had to exceed 1 case per 54 patient-years of follow-up for surveillance of Barrett's esophagus without dysplasia every 5 years to have an incremental cost-effectiveness ratio of less than $50,000 per QALY saved.

Conclusions.—The screening of 50-year-old white men with GERD symptoms to detect adenocarcinoma associated with Barrett's esophagus appears to be cost effective. Subsequent surveillance of patients with Barrett's esophagus without dysplasia is costly, even at 5-year intervals.

▶ The complications of GERD are divided into local (esophagitis, Barrett's esophagus) and extraesophageal, which include airway and laryngeal effects. Barrett's esophagus is columnar cell metaplasia that replaces native squamous cell esophageal epithelium. This is felt to result from acid/pepsin reflux. Barrett's has a propensity to develop dysplasia and adenocarcinoma; the latter has been increasing in frequency. Adenocarcinoma of the esophagus occurs more frequently in white men older than 50 years. Therefore, screening for the presence of Barrett's epithelium and surveillance of those patients who are found to have Barrett's esophagus is recommended.[1]

Inadomi et al used a decision analysis to determine whether current, one-time screening recommendations in white men older than 50 years, with symptoms of GERD and subsequent surveillance, represents cost-effective care if Barrett's is found. They demonstrated potential benefit of strategies of screening and then surveillance for Barrett's esophagus and associated adenocarcinoma of the esophagus among white men with symptoms of GERD. They also found that performing this screening and limiting surveillance to patients with Barrett's esophagus and dysplasia is associated with a cost-effectiveness ratio of more than $10,000 compared with no screening or surveillance. Thus, reinforcing that screening in this high-risk patient group with GERD is, in their model, cost effective. What about those found to have Barrett's esophagus but no dysplasia? They found that it may increase the total number of QALYs saved, but it was expensive.

J. S. Barkin, MD

Reference

1. Sampliner RE: Updated guidelines for the diagnosis, surveillance and therapy of Barrett's esophagus. *Am J Gastroenterol* 97:1888-1895, 2002.

A Case-Control Study of Endoscopy and Mortality From Adenocarcinoma of the Esophagus or Gastric Cardia in Persons With GERD
Kearney DJ, Crump C, Maynard C, et al (VA Puget Sound Health Care System, Seattle; Univ of Washington, Seattle; Veterans Affairs Epidemiologic Research and Information Ctr, Seattle)
Gastroenterology 57:823-829, 2003   58–4

Background.—In the past 30 years, the incidence of adenocarcinoma of the esophagus and gastric cardia has increased markedly in the United States. A major risk factor for this cancer are gastroesophageal reflux disease symptoms. Some authorities have advocated an esophagogastroduodenoscopy (EGD) to detect Barrett's esophagus for patients with GERD when heartburn is the main symptom, when GERD is longstanding, or as a single lifetime examination. Whether EGD decreases mortality rates from adenocarcinoma of the esophagus or gastric cardia for patients with GERD was studied.

Methods.—Two hundred forty-five patients who had had reflux and who died of adenocarcinoma of the esophagus or gastric cardia between 1995 and 1999 were compared with 980 patients with reflux who had not died of adenocarcinoma. The 2 groups were frequency matched for age and race. All patients were men identified from Veterans Health Administration databases.

Findings.—Case patients were significantly less likely than control patients to have had an EGD. This negative relation was as strong for any EGD performed 1 to 8 years before diagnosis as for more recent EGD. However, EGD and decreased mortality rate were not shown to be causally linked. The risk of dying of adenocarcinoma was significantly lower for men diagnosed with GERD as inpatients than for those diagnosed as outpatients.

Conclusions.—Performing an EGD is associated with decreased mortality rate from adenocarcinoma of the esophagus or gastric cardia among patients with GERD. Whether this association is causative has yet to be established.

▶ Unfortunately, endoscopy with biopsy is not an ideal modality to detect dysplasia. Yield depends on the number and location of biopsies and histologic interpretation. Therefore, not performing surveillance in these patients is a path fraught with dangers. Should once-in-a-lifetime endoscopy be performed in all subgroups of patients with GERD who have prolonged (>7 years) symptoms of GERD requiring medication, but who lack the alarm symptoms of dysphagia, odynophagia, hemoptysis, or extra esophageal symptoms? This is not cost effective but seems to be reasonable medical care to both reassure the patient and yourself and to diagnose other causes of symptoms. Kearny et al reported another benefit of endoscopy in these patients.

In a case-control study, the authors reported that endoscopy reduced mortality rates from adenocarcinoma of the esophagus or gastric cardia for patients with GERD. There is early evidence that the use of proton-pump inhibitors in patients with Barrett's may reduce the risk of adenocarcinoma, thus partially reaffirming our belief that decreasing injury is a good therapeutic aim in patients with Barrett's esophagus. The chemopreventive potential of nonsteroidal anti-inflammatory drugs is important, as there has been a 7-fold increase in the incidence of esophageal adenocarcinoma among US men since the mid 1970s.[1]

J. S. Barkin, MD

Reference

1. Institute NC SEER Program public use data tapes, 1973-1999, vol 2002. DCCPS, Surveillance Research Program.

Protective Association of Aspirin/NSAIDs and Esophageal Cancer: A Systematic Review and Meta-analysis

Corley DA, Kerlikowske K, Verma R, et al (Univ of California, San Francisco; Department of Veterans Affairs Med Ctr, San Francisco; Univ of California, Berkeley)

Gastroenterology 124:47-56, 2003   58–5

Background.—The high fatality rates associated with esophageal carcinomas make chemoprevention a desirable strategy. A meta-analysis of observational studies was performed to assess the association of aspirin and nonsteroidal anti-inflammatory drug (NSAID) use with esophageal cancer.

Methods.—Studies published between 1980 and 2001 were included in the meta-analysis if they assessed exposure to NSAIDs or aspirin, evaluated esophageal cancer, and reported relative risks or odds ratios or provided data by calculation. The 9 publications included were 2 cohort and 7 case-control studies presenting data on a total of 1813 patients with cancer. Two investigators independently abstracted data. Primary and sensitivity analyses were performed by using fixed and random-effects models.

Findings.—Statistical pooling demonstrated a protective relation between any aspirin or NSAID use and esophageal cancer. Intermittent and frequent medication use were both protective, with more frequent use being more so. When data were stratified by medication type, aspirin use showed a protective effect and NSAID use showed a borderline protective effect. Any use protected against esophageal adenocarcinoma and squamous cell carcinoma.

Conclusions.—Pooled data support the notion that aspirin or NSAID use protects against esophageal cancer. Current evidence suggests a dose effect. Clinical trials of these agents in high-risk patients are warranted.

▶ The rationale for use of NSAIDs is that there is an association between increased cyclooxygenase-2 expression and the development and malignant progression of Barrett's esophagus. In addition, NSAIDs/aspirin may decrease the incidence of esophageal squamous cell carcinoma. Corley et al performed a review and meta-analysis of observational studies to search for an association between aspirin/NSAIDs ingestion and esophageal cancer. They found a protective association between aspirin/NSAID ingestion and esophageal adenocarcinoma and squamous cell carcinoma. They also found a dose effect; a higher intake had the most effect. However, dosage levels were not available. Overall, persons who report any use of aspirin/NSAIDs have approximately a 40% lower annual risk of esophageal cancer than those who do not take aspirin/NSAIDs. This effect is similar to the aspirin/NSAIDs protective effect against colorectal cancer. Therefore, it seems reasonable to ensure that our patients who are at least 40 years of age ingest aspirin/NSAIDs as a chemoprotective agent.

J. S. Barkin, MD

59 Stomach

Gastro-protective Treatment in Patients Using NSAIDs: Development of Appropriateness Criteria by a Multidisciplinary Expert Panel
Stoevelaar HJ, for the Belgian Expert Panel on Gastro-protective Treatment in NSAID Users (Erasmus Univ, Rotterdam; et al)
Scand J Rheumatol 32:162-167, 2003   59–1

Background.—Up to 20% of patients who regularly use nonsteroidal anti-inflammatory agents (NSAIDs) have gastrointestinal symptoms such as dyspepsia, heartburn, nausea, gastroduodenal ulcer, bleeding ulcer, and perforated ulcer. Many researchers advocate the use of gastroprotective drugs to prevent NSAID-associated gastrointestinal complications. A computer model was developed to assist in deciding the appropriateness of gastroprotective drug use in patients taking NSAIDs.

Methods.—The model is based on the RAND Appropriateness Method, with the underlying assumption that preventive treatment with a proton pump inhibitor is associated with the best benefit-to-risk ratio in patients taking NSAIDs. A literature search identified relevant articles, which were reviewed by a multidisciplinary team of experts in NSAID-related upper gastrointestinal complications. This panel rated the appropriateness of gastroprotective drug use in 4608 different clinical scenarios on a 9-point scale (1, extremely inappropriate; 5, equivocal or uncertain; 9, extremely appropriate). These initial responses were combined for each case and condensed into 3 categories (appropriate, inappropriate, or uncertain). These ratings were reviewed by the entire panel, who decided the appropriateness of therapy in each case by consensus. Logistic regression analysis was used to identify factors for helping physicians decide whether a gastroprotective drug should be used in a given patient.

Results.—After the initial round of responses (the 1-9 scale), the panelists agreed completely in 79% of the 4608 cases and disagreed in only 3%. After the second round of responses (3-option scale), there was 100% agreement regarding the appropriateness of gastroprotective drugs in patients with a history of peptic ulcer, whether complicated or uncomplicated. There was only 39% agreement, however, regarding the appropriateness of gastroprotective drug use in patients without a history of peptic ulcer. Regression analyses showed disagreements were related to the patient's age, the type and dose of NSAID, expected frequency of NSAID use, comorbid conditions, the use of other drugs (corticosteroids, coagulation-influencing drugs, aspirin), and whether the patient had previously had a reaction. Combining 3 to 6 of these variables resulted in a 90% probability of agreement on the appropriateness of gastroprotective drug use in a given patient without peptic ulcer disease.

Conclusion.—This computer program was developed to assist physicians in the appropriate use of gastroprotective drugs in patients taking NSAIDs. The program can store information on outcomes, too, which will assist in validating the utility of the expert panel's criteria in real-life practice.

▶ NSAIDs remain one of the most frequently ingested medications that commonly result in gastrointestinal side effects. Ten to 20 percent of patients who ingest NSAIDs on a daily basis have dyspepsia, heartburn, and nausea.[1] Gastrointestinal ulcers occur in 15% of regular users of NSAIDs and may be complicated by perforation, obstruction, or bleeding.[2,3] Patient and medication characteristics that put patients at an increased risk for these complications are listed in Table 1.

TABLE 1.—Factors for Increased Risk of GI
Ulcer Complications

- Dosage and frequency of NSAIDs
- Advanced age
- History of gastrointestinal ulcers
- Concomitant use of ASA or anticoagulants

Abbreviations: GI, Gastrointestinal; *NSAIDs*, nonsteroidal anti-inflammatory drugs; *ASA*, acetylsalicylic acid.

Stoevelaar et al developed a decision support model combining evidence from clinical studies with expert collective judgment. They included more than 4000 patient scenarios, and there was agreement in 79% of cases and disagreement in only 3%. This was due to acceptance of the usefulness of gastroprotective drugs in patients who have a history of uncomplicated or complicated peptic ulcer disease (PUD). However, there was marked variability on the acceptance of the usefulness of gastroprotective drugs in patients with no history of PUD. There was significant agreement by the experts on the use of gastroprotective treatment in the patient with no history of PUD if at least 3 of 5 variables were present, including regular use of NSAIDs, severe comorbidity, use of corticosteroids, aspirin intake, or age greater than 60 years.

In high-risk patients, our strategies to decrease gastrointestinal complications can be use of gastroprotective medications or use of the more expensive selective cyclooxygenase (COX)-2 inhibitor drugs. Chan et al[4] have previously compared use of a COX-2–specific inhibitor (celecoxib) with the use of diclofenac, a nonselective NSAID, along with intake of a proton pump inhibitor (PPI). They found that celecoxib was associated with a 4.9% rate of recurrent ulcer bleeding, compared with a 6.4% rate for diclofenac plus omeprazole (not significantly different). Unfortunately, even intake of selective COX-2 drugs is associated with gastrointestinal bleeding; therefore, in the high-risk patient as defined above, a COXIB should be combined with a PPI.

J. S. Barkin, MD

References

1. Lanza FL: A guideline for the treatment and prevention of NSAID-induced ulcers. Members of the Ad Hoc Committee on Practice Parameters of the American College of Gastroenterology. *Am J Gastroenterol* 93:2037-2046, 1998.
2. Wolfe MM, Lichtenstein DR, Singh G: Gastrointestinal toxicity of nonsteroidal anti-inflammatory drugs. *N Engl J Med* 340:1888-1899, 1999.
3. Silverstein FE, Graham DY, Senior JR, et al: Misoprostol reduces serious gastrointestinal complications in patients with rheumatoid arthritis receiving nonsteroidal anti-inflammatory drugs. *Ann Intern Med* 123:241-249, 1995.
4. Chan FK, Hung LC, Suen BY, et al: Celecoxib versus diclofenac and omeprazole in reducing the risk of recurrent ulcer bleeding in patients with arthritis. *N Engl J Med* 347:2104-2110, 2002.

SUGGESTED READING

Lydeard S, Jones R: Factors affecting the decision to consult with dyspepsia comparison of consulters and non-consulters. *J R Coll Gen Pract* 39:495-498, 1989.)

Rates of Dyspepsia One Year After *Helicobacter pylori* Screening and Eradication in a Danish Population
Wildner-Christensen M, Møller Hansen J, Schaffalitzky de Muckadell OB
(Odense Univ, Denmark)
Gastroenterology 125:372-379, 2003   59–2

Background.—Dyspepsia is a common condition that affects 25% to 50% of the general population annually, placing a significant clinical and financial burden on health services. Dyspepsia also results in lost work time and has an adverse effect on the quality of life. *Helicobacter pylori* has been shown to be strongly correlated with peptic ulcer disease, and the elimination of *H pylori* cures the condition. It is now generally accepted that *H pylori* infection is a contributing risk factor for distal gastric cancer. However, the significance of *H pylori* in functional dyspepsia would appear to be limited. Whether screening and eradication of *H pylori* in a general population would reduce the prevalence of dyspepsia and the incidence of peptic ulcer was investigated.

Methods.—This study was conducted among the population of 1 Danish city and the surrounding municipalities. A total of 20,000 persons aged 40 to 65 years were randomly assigned to screening and eradication for *H pylori* or to a control group. *H pylori* status was determined by a whole blood *H pylori* test, and a positive result was confirmed by a ^{13}C-urea breath test. Persons who tested positive for *H pylori* were offered eradication therapy. A mailed questionnaire was used to assess the prevalence of dyspepsia and the quality of life. Data regarding the use of endoscopy and prescription medication were obtained from registers.

Results.—The rate of response was 62.6%. The prevalence of *H pylori* was 17.5%, and the rate of eradication was 95%. In the intervention group, the prevalence of dyspepsia decreased from 24.3% at inclusion to 20.5% at 1 year of follow up. A similar reduction was seen in *H pylori*–negative and *H pylori*–positive persons. Dyspepsia in the control group increased from 20.3% to 21.5%. There was a modest improvement in the symptoms of gastroesophageal reflux in *H pylori*–eradicated participants. However, with the exception of a decreased rate of consultation for dyspepsia, there were no apparent savings in health care.

Conclusions.—This study found a modest reduction in the prevalence of dyspepsia after the screening and treatment procedure, but the result did not significantly affect health care use or improve the quality of life.

▶ Dyspepsia is defined as upper abdominal discomfort or pain, often accompanied by fullness, bloating, or early satiety. This symptom complex affects at least 25% of the general population in 1 year, of which 2% to 5% seek medical attention.[1] The therapeutic approaches that have been advocated include (1) empiric therapy with short course of a proton-pump inhibitor, (2) referral for endoscopy, or (3) test for *H pylori* and treat if present. Unfortunately, this latter treatment regimen for dyspepsia has failed to prove efficacious in US trials.

Wildner-Christensen et al presented their 1-year follow-up of a program on *H pylori* screening and eradication in a Danish population. They found a reduction in dyspepsia; however, *H pylori*–negative participants also experienced a reduction in dyspepsia, which was similar to *H pylori*–positive patients. While effective treatment exists for *H pylori* and prevention of its complications, the role of *H pylori* in functional dyspepsia is limited.

J. S. Barkin, MD

Reference

1. Westbrook JI, McIntosh JH, Talley NJ: The impact of dyspepsia definition on prevalence estimates: Considerations for future researchers. *Scand J Gastroenterol* 35:227-233, 2000.

The Relationship Among Previous Antimicrobial Use, Antimicrobial Resistance, and Treatment Outcomes for *Helicobacter pylori* Infections
McMahon BJ, Hennessy TW, Bensler JM, et al (Ctrs for Disease Control and Prevention, Anchorage, AK; Alaska Native Med Ctr, Anchorage, AK)
Ann Intern Med 139:463-469, 2003   59–3

Background.—*Helicobacter pylori* has been reported to infect the gastric mucosa of 40% of persons in developing countries and 90% of persons living in developing countries. *H pylori* infection has been shown to be a major cause of gastric and duodenal ulcers and has also been associated with chronic gastritis, mucosa-associated lymphoid tissue lymphoma, and adenocarcinoma of the stomach. Eradication of *H pylori* has been reported in up to 95% of patients treated with a combination of antimicrobial agents.

However, lower cure rates have been reported in patients with clarithromycin-resistant or metronidazole-resistant *H pylori* when they are treated with these agents. Whether previous use of antimicrobial agents is predictive of subsequent antibiotic resistance of *H pylori* and whether treatment outcome is affected by this resistance were investigated.

Methods.—This retrospective cohort analysis was conducted among adults recruited sequentially from a referral hospital in Alaska. The study group was composed of 125 adults infected with *H pylori*. Medical records were reviewed for antimicrobial agents prescribed in the 10 years before diagnosis with *H pylori* infection. *H pylori* isolates were obtained by endoscopic gastric biopsy, and the antimicrobial susceptibility of these isolates was determined by the urea breath test 2 months after antimicrobial treatment.

Results.—Nearly one third (30%) of patients were found to have *H pylori* isolates resistant to clarithromycin, and two thirds (66%) were found to have *H pylori* isolates resistant to metronidazole. Resistance to clarithromycin was associated with previous use of any macrolide antibiotic, and resistance to metronidazole was associated with previous use of metronidazole. The odds of isolates being resistant to clarithromycin increased in relation to the number of courses of macrolides received. Of the 53 patients treated with clarithromycin-based regimens, treatment was unsuccessful in 77% of patients with clarithromycin-resistant *H pylori* and in 13% of those with clarithromycin-susceptible strains of *H pylori*.

Conclusions.—The previous use of macrolides and metronidazole is associated with *H pylori* resistance to those agents. Clarithromycin resistance was found to be associated with a greater risk of failure with clarithromycin-based treatments.

▶ If testing is not available, then one must be aware of factors that predispose to *H pylori* resistance; if these are present, use another regime. McMahon et al sought to determine whether past antimicrobial use was associated with antimicrobial resistance among *H pylori* isolates. This study was performed in a native Alaskan population, in whom they found *H pylori* resistant to clarithromycin in 30% and to metronidazole in 66%. They found a relatively significant relationship between a patient's previous use of metronidazole or a macrolide antimicrobial agent and subsequent isolation of *H pylori* resistant to these medications. Infection with *H pylori* resistant to clarithromycin was associated with a 6-fold increased risk for treatment failure in persons receiving a clarithromycin-containing regimen. They also found that in women metronidazole resistance was associated with previous metronidazole use.

Clinically, if we are going to empirically treat *H pylori*, we should not use a clarithromycin regimen if the patients have been treated with clarithromycin in the past. If we add a proton-pump inhibitor to the regimen, we can use metronidazole, even in patients with a history of previous use that may have resulted in *H pylori* metronidazole resistance. The use of antibiotics per person in the lower 48 states is less and therefore, as expected, resistant strains are less frequent. Resistance rates vary by geographical areas. If we practice in areas where *H pylori* drug resistance is common, then we need to consider having documentation of eradication.

J. S. Barkin, MD

Impact of Upper Endoscopy on Satisfaction in Patients With Previously Uninvestigated Dyspepsia

Rabeneck L, Wristers K, Souchek J, et al (Baylor College of Medicine, Houston)

Gastrointest Endosc 57:295-299, 2003   59–4

Background.—There is pressure from payers on gastroenterologists in the United States to defend the widespread use of endoscopic procedures, which account for a significant amount of health care expenditures. Upper endoscopy is the most frequently performed of endoscopic procedures, and although evaluation of uninvestigated dyspepsia is the most common indication for endoscopy, no gross abnormality is detected in two thirds of these patients. Thus, the value of the procedure has been investigated in this large group of patients with negative findings on endoscopy. The impact of endoscopy on patient satisfaction was evaluated in patients with previously uninvestigated dyspepsia.

Methods.—This study was conducted as a secondary analysis of data from a previous randomized, double-blind, placebo-controlled trial evaluating a 6-week course of omeprazole versus placebo in 140 patients with uninvestigated dyspepsia. The patients were followed up for 1 year. Study participants were recruited from primary care outpatient clinics at a Veterans Affairs hospital. The patients were 18 years of age or older with at least a 1-week history of dyspepsia (epigastric discomfort) without alarm features. Patient satisfaction was measured at each of 5 visits with the Severity of Dyspepsia Assessment. Endoscopy was performed in patients who were unresponsive to empiric therapy with omeprazole or placebo.

Results.—Data on all 5 follow-up visits were available in 62 patients, of whom 36 had a negative endoscopy. The mean scores for all patients for times 2 and 3 were significantly lower than those for time 4 and time 5. The mean score for time 1 was significantly lower than the mean score for time 5. Similar significant improvements in satisfaction scores were observed in subgroups with negative and positive findings.

Conclusions.—This study found that endoscopy in patients with previously uninvestigated dyspepsia results in improved patient satisfaction regardless of endoscopic findings.

▶ There are 3 appropriate therapeutic roads to take after seeing a patient younger than 45 years with dyspepsia and no alarm symptoms or exposure to nonsteroidal anti-inflammatory drugs. These include an empirical course of a proton-pump inhibitor, test and treat for *H pylori,* and upper endoscopy. The reason that most patients with dyspepsia seek medical care is not severity of symptoms, but concern about the possible seriousness of symptoms, or what caused them.[1] While most of these endoscopy results will be negative, they are of benefit because they reduce diagnostic uncertainty, alleviate patient anxiety, and result in patient satisfaction.

Rabeneck et al reported on the effect of upper endoscopy on satisfaction in patients with previously uninvestigated dyspepsia. They found a significant improvement in satisfaction with dyspepsia-related health for all patients regardless of whether the endoscopy was positive or negative. Thus, its key benefit is reassurance—something each of us practices daily. Thus, it seems that this course or a short therapeutic trial with a proton-pump inhibitor should be utilized in dyspeptic patients with low-risk of "organic" disease.

J. S. Barkin, MD

Reference

1. Lydeard S, Jones R. Factors affecting the decision to consult with dyspepsia comparison of consulters and non-consulters. *J Coll Gen Pract* 39:495-498, 1989.

Randomized Trial of Medical and Endoscopic Therapy to Prevent Recurrent Ulcer Hemorrhage in Patients With Adherent Clots
Jensen DM, Kovacs TOG, Jutabha R, et al (Univ of California, Los Angeles; Northridge Hosp, Van Nuys, Calif; Univ of California, San Diego; et al)
Gastroenterology 123:407-413, 2002   59–5

Background.—Stigmata of peptic ulcer hemorrhage have been used for more than a decade for the stratification of patients according to the risk of recurrent hemorrhage with medical treatment. Endoscopic therapies have also been recommended for patients with major stigmata of ulcer hemorrhage, such as active bleeding or nonbleeding visible vessels. In contrast, other stigmata of ulcer hemorrhage, such as adherent clots, have not been recommended for endoscopic therapy. A previous randomized trial found no benefit to endoscopic therapies compared with medical therapy for the prevention of ulcer rebleeding. The hypothesis that treatment with combination endoscopic therapy would result in significantly lower rebleeding rates compared with medical therapy in patients with recurrent ulcer hemorrhage was tested.

Methods.—The study group for this randomized controlled trial was composed of 32 high-risk patients with severe ulcer hemorrhage and nonbleeding adherent clots resistant to target irrigation. The patients were randomly assigned to medical therapy or to combination endoscopic therapy with epinephrine injection, shaving of the clot with cold guillotining, and bipolar coagulation of the underlying stigmata. All patients were managed by physicians blinded to the endoscopic therapy.

Results.—The patients in both groups were similar at study entry, with the exception of older age in the medical group and lower platelet count in the endoscopic group. At hospital discharge, significantly more medically treated patients than endoscopically treated patients had rebleeding (35.3% vs 0%). There were no complications from endoscopic treatment.

Conclusions.—It would appear from these findings that combination endoscopic therapy for the treatment of nonbleeding adherent clots was safe and effective in significantly reducing early ulcer rebleeding rates in high-risk patients compared with medical therapy alone.

The Effect of Endoscopic Therapy in Patients Receiving Omeprazole for Bleeding Ulcer With Nonbleeding Visible Vessels or Adherent Clots: A Randomized Comparison
Sung JJY, Chan FKL, Lau JYW, et al (Chinese Univ of Hong Kong)
Ann Intern Med 139:237-243, 2003   59–6

Background.—Endoscopic hemostasis is effective in controlling bleeding from peptic ulcers, but the optimal treatment of ulcers with nonbleeding visible vessels and adherent clots is unclear. The source of this uncertainty is the variability in endoscopic diagnosis and in the standard treatment strategies used by endoscopists for ulcers with adherent clots. Clots and protuberant vessels are the most difficult stigmata of hemorrhage to differentiate. A recent study has reported on the effectiveness of endoscopic therapy in combination with IV omeprazole infusion in a small group of patients who were at high risk for ulcer hemorrhage. IV omeprazole infusion plus endoscopic therapy was compared with IV omeprazole infusion alone for the prevention of recurrent bleeding from ulcers with nonbleeding visible vessels or adherent clots.

Methods.—A total of 156 persons with upper gastrointestinal bleeding and ulcers showing nonbleeding visible vessels or adherent clots were enrolled in this blinded randomized study. The patients were treated with combination endoscopic therapy and omeprazole infusion (78 patients) or sham endoscopic therapy and omeprazole infusion (78 patients). The main outcome measurement was comparison of recurrent ulcer bleeding before discharge and within 30 days.

Results.—Ulcer bleeding recurred before discharge in 7 patients who received IV omeprazole alone (9%) and in no patients who received combination therapy. The probability of recurrent bleeding within 30 days was 11.6% (9 patients) in the omeprazole-only group and in 1.1% (1 patient) in the combined therapy group. In addition, patients in the combined therapy group needed fewer transfusions. One patient in the combined therapy group underwent surgery for ulcer perforation. There were 4 deaths within 30 days, 2 in each group.

Conclusions.—The combination of endoscopic therapy and omeprazole infusion is superior to omeprazole infusion alone for the prevention of recurrent bleeding in patients with ulcers with nonbleeding visible vessels and adherent clots.

▶ The overwhelming majority of patients with upper gastrointestinal bleeding have spontaneous cessation; however, approximately 20% have recurrent bleeding. We have identified clinical criteria and endoscopic findings that predispose the patient to have recurrent bleeding. These endoscopic findings in an ulcer include the presence of active bleeding ulcer or a visible vessel in the ulcer base. The reason for the recurrent bleeding is erosion of the exposed artery or lysis of the sealed clot at the ulcer base caused by acid and pepsin. Therefore, medical therapy with proton-pump inhibitors (PPIs) has been proposed as a therapeutic regime for ulcers that have bled. The basis of this recommendation is that high pH can inactivate pepsin and prevent platelet dysfunction observed at low pH levels. Two studies performed in India supported this proposal. A 5-day course of oral omeprazole, 40 mg twice daily, reduced recurrent bleeding even without endoscopic therapy[1]; however, is medical therapy alone adequate? The study by Jensen et al[2] compared medical therapy and medical therapy combined with endoscopic therapy and showed that the combined regimen was statistically superior, although in a small number of patients. Sung et al (Abstract 59–6) expanded our knowledge of therapy of bleeding peptic ulcers. When actively bleeding lesions are encountered at endoscopy, our initial approach is endoscopic hemostasis, but what should we do if a nonbleeding visible vessel or nonbleeding clot that has a high likelihood to rebleed is encountered at endoscopy? In this randomized trial, patients with these endoscopic findings were treated with combined endoscopic hemostatic methods—thermocoagulation and epinephrine injection followed by omeprazole or omeprazole alone. The group that received endoscopic therapy and omeprazole had significantly less rebleeding within 30 days than those who received only medical therapy. This combined benefit of medical and endoscopic therapy is similar to this group's findings in patients who had actively bleeding ulcers. The take-away message for patient care is to have a very technically competent endoscopist treat the hemorrhage site in the ulcer base and initiate endoscopic hemostasis. This should be followed by PPI infusion in an attempt to prevent recurrent ulcer bleeding. This study utilized an 80-mg bolus followed by continuous infusion of omeprazole, 8 mg/d for 72 hours. This PPI is currently unavailable in the United States; therefore, we use another IV PPI preparation. The analysis by Lee et al[3] of this method found that the use of IV omeprazole was cost effective. Hence, we need to make sure that patients receive IV infusion of a PPI for 72 hours after bleeding, followed by oral PPI therapy. In addition, we need to determine their *H pylori* status and, if positive, initiate treatment and document elimination by fecal or breath hydrogen testing.

J. S. Barkin, MD

References

1. Lau JY, Chung SC, Leung JW, et al: The evolution of hemorrhage in bleeding peptic ulcers: A sequential endoscopic study. *Endoscopy* 30:513-518, 1998.
2. Jensen DM, Kovacs TOG, Jutabha R, et al: Final results and cost assessment of endoscopic vs. medical therapies for prevention of recurrent ulcer hemorrhage from adherent clots in a randomized controlled trial [abstract]. *Gastrointest Endosc* 41:279, 1995.
3. Lee KKC, You JHC, Wong ICK, et al: Cost-effectiveness analysis of high-dose omeprazole infusion as adjuvant therapy to endoscopic treatment of bleeding peptic ulcer. *Gastrointest Endosc* 57:160-164, 2003.

Use of Selective Serotonin Reuptake Inhibitors and Risk of Upper Gastrointestinal Tract Bleeding: A Population-Based Cohort Study

Dalton SO, Johansen C, Mellemkjaer L, et al (Danish Cancer Society, Copenhagen; Univ of Aarhus, Denmark; Aarhus Univ Hosp, Denmark)

Arch Intern Med 163:59-64, 2003   59–7

Background.—The use of newer, more receptor-selective antidepressive agents increased during the last decade, in part because of the relatively few adverse effects and low toxicity associated with these agents. Several clinical reports have indicated an association between selective serotonin reuptake inhibitors (SSRIs) and bleeding disorders ranging from prolonged bleeding time, ecchymoses, purpura, and epistaxis to more serious conditions such as gastrointestinal tract, genitourinary tract, and intracranial bleeding. The risk of upper gastrointestinal tract bleeding with the use of antidepressant medication was examined.

Methods.—The study was conducted among all users of antidepressants in 1 county in Denmark from January 1991 to December 1995. Study participants were identified in the Pharmaco-Epidemiologic Prescription Database of North Jutland. Hospitalizations for upper gastrointestinal bleeding were searched among 26,005 users of antidepressant medications and compared with the number of hospitalizations in that county that did not involve prescriptions for antidepressant medications.

Results.—The rate of upper gastrointestinal bleeding episodes was 3.6 times higher than expected, corresponding to a rate difference of 3.1 per 1000 treatment-years, during periods of SSRI use without the use of other drugs associated with upper GI bleeding. When the use of an SSRI was combined with nonsteroidal anti-inflammatory drugs or low-dose aspirin, the risk of upper gastrointestinal bleeding was increased to 12.2 and 5.2, respectively. The use of non-SSRIs increased the risk of upper gastrointestinal bleeding to 2.3, whereas the use of antidepressants without action on the serotonin receptor had no significant effect on the risk of upper gastrointestinal bleeding. The risk associated with SSRI use returned to unity after termination of SSRI treatment, whereas the risks were similarly increased during periods of use and nonuse of non-SSRI agents.

Conclusions.—There is an increased risk of upper gastrointestinal bleeding associated with the use of SSRIs. This study indicated that this effect is potentiated by concurrent use of nonsteroidal anti-inflammatory drugs or low-dose aspirin; an increased risk of upper gastrointestinal bleeding could not be associated with non-SSRI antidepressants.

Combined Use of SSRIs and NSAIDs Increases the Risk of Gastrointestinal Adverse Effects

de Jong JCF, van den Berg PB, Tobi H, et al (Univ Centre for Pharmacy, Groningen, The Netherlands)

Br J Clin Pharmacol 55:591-595, 2003   59–8

Background.—Several studies have indicated an association between the use of selective serotonin reuptake inhibitors (SSRIs) and an increase in the risk of gastrointestinal bleeding. The risks of gastrointestinal adverse effects in association with nonselective tricyclic antidepressants have not been described. In addition to the anti-inflammatory, analgesic, and antipyretic actions of nonsteroidal anti-inflammatory drugs (NSAIDs), these agents are known to exert serious adverse effects on the thrombocytes, the kidneys, and the gastrointestinal tract. The most frequently reported adverse effect is subjective atrophy, which has been reported in up to half of all NSAID users. There is also a high prevalence of ulcers associated with NSAID use. The relation between the use of antidepressants with or without NSAIDs and the risk of gastrointestinal side effects was investigated.

Methods.—This population-based cohort study used medication data for 180,000 patients from 16 pharmacies in The Netherlands. The study group was composed of 15,445 new users of antidepressants with or without NSAIDs. A review of patient profiles was conducted for cases of gastrointestinal adverse effects caused by first-time use of antidepressants with or without NSAIDs. The main outcome measure was the number of first prescriptions for peptic ulcer drugs in the period from day 2 after starting antidepressants with or without NSAIDs until 10 days after the last dose.

Results.—The incidence of first prescriptions for peptic ulcer drugs in the reference group of 619 new users of nonselective antidepressants was 0.051. The use of SSRIs caused a slightly higher incidence rate ratio of 1.2. The incidence rate ratio was increased to 12.4 with the combined use of SSRIs and NSAIDs, whereas the combination of nonselective antidepressants and NSAIDs increased the incidence rate ratio to 2.5.

Conclusions.—This study found that the risk of gastrointestinal adverse effects was increased in first-time users of SSRIs compared with nonselective antidepressants. The risk was strongly increased with the combined use of SSRIs and NSAIDs, and this combination should be avoided. However, the combination of nonselective antidepressants and NSAIDs was not found to strongly increase the risk of gastrointestinal adverse effects.

▶ The usual drugs that result in gastrointestinal damage are aspirin, NSAIDs, potassium chloride, and toxins, such as alcohol. Selective serotonin reuptake inhibitors (SSRIs) have been associated with bleeding disorders. This is felt to be secondary to their effects on platelets, whose release of serotonin is important in hemostasis. Platelets are unable to synthesize serotonin, and depletion of serotonin stores because of SSRI effects could therefore induce a hemorrhagic complication. These effects may induce prolonged bleeding time or ecchymosis and result in organ bleeding from gastrointestinal or genitourinary tract disease. Unfortunately, these effects on hemostasis have not been confirmed in healthy volunteers.

Dalton et al, a Danish group (Abstract 59–7), investigated the risk of upper gastrointestinal bleeding in users of SSRIs and other antidepressants in a population-based cohort study. They found that users of SSRIs were hospitalized with upper gastrointestinal bleeding at a rate of 3.6 times greater than persons of a similar sex and age for whom these medications had not been prescribed. This effect was the same for different types of SSRIs; therefore, it is a class effect. As one would expect, this effect was potentiated by concurrent use of NSAIDs and aspirin. We do not have information on smoking and alcohol use in this population, which influences the risk of upper gastrointestinal bleeding. This increased risk of upper gastrointestinal bleeding is most likely secondary to these or other confounding factors. Clinically, we need to consider patients' use of an SSRI as an added risk for upper gastrointestinal bleeding and be cautious in our use of NSAIDs in patients taking SSRIs.

De Jong et al (Abstract 59–8) have shown that the combination of SSRIs and NSAIDs increased the incidence rate ratio of upper gastrointestinal bleeding from 1.2 in SSRI users alone to 12.4. Interestingly, the incident rates only increased from 1.2 to 2.5 with the combination of nonselective antidepressants and NSAIDs.

J. S. Barkin, MD

Acquired von Willebrand Syndrome in Aortic Stenosis
Vincentelli A, Susen S, Le Tourneau T, et al (Univ of Lille II, France; Clinique de Chirugie Cardiovasculaire, Lille, France; Institut d'Hématologie Biologique et d'Hémobiologie-Transfusion, Lille, France; et al)
N Engl J Med 349:343-349, 2003   59–9

Background.—Aortic valve stenosis can be complicated by Heyde's syndrome (gastrointestinal angiodysplasia). Heyde's syndrome is associated with acquired type 2A von Willebrand's syndrome, which is characterized by the loss of the largest multimers of von Willebrand factor. One of the proposed causes of the bleeding is proteolysis of von Willebrand factor as it passes through the stenotic valve. Structural changes in the shape of the von Willebrand factor molecule can be induced by high shear forces, resulting in exposure of the bonds between amino acids 842 and 843, which are sensitive to the action of a specific von Willebrand protease. Proteolysis of the highest molecular weight multimers of von Willebrand factor is the result; these multimers are the most effective in platelet-mediated hemostasis under conditions of high shear stress. The fact that these biologic abnormalities can be corrected by valve replacement provides further support of this concept. The prevalence and cause of hemostatic abnormalities in patients with aortic stenosis as well as their clinical consequences were determined.

Methods.—A consecutive series of 50 patients with aortic stenosis were enrolled in this study, and each patient completed a standardized screening questionnaire to detect a history of bleeding. Valve replacement was performed in 42 patients with severe aortic stenosis. Platelet function under high shear stress, von Willebrand factor collagen-binding activity and antigen levels, and the multimeric structure of von Willebrand factor were assessed at baseline and at 1 and 7 days and 6 months postoperatively.

Results.—Skin or mucosal bleeding occurred in 21% of patients with severe aortic stenosis. High shear stress–induced platelet function abnormalities, decreased von Willebrand factor collagen-binding activity, and the loss of the largest multimers, or a combination of these conditions, was present in 67% to 92% of patients with severe aortic stenosis and correlated significantly with the severity of valve stenosis. Primary hemostatic abnormalities were completely corrected on the first day after surgery but tended to recur at 6 months, particularly when there was a mismatch between patient and prosthesis.

Conclusions.—Type 2A von Willebrand syndrome is a common finding in patients with severe aortic stenosis. Von Willebrand factor abnormalities are directly associated with the severity of aortic stenosis, and these abnormalities are improved by replacement of the valve in the absence of mismatch between patient and prosthesis.

▶ Patients with aortic valve stenosis have an increased risk of gastrointestinal bleeding from angiodysplasia (Heyde's syndrome).[1] This is due to acquired type 2A von Willebrand syndrome resulting from proteolysis of the highest molecular weight multimers of von Willebrand factor, which are the most effective in platelet-mediated hemostasis under conditions of high shear stress.[2] Vincentelli et al calculated the prevalence of hemostatic abnormalities in patients with aortic stenosis and their clinical consequences. Bleeding mostly arises from the skin, nose, and gastrointestinal mucosa and occurred in 20% of patients with severe aortic stenosis. Abnormalities of von Willebrand factor are related to the severity of aortic stenosis. Bleeding is best controlled by valve replacement. The authors point out that we must now consider that acquired von Willebrand syndrome with hemostatic abnormalities and bleeding are indications for aortic valve replacement.

J. S. Barkin, MD

References

1. Heyde EC: Gastrointestinal bleeding in aortic stenosis. *N Engl J Med* 259:196, 1958.
2. Sugimoto M, Matsui H, Mizuno T, et al: Mural thrombus generation in type 2A and 2B von Willebrand disease under flow conditions. *Blood* 101:915-920, 2003.

60 Small Bowel

Prevalence of Celiac Disease in At-Risk and Not-At-Risk Groups in the United States: A Large Multicenter Study
Fasano A, Berti I, Gerarduzzi T, et al (Univ of Maryland, Baltimore; Istituto per l'Infanzia Burlo Garofalo, Trieste, Italy; Univ of Vermont, Burlington; et al)
Arch Intern Med 163:286-292, 2003   60–1

Background.—The ingestion of grains containing gluten (eg, wheat, barley, rye) can trigger celiac disease (CD) in genetically susceptible persons. Early treatment of this immune-mediated enteropathy can prevent potentially life-threatening complications. CD is relatively common in Europe, occurring in 1 of 130 to 1 of 300 persons. The frequency of CD in the United States was examined.

Methods.—Blood samples from 9019 persons at risk of CD and 4126 persons not at risk of CD from 32 US states were analyzed. Persons at risk of CD were either first-degree relatives (n = 4508) or second-degree relatives (n = 1275) of patients with biopsy-proven CD, or were experiencing CD-associated symptoms (diarrhea, abdominal pain, or constipation) or disorders (diabetes mellitus type 1, Down syndrome, anemia, arthritis, osteoporosis, infertility, or short stature; n = 3236). Blood samples were analyzed for serum antigliaden antibodies and anti–endomysial antibodies (EMAs). HLA-DQ2/DQ8 haplotyping and (when possible) intestinal biopsy were performed in EMA-positive persons. In addition, human tissue transglutaminase (hTTG) IgA antibodies were assayed in EMA-positive samples, and values higher than 13% (in comparison with those in a control group of 100 healthy persons) were taken as positive.

Results.—Of the 13,145 blood samples screened, 350 (3.7%) were EMA positive. All EMA-positive persons were also positive for hTTG and had an HLA-DQ2/DQ8 haplotype. The prevalence of CD was 1:22 in first-degree relatives of patients with CD, 1:39 in second-degree relatives, and 1:56 in persons with symptoms or disorders associated with CD. The prevalence of CD in persons with CD-associated symptoms or disorders was significantly higher in children (1:25) than in adults (1:68). Among the not-at-risk persons, the prevalence of CD was 1:333 overall, and was significantly higher in adults (1:105) than in children (1:320). Multivariate analyses indicated being a first-degree relative of a patient with CD significantly increased the risk of CD compared with being a second-degree relative (odds ratio, 1.7). Among persons who were not relatives of patients with CD, being symptom-

491

atic significantly increased the likelihood of CD (odds ratio, 2.1). In both at-risk and not-at-risk groups, all EMA-positive patients who underwent intestinal biopsy (78 total) had findings consistent with CD.

Conclusion.—Compared with the not-at-risk population, the prevalence of CD is much higher in relatives (especially first-degree relatives) of patients with CD and in patients with CD-associated symptoms or disorders. In particular, the prevalences of CD in persons with CD-associated symptoms or disorders and in not-at-risk persons are similar to those reported in Europe. Serologic testing of at-risk US persons should be encouraged to allow early diagnosis and improve the quality of life of patients with CD.

▶ Gluten sensitive enteropathy (so-called CD) is immune mediated by gluten in genetically predisposed individuals. CD is the most common hereditary gastrointestinal disease, occurring in 1 of 130 to 1 of 300 European individuals.[1] Fasano et al determined the prevalence of CD in the United States to be 4.5% among first-degree relatives of patients with CD, and 0.75% in not-at-risk persons. Diagnosis was established by EMA-positive and also tissue transglutaminase–positive findings.

Maki et al[2] has reported that the presence of serum tissue transglutaminase and EMAs is predictive of small bowel abnormalities indicative of CD. If CD is so common, why is it not diagnosed more frequently? This is because of its wide spectrum of gastrointestinal manifestations, presentation of nonluminal manifestations, and use of less-specific antigliaden antibody testing as opposed to EMA and tissue transglutaminase.[3]

In addition, as Fasano points out, small bowel biopsy may not be obtained at endoscopy, and even when obtained, it may be pathologically misinterpreted, as only a third of patients have classic flat small intestinal mucosa. These factors translate into over a decade delay in diagnosis of CD.[4] Thus, we need to consider the diagnosis of CD in first- and second-degree relatives of patients with CD as well as in patients with gastrointestinal and nongastrointestinal symptoms that can be caused by CD. While CD was initially described in children, we are now finding a large proportion of CD patients to be adults, who have nonspecific or atypical symptoms and are in the fifth or sixth decade of life.[5]

J. S. Barkin, MD

References

1. Ascher H, Krantz I, Kristiansson B: Increasing incidence of coeliac disease in Sweden. *Arch Dis Child* 66:608-611, 1991.
2. Maki M, Mustalahti K, Kokkonen J, et al: Prevalence of celiac disease among children in Finland. *N Engl J Med* 348:2517-2524, 2003.
3. Fasano A. Catassi C: Current approaches to diagnosis and treatment of celiac disease: An evolving spectrum. *Gastroenterology* 120:636-651, 2001.
4. Green P, Stavropoulos S, Panagi S, et al: Characteristics of adult celiac disease in the USA: Results of a national survey. *Am J Gastroenterol* 96:126-131, 2001.
5. Farrell RJ, Kelly CP: Current concepts: Celiac sprue. *N Engl J Med* 346:180-188, 2002.

Presentations of Adult Celiac Disease in a Nationwide Patient Support Group

Zipser RD, Patel S, Yahya KZ, et al (Harbor-UCLA Med Ctr, Torrance, Calif; Celiac Disease Found, Studio City, Calif)
Dig Dis Sci 48:761-764, 2003   60–2

Background.—Celiac disease (CD) typically presents in children and causes steatorrhea, weight loss, and failure to thrive. Yet CD can present in adults without these classic childhood symptoms. The prevalence of adult-onset CD in the United States and its associated symptoms were investigated.

Methods.—A total of 1032 members of the Celiac Disease Foundation were surveyed from 1993 through 2001. Demographic and clinical characteristics were determined in all patients. In addition, a subset of 134 adults responded to an Internet-based survey regarding presenting signs and symptoms and their initial diagnoses.

Results.—The total cohort included 248 men (24%) and 784 women (76%), with a median age at diagnosis of 46 years. Only 166 patients (16%) had received a diagnosis of CD before 18 years. Patients had consulted an average of 3 physicians before their CD was diagnosed, and the median time from their initial physician evaluation until a biopsy confirmed CD was 12 months. Twenty-one percent of patients had symptoms for longer than 10 years before CD was diagnosed. Of the 583 patients for whom height and weight data were available, 54% had a normal body mass index (BMI) and only 32% were underweight (BMI ≤ 18.5 kg/m^2). The Internet cohort included 109 women (81.3%) and 25 men (18.7%), with a mean age at diagnosis of 44 and 48 years, respectively. The most common presenting signs of CD in this subset were fatigue (82%), abdominal pain (77%), gas or bloating (73%), and anemia (63%). The most common initial diagnoses were irritable bowel syndrome (37%), psychological disorders (29%), and fibromyalgia (9%).

Conclusion.—Presenting signs and symptoms of adult-onset CD are often nonspecific, and they differ from those of CD in childhood, as only about 50% of adults with CD have weight loss or frequent diarrhea. Almost 40% of these patients were initially misdiagnosed as having irritable bowel syndrome. These characteristics are similar to those reported in adult-onset CD in European and Brazilian studies.

Associations of Adult Coeliac Disease With Irritable Bowel Syndrome: A Case-Control Study in Patients Fulfilling ROME II Criteria Referred to Secondary Care

Sanders DS, Carter MJ, Hurlstone DP, et al (Royal Hallamshire Hosp, Sheffield, England; Univ of Sheffield, England; Northern Gen Hosp, Sheffield, England)
Lancet 358:1504-1508, 2001   60–3

Background.—The ROME II criteria were developed by consensus to aid in the diagnosis of functional gastrointestinal disorders, including irritable bowel syndrome (IBS). Many patients with celiac disease (CD) are misdiagnosed as having IBS, but it is not known how many patients with IBS have CD. Patients meeting ROME II criteria for IBS were investigated to determine the incidence of CD in this population.

Methods.—A total of 300 patients (86 men and 214 women; median age, 56 years) meeting the ROME II criteria for IBS and 300 healthy age- and sex-matched controls were studied. Blood samples were analyzed to detect serum IgA and IgG antigliadin antibodies and endomysial antibodies (EMAs). EMA-positive persons were offered duodenal biopsy to check for lesions of CD.

Results.—In all, 66 patients with IBS and 44 controls had positive antibody results. Of the 66 cases, 43 had normal histologic findings, 9 were lost to follow-up or declined biopsy, and 14 had biopsy evidence of CD. Of those with CD, 11 were EMA positive but 3 were EMA negative. Of the 44 controls, only 2 had biopsy-proven CD (both were EMA positive). After excluding cases lost to follow-up, CD was significantly more common in the cases than in the controls (odds ratio, 7.0).

Conclusion.—Patients meeting ROME II criteria for IBS are at greatly increased risk of CD. Thus, immunologic testing (including IgA and IgG antigliadins and EMAs) should be performed in all patients with IBS who are referred for secondary care.

▶ Zipser et al (Abstract 60–2) surveyed the adult presentations of CD. They found that only approximately one half of adult celiac patients reported frequent diarrhea, with only one third underweight. Thus, classic symptoms of CD are uncommon in adult CD patients. Their most frequent symptoms were nonspecific, including fatigue, abdominal discomfort or pain, gas and bloating, psychological symptoms, and muscle and joint pain. As one would expect, the physician diagnoses included IBS, fibromyalgia, anxiety, and depression. These results confirm the finding of Sanders et al (Abstract 60–3) of a significant increase in the incidence of CD in European patients with IBS, who fulfilled the Rome II diagnostic criteria.

J. S. Barkin, MD

Celiac Disease in Patients With Severe Liver Disease: Gluten-Free Diet May Reverse Hepatic Failure
Kaukinen K, Halme L, Collin P, et al (Univ of Tampere, Finland; Helsinki Univ Hosp; Finnish Red Cross Blood Transfusion Service, Helsinki)
Gastroenterology 122:881-888, 2002   60–4

Background.—Up to 55% of patients with untreated celiac disease (CD) have modestly elevated serum aminotransferase levels. These liver abnormalities usually resolve with the institution of a gluten-free diet. The utility of a gluten-free diet in patients with untreated CD who have more severe liver impairment was investigated.

Methods.—The medical records of 4 patients with severe liver disease who had untreated CD were reviewed. Also, 185 patients (67 men and 118 women; median age, 52 years) who had undergone liver transplantation were screened to determine the incidence of CD. These patients provided blood samples for determining serum IgA endomysial antibodies and tissue transglutaminase antibodies.

Results.—Liver diseases in the 4 patients with concomitant CD were congenital liver fibrosis (1 case), massive hepatic steatosis (1 case), and progressive hepatitis of unknown cause (2 cases). Three patients were being considered for liver transplantation. Yet, each patient's hepatic dysfunction reversed after adopting a gluten-free diet, and the 2 patients who maintained a strict gluten-free diet had improved or even normal bowel mucosa at last follow-up. Among the 185 patients with a liver transplant, 8 (4.3%) had biopsy-proven CD. In 6 patients, CD had been diagnosed before transplantation; 3 of these patients had primary biliary cirrhosis, 1 had autoimmune hepatitis, 1 had primary sclerosing cholangitis, and 1 had congenital liver fibrosis. In 5 of these 6 patients, the liver disorder developed before CD was diagnosed. Only 1 of these patients had strictly maintained a gluten-free diet since diagnosis. Screening uncovered 2 patients with CD; 1 had autoimmune hepatitis and 1 had secondary sclerosing cholangitis.

Conclusion.—Liver function in all 4 patients with severe liver disease who had CD improved on a gluten-free diet, and disease resolved in both patients who maintained this diet. Also, 8 patients who had undergone liver transplantation had CD, including 2 patients with unrecognized CD. Thus, all patients with autoimmune hepatitis or hepatitis of unknown cause should be screened for CD and, if necessary, adopt a gluten-free diet to prevent the progression to end-stage liver failure.

▶ We do not associate CD with liver function test abnormalities; however, 15% to 55% of untreated CD patients have elevation of serum aminotransferase levels.[1] These elevations may be secondary to CD-associated liver diseases, including autoimmune liver disorders such as primary biliary cirrhosis, autoimmune hepatitis, and primary sclerosing cholangitis. Elevation of liver function tests may be the sole presentation of CD, which often resolves with institution of a gluten-free diet.

Kaukinen et al described patients with advanced liver disease, whose pathology reversed with a gluten-free diet. In addition, they screened a population of liver transplant patients and found an increased incidence of CD. Thus, we agree with Kaukinen that there is a need to screen for CD in all patients with hepatitis of unknown etiology as well as those with autoimmune hepatitis.

J. S. Barkin, MD

Reference

1. Hagander B, Berg N, Brandt L, et al: Hepatic injury in adult coeliac disease. *Lancet* 1:270-272, 1977.

Cancer Incidence in a Population-based Cohort of Individuals Hospitalized With Celiac Disease or Dermatitis Herpetiformis

Askling J, Linet M, Gridley G, et al (Karolinska Inst/Hosp, Stockholm; Natl Cancer Inst, Bethesda, Md; Univ of Oslo, Norway)

Gastroenterology 123:1428-1435, 2002   60–5

Background.—Celiac disease and dermatitis herpetiformis are 2 interrelated conditions of abnormal gluten sensitivity and occur primarily in genetically predisposed persons. Studies of cancer risk in patients with celiac disease or dermatitis herpetiformis indicate that they are at an increased risk for malignant lymphoma and occasionally other neoplasms, but these studies have been limited by small numbers of study subjects, lack of systematic cancer assessment, and subjects identified from referral institutions. The cancer profiles among patients with celiac disease or dermatitis herpetiformis were assessed.

Methods.—Swedish population-based inpatient and cancer registry data were used to follow up 12,000 patients with celiac disease or dermatitis herpetiformis. Cancer incidence was determined with the use of standardized incidence ratios.

Results.—Adults with celiac disease (but not children or adolescents) had an elevated overall risk for cancer (standardized incidence ratios = 1.3) that decreased with time and eventually reached unity. Elevated risks were also identified for malignant lymphomas, small-intestinal, oropharyngeal, esophageal, large intestinal, hepatobiliary, and pancreatic carcinomas. The excess occurrence of malignant lymphomas was confined to adults, and there was a decrease in occurrence with the time of follow-up evaluation and over successive calendar periods. Decreased risks were identified for breast cancer. Patients with dermatitis herpetiformis had a slightly increased overall cancer risk, which resulted from excesses of malignant lymphoma and leukemia. There were no increases in gastrointestinal carcinomas in these patients.

Conclusions.—The relative risks for lymphomas and gastrointestinal cancers in this study, although increased, are lower (and declining) than in most previous reports. The risk is only moderately increased in adult patients with celiac disease or dermatitis herpetiformis. The risk is not elevated at all in childhood or adolescence.

No Harm From Five Year Ingestion of Oats in Coeliac Disease

Janatuinen EK, Kemppainen TA, Julkunen RJK, et al (Univ of Kuopio, Finland; Univ of Tampere, Finland)

Gut 50:332-335, 2002   60–6

Background.—In a previous study, these authors showed that up to 12 months of ingesting moderate amounts of oats does not have harmful effects in adults with celiac disease (CD) who follow an otherwise gluten-free diet.

The follow-up of these patients was extended to 5 years, to study the long-term effects of oat intake on CD.

Methods.—The initial trial involved 92 adults with CD who were randomly assigned to follow either a conventional gluten-free diet (47 patients) or a diet that was gluten free except for 50 to 70 g per day of oats (45 patients) for 6 to 12 months. At the end of that study, 39 patients in the oats group elected to continue their diet, as did 42 patients in the control group. After an additional 5 years, 23 patients (66%) who were still following their modified gluten-free diet and 28 of 42 controls (66%) who were still following their strict gluten-free diet agreed to participate in the current study. Assessments at the 5-year follow-up included clinical and nutritional evaluations, biopsies of duodenal specimens, and assays for antiendomysial, antireticulin, and antigliadin antibodies.

Results.—About 75% of patients in each group followed their prescribed diet strictly. At 5 years, the 2 groups did not differ significantly in body mass index or change in body mass index, nutritional status, or routine laboratory data. Histologic and histomorphometric variables, including duodenal villous architecture and inflammatory cell infiltrates in the duodenal mucosa, improved significantly and to a similar extent in the 2 groups. Antibody titers were also similar in the 2 groups at 5 years.

Conclusion.—Allowing a limited amount of oats (50-70 g/d) into an otherwise gluten-free diet does not adversely affect disease control in adults with CD. Being able to include oats in the diet gives more choice to the patient with CD, and this might improve compliance.

▶ Unfortunately, CD patients alone and patients with dermatitis herpetiformis (DH) have an increased risk of developing non-Hodgkin lymphoma. Askling et al (Abstract 60–5) reported on cancer risk in CD/DH patients who were hospitalized, and then followed up this select severe group. Cancer risk was found to be increased by 30% in CD and included malignant lymphomas, as well as oropharyngeal, esophageal, and small bowel carcinomas. This risk may be decreased by adherence to a gluten-free diet, as Askling et al have observed a decreasing relative risk over calendar time for these tumors.

Our therapeutic goal is to reinforce to our patients the necessity to maintain a gluten-free diet. This has included avoidance of wheat, rye, and oats.[1,2] Obviously, this severity limits their diet.

Janatuinen et al (Abstract 60–6), expanded their initial 6- to 12-month study on the lack of harmful effects of oats ingestion on CD. If this were not harmful, it would significantly expand the diet of patients with CD and improve their quality of life. They followed up their patients and after 5 years found definite improvement on a gluten-free diet both with and without oats. This may allow increased compliance to a gluten-free diet.

J. S. Barkin, MD

References

1. Dicke WK: Coeliakie. Een onderzoek nor de nadelige invloed van sommige groonsoorten op de lijder oon coeliake. Thesis Utrecht. Netherlands, 1950.

2. Van de Kamer JH, Weijers HA, Dicke WK: Celiac disease IV. An investigation into the injurious constituents of wheat in connection with their action on patients with celiac disease. *Acta Paediatr* 42:223-231, 1953.

Diarrhea Caused by Enterotoxigenic *Escherichia coli* Infection of Humans Is Inhibited by Dietary Calcium

Bovee-Oudenhoven IMJ, Lettink-Wissink MLG, Van Doesburg W, et al (Wageningen Ctr for Food Sciences/NIZO Food Research, Ede, The Netherlands; Gelderse Vallei Hosp, Ede, The Netherlands)
Gastroenterology 125:469-476, 2003   60–7

Background.—Infectious diarrhea is a common cause of morbidity among travelers, and worldwide is second only to cardiovascular disease as a cause of mortality. One of the strategies endorsed by the World Health Organization to decrease morbidity and mortality from infectious diarrhea is to improve host resistance to infection. Experiments in rats show dietary calcium inhibits colonization and translocation of invasive salmonella. Whether calcium supplementation can protect humans against enterotoxigenic *Escherichia coli* (ETEC) infections was examined.

Methods.—Participants were 32 healthy men aged 20 to 55 years who were screened to ensure the absence of colonization factor antigen type II in serum and of *E coli* in feces. They were randomly assigned to consume either low-calcium (60 mg/d) or high-calcium (1100 mg/d) milk products for 3 weeks. They otherwise consumed their normal diet, but other high-calcium foods were forbidden. On day 10, the men ingested a live but attenuated strain of ETEC (strain E1392/75-2A), which has been shown to cause mild diarrhea of 1 to 3 days' duration in humans. Before (days 7 and 8) and after (days 11-13, 15, and 17), 24-hour fecal samples were collected, and total fecal output, relative fecal dry weight, and fecal mucin excretion were compared between the 2 groups.

Results.—ETEC infection induced diarrhea in both groups, as indicated by a doubling in total fecal output, a decrease in the mean relative fecal dry weight, and increased mucin production. In the high-calcium group, all of these parameters were completely normalized by the second day after ETEC administration. In contrast, in the low-calcium group, these parameters did not normalize until the third day after ETEC ingestion.

Conclusion.—Calcium supplementation with high-calcium milk products significantly reduced the severity of ETEC-induced diarrhea in these healthy men. Inadequate calcium intake appears to decrease resistance to food-borne intestinal infections, and efforts to increase calcium intake to recommended levels (1000-1200 mg/d in adults in Western countries) might improve intestinal health.

▶ Tourism is significant to the economic stability of many nations, and with our graying population, an ever-increasing segment of our population is seeking new lands to explore. Almost two thirds of tourists develop traveler's diarrhea during visits in Asia, Africa, or South America. The leading pathogen is

ETEC, which is a food and water contaminant. Bovee-Oudenhoven et al evaluated whether dietary calcium could increase host resistance. They found that dietary calcium supplementation was effective in reducing the severity of ETEC-induced diarrhea. Persons in the high-calcium group ingested about 1500 mg of calcium per day—this intake will not only improve gastrointestinal problems but also bone health. This intake should be emphasized in the very young, the elderly, and those with comorbid disease, groups who have the greatest danger from ETEC infection.

J. S. Barkin, MD

61 Irritable Bowel Syndrome

Influence of Body Posture on Intestinal Transit of Gas
Dainese R, Serra J, Azpiroz F, et al (Hosp General Vall d'Hebron, Barcelona)
Gut 52:971-974, 2003   61–1

Background.—Body posture may influence abdominal bloating, distension, and flatulence. Whether changes in position have effects that can be objectively demonstrated has not been studied. The effect of body posture on intestinal transit of gas loads was investigated.

Methods.—Eight healthy persons without gastrointestinal symptoms participated in the study. A gas mixture was continuously infused into the jejunum, 12 mL/min, for 3 hours. Gas evacuation, clearance of a nonabsorbable gaseous marker, perceptions, and abdominal girth were recorded. Paired studies were then randomly performed on separate days in each participant in the upright and supine positions.

Findings.—Intestinal gas retention was much lower in the upright than in the supine position. Clearance of the gas marker was also expedited in the upright position. Participants tolerated the gas challenge well in both positions, with no abdominal distension.

Conclusions.—These data show that body posture significantly influences intestinal gas propulsion. Transit is faster in the upright position than in the supine position.

► Bloating is a common complaint of patients and is defined as a feeling of distension without an increase in abdominal girth. It is associated with abdominal discomfort or pain and is part of the spectrum of symptoms that we commonly characterize as part of the irritable bowel syndrome.

Bloating may result from a variety of causes, including (1) intake of gas-producing food, including beans, broccoli, cauliflower, and cabbage; (2) intake of nonabsorbable foods, such as lactose-containing foods; (3) aerophagia with swallowing of air caused by anxiety or gastroesophageal reflux disease; and (4) intestinal motility disorders (slowing of motility can be induced by endoluminal lipids).[1]

Our approaches have included restrictive dietary counseling, treatment of reflux, and medications that increase intestinal motility. A novel therapeutic approach to gas within the abdominal cavity is to change body position to facilitate intestinal transit. Dainese et al compared intestinal gas transit in 8 healthy individuals. They found that in the upright body position, gas transit and evacuation are faster compared with the supine position. Whether these results in healthy individuals are applicable to patients complaining of abdominal pain, bloating, and distension is unclear. However, it is a logical extension of this study not to have our patients with bloating lie postprandially.

J. S. Barkin, MD

Reference

1. Serra J, Azpiroz F, Malagelada KR: Gastric distension and duodenal lipid infusion modulate intestinal gas transit and tolerance in humans. *Am J Gastroenterol* 97:2225-2230, 2002.

An Asia-Pacific, Double Blind, Placebo Controlled, Randomised Study to Evaluate the Efficacy, Safety, and Tolerability of Tegaserod in Patients With Irritable Bowel Syndrome

Kellow J, Lee OY, Chang FY, et al (Novartis Pharma AG, Basel, Switzerland)
Gut 52:671-676, 2003   61–2

Background.—In Western populations, tegaserod has been an effective treatment for the multiple symptoms of irritable bowel syndrome (IBS). Few data are available on the use of this agent in Asian-Pacific populations.

Methods.—A total of 520 patients with IBS from the Asia-Pacific region were included in the study. None had diarrhea-predominant IBS. By random assignment, patients received tegaserod 6 mg twice daily or placebo for 12 weeks.

Findings.—During weeks 1 to 4, 56% of patients in the tegaserod group and 35% in the placebo group had overall satisfactory relief. During weeks 1 to 12, these proportions were 62% and 44%, respectively. A clinically relevant effect was seen as early as week 1 and maintained throughout the 12-week period of treatment. Compared with placebo recipients, tegaserod recipients had greater reductions in number of days with at least moderate abdominal pain and discomfort, bloating, no bowel movements, and hard or lumpy stools. The most commonly reported adverse event was headache, occurring in 12% of the tegaserod group and in 11.1% of the placebo group. Diarrhea prompted 2.3% of the tegaserod recipients to quit treatment. Serious adverse effects were uncommon.

Conclusions.—This dose of tegaserod appears to be an effective treatment for IBS in Asian-Pacific patients whose main bowel symptom is not diarrhea. The patients in this study tolerated tegaserod well, and serious adverse events were infrequent.

▶ The symptoms of IBS—altered bowel habits with abdominal pain or bloating—are felt to result from bowel motility as well as a decrease in sensory threshold. Constipation-predominant IBS is associated with decreased small bowel motility. Tegaserod (Zelmac, Novartis, Switzerland; Zelnorm, Novartis USA) partially inhibits the 5-HT$_4$ receptor that inhibits motility and modulates function in visceral pain. Studies on the use of this drug in the United States is for constipation-predominant IBS patients, whereas this study from Asia excluded only those with diarrhea-predominant IBS. Thus, including patients with alternating constipation with diarrhea, tegaserod led to significant improvement of symptoms over placebo. Importantly, this and other studies have shown that with placebo the response rate is approximately 35%. Consequently, health care–giver effect has an important therapeutic office. This study emphasizes the need to broadly classify patients with IBS as diarrhea or constipation predominant and not as alternators. When the group of patients that are treated is increased by this definition, they still only had a 10% incidence of diarrhea (a common effect of tegaserod), which led to discontinuation in only 2.5%. Physicians often relate that they do not have patients with constipation-predominant IBS. I feel that we are seeing patients with constipation and ascribe their associated symptoms to the constipation rather than labeling them with constipation-predominant IBS.

J. S. Barkin, MD

62 Colon Cancer and Screening

Screening for Colorectal Cancer on the Front Line
Lemon SC, Zapka JG, Estabrook B, et al (Univ of Massachusetts, Worcester)
Am J Gastroenterol 98:915-923, 2003   62–1

Background.—Several options are available for colorectal cancer screening. However, the rate of screening in the general population remains low. Primary care clinicians' knowledge of, beliefs about, and practices in colorectal cancer screening were evaluated.

Methods and Findings.—Seventy-seven primary care providers in 6 clinics in central Massachusetts were surveyed. Ninety-seven percent agreed with guidelines for fecal occult blood testing and 87% with guidelines for sigmoidoscopy. Both were commonly reported as usual practice. Eighty-six percent recommended colonoscopy as a colorectal cancer screening test, but this was reported infrequently as usual practice. Thirty-six percent of the clinicians considered barium enema as a colorectal cancer screening option, which was rarely reported as usual practice. Digital rectal examinations and in-office fecal occult blood testing were commonly cited as usual practice, though evidence supporting the efficacy of these approaches is lacking. Typically, these practices were reported in combination with a guideline-endorsed testing option. Ten percent of clinicians reported that patients frequently refused fecal occult blood testing at home. However, 60% of clinicians said patients frequently refused sigmoidoscopy. Barriers to compliance with sigmoidoscopy included patients' fears that the procedure would hurt and assumptions that, if there is a problem, symptoms will occur.

Conclusions.—This survey indicates that most primary care providers recommend guideline-endorsed colorectal cancer screening. However, patients commonly refused sigmoidoscopy. Multiple levels of intervention, including patients and provider education and systems strategies, are needed to improve the prevalence of colorectal cancer screening.

▶ Colorectal cancer is the second leading cause of cancer death in the United States. Overall it is preventable and curable when detected at an early stage. To accomplish this goal, screening is mandatory; however, rates of screening are still below 50%. Lemon et al reported the usual colorectal cancer screening practices of primary care providers, including assessment of colorectal cancer risk and agreement with and adherence to guidelines. The primary care providers at the time of this study were utilizing fecal occult blood testing and sigmoidoscopy—both of which previously fit colorectal cancer screening guidelines. Clinicians felt that the patients had 2 barriers to undergo a colonic diagnostic study. One was fear that the procedure would hurt and the second was the belief that without symptoms screening for colorectal cancer is not needed. Therefore, providers need to educate their patients regarding these and other commonly cited barriers to sigmoidoscopy screening and presently colonoscopy. Conversely, to implement CRC screening, there needs to be a strong physician's recommendation.

J. S. Barkin, MD

Physician and Patient Factors Associated With Ordering a Colon Evaluation After a Positive Fecal Occult Blood Test
Turner B, Meyers RE, Hyslop T, et al (Univ Pennsylvania, Philadelphia; Thomas Jefferson Univ, Philadelphia)
J Gen Intern Med 18:357-363, 2003   62–2

Background.—For colorectal cancer screening to be effective, clinicians must order a complete diagnostic evaluation (CDE) of the colon with colonoscopy or barium enema along with sigmoidoscopy after a positive finding on screening fecal occult blood testing (FOBT). Primary care physicians were surveyed about their colorectal cancer screening practices, beliefs, and intentions.

Methods.—Surveys were sent to 413 primary care practices affiliated with a managed care organization offering a mailed FOBT program for patients aged 50 years and older. At least 1 physician in 318 (77%) of 413 practices responded to the survey. Sixty-seven percent of responding practices had a total of 602 FOBT-positive patients from August through November 1998. After excluding practices judged ineligible for a CDE or lacking demographic data, 184 practices were included in the analysis. Three months after notification of the positive FOBT finding, physicians were asked by audit form whether they ordered CDEs.

Findings.—Physicians reported ordering CDEs for only 69.5% of the 490 FOBT-positive patients. After adjustment in a logistic regression analysis, physicians were found to be more likely to order CDEs for men than for women. Physicians who reported an intermediate or high intention to evaluate FOBT-positive patients by CDE had a nearly 2-fold greater adjusted odds of actually initiating a CDE for such patients compared with physicians reporting low intention.

Conclusions.—These data suggest that primary care physicians often fail to order CDEs for FOBT-positive patients. Physician initiation of a CDE was influenced by the patient's sex and physician's beliefs about CDEs.

▶ Screening for colorectal cancer requires that we improve practitioners' clinical knowledge and practice. In these multiple intervention strategies, it is also important to educate and remind patients of their screening needs. Turner et al reported the magnitude of this reluctance by health care providers to order a CDE (ie, colonoscopy and/or sigmoidoscopy with barium enema). They surveyed physicians regarding suggested follow-up of patients older than 50 years with positive FOBT as determined by a central laboratory. Of the 490 patients with a positive FOBT, in only 341 (69.5%) was a CDE ordered. They found that women were one third less likely than men to have a CDE initiated by their primary care physicians. Whether this is from physician approach to gender or to a woman's incorrect belief that she has a lower risk of CRC than men is unclear.

The point of this article is not whether FOBT is a good screening test, but if found to be positive—irrespective of the number of positive hemoccult tests, patient gender or medication intake—it is standard care in 2004 to have the patient then undergo a follow-up colonoscopy.

J. S. Barkin, MD

Colorectal Neoplasms: Prospective Comparison of Thin-section Low-dose Multi-detector Row CT Colonography and Conventional Colonoscopy for Detection
Macari M, Bini EJ, Xue X, et al (New York Univ; Siemens Med Systems, Forcheim, Germany)
Radiology 224:383-392, 2002   62–3

Background.—Screening for colorectal cancer reduces the morbidity and mortality associated with this disease, but many patients are reluctant to undergo the current screening procedures. This is one factor that contributes to the 50,000 deaths from colon cancer each year in the United States. CT colonography is a safe, noninvasive technique for the evaluation of the entire colonic surface and for detection of polyps or cancers. Thin-section low-dose multidetector row CT colonography was compared with conventional colonoscopy for the detection of colorectal neoplasms in this prospective study.

Methods.—A series of 105 patients underwent CT colonography immediately before colonoscopy. Supine and prone CT colonographic acquisitions to image the region during a 30-second breath hold were performed. The CT colonographic images were interpreted for the presence, location, size, and morphological features of polyps. The time of image interpretation was noted. The sensitivity, specificity, and positive and negative predictive values of CT colonography were calculated, with 95% confidence intervals, with colonoscopic findings as the reference standard.

The weighted CT dose index was calculated on the basis of measurements in a standard body phantom. Commercially available software was used to calculate the effective dose.

Results.—The median CT data interpretation time was 12 minutes. Colonoscopy identified 132 polyps in 59 patients. In 46 patients, there were no polyps detected. Sensitivities for the detection of polyps were 12% for polyps smaller than 5 mm in diameter, 70% for polyps 6 to 9 mm, and 93% for polyps larger than 10 mm. The estimated overall specificity was 97.7%. The total weighted CT dose index for combined supine and prone CT colonography was 11.4 mGy. The effective doses for combined CT colonography were 5.0 mSv and 7.8 mSv for men and women, respectively.

Conclusion.—Low-dose multidetector row CT colonography has excellent sensitivity and specificity for the detection of large colorectal neoplasms (10 mm diameter or greater).

▶ While colonoscopy remains the gold standard for screening for colorectal cancer, it is not applicable to, or acceptable for all patients. CT colonography could be an alternative screening method in these patients. A change in CT technique with adaptation of thin-section protocols used for standard abdominal CT gives patients increased exposure to ionizing radiation. In addition, bowel preparation similar to colonoscopy was used by Macari et al in this study that compared this modified technique with colonoscopy. Unfortunately, these modifications still did not overcome the inability of CT colonography to detect small polyps (< 5 mm), as evidenced by a 12% detection rate, whereas in those between 6 and 9 mm, there was a 70% detection rate, and the rate was 93% for polyps larger than 1 cm. In addition, false-positive CT colonographic results occurred 12 times in 9 patients (8.5%). This technique resulted in a decreased false-positive rate, which is reported in up to 37% with the conventional technique, thus leading to many unnecessary colonoscopies. Variability in interpretation is also a significant problem with this as well as any new procedures. This technique is undergoing technical improvements, but is not ready for "prime time" screening. These results from an experienced tertiary center of expertise are certainly not transportable to our local x-ray diagnostic centers. We should, therefore, use this procedure in patients who have incomplete colonoscopies or who cannot or will not undergo colonoscopy.

J. S. Barkin, MD

Aspirin and the Prevention of Colorectal Cancer
Imperiale TF (Indiana Univ, Indianapolis)
N Engl J Med 348:879-880, 2003   62–4

Background.—Colorectal cancer is associated with substantial rates of morbidity and mortality. Thus, early detection and prevention have been major areas of interest to clinicians and researchers. The possibility that aspirin has a protective effect against colorectal cancer was discussed.

Discussion.—A protective effect of aspirin is plausible biologically, but the only randomized trial of the association between aspirin and colorectal cancer reported no reduction in the incidence of such cancer. Because of the large sample sizes and long-term follow-up required, there will probably not be a definitive clinical trial of aspirin or NSAIDs for the primary or secondary chemoprevention of colorectal cancer in which such cancer is the outcome. However, the development of most colorectal cancers is believed to follow a sequence from adenoma to carcinoma; thus, clinical studies finding that aspirin decreases the rate of recurrent adenomas would suggest that aspirin protects against colorectal cancer. Two such trials were published in *The New England Journal of Medicine* on March 6, 2003. Both studies showed that aspirin decreased the risk of adenoma recurrence among persons with a history of colorectal cancer or adenomas. These well-conducted trials provided proof that aspirin moderately decreases the risk of colorectal neoplasia recurrence and support for assumptions and probabilities used in analyses of cost-effectiveness.

Conclusions.—Aspirin appears to be of some benefit in preventing colorectal cancer. However, further research is needed before it can be recommended for this indication. Aspirin use is not a substitute for screening and surveillance.

▶ Sandler et al[1] also reported the beneficial effects of aspirin in preventing adenomas in patients who had undergone curative colorectal cancer surgery. Overall, 325 mg of enteric-coated aspirin compared with placebo delayed the development of adenomas. Aspirin intake therefore decreases the occurrence of polyps, but as Imperiale points out, its clinical significance may not be all that significant as most adenomas do not progress to cancer and aspirin has adverse effects. Overall, the true clinical benefit is avoidance or delay of polypectomy for 1 of every 10 or 19 patients treated with aspirin, which I feel is significant. However, cost effectiveness analysis of aspirin as primary chemoprophylaxis showed that it saves fewer lives at higher costs than does screening for colorectal cancer by any method. However, this assumes that screening for colorectal cancer will take place.

The importance of this study is that aspirin is beneficial, albeit in a small way, in preventing colorectal cancer. It should be utilized in patients with familial adenomatous polyposis and in those who have had an adenomatous polyp or colorectal cancer. It does not need to be used in average-risk patients.

J. S. Barkin, MD

Reference

1. Sandler RS, Halabi S, Baron JA, et al: A randomized trial of aspirin to prevent colorectal adenomas in patients with previous colorectal cancer. *N Engl J Med* 348:883-890, 2003.

Ursodeoxycholic Acid as a Chemopreventive Agent in Patients With Ulcerative Colitis and Primary Sclerosing Cholangitis

Pardi DS, Loftus EV Jr, Kremers WK, et al (Mayo Clinic and Found, Rochester, Minn)

Gastroenterology 124:889-893, 2003   62–5

Background.—Preclinical studies have shown that ursodeoxycholic acid (UDCA) is an effective chemoprevention for colon cancer. A recent report suggested that this agent may also reduce the risk for colorectal dysplasia in patients with ulcerative colitis (UC) and primary sclerosing cholangitis (PSC). The effect of UDCA on colorectal neoplasia in patients with UC and PSC enrolled in a randomized, placebo-controlled study was evaluated.

Methods.—Fifty-two patients previously enrolled in a trial of UDCA therapy in PSC at the authors' center were followed up for a total of 355 person-years. The patients in the current analysis had concomitant UC.

Findings.—Patients initially given UDCA had a 0.26 relative risk for colorectal dysplasia or cancer development. Many patients initially given placebo subsequently received UDCA in an open-label fashion. Assigning these patients to UDCA from the time they began active treatment did not alter the magnitude of the protective effect.

Conclusions.—These results must be interpreted with caution, yet the study showed that UDCA treatment decreased the risk of colorectal neoplasia by 74%. Further research is needed to determine the mechanisms involved in the chemoprotective effects of UDCA and to identify which patients are most likely to benefit from such treatment.

▶ Overall, patients with UC have an increased risk of colorectal cancer. A subgroup of patients with UC develop PSC. Clinically, PSC presents as a cholestatic liver disease with elevated bilirubin levels from inflammation with scarring of the bile ducts. This subgroup of patients with UC and PSC seems to be at a higher risk for development of colorectal cancer than other UC patients. Pardi et al presented a chemoprotective study of 52 patients with UC and PSC, 23 of whom received placebo versus 29 who were treated with UDCA for a median of 42 months. UDCA is a bile acid used for decreasing LFTs in patients with PSC.

They found that the protective effect in colon tumor genesis for UDCA was strong. Thus, we have a relatively nontoxic drug that is an effective chemopreventive agent and should be used in patients with UC and PSC. Its chemoprotective efficacy in UC patients without PSC needs to be determined.

J. S. Barkin, MD

Association Between Physical Activity, Fiber Intake, and Other Lifestyle Variables and Constipation in a Study of Women

Dukas L, Willett WC, Giovannuci EL (Harvard School of Public Health, Boston; Harvard Med School, Boston; Univ Hosp, Basel, Switzerland)
Am J Gastroenterol 98:1790-1796, 2003   62–6

Background.—The risk factors for constipation in the general population are not clearly defined. The relation between the prevalence of constipation and age, body mass index, lifestyle factors, and dietary factors in women was investigated.

Methods.—A total of 62,036 participants in the Nurses' Health Study completed questionnaires in 1980 and 1982 assessing bowel movement frequency, dietary factors, and lifestyle factors. The women were aged 36 to 61 years and free of cancer at the time of the survey. Constipation was defined as no more than 2 bowel movements per week.

Findings.—Overall, 5.4% of the women were classified as having constipation. Constipation was inversely correlated with age and body mass index. In a multivariate analysis, the prevalence of constipation was lower in women reporting daily physical activity. Compared with women in the lowest quintile of dietary fiber intake, women in the highest quintile were less likely to have constipation. Women reporting daily activity and who were in the highest quintile of fiber intake had a 0.32 prevalence ratio of constipation compared with women reporting physical activity less than once a week and in the lowest quintile of fiber intake. The prevalence of constipation increased with a greater frequency of aspirin use. Constipation was inversely associated with current smoking and alcohol use.

Conclusions.—The prevalence of constipation in Nurses' Health Study participants was 5.4%. Moderate physical activity and increased fiber intake appear to be associated with a marked decrease in the prevalence of constipation in women.

▶ Constipation has 3 components, including infrequent passage of stool with fewer than 3 bowel movements per week, passage of hard stools, and excessive straining during passage of stool. It is one of the most frequent of patients' complaints and occurs in 10% to 20% of adults, of which only a minority seek medical care. The greatest number of physician visits for evaluation and therapy of constipation occurs in adult women who are 65 years of age and older.[1] We do not know what, if any, lifestyle factors contribute to constipation. Dukas et al investigated the associations among age, body mass index, physical activity, dietary fiber intake, and other selected lifestyle variables with prevalence of constipation. This study is important as it confirms our belief that regular physical exercise and a higher level of fiber intake were associated with reduced risk of constipation. This benefit occurred even though the higher intake of fiber was a mere 20 g/day, which is below the daily recommended fiber intake of 30 g/day. They also confirmed that age was inversely associated with bowel movement frequency; therefore, laxative use, as expected, increases with age. They also found an association between physical activity and bowel movement frequency. The combination of a high-fiber diet and a high level of physical activity would tend to lead to the lowest risk for constipation. Interestingly, they also found that constipation is a side effect of nonsteroidal anti-inflammatory drugs (NSAIDs). Whether this is a direct cause and effect or is related to the fact that older people take NSAIDs, especially those older people with coexistent diseases who take increased NSAIDs, is unclear. It is important for us to include this class of drugs when we obtain a history in patients with constipation. This study reinforces our role as health care advisors to stress increasing or maintaining regular exercise, eating healthy, including fiber, and recognizing drugs, including NSAIDs, that can result in constipation.

J. S. Barkin, MD

Reference

1. Sonnenberg A, Koch TR: Physician visits in the United States for constipation: 1958 to 1986. *Dig Dis Sci* 34:606-611, 1989.

Risk Factors for Chronic Constipation Based on a General Practice Sample

Talley NJ, Jones M, Nuyts G, et al (Univ of Sydney, Pernith NSW, Australia; Janssen Research Found, Beerse, Belgium)
Am J Gastroenterol 98:1107-1111, 2003   62–7

Background.—Poor diet and a lack of exercise are among the many factors correlated with constipation. The roles of medications and medical illnesses are less clear. Clinical, therapeutic, and demographic risk factors for constipation were identified.

Methods.—Data on 7251 patients with chronic constipation, 6441 with constipation of unspecific chronicity, and 7103 healthy persons were analyzed. The information was obtained from a general practice research database representing more than 10 years of data collection.

Findings.—After adjustment for age and sex, a large number of clinical and treatment variables correlated independently with chronic constipation. Primary neurologic diseases correlated strongly with constipation, although they accounted for few cases. Among medications associated with constipation, those with the highest risk were opioids, diuretics, antidepressants, antihistamines, antispasmodics, anticonvulsants, and aluminum antacids.

Conclusions.—Multiple medications appear to contribute to the risk of constipation. Concurrent diseases are also related to this risk, but most account for only a minority of cases.

▶ The causes of constipation may vary, and we as practitioners must identify those reversible factors of chronic constipation. Talley et al aimed to identify the relevant medication and disease risk factors for chronic constipation. They found that age greater than 25 years, female gender, pregnancy, and a number of diverse diseases including multiple sclerosis, parkinsonism, diabetes mellitus, and multiple medications, including opioid analgesics, diuretics, antipsychotics, antidepressants, iron supplements, antispasmodics, antihistamines, β-blockers, and aluminium antacids, were independently associated with chronic or unspecified constipation (see Abstract 62–6). It is the identification of this group of medications that enabled us as clinicians to make the greatest impact in improving the symptoms of our patients. The use of these drugs is associated with a 2- to 3-fold increased risk of constipation. Once recognized, we have the opportunity to change or discontinue those medications. Conversely, we make little impact on patients' neurologic, endocrine, or metabolic disease or psychologic factors.

J. S. Barkin, MD

63 Liver

Serum Ferritin Level Predicts Advanced Hepatic Fibrosis Among U.S Patients With Phenotypic Hemochromatosis
Morrison ED, Brandhagen DJ, Phatak PD, et al (Univ of Washington, Seattle; Mayo Clinic, Rochester, Minn; Univ of Rochester, NY; et al)
Ann Intern Med 138:627-633, 2003   63–1

Background.—In most people of Northern European descent, DNA-based *HFE* gene testing can verify hereditary hemochromatosis. However, detection of cirrhosis generally requires liver biopsy. Noninvasive criteria were developed to predict the presence or absence of advanced hepatic fibrosis or cirrhosis in patients with hemochromatosis.

Methods.—A total of 182 patients with phenotypically defined hemochromatosis were enrolled in the cross-sectional study. Liver histopathology and serum ferritin, aspartate aminotransferase, and alanine aminotransferase concentrations were assessed.

Findings.—Twenty-two percent of the patients had cirrhosis. Twenty-four percent of C282Y homozygotes had cirrhosis. Of 93 patients with a serum ferritin concentration of less than 1000 µg/L, only 1 had cirrhosis compared with 39 of 89 patients with serum ferritin concentrations exceeding 1000 µg/L. Cirrhosis was not present in any of the C282Y homozygotes or C282Y/H63D compound heterozygotes with serum ferritin concentrations of less than 1000 µg/L. Factors independently correlated with cirrhosis included increased serum aminotransferase levels and serum ferritin levels exceeding 1000 µg/L, but not age older than 40 years. A multivariate model indicated a 7.4% probability of cirrhosis among patients with serum ferritin concentrations of less than 1000 µg/L compared with 72% among patients with serum ferritin levels exceeding 1000 µg/L, after adjusting for age and increased serum liver enzyme levels.

Conclusions.—Cirrhosis is unlikely in patients with hemochromatosis and serum ferritin concentrations of less than 1000 µg/L. Thus, liver biopsy may be unnecessary to screen for cirrhosis in such patients, irrespective of age or serum liver enzyme levels.

▶ The initial decision when evaluating a patient with elevated liver enzymes is to determine the etiology. First, it should be determined if the elevation of these enzymes is due to hepatotoxicity and not extrahepatic causes such as rhabdomyolysis or high-calorie and high-carbohydrate diets. Realizing that they may be raised from a multitude of causes, including heredity (hemochromatosis), infection (hepatitis A, B and C), toxins (alcohol and drugs), metabolism (fatty liver), or any combination of the above.

Hereditary hemochromatosis is the most common congenital liver disease, with an estimated carrier frequency of 10% in individuals of northern European descent.[1] It should be sought in all patients with elevated liver enzymes, especially those with concurrent organ system abnormalities in the pancreas and who may also have diabetes mellitus, cardiac disease, congestive heart failure, joint involvement with arthropathy, endocrine disorders such as dysmenorrhea, or impotence. Diagnosis is suggested by increased iron saturation and is established by detection of the hemochromatosis gene (*HFE*) mutation [C282Y and H63D] and liver biopsy with iron stains and quantitative iron measurement. Once the diagnosis is established, the next clinical question is whether fibrosis is present. Liver has been used to ascertain its presence and, if found, screening for hepatocellular carcinoma is begun. The clinical features that suggest the presence of severe fibrosis in European patients include hepatomegaly, elevated aspartate aminotransferase levels, severe ferritin level more than 1000 mg/L, and age less than 40 years.[2,3] Morrison et al determined whether these were applicable to the US population. They compared patients with hemochromatosis with bridging fibrosis or cirrhosis with patients without fibrosis or cirrhosis and found 3 factors that significantly predicted fibrosis, including age greater than 40 years, abnormal serum liver enzyme levels, and serum ferritin 1000 mg/L or greater. Serum ferritin levels less than 1000 mg/L and normal aspartate aminotransferase and alanine aminotransferase levels highly suggest that liver biopsy is not necessary for prognosis.

J. S. Barkin, MD

References

1. Edwards CQ, Griffen LM, Goldgar D, et al: Prevalence of hemochromatosis among 11,065 presumably healthy blood donors. *N Engl J Med* 318:1355-1362, 1998.
2. Guyader D, Jacqueliner C, Moirand R, et al: Noninvasive prediction of fibrosis in C282Y homozygous hemochromatosis. *Gastroenterology* 115:929-936, 1998.
3. Bacon BR, Olynyk JK, Brunt EM, et al: HFE genotype in patients with hemochromatosis and other liver diseases. *Ann Intern Med* 130:953-962, 1999.

The Prevalence and Etiology of Elevated Aminotransferase Levels in the United States
Clark JM, Brancati FL, Diehl AM (Johns Hopkins Univ, Baltimore, Md)
Am J Gastroenterol 98:960-967, 2003   63–2

Background.—Increased aminotransferase levels are often used to detect liver disease. However, the prevalence and cause of increased aminotransferase levels are not known.

Methods.—Data were obtained on 15,676 adults participating in the Third National Health and Nutrition Examination Survey between 1988 and 1994. Participants were classified as having increased aminotransferase concentrations if aspartate or alanine aminotransferase levels were above normal. Increases in aminotransferase levels were considered "explained" if laboratory evidence showed hepatitis B or C infection or iron overload or if patient history included alcohol consumption. Analyses were then weighted to produce national estimates.

Findings.—The US national prevalence of increased aminotransferase concentrations was 7.9%. Such increases were more common in men than in women: 9.3% and 6.6%, respectively. Increases were also more common in Mexican Americans (14.9%) and in non-Hispanic blacks (8.1%) than in non-Hispanic whites (7.1%). Only 31% of persons with elevated aminotransferase levels had high alcohol intakes, hepatitis B or C infection, or high transferring saturation. Thus, in 69% of cases increased aminotransferase levels were unexplained. In men and women, unexplained increases in aminotransferases correlated significantly with higher body mass index, waist circumference, triglycerides, fasting insulin, and lower HDL. In women, increased aminotransferases were also associated with type 2 diabetes and hypertension.

Conclusions.—Increased aminotransferase levels are common in the US population. Most cases cannot be explained by alcohol intake, viral hepatitis, or hemochromatosis. Unexplained increases were strongly associated with adiposity and other features of the metabolic syndrome, possibly representing nonalcoholic fatty liver disease.

▶ In all probability, nonalcoholic fatty liver disease (NAFLD) is the most common cause of elevated liver enzymes that we will encounter. It may account for up to 80% of patients with elevated liver function test results. This is a reflection of the increasing prevalence of obesity in our population and its accompanying risk factors for NAFLD, including diabetes, insulin resistance, and hyperlipemia. NAFLD may progress to steatohepatitis (NASH) in 20% to 30% of patients.[1-4] When should we suspect the presence of NAFLD? Clark et al found that the prevalence of aminotransferase elevation in the general US adult population was 7.9% and that approximately 70% was unexplained. This unexplained elevation was strongly associated with central obesity and related features of hyperlipidemia, higher insulin levels, diabetes, and hypertension, which is suggestive of NAFLD presence. Although no liver biopsies were obtained, they excluded chronic liver disease from alcoholism, hepatitis B or C, and heme chromatosis. Clinically, we should evaluate the patient with a singularly elevated aminotransferase level of which the source is not readily apparent and that coincides with the presence of NAFLD.

J. S. Barkin, MD

References

1. Bacon BR, Farahvash MJ, Janney CG, et al: Nonalcoholic steatohepatitis: An expanded clinical entity. *Gastroenterology* 107:1103-1109, 1994.
2. Diehl AM, Goodman Z, Ishak KG: Alcohol-like liver disease in nonalcoholics. A clinical and histologic comparison with alcohol-induced liver injury. *Gastroenterology* 95:1056-1062, 1988.

3. Powell EE, Cooksley WG, Hanson R, et al: The natural history of nonalcoholic steatohepatitis: A follow-up study of forty-two patients for up to 21 years. *Hepatology* 11:74-80, 1990.
4. Matteoni CA, Younossi ZM, Gramlich T, et al: Nonalcoholic fatty liver disease: A spectrum of clinical and pathological severity. *Gastroenterology* 116:1413-1419, 1999.

Nonalcholic Fatty Liver, Steatohepatitis, and the Metabolic Syndrome

Marchesini G, Bugianesi E, Forlani G, et al (Univ of Bologna, Italy; Univ of Turin, Italy)
Hepatology 37:917-923, 2003

63–3

Introduction.—Nonalcoholic fatty liver disease (NAFLD) may account for approximately 80% of cases with elevated liver enzyme levels in the United States. Between 20% and 30% of such patients have histologic signs of fibrosis and necroinflammation, indicating the presence of nonalcoholic steatohepatitis (NASH). An association has also been found between NAFLD and the metabolic syndrome. The prevalence of the metabolic syndrome and the risk for potentially progressive NASH was examined in patients with NAFLD.

Methods.—In the period from January 1999 to June 2002, 304 patients with NAFLD and without a previous diagnosis of diabetes mellitus were studied. All patients had chronic hypertransaminasemia and negative or negligible alcohol consumption. Those with at least 3 of the 5 components of the metabolic syndrome were considered to have the syndrome. Patients underwent clinical, anthropometric, and laboratory studies, and some had liver US.

Results.—Patients were 252 men (mean age, 39.5 years) and 52 women (mean age, 54.7 years). Men had a higher body mass index (BMI) than women and higher blood glucose, arterial pressure, and transaminase levels. The prevalence of the metabolic syndrome increased with increasing BMI, from 18% in those with normal weight to 67% in obesity. There was a significant association between insulin resistance and the metabolic syndrome (odds ratio [OR], 2.5). Liver biopsy findings, available in 163 cases, classified 120 patients as having NASH. Fifty-three percent of patients with pure fatty liver had a metabolic syndrome, but the proportion was 88% in those with NASH. Logistic regression analysis adjusting for age, sex, and BMI confirmed that the presence of metabolic syndrome carries a high risk of NASH (OR, 3.2) among patients with NAFLD. The presence of the metabolic syndrome did not increase the risk of severe steatosis or severe necroinflammatory activity, but it was associated with a high risk of combined grade 3 or 4 fibrosis.

Conclusion.—The increasing prevalence of obesity in the western world, together with diabetes, dyslipidemia, hypertension, and the metabolic syndrome, places a large population at risk in coming years for the development of liver failure.

▶ Marchesini et al sought to determine the prevalence and prognosis of patients with NAFLD and the metabolic syndrome. The definition of the metabolic syndrome from the Adult Treatment Panel III included central obesity, hypertension, hypertriglyceridemia, low levels of high-density lipoprotein cholesterol, and hyperglycemia. They found the presence of the metabolic syndrome in 88% of NASH patients versus 53% of patients with NAFLD. The importance of this study was to focus on the obesity epidemic, particularly on its liver complications. Presently, chronic liver disease and cirrhosis are the 10th leading causes of death overall, and this is likely to increase unless we address obesity and its complications.

J. S. Barkin, MD

Hepatic Injury in 12 Patients Taking the Herbal Weight Loss Aids Chaso or Onshido

Adachi M, Saito H, Kobayashi H, et al (Keio Univ, Tokyo)
Ann Intern Med 139:488-492, 2003   63–4

Introduction.—Dietary supplements for weight loss have become popular in Japan, despite a lack of evidence for their efficacy and a known potential for adverse effects. Twelve Japanese patients were described who had acute liver injury diagnosed after taking the Chinese herbal weight loss aids Chaso and Onshido.

Methods.—Records of the 12 patients, 6 who took Chaso and 6 who took Onshido, were reviewed. Ingredients in these products ingested by 5 of the patients were analyzed with the Agilent 1100 Series Liquid Chromatograph/Mass Selective Detector. A spectrophotometer assessed contamination with heavy metals.

Results.—None of the 12 patients had taken other over-the-counter or prescription medications or alternative therapies, and all had viral infection, autoimmune diseases, alcoholic liver diseases, or other metabolic liver diseases ruled out as a cause of liver injury. Their clinical symptoms, which included fatigue and appetite loss, appeared 5 to 40 days after ingesting the weight loss aid. Two patients had hepatic encephalopathy and met diagnostic criteria for fulminant hepatic failure. Ten patients improved after discontinuing the products and had normal liver test results after hospital discharge. One patient died, however, and another required liver transplantation. Both Chaso and Onshido were found to contain N-nitroso-fenfluramine, a variant of fenfluramine, which was withdrawn from the market because of cardiac complications. N-nitroso compounds have been linked with carcinogenesis in the liver.

Discussion.—Dietary supplements are often considered "health foods," despite their potential risks. After these patients' acute liver injury was linked to Chaso and Onshido, the Japanese public was warned, and 156 additional cases of hepatotoxicity related to the products were identified. The severity of hepatotoxicity showed no apparent correlation with the duration of use or the amount of product ingested. Persons may differ in their susceptibility to these agents, and the lack of regulations may result in variation from one batch to another in the amount of toxic ingredients.

▶ Dietary supplements are used weekly by up to 40 million Americans. Complementary, alternative medications are commonly ingested by up to 40% of patients attending a clinic for liver diseases. The intake of these supplements is commonly not reported by these patients. Therefore, in our history taking, we need to focus on patients' use of dietary supplements, as they are important potential sources of hepatotoxicity. Adachi et al reported on hepatic injury from the intake of the herbal weight loss aids Chaso or Onshido. Interestingly, both of these products contained a synthetic fenfluramine, a weight loss product that was withdrawn from the US market because of its cardiac complications. This, potentially, is a significant public health issue with increasing obesity and search for natural cures.

J. S. Barkin, MD

High Prevalence of Potentially Hepatotoxic Herbal Supplement Use in Patients With Fulminant Hepatic Failure
Estes JD, Stolpman D, Olyaei A, et al (Oregon Health & Sciences Univ, Portland)
Arch Surg 138:852-858, 2003   63–5

Introduction.—Fulminant hepatic failure (FHF) affects approximately 2000 patients annually in the United States, where most cases result from acetaminophen toxicity and idiosyncratic drug reactions. But the increasing use of dietary and herbal supplements, some of which are potentially hepatotoxic, is also linked to FHF. Patients with FHF who were referred for liver transplantation were retrospectively reviewed for supplement use and rate of survival.

Methods.—During the study period, January 2001 through October 2002, 20 patients wih FHF were referred to the liver transplantation service. All patients were evaluated to determine the cause of liver injury and the identity and duration of medication or supplement use. Histologic specimens, obtained via core biopsy, liver explantation, or autopsy, were also examined.

Results.—Ten of the 20 patients referred with FHF during the study period had a recent history of ingesting a dietary supplement or herb with documented hepatotoxic potential. Seven of these 10 patients had no other cause of FHF identified, whereas 3 had an additional cause found. Liver specimens in all 10 patients showed significant hepatic necrosis. Acetaminophen toxicity was the leading cause of FHF in patients without a history of supplement use. Supplement users did not differ from nonusers in age, sex, overall survival, rate of liver transplantation, recovery rates with or without orthotopic liver transplantation, mortality without transplantation, or mortality after transplantation.

Discussion.—There was a high prevalence of dietary supplement use in this series of patients with FHF. The duration of the use of supplements with known hepatotoxic potential ranged from several days to 15 years. Five of the 10 patients died. The 4 major agents used were LipoKinetix, kava, chaparral, and ma huang. Regulatory oversight of these commonly used agents is recommended, together with campaigns to warn the public of the potential for serious toxicity.

▶ Hepatotoxin agents can cause a wide spectrum of liver diseases ranging from asymptomatic elevation of liver enzymes to acute hepatic failure. Estes et al found that patients with FHF have a high rate of ingesting these agents, which include LipoKinetix, kava, chaparral, and ma huang. A plethora of hepatotoxic herbal supplements has been identified and among them, germander and mixtures of valerian and skullcap are included.

J. S. Barkin, MD

SUGGESTED READING

Pratt DS, Kaplan MM: Evaluation of abnormal liver-enzyme results in asymptomatic patients. *N Engl J Med* 342:1266-1271, 2000.

Identification and Management of Hepatitis C Patients in Primary Care Clinics
Shehab TM, Orrego M, Chunduri R, et al (Univ of Michigan, Ann Arbor)
Am J Gastroenterol 98:639-644, 2003   63–6

Introduction.—Approximately 75% of the 4 million Americans with antibodies to the hepatitis C virus are chronically infected, and chronic hepatitis C infection is the most common cause of end-stage liver disease. Early diagnosis can allow the patient to be evaluated for therapy and prevent transmission of the infection to others. But in the primary care setting, many patients with hepatitis C are undiagnosed or fail to be referred to a specialist. The actual level of care received by patients with hepatitis C in primary care clinics was examined.

Methods.—The University of Michigan's clinical laboratory database was used to identify patients aged 18 years or older who were seen in a primary care clinic and tested positive for hepatitis C virus antibody (anti-HCV) using enzyme immunoassay from January 1990 through December 1999. Two control groups were included: patients who tested negative for anti-HCV during the same period and were matched for age, sex, and clinic site; and similarly matched patients who were not tested for hepatitis C. Each group included 229 patients and had similar demographics.

Results.—Only 16% of anti-HCV–positive and 10% of anti-HCV–negative patients had been tested for hepatitis C on the basis of physician-identified risk factors. Yet at least 95% of patients in both groups had a documented indication for hepatitis C testing. And only 1% of those not tested had a documented discussion of hepatitis C risk factors during their initial visit with the primary care physician. Overall, 139 (59%) of anti-HCV–positive patients were referred for further evaluation: 77% of those who were HCV RNA positive with elevated alanine aminotransferase (ALT) levels, and 39% who were HCV RNA positive with normal ALT. Of 59 anti-HCV–positive patients who underwent liver biopsy, 40% had bridging fibrosis or cirrhosis.

Conclusion.—There has been concern that hepatitis C, a significant health problem in the United States, is underdiagnosed in primary care clinics. This survey found that testing for hepatitis C in these clinics is seldom initiated because of physician-identified risk factors, and few patients are asked about potential risk factors at their initial visit. Because the disease may be asymptomatic, better strategies for early diagnosis are needed.

▶ Chronic hepatitis C infection is the most common cause of end-stage liver disease and the leading indication for liver transplantation in the United States.[1] It has been estimated that 3.9 million Americans have been infected, and this represents 1.8% of the population. In the United States, an estimated 8000 to 10,000 deaths each year result from HCV-associated liver disease. Therefore, it is critical to identify these patients, counsel them, and initiate treatment. They must be advised against alcohol ingestion, which causes progression of the disease as well as behaviors that may transmit infection, and must be vaccinated against other hepatotropic viruses such as hepatitis A and B.

The burden of identification of these individuals falls on the primary care physician. Shehab et al found that less than 10% of patients attending a primary care clinic were asked about IV drug use and blood transfusion before 1992—the 2 most common risk factors for hepatitis C—during their initial visit, and less than 15% ordered an acute HCV test because of physician-identified risk factors. This suggests that hepatitis C is grossly underdiagnosed in the primary care clinics.

In addition, patients with elevated ALT levels were not intensely tested for hepatitis C, and conversely, patients who were acutely HCV positive with normal aminotransferase levels were not referred for therapy evaluation. Perhaps this was because of the misconception that patients with hepatitis C who have normal liver enzyme levels are not at risk for progressive liver disease and that therapy should not be given to those patients. Indeed, as Jamal and Abdelkarim[2] note, it has been shown that despite having repeatedly normal ALT levels, a significant number of patients have moderate to severe fibrosis, and a few will have cirrhosis on liver biopsy. Besides, according to Bruce Bacon and the last NIH consensus statement for the management of hepatitis C in patients with normal serum aminotransferase levels, treatment of these patients has demonstrated response rates that are almost identical to those achieved for patients with abnormal aminotransferase levels.

Hepatitis C infection is associated with a wide array of complications (Table 1).

TABLE 1.—Hepatitis C Extrahepatic Manifestations

Eye	Mooren's corneal ulcers
Mouth	Lichen planus
Serum	Essential mixed cryoglobulinemia (EMC) type II and III nonspecific autoantibodies (rheumatoid factor, antinuclear and smooth muscle antibodies, antibodies to liver/kidney microsome type I [anti-LKM-I], organ-specific antibodies (autoantibodies against the thyroid gland)
Renal	Cryoglobulinemic glomerulonephritis (CGN) non-cryoglobulinemic glomerulonephritis
	Membranoproliferative glomerulonephritis
	Acute proliferative glomerulonephritis
	Membranous glomerulonephritis
Cutaneous	Cutaneous vasculitis (leukocytoclastic vasculitis)
	Lichen planus
	Porphyria cutanea tarda
	Polyarteritis nodosa (questionable association with erythema nodosum, erythema multiform, urticaria, Adamantiades–Behçet syndrome, and vitiligo)
Respiratory	Intestinal pneumonitis
Endocrine	Diabetes mellitus (genotype 2-a)
Lymphoproliferative disorders	Non-Hodgkin B-cell lymphoplasmatocytoid immunocytomas

J. S. Barkin, MD

References

1. Powell DW, for the Hepatitis C Consensus Development Panel: National Institutes of Health consensus development conference panel statement: Management of hepatitis C. *Hepatology* 26:2S-10S, 1997.
2. Jamal MM, Abdelkarim BZ: Chronic hepatitis C with persistently normal aminotransferase levels: Do we have an adequate definition? *Am J Gastroenterol* 98:1455-1456, 2003.

Association Between Hepatitis C, Diabetes Mellitus, and Race: A Case-Control Study

Thuluvath PJ, John PR (Johns Hopkins Univ, Baltimore, Md)
Am J Gastroenterol 98:438-441, 2003   63–7

Introduction.—Patients with liver disease appear to have an increased prevalence of glucose intolerance, and there are also reports of an association between hepatitis C virus (HCV) infection and type II diabetes mellitus (DM). A case-control study was designed to compare the prevalence of type II DM in patients with HCV cirrhosis with that of a population matched for age, sex, body mass index (BMI), and severity of liver disease.

Methods.—Both cases and controls were selected from the liver transplant registry at the Johns Hopkins Hospital. Cases were 97 patients with cirrhosis and HCV; controls were 194 HCV-negative patients with cirrhosis from other causes. All patients had a Child-Pugh score greater than 7. Pretransplantation data gathered included race, albumin, total bilirubin, direct bilirubin, and BMI.

Results.—Compared with the control group, the HCV group had a higher proportion of blacks and a higher mean BMI. Among black patients, the mean BMI was similar in HCV and control groups. The proportion of patients with obesity (BMI >30) did not differ statistically between black and white patients. The prevalence of pretransplant DM was higher in the HCV group, and blacks with HCV were significantly more likely than whites with HCV to have pretransplant DM (33.3% vs 13.2%). In logistic regression analysis, however, age was found to be the only independent predictor for pretransplant DM, and black race was an independent predictor for the development of new-onset DM.

Discussion.—Compared with matched controls with cirrhosis but without HCV infection, patients with cirrhosis and HCV infection had a higher prevalence of type II DM. The difference was attributed primarily to the higher prevalence of type II DM in black patients with HCV infection. Whereas a third of black patients with HCV had DM, only 6.3% of black patients without HCV had DM.

▶ HCV infection has been associated with the development of type II diabetes mellitus. Thuluvath and John reported on a case-controlled study that examined this association. They looked at the presence of the known risk factors for type II DM in HCV cirrhotic patients versus non-HCV cirrhotic patients. They confirmed a higher prevalence of type II DM in cirrhotic patients with HCV infection compared with a non-HCV group. They found a very high prevalence of DM in African Americans with HCV versus non-HCV cirrhosis (33% vs 6%).

Mason and Nair,[1] in the accompanying editorial, postulated that HCV mediates type II DM in genetically susceptible individuals. While liver disease per se has a role in glucose intolerance, HCV infection seems to provide an additional risk factor.

J. S. Barkin, MD

Reference

1. Mason A, Nair S: Is type II diabetes another extrahepatic manifestation of HCV infection (editorial)? *Am J Gastroenterol* 98:243-246, 2003.

Infection and the Progression of Hepatic Encephalopathy in Acute Liver Failure
Vaquero J, and the US Acute Liver Failure Study Group (Northwestern Univ, Chicago; et al)
Gastroenterology 125:755-764, 2003   63–8

Introduction.—Predictive factors for the progression to deep hepatic encephalopathy (HE) in patients with acute liver failure (ALF) have not been defined fully. The findings of a previous study, however, highlighted an association between the systemic inflammatory response syndrome (SIRS), infection, and progressive encephalopathy. Patients prospectively included in the US Acute Liver Failure Study Group Registry from January 1998 to June 2002 were evaluated for factors predictive of progression to stage III-IV HE in ALF, and to characterize the relationship between SIRS, infection, and HE.

Methods.—During the study period, 448 patients with ALF were included in the registry. Upon admission to the study, 227 had stage I-II HE and 221 had stage III-IV HE. Those in the former group were divided according to etiology; 96 patients had acetaminophen-induced ALF and 131 had non–acetaminophen-induced ALF. Twenty-seven qualitative and quantitative variables were examined for their ability to predict progression to stage III-IV HE.

Results.—Patients in the acetaminophen group were younger, more likely to be white and to have a history of alcohol consumption, and had significantly lower bilirubin levels and higher pulse, prothrombin time, and serum sodium and transaminase levels at admission than patients in the nonacetaminophen group. The proportion of patients who progressed to stage III-IV HE was similar in acetaminophen (33/96) and nonacetaminophen (58/131) groups, but progression occurred more rapidly in the acetaminophen group (mean, 2.4 vs 4.1 days). Multivariate analysis identified acquisition of infection during stage I-II HE, increased leukocyte levels at admission, and decreased platelet count as predictors of worsening HE in the acetaminophen group. The only predictive variables in the nonacetaminophen group were increased pulse rate and aspartate aminotransferase levels. More patients in the acetaminophen group (15/19) than in the nonacetaminophen group (12/23) had an infection detected before progression to stage III-IV HE. A higher number of components of SIRS at admission was associated with more frequent worsening of HE in patients without positive microbiologic cultures.

Conclusion.—The acquisition of infection and development of the related systemic inflammatory response may contribute to the worsening of HE in patients with ALF, mainly in cases of acetaminophen-induced disease. Monitoring of such patients for infection and early antimicrobial treatment may be beneficial.

▶ In addition to identifying the causes of both acute and chronic liver disease, our goal as physicians is to prevent their complications. ALF in the United States usually results from drug ingestion (acetaminophen); N-acetylcysteine has been shown to improve the outcome and spare these patients from liver transplantation. Vaquero et al prospectively analyzed the factors that influence the progression of HE in ALF. They found a temporal relationship between acquisition of infection and subsequent progression of HE, especially in acetaminophen-induced ALF. In addition, they found that a decreased platelet count on admission, which may reflect undiagnosed sepsis, was also associated with progression. They also found and confirmed that patients with a higher number of components of SIRS (ie, white blood cell count <4000 or >12,000, pulse >90/min, and temperature <36°C or >38°C) have an increased risk of subsequent worsening of HE and presence of brain edema.

Clinically, does this call for prophylactic antibiotic administration? Two previous studies have evaluated antibiotic prophylaxis in patients with HE, one of which reported that a higher number of patients could undergo transplantation in the treated group,[1] and the other reported a decrease in infections.[2] Thus, it seems reasonable to use prophylactic broad-spectrum and antifungal antibiotics in these severely ill patients.

J. S. Barkin, MD

References

1. Rolando N, Gimson A, Wade J, et al: Prospective controlled trial of selective parenteral and enteral antimicrobial regimen in fulminant liver failure. *Hepatology* 17:196-201, 1993.
2. Salmeron JM, Tito L, Rimola A, et al: Selective intestinal decontamination in the prevention of bacterial infection in patients with acute liver failure. *J Hepatol* 14:280-285, 1992.

Spontaneous Bacterial Peritonitis in Asymptomatic Outpatients With Cirrhotic Ascites

Evans LT, Kim WR, Poterucha JJ, et al (Mayo Clinic, Rochester, Minn)
Hepatology 37:897-901, 2003   63–9

Background.—Spontaneous bacterial peritonitis (SBP) in hospitalized patients with cirrhosis is associated with renal failure, sepsis, and death. Whether SBP is also associated with poorer outcomes in asymptomatic outpatients with cirrhotic ascites was examined.

Methods.—The medical records of 427 asymptomatic outpatients with cirrhotic ascites evaluated between July 1994 and December 2000 were reviewed. Patients with SBP, defined as an absolute neutrophil count of at least 250 cells/mm^3 (ie, neutrocytic ascites) were identified for further study.

Results.—Fifteen patients (3.5%) had SBP; culture results were positive in 6 (1.4% of total) and negative in 9 (2.1% of total). Another 8 patients (1.9%) had bacterascites (ie, positive ascitic fluid culture results but no neutrocytic ascites). Most of the isolates from the 14 patients with positive ascites culture results (both culture-positive SBP and bacterascites) were gram-positive organisms, especially *Streptococcus viridans* (4 cases) and *Staphylococcus aureus* (3 cases). Of the 15 patients with SBP, 10 were hospitalized for antibiotic therapy, 1 received antibiotics as an outpatient, and 4 patients whose neutrophil counts were less than 500 cells/mm^3 were not treated. Yet none of these 15 patients had type I hepatorenal syndrome develop. One-year follow-up information was available for 12 patients, of whom 3 had died (67% survival). Of the 8 patients with bacterascites, 1 was treated as an outpatient, whereas the rest were not treated. At 1 year, 1 patient had died (87% survival).

Conclusion.—Only 3.5% of these asymptomatic outpatients with cirrhotic ascites had SBP develop. Patients with SBP who did not receive antibiotics had outcomes similar to those in treated patients. The 1-year mortality rate of 33% in these outpatients is better than that in inpatients with SBP (50%-70%). The pathogens involved also differed between outpatients (primarily gram-positive isolates) and inpatients (primarily gram-negative isolates). Because the characteristics and outcomes of SBP in asymptomatic outpatients with cirrhotic ascites differ from those in their hospitalized counterparts (particularly in the occurrence of spontaneous reversal of infection), the criteria used to diagnose SBP in outpatients may need to be revisited.

Rapid Diagnosis of Spontaneous Bacterial Peritonitis by Use of Reagent Strips
Castellote J, López C, Gornals J, et al (L'Hospitalet d Llobregat, Barcelona)
Hepatology 37:893-896, 2003   63–10

Background.—The development of spontaneous bacterial peritonitis (SBP) in cirrhotic inpatients with ascites can be life threatening. Currently, SBP is diagnosed by a polymorphonuclear (PMN) cell count of at least 250 cells/mm^3 in ascitic fluid, but PMN counts are not always routinely available. The utility of reagent strip testing for the rapid diagnosis of SBP in hospitalized patients with cirrhotic ascites was investigated.

Methods.—A total of 128 patients with cirrhosis (71% men; median age, 59 years) who underwent 228 paracenteses for suspected SBP were studied. Immediately after collection, ascitic fluid was tested by a reagent strip sensitive to leukocyte esterase. Results were read at 90 seconds by 2 blinded investigators; scores of 2 or higher (on a scale of 0-4) were taken as positive. Culture and PMN counts were also performed.

Results.—According to classic criteria (including cultures and PMN counts), 52 samples showed SBP and 5 revealed secondary bacterial peritonitis. Reagent strips were positive in 55 of these 57 cases (sensitivity, 96%), and negative in 152 of the 171 culture- and PMN-negative cases (specificity, 89%). Positive and negative predictive values were 74% and 99%, respectively. The overall accuracy of a score of 2 or higher on the reagent strip in identifying cases of SBP or secondary bacterial peritonitis was 91%.

Conclusion.—The use of a reagent strip developed to detect leukocyte esterase in ascitic fluid is a rapid (90 seconds), easy, and inexpensive (about 16 euros per strip) method for diagnosing SBP in hospitalized patients with cirrhotic ascites. Patients with a positive score on the reagent strip should be treated empirically with antibiotics pending culture results. Conversely, SBP can safely be excluded in patients with negative strip results.

▶ In patients who have cirrhosis with ascites, SBP may result in renal failure, systemic sepsis, and decreased survival. SBP is sought in all hospitalized patients with ascites, as an aspirate is sent for cell count with culture and sensitivity (C & S), whereas in outpatients, C & S is only performed if the PMN count is at least 250/mm^3—so-called neutrocytic ascites. Evans et al (Abstract 63–9) determined that there was a 3.5% prevalence of SBP among cirrhotic outpatients undergoing paracentesis and that the predominant organisms are gram positive. This included patients with a PMN count of at least 250/mm³ (neutrocytic ascites) as well as patients with a PMN count of less than 250/mm³, who also had positive cultures—so-called bacteritic ascites. However, if the PMN count is greater than 250/mm³, antibiotics are often begun before culture results are available. Urine "dipsticks," which detect leukocyte esterase, indicative of neutrophils in ascitic fluid, can now routinely determine an estimate of this count. Castellote et al (Abstract 63–10) found a sensitivity of 96%, specificity of 89%, and a negative predictive value of 99% for determining SBP based on "dipstick" findings. When the reagent strip result of 2 or more by visual determination of color was found, the test was considered positive. Therefore, in addition to sending the aspirate for cell count and C & S, use a urine dipstick to determine whether 2+ leukocyte esterase is present and if so, institute empirical antibiotic therapy.

J. S. Barkin, MD

The North American Study for the Treatment of Refractory Ascites
Sanyal AJ, and the Nastra Group (Virginia Commonwealth Univ, Richmond; et al)
Gastroenterology 124:634-641, 2003   63–11

Background.—Ascites has a poor prognosis, especially when it is refractory to medical treatment. Total paracentesis is the current treatment of choice for refractory ascites; recent reports have described the use of transjugular intrahepatic portosystemic shunts (TIPS). A randomized controlled trial was performed to compare the outcomes of methods including total paracentesis versus the use of TIPS for the treatment of refractory ascites.

Methods.—The study included 109 patients with refractory ascites at 6 US and Canadian centers who were randomly placed into 2 treatment groups. One group received medical therapy, consisting of sodium restriction, diuretic medications, and repeated total paracentesis, as necessary. The other group received medical therapy plus TIPS. The mortality rates and the rates of recurrent tense symptomatic ascites were compared for the 2 groups.

Results.—In the TIPS group, the technical success rate was 94%. The rate of recurrent tense ascites was 84% in the medical therapy group compared with 42% in the TIPS group. The risk of initial treatment failure was 4 times higher with medical therapy than with TIPS. Overall mortality and transplant-free survival rates were similar between groups. Moderate to severe encephalopathy was less frequent with medical therapy: 21%, compared to 38% with TIPS. Rates of complications, including liver failure, variceal hemorrhage, or acute renal failure, were similar between groups. Other outcomes were also similar, including emergency department visits, hospitalization rate, and quality of life.

Conclusions.—For patients with ascites that does not respond to initial medical treatment, a strategy of TIPS plus medical therapy yields better control of ascites than medical therapy plus total paracentesis. TIPS reduces the rate of recurrent ascites, yet other outcomes are similar between these 2 strategies, including survival and hospitalization rates, and quality of life. The findings suggest that TIPS is best reserved as a second-line therapy for refractory ascites.

▶ The most common complication of portal hypertension is ascites. Its presence portends a poor prognosis if it becomes infected—so-called spontaneous bacterial peritonitis—or if it becomes refractory to medical therapy. Refractory ascites is approached with repeated large-volume paracentesis with concomitant use of albumin to prevent postparacentesis circulatory dysfunction, and dietary sodium restriction. In most patients, this is for their comfort and does not affect survival. Sanyal et al reported the results of a prospective, randomized multicenter trial comparing medical therapy with total paracentesis, sodium restriction, and treatment with diuretics versus medical therapy plus TIPS. TIPS are performed by interventional radiologists; the stent is passed through the right hepatic vein to the liver parenchyma and reaches the right branch of the portal vein and, therefore, decompresses the portal circulation and corrects the portal hypertension. Its major complications are development of portasystemic encephalopathy and stent occlusion. TIPS were found to be superior to conventional medical therapy for control of ascites, which confirms previous studies. However, it fails in the most important aspects—no improvement in quality of life or improved survival. Even after TIPS, we need to continue medical therapy with sodium restriction and, sometimes, diuretics. Therefore, in the patient whose only complication is refractory ascites, it is most reasonable to continue intense medical therapy, keeping in mind that its only cure is liver transplantation.

J. S. Barkin, M.D.

SUGGESTED READING

Pyrsopoulos NT, Reddy RK: Extrahepatic manifestations of chronic viral hepatitis. *Curr Gastroenterol Rep* 3:71-78, 2001.

PART EIGHT

ENDOCRINOLOGY, DIABETES, AND METABOLISM

ERNEST L. MAZZAFERRI, MD

Introduction

Last year, many important articles were published concerning the basic science, prevention, diagnosis, and treatment of endocrine disorders. The articles for the Endocrinology section of the YEAR BOOK OF MEDICINE were selected from over 200 articles that our editors thought would have a substantial impact on our understanding of endocrine disorders and the practice of endocrinology. From this group, 45 articles were chosen that should be of particular importance to internists because they emphasize prevention of important clinical problems such as diabetes mellitus and coronary artery disease and early diagnosis and treatment of ubiquitous disorders such as osteoporosis and thyroid nodules. During the past year, new and important information has been added to our growing understanding of subclinical thyroid dysfunction, including new information concerning its effects on the pregnant woman and the fetus. The articles, which have been grouped according to several broad categories, are each accompanied by comments from the section editors of the YEAR BOOK OF ENDOCRINOLOGY.

We hope these articles and their accompanying editorial comments give the reader fresh insight into these common endocrine problems encountered in everyday practice.

Ernest L. Mazzaferri, MD

64 Lipoproteins and Atherosclerosis

Adherence to a Mediterranean Diet and Survival in a Greek Population
Trichopoulou A, Costacou T, Bamia C, et al (Univ of Athens, Greece; Harvard School of Public Health, Boston)
N Engl J Med 348:2599-2608, 2003   64–1

Background.—Many believe that adhering to a Mediterranean diet will increase longevity, but few relevant data have been published. The relationship of adherence to a Mediterranean diet and survival in a Greek population was examined in a population-based prospective study.

Methods.—A total of 22,043 adults in Greece completed an extensive, validated food-frequency questionnaire at baseline. A 10-point scale was used to determine adherence to the traditional Mediterranean diet, with higher scores indicating greater adherence. Analyses were conducted with adjustment for age, sex, body mass index, physical activity level, and other potential confounding factors. The study population was followed up for a median of 44 months.

Findings.—Two hundred seventy-five persons died during the follow-up period. Greater adherence to the Mediterranean diet correlated with a decrease in total mortality rate. Greater adherence to the diet was inversely associated with death due to coronary heart disease (adjusted hazard ratio, 0.67) and due to cancer (adjusted hazard ratio, 0.76). In general, associations between individual food groups in the Mediterranean diet score and total mortality rate were nonsignificant.

Conclusions.—Greater adherence to a traditional Mediterranean diet is significantly associated with a decrease in the overall mortality rate. The substantial magnitude of this reduction is consistent with findings from other research.

▶ We have known about and have recommended Mediterranean diets for years. What is so special about this report that warrants publication as the lead article in the June 26, 2003, issue of this prestigious journal? There is more to this diet than just olive oil. It entails a high intake of vegetables, legumes, fruits, nuts, and fish in addition to olive oil and a low intake of meat, poultry, and dairy products. In addition, there is regular moderate exercise and of course ethanol, primarily wine, with meals.

The authors prospectively graded the intensity of the diet and related the score to outcome in a large population. The scoring technique divided the population into 3 groups: low, intermediate, and high relative to the intensity of following a Mediterranean diet. Only the intake of fruits and nuts and the ratio of monounsaturated to saturated lipids were related to total mortality.

Overall, the benefit of a high-score Mediterranean diet was observed despite age, body mass index, visceral obesity, or level of physical activity. Unfortunately, detailed data concerning body mass index, blood pressure, lipid/lipoprotein levels, and insulin resistance were not provided but will no doubt appear in the future from this large population. Without knowing why but knowing that it is associated with a survival advantage, we could easily adopt its essential features.

Diet is always a popular topic. Much is said but little is done about it. Consumption of trans fatty acids not only increases low-density lipoprotein cholesterol (LDL-C) but also increases small dense LDL particles.[1] Replacement of trans fatty acids with unsaturated fatty acids has a better impact on blood lipids and the ratio of total cholesterol to high-density lipoprotein cholesterol than does replacement by carbohydrate.[2] Replacement of saturated fatty acids by cis monounsaturated fatty acids 21b reduces coronary heart disease risk.[2] These findings suggest considerable benefit from changing the dietary distribution of fat without necessarily changing the content of fat in the diet, provided that the latter is not excessive.

I am beginning to think heretically that we should follow diets that are basically healthy and be careful to just consume the right amount to maintain optimum weight. Unfortunately, some people believe that they can eat as much as they want if it is "heart healthy."

A fascinating article demonstrated that the lipid response of patients entered in the Dietary Approach to Stop Hypertension (DASH) trial was related to the C-reactive protein (CRP) level.[3] This trial employed the use of a 2100 K calorie diet with 3 levels of sodium intake (50, 100, and 150 mmol/d). The diet provided 27% of calories from fat and 150 mg cholesterol daily, whereas the control diet provided 37% of calories from fat and 300 mg cholesterol daily. The diet reduced cholesterol by approximately 13 mg/dL, LDL-C by about 11 mg/dL, and high-density lipoprotein cholesterol by about 5 mg/dL without any change in triglyceride. However, when the CRP level was low—that is, less than the median—the reduction in LDL-C was about 15 mg/dL and when it was greater than the median, it was only approximately 4mg/dL. Furthermore, the triglyceride was unchanged in those with CRP less than the median, and it increased by about 20% in those above the median.

Although the study is small and could be wrong, it raises the possibility that the CRP could be used to identify patients who would or would not respond optimally to diet. It would have been helpful to know more about the patients with CRP above the median with regard to body mass index and glucose or insulin parameters. Baseline lipids did not suggest the metabolic syndrome, but the subjects all had hypertension and, as a group, had a body mass index of approximately 30 kg/m².

R. A. Kreisberg, MD

References

1. Mauger J-F, Lichtenstein AH, Ausman LM, et al: Effect of different forms of dietary hydrogenated fats on LDL particle size. *Am J Clin Nutr* 78:370-375, 2003.
2. Mensink RP, Zock PL, Kester ADM, et al: Effects of dietary fatty acids and carbohydrates on the ratio of serum total to HDL cholesterol and on serum lipids and apolipoproteins: A meta-analysis of 60 controlled trials. *Am J. Clin Nutr* 77:1146-1155, 2003.
3. Erlinger TP, Miller ER III, Charleston J, et al: Inflammation modifies the effects of a reduced-fat low-cholesterol diet on lipids. Results from the DASH-Sodium Trial. *Circulation* 108:150-154, 2003.

Use of Antioxidant Vitamins for the Prevention of Cardiovascular Disease: Meta-analysis of Randomised Trials

Vivekananthan DP, Penn MS, Sapp SK, et al (Cleveland Clinic Foundation, Ohio)
Lancet 361:2017-2023, 2003   64–2

Background.—The study of antioxidant vitamins in the prevention of the initiation and progression of cardiovascular disease has been prompted by the oxidative-modification hypothesis of atherosclerosis. Several large prospective cohort studies in humans have found significant reductions in mortality and in the incidence of cardiovascular events in men and women taking antioxidant vitamins. However, several large randomized trials of antioxidant vitamins have shown no such reduction in mortality. Specifically, tocopherol (vitamin E), β-carotene, or both has been associated with reductions in cardiovascular events in observational studies but not in clinical trials. The effect of vitamin E and β-carotene on long-term cardiovascular mortality and morbidity was assessed.

Methods.—Seven randomized trials of vitamin E treatment and 8 randomized trials of β-carotene treatment were reviewed. All of these trials included 1000 or more patients. The dose range for vitamin E was 50 to 800 IU; for β-carotene, the dose range was 15 to 50 mg. Follow-up ranged from 1.4 to 12.0 years.

Results.—A total of 81,788 patients from the vitamin E trials and 138,113 patients from the β-carotene trials were involved in the all-cause mortality analyses. Vitamin E provided no benefit in mortality compared with control treatment and did not significantly decrease the risk of cardiovascular death or cerebrovascular accident. β-Carotene was associated with a small but significant increase in all-cause mortality and a slight increase in cardiovascular death. There was no significant heterogeneity noted in any analysis.

Conclusion.—The routine use of vitamin E is not supported for prevention of cardiovascular disease as no salutary effect of vitamin E was seen at a variety of doses in diverse populations.

▶ The theory that antioxidant vitamin supplements are cardioprotective appears to be nearly dead, although articles continue to be published that prevent the concept from dying. This is one of those areas where epidemiologic studies, observational studies, and bench research strongly supported the concept that antioxidant vitamins would be beneficial.

This meta-analysis finds no support for using vitamin E or β-carotene for preventing cardiovascular disease. The US Preventive Services Task Force finds insufficient evidence to recommend the use of vitamins A, C, or E with folic acid, alone or in combination, for prevention of cancer or cardiovascular disease.[1] Furthermore, in heavy smokers, β-carotene supplementation is associated with a higher incidence of lung cancer and all-cause mortality.[2]

The adverse effects of β-carotene disappear after it is stopped.[2] Vitamin E has no effect on cardiovascular outcomes or nephropathy in patients with diabetes.[3] Yet vitamins C and E restore endothelial function in hyperlipidemic children,[4] slow the progression of atherosclerosis in patients with hypercholesterolemia,[5] and prevent the increase in C-reactive protein that occurs with a McDonalds's Big Mac meal.[6]

We need to move on. The general take on antioxidant vitamins is that they don't work to prevent cardiovascular events in patients with high risk of coronary heart disease. On the contrary, we should encourage all persons to consume a diet that is high in fruits, vegetables, and antioxidant vitamins.

R. A. Kreisberg, MD

References

1. U.S. Preventive Services Task Force: Routine vitamin supplementation to prevent cancer and cardiovascular disease: Recommendations and rationale. *Ann Intern Med* 139:51-55, 2003.
2. ATBC Study Group: Incidence of cancer and mortality following α-tocopherol and β-carotene supplementation: A postintervention follow-up. *JAMA* 290:476-485, 2003.
3. Lonn E, on behalf of the Heart Outcomes Prevention Evaluation (HOPE) Investigators: Effects of vitamin E on cardiovascular and microvascular outcomes in high-risk patients with diabetes. *Diabetes Care* 25:1919-1927, 2002.
4. Engler MM, Engler MB, Malloy MJ, et al: Antioxidant vitamins C and E improve endothelial function in children with hyperlipidemia: Endothelial Assessment of Risk From Lipids in Youth (EARLY) Trial. *Circulation* 108:1059-1063, 2003.
5. Salonen RM, Nyyssonen K, Kaikkonen J, et al: Six-year effect of combined vitamin C and E supplementation on atherosclerotic progression. The Antioxidant Supplementation in Atherosclerosis Prevention (ASAP) Study. *Circulation* 107:947-953, 2003.
6. Carroll MF, Schade DS: Timing of antioxidant vitamin ingestion alters postprandial proatherogenic serum markers. *Circulation* 108:24-31. 2003.

Major Risk Factors as Antecedents of Fatal and Nonfatal Coronary Heart Disease Events

Greenland P, Knoll MD, Stamler J, et al (Northwestern Univ, Chicago; Univ of Minnesota, Minneapolis; Boston Univ)
JAMA 290:891-897, 2003   64–3

Background.—There has been extensive study of the precursors of coronary heart disease (CHD), and causal risk factors for CHD have been identified. The most significant of these risk factors are unfavorable levels of blood cholesterol, high blood pressure, cigarette smoking, diabetes, and adverse dietary habits. Yet it has frequently been noted that individual major CHD risk factors are perhaps not present in more than 50% of patients with CHD. However, previous studies of CHD risk factors have not included systematic evaluations of the degree to which these patients have had previous exposure to at least 1 of the major risk factors cited above. The frequency of exposure to major risk factors for CHD was investigated.

Methods.—This analysis utilized 3 prospective cohort studies—The Chicago Heart Association Detection Project in Industry, the Multiple Risk Factor Intervention Trial, and a sample from the Framingham Heart Study. The Chicago Heart Association Detection Project in Industry comprised a population sample of 35,642 employed men and women aged 18 to 59 years. The Multiple Risk Factor Intervention Trial included 347,978 men aged 35 to 57 years. A population sample from the Framingham Heart Study included 3295 men and women aged 34 to 59 years.

The follow-up period across the 3 studies ranged from 21 to 30 years. The main outcome measures were fatal CHD in all cohorts and nonfatal myocardial infarction in the Framingham Heart Study, compared by exposure to major CHD risk factors. The risk factors were defined as total cholesterol of at least 240 mg/dL, systolic blood pressure of at least 140 mm Hg, diastolic blood pressure of at least 90 mm Hg, cigarette smoking, and the presence of diabetes. Study participants were stratified by age and sex.

Results.—Among the 20,995 persons with fatal CHD, exposure to at least 1 clinically relevant major CHD risk factor ranged from 87% to 100%. Among persons aged 40 to 59 years at baseline with fatal CHD, exposure to at least 1 major risk factor ranged from 87% to 94%. Among patients with nonfatal myocardial infarction, prior exposure to at least 1 major risk factor was documented in 92% of men and 87% of women aged 40 to 59 years at baseline.

Conclusion.—In this study, prior exposure to major risk factors for CHD was quite common in persons who had the condition develop. All major risk factors should be considered in determining CHD risk estimates and for working to prevent clinical CHD. Finally, these findings call into question the frequently cited concept that CHD events are common among persons with no prior exposure to at least 1 major risk factor for CHD.

▶ This is one of several recently published articles concluding that more than 80% of CHD events in men and women are directly attributable to the standard risk factors of smoking, diabetes, hyperlipidemia, and hypertension.[1,2] This is not a new concept. An editorial in 2001 refuted the traditional wisdom that only 50% of the CHD risk was attributable to standard risk factors.[3] In 1999, Stamler and associates concluded that patients with cholesterol of less than 200 mg/dL, blood pressure of less than 120/80 mm Hg, nonsmoking, and without diabetes are at very low risk of CHD mortality (relative risk, less than 0.2 vs all others with 1 or more CHD risk factors).[4]

A recent article suggested that the use of a single pill ("polypill") containing a statin, 3 blood pressure–lowering drugs, folate, and aspirin could reduce cardiovascular disease by 80%.[5] While a lot of cardiologists got "bent out of shape" by the proposal, it speaks to the importance of standard CHD risk factors. I actually believe the polypill authors had their "tongue in cheek" when they made their provocative suggestion and did so to draw attention to the need for better medical therapy for common risk factors.

Another important issue is, if 80% to 90% of CHD is related to standard risk factors, where do "emerging" risk factors fit? Many physicians that I meet are more concerned about lipoprotein(a), low-density lipoprotein cholesterol and high-density lipoprotein cholesterol size, homocysteine, C-reactive protein, and probably now myeloperoxidase, compared with appropriate therapy of standard risk factors. Many physicians are measuring the poorly understood "emerging" risk factors and using therapies that have not yet been proven to be effective. They attribute precision to something that is not only not precise, but highly speculative. It is very likely that much of the residual CHD risk of approximately 65% observed in statin studies is due to continued smoking, suboptimally treated hypertension, poor diabetic control, and persisting dyslipidemia. We need to get "real." Traditional wisdom in medicine has often been wrong; examples are cardioprotection from hormone replacement therapy, heart disease prevention with antioxidant vitamins, and the contraindication to the use of β-blockers in patients with heart failure. Although my mother has been known to say "It couldn't hurt," this is also wrong when β-carotene supplements are used by cigarette smokers.

R. A. Kreisberg, MD

References

1. Khot UN, Khot MB, Bajzer CT, et al: Prevalence of conventional risk factors in patients with coronary heart disease. *JAMA* 290:898-904, 2003.
2. Emberson JR, Whincup PH, Morris RW, et al: Re-assessing the contribution of serum total cholesterol, blood pressure and cigarette smoking to the aetiology of coronary heart disease: Impact of regression dilution bias. *Eur Heart J* 24:1719-1727, 2003.
3. Magnus P: The real contribution of the major risk factors to the coronary epidemics: Time to end the "only-50%" myth (commentary). *Arch Intern Med* 161:2657-2660, 2001.
4. Stamler J, Stamler R, Neaton JD, et al: Low risk-factor profile and long-term cardiovascular and noncardiovascular mortality and life expectancy: Findings for 5 large cohorts of young adult and middle-aged men and women. *JAMA* 282:2012-2018, 1999.
5. Wald NJ, Law MR: A strategy to reduce cardiovascular disease by more than 80%. *BMJ* 326:1419, 2003.

Prevention of Coronary and Stroke Events With Atorvastatin in Hypertensive Patients Who Have Average or Lower-Than-Average Cholesterol Concentrations, in the Anglo-Scandinavian Cardiac Outcomes Trial— Lipid Lowering Arm (ASCOT-LLA): A Multicentre Randomised Controlled Trial

Sever PS, for the ASCOT Investigators (Imperial College, London; et al)
Lancet 361:1149-1158, 2003 64–4

Background.—The benefits of statins for the prevention of major fatal and nonfatal cardiovascular events have been demonstrated in several large randomized trials. Patients at high risk of cardiovascular disease as a result of hypertension have improved outcomes as a result of the lowering of their cholesterol concentrations. However, no study has determined the benefits of cholesterol lowering in the primary prevention of coronary heart disease (CHD) in hypertensive patients who are not considered to be dyslipidemic. The long-term effects of statin plus antihypertensive treatment on nonfatal and fatal myocardial infarction (MI) were evaluated.

Methods.—As part of the Anglo-Scandinavian Cardiac Outcomes Trial, a total of 19,342 patients (aged 40-79 years) with at least 3 other cardiovascular risk factors were randomly assigned to 1 of 2 antihypertensive regimens. In the lipid-lowering arm of the trial, 10,305 patients with nonfasting total cholesterol concentrations of 6.5 mmol/L or less were randomly assigned to additional atorvastatin, 10 mg, or placebo. An average of 5 years of follow-up was planned, with the primary end point of nonfatal MI and fatal CHD. Data were analyzed by intention to treat.

Results.—Treatment was halted after a median follow-up of 3.3 years. A total of 100 primary events had occurred in the atorvastatin group by that time, compared with 154 events in the placebo group. In addition, fatal and nonfatal stroke (89 atorvastatin vs 121 placebo), total cardiovascular events (389 vs 486), and total coronary events (178 vs 247) were also significantly lowered. There were 185 deaths in the atorvastatin group and 212 deaths in the placebo group. Atorvastatin provided a reduction at 12 months of about 1.3 mmol/L in total serum cholesterol compared with placebo and a reduction of 1.1 mmol/L after 3 years of follow-up.

Conclusion.—There was a significant reduction in major cardiovascular events with atorvastatin, even with a short follow-up.

▶ This is an article addressing the use of statins to reduce cholesterol in hypertensive patients. The topic is important because of the high probability that a patient will have both risk factors, plus the realization that hypercholesterolemia interacts synergistically with hypertension to produce endothelial dysfunction.[1]

These patients were at high risk for CHD but did not have known CHD as represented by previous MI, angina, or a recent cerebrovascular event. The mean LDL-cholesterol (LDL-C) was approximately 150 mg/dK; HDL-cholesterol (HDL-C) approximately 49 mg/dL; and triglyceride, approximately 150 mg/dL. The 10-mg dose of atorvastatin reduced the LDL-C by 33% to 88 mg/dL and reduced the risk of major CHD events by 36% within a median of 3.3 years. The study was planned to last 5 years. The absolute risk reduction was 1.1% (3.0% to 1.9%), indicating that the baseline risk was relatively low, perhaps because of concomitant therapy of hypertension.

The number needed to treat for 3 years to prevent 1 major CHD event is about 100, placing this result in the upper range of values seen in other statin trials. Many of these patients had the metabolic syndrome (hypertension, overweight/obesity, fasting glucose greater than 110 mg/dL, triglyceride more than 150 mg/dL) and about 25% had diabetes, thereby demonstrating the additional benefit of using statins in patients with this general profile whose mean baseline LDL-C was only slightly higher than optimal.

Some have said that atorvastatin did not reduce the cardiovascular event rate in diabetics. This is not an appropriate conclusion since there were only 84 events among patients with diabetes (38 in the atorvastatin group and 46 in the placebo group), too few to get reliable data. It should be pointed out that about 95% of the patients were white and about 80% were men.

In contrast, the Antihypertensive and Lipid-Lowering Treatment to Prevent Heart Attack Trial concluded that pravastatin did not prevent CHD events in moderately hypercholesterolemic and hypertensive patients.[2] This was also a large trial (about 10,000 patients), with many differences from the ASCOT-LLA. The patients were slightly older, women represented approximately 50% of the subjects, only 40% were white, the subjects were heavier (about 40% had a body mass index greater than 30 kg/m²), and approximately 35% had diabetes.

By the end of the study, only 77% of the experimental group were taking pravastatin and 26% of the usual care group had started a statin. Consequently, the difference in LDL-C between the 2 groups was small, about 17 mg/dL, and had decreased 29% from baseline in the atorvastatin group and 17% from baseline in the pravastatin group. The LDL-C difference between the 2 groups was only 12%, a difference that was marginally associated with cardioprotection in trials conducted prior to the statin era. Despite the absence of cardioprotection, the 9% reduction in CHD events was consistent with that expected when related to the percentage difference in cholesterol between control and treatment arms of other statin trials.

Another serious problem with this study was that lipid follow-up data (LDL-C, HDL-C and triglyceride levels) were available on 20% or less of the patients at intervals of 2.4 and 6 years. A fascinating comment by the author of the accompanying editorial relates to putative pleiotropic properties.[3] If pleiotropic properties were important in cardioprotection, they were not observed in this trial at any time point with pravastatin, 40 mg daily—again emphasizing that the reason to use statins is to reduce LDL-C and not the publicized pleiotropic properties.

R. A. Kreisberg, MD

References

1. Rodriquez-Porcel M, Lerman LO, Herrmann J, et al: Hypercholesterolemia and hypertension have synergistic deleterious effects on coronary endothelial function. *Arterioscler Thromb Vasc Biol* 23:885-891, 2003.
2. ALLHAT Officers and Coordinators for the ALLHAT Collaborative Research Group: Major outcomes in moderately hypercholesterolemic, hypertensive patients randomized to pravastatin vs usual care. The Antihypertensive and Lipid-Lowering Treatment to Prevent Heart Attack Trial (ALLHAT-LLT).*JAMA* 288:2998-3007, 2002.
3. Pasternak RC: The ALLHAT lipid-lowering trial—Less is less. *JAMA* 288:3042-3044, 2002.

Comparison of the Efficacy and Safety of *Rosuvastatin* Versus *Atorvastatin, Simvastatin,* and *Pravastatin* Across Doses (STELLAR Trial)

Jones PH, for the STELLAR Study Group (Baylor College of Medicine, Houston; et al)

Am J Cardiol 93:152-160, 2003   64–5

Background.—Studies have shown that, at usual starting doses, rosuvastatin is more efficacious in reducing plasma LDL-cholesterol and in achieving LDL-cholesterol goals than atorvastatin, simvastatin, or pravastatin. A previous trial compared atorvastatin across its dose range with other statins, but the patient number in this study was small, and pairwise comparisons were not prospectively planned.

The goal of the present large trial was to compare the efficacy of rosuvastatin for reduction of LDL cholesterol across the dose range with that of the Food and Drug Administration approved dose ranges of atorvastatin, simvastatin, and pravastatin, the 3 most widely prescribed statins. Secondary goals included stepwise multiple, pairwise comparisons; safety assessments; and comparisons of the efficacy for modifying other lipids and achieving the objectives of the National Cholesterol Education Program (NCEP) Adult Treatment Panel III and the Joint European Task Force LDL cholesterol objectives.

Methods.—After a dietary lead-in period, 2431 adults with hypercholesterolemia (defined as LDL-cholesterol of 160 or greater and less than 250 mg/dL; triglycerides less than 400 mg/dL) were randomly assigned to receive rosuvastatin at 10, 20, 40, or 80 mg; atorvatatin 10,20, 40, or 80 mg; simvastatin at 10, 20, 40, or 80 mg; or pravastatin at 10, 20, or 40 mg.

Results.—Across-dose analyses at 6 weeks showed that rosuvastatin at 10 to 80 mg reduced LDL-cholesterol by a mean of 8.2% more than atorvastatin 10 to 80 mg, 26% more than pravastatin 10 to 40 mg, and 12% to 18% more than simvastatin 10 to 80 mg. The mean percentage of changes in HDL cholesterol in the rosuvastatin groups were +7.7% to +9.6%, compared with +2.1% to +6.8% in all other groups. Rosuvastatin reduced total cholesterol significantly more across all dose ranges than all comparators and reduced triglycerides significantly more than simvastatin and pravastatin. Analysis of the secondary study objectives found that the NCEP Adult Treatment Panel III goals were met by 82% to 89% of patients treated with rosuvastatin 10 to 40 mg, compared with 69% to 85% of patients treated with atorvastatin 10 to 80 mg. The European LDL-cholesterol goal was attained by 79% to 92% of patients in the rosuvastatin groups, compared with 52% to 81% of patients in the atorvastatin groups. Similar drug tolerability was seen across treatments.

Conclusion.—This large multicenter trial comparing the lipid-modifying efficacy of statins found that rosuvastatin provided greater efficacy in the reduction of LDL-cholesterol, compared with atorvastatin, simvastatin, and pravastatin across dose ranges.

▶ We now have a bigger and better statin for reducing the concentration of LDL-cholesterol. Equipotent doses of the statins are as follows: 5 mg rosuvastatin = 10 mg atorvastatin = 20 mg simvastatin = 40 mg lovastatin or pravastatin = 80 mg fluvastatin. However, since the maximum doses of rosuvastatin and atorvastatin are 40 and 80 mg, respectively, the maximum LDL-cholesterol lowering is roughly equivalent. The dose of rosuvastatin was "capped" at 40 mg because of FDA concern about interstitial nephritis. Some increased risk of this adverse effect was observed at this 40-mg dose. Rosuvastatin has cleared the first hurdle by showing efficacy in reducing LDL-cholesterol but has an important second hurdle to clear by showing it reduces cardiovascular events.

The issue about whether drugs of the same class have equivalent effects is controversial.[1] A theoretic advantage of rosuvastatin over all other available statins is that it is twice as effective in increasing HDL-cholesterol (approximately 9% vs approximately 5%) and that it is somewhat more likely to get patients to ATP III targets than atorvastatin. This is only true for the lowest dose(s). Given these small incremental benefits, why would one chose rosuvastatin, which has no clinical end point data, over somewhat less potent statins with extensive clinical data?

I think it is premature to switch patients to or even start new patients on rosuvastatin. There may be an occasional patient where such a decision is justified, but my own preference for a patient who is not at target is to add another drug with a complementary mechanism of action to further lower LDL- cholesterol and/or treat an increased non–HDL-cholesterol. With most drugs, adverse effects parallel potency. Why would Astra-Zeneca get into the statin market as Bayer (cerivastatin, Baycol) was getting out of it? It's the money! Each 1% of the statin market is worth about $100 to $125 million; you don't need much of the market to have a formidable asset. Atorvastatin (Lipitor) currently has approximately 60% of the market in the United States and greater than $6.3 billion in annual sales.

All kinds of interesting observations concerning statins continue to appear. Atorvastatin and simvastatin increase fibrinogen but do not influence changes in carotid internal medial thickness,[2] and coronary artery calcification scores progress equally in patients treated with either of these statins.[3] At the 2003 annual American Heart Association meeting, atorvastatin (80 mg) was shown to reduce atheroma size while pravastatin (40 mg) did not.[4] Perhaps of greater interest is the observation that statin treatment after focal cerebral ischemia in rats reduces the extent of brain damage.[5] In other words, the use of statins in patients with acute stroke may reduce the size of the infarct; this should be evaluated in a randomized trial. Articles continue to appear suggesting that statins reduce the risk of cognitive impairment.[6] A case-control study observed that perioperative mortality was reduced by statin use in patients undergoing noncardiac vascular surgery.[7]

R. A. Kreisberg, MD

References

1. Kereiakes DJ, Willerson JT: Therapeutic substitution. Guilty until proven innocent. *Circulation* 108:2611-2612, 2003.
2. Trip MD, van Wissen S, Smilde TJ, et al: Effect of atorvastatin (80 mg) and simvastatin (40 mg) on plasma fibrinogen levels and on carotid intima media thickness in patients with familial hypercholesterolemia. *Am J Cardiol* 91:604-606, 2003.
3. Hecht HS, Harman SM: Comparison of the effects of atorvastatin versus simvastatin on subclinical atherosclerosis in primary prevention as determined by electron beam tomography. *Am J Cardiol* 91:42-45, 2003.
4. Nissin S: A study comparing the effects of atorvastatin versus pravastatin on progression of coronary atherosclerotic lesions as measured by intravascular ultrasound (REVERSAL). Presented at the American Heart Association Plenary Session XI, November 12, 2003.
5. Sironi L, Cimino M, Guerrini U, et al: Treatment with statins after induction of focal ischemia in rats reduces the extent of brain damage. *Arterioscler Thromb Vasc Biol* 23:322-327, 2003.
6. Etminan M, Gill S, Samii A: The role of lipid-lowering drugs in cognitive function: A meta-analysis of observational studies. *Pharmacotherapy* 23:726-730, 2003.
7. Poldermans D, Bax JJ, Kertai MD, et al: Statins are associated with a reduced incidence of perioperative mortality in patients undergoing major noncardiac vascular surgery. *Circulation* 107:1848-1851, 2003.

65 Diabetes Mellitus

Intensive Diabetes Therapy and Carotid Intima–Media Thickness in Type 1 Diabetes Mellitus

Nathan DM, for the Diabetes Control and Complications Trial/Epidemiology of Diabetes Interventions and Complications Research Group (Albert Einstein College of Medicine, New York; et al)

N Engl J Med 348:2294-2303, 2003   65–1

Background.—Patients with diabetes mellitus have a significantly increased risk of cardiovascular disease. Most deaths among patients with type 2 diabetes (70%) are attributable to cardiovascular disease, and most epidemiologic and clinical trial data have been obtained from studies of type 2 diabetes. Much less is known about cardiovascular disease in patients with type 1 diabetes. Patients with type 1 disease have a lower absolute risk of cardiovascular disease than those with type 2 diabetes, but the relative risk as compared with that of nondiabetic persons of similar age may be 10-fold higher. The progression of carotid intima–media thickness, a known measure of atherosclerosis, in a group of patients with type 1 diabetes was investigated.

Methods.—This study was conducted as part of the Epidemiology of Diabetes Interventions and Complications (EDIC) study, a long-term follow-up of the Diabetes Control and Complications Trial (DCCT). A total of 1229 patients with type 1 diabetes underwent B-mode US of the internal and common carotid arteries in 1994 to 1996 and again in 1998 to 2000. This study assessed the intima–media thickness in 611 subjects who had been randomly assigned to undergo conventional diabetes treatment during the DCCT and in 618 subjects who were assigned to undergo intensive diabetes treatment.

Results.—At year 1 of the EDIC study, the carotid intima–media thickness was similar to that in an age- and sex-matched nondiabetic population. After 6 years, the intima–media thickness was significantly greater in the diabetic patients than in the control subjects. The mean progression of the intima–media thickness was significantly less in patients who received intensive therapy during the DCCT than in patients who received conventional therapy. The progression of carotid intima–media thickness was associated with age, and the EDIC baseline systolic blood pressure, smoking, the ratio of low-density lipoprotein to high-density lipoprotein cholesterol, and urinary albumin excretion rate as well as the mean glycosylated hemoglobin value during the mean duration of the DCCT (6.5 years).

Conclusions.—Intensive diabetes treatment during the DCCT resulted in a slowing of the progression of carotid intima–media thickness 6 years after the end of that trial.

▶ It has been more than 10 years since the publication of the major findings of DCCT.[1] One of the minor frustrations of the original trial, in which 1441 type 1 diabetic patients were randomized to either conventional or intensive management, was that insufficient time would elapse to permit an evaluation of the effect of intensive treatment on macrovascular disease. Although a sufficient number of microvascular end points were reached to demonstrate unequivocally the benefits of good glycemic control in the prevention and progression of retinopathy, neuropathy, and early nephropathy, there were simply not enough macrovascular events for meaningful analysis, though there was a trend toward a reduction in events in the intensive group.

The foresight of the investigators in recognizing the potential benefit of "keeping tabs" on the original cohort of type 1 diabetic patients long after the end of the original trial is to be applauded. More than 95% of the surviving DCCT pateints volunteered to participate in the follow-up EDIC study. Essentially, the randomization to intensive or conventional care ended, with all patients being recommended to follow the intensive treatment plan under the supervision of their own physicians, but free to choose whether to do so. They agreed to have periodic investigations under the auspices of EDIC. The difference in HbA1c levels between the 2 groups at the end of DCCT—intensive, 7.2% and conventional, 9.1%—began to narrow until, 5 years after DCCT ended, it was insignificant. Therefore, the influence of glycemia, if any, on findings beyond that point owes more to differences in control long in the past rather than to recent control. And naturally, as time passes and the subjects age, it becomes possible to examine the effect of enhanced early glycemic control on the later development of macrovascular disease in type 1 diabetes.

Table 2 of this paper demonstrates that over a 4-year period (from approximately 8 to 12 years after the start of DCCT), during which the difference in HbA1c between the 2 groups effectively disappeared, carotid intima–media thickness, a surrogate marker of evolving macrovascular change, progressed to a much greater extent in those who had received conventional treatment than in those who had been treated intensively. Two previous studies had found increased carotid intima–media thickness in type 1 diabetic patients compared with nondiabetic control subjects.[2,3] The EDIC study highlighted here is the first to demonstrate convincingly, in a prospective study, that emphasis on glycemic control early in the course of type 1 diabetes may reduce the risk of eventual macrovascular disease.

Two other EDIC reports emphasize how the benefits of early intensive treatment of type 1 diabetes extend well beyond the period of its most intensive implementation with respect to progression of retinopathy and early nephropathy.[4,5] It is difficult to disagree with the conclusion of the EDIC investigators that "intensive treatment should be started as soon as safely possible after the onset of type 1 diabetes and maintained thereafter."[5] I have a feeling that

EDIC will be a rich seam mined over the next few years for more insights into the development of diabetic complications.

A final and purely speculative thought on my part—could it be that there is something about the earliest period after the onset of type 1 diabetes that makes good glycemic control at that time particularly critical for protection against complications? Is there some protective mechanism that can be imprinted early in the course of the disease?

L. Kennedy, MD, FRCP

References

1. The DCCT Research Group: The effect of intensive treatment of diabetes on the development and progression of long-term complications in insulin-dependent diabetes mellitus. *N Engl J Med* 329:977-986, 1993.
2. Yamasaki Y, Kawamori R, Matushima H, et al: Atherosclerosis in carotid artery of young IDDM patients monitored by ultrasound high-resolution B-mode imaging. *Diabetes* 43:634-639, 1994.
3. Giannattasio C, Failla M, Grappiolo A, et al: Progression of large artery structural and fucntional alterations in type 1 diabetes. *Diabetologia* 44:203-208, 2001.
4. DCCT/EDIC Research Group: Beneficial effects of intensive therapy of diabetes during adolescence: Outcomes after the conclusion of the Diabetes Control and Complications Trial (DCCT). *J Pediatr* 139:804-812, 2001.
5. The Writing Team for the Diabetes Control and Complications Trial/Epidemiology of Diabetes Interventions and Complications Research Group: Effect of intensive therapy on the microvascular complications of type 1 diabetes. *JAMA* 287:2563-2569, 2002.

Pregnancy in Women With Type 2 Diabetes: 12 Years Outcome Data 1990-2002
Dunne F, Brydon P, Smith K, et al (Univ of Birmingham, England)
Diabetic Med 20:734-738, 2003   65–2

Background.—Women with type 2 diabetes comprise a significant portion of those attending prepregnancy/antenatal diabetes clinics. Pregnancy outcomes in women with type 2 diabetes in a multiethnic, geographically defined region were reported.

Methods and Findings.—One hundred eighty women having babies between 1990 and 2002 were included in the analysis. All pregnancies were singleton. Eighty-eight percent of the pregnancies resulted in live births. Spontaneous miscarriage occurred in 8.8% of the women and stillbirths in 1.2%. Pregnancies were terminated electively in 1.6%. Eighteen infants had congenital malformations. Two early and 1 late neonatal deaths occurred, with another 2 infants dying in the postnatal period. Twenty-eight percent of the infants were large for their gestational age. Fifty-three percent were delivered by cesarean section. Thirty-seven percent of the neonates were admitted to the neonatal unit. Hypertension and preeclampsia were twice as common in diabetic women than in nondiabetic women. Polyhydramnios was 3 times more common in the diabetic group, and postpartum hemorrhage 6 times more common.

Conclusions.—Pregnancy outcomes in women with type 2 diabetes are less satisfactory than in the general population. The infants of these diabetic women have a 2-fold higher risk of stillbirth and a 2.5-fold greater risk of perinatal death. The risk of infant death within the first month of life is increased 6-fold, and the risk of death up to 1 year is 6-fold greater. In addition, the infants of women with type 2 diabetes are 11 times more likely to have congenital malformations.

▶ When I first got interested in diabetes in the mid 1970s (in the United Kingdom), pre-existing diabetes in pregnancy was almost always type 1. Now maternal type 2 diabetes at the time of booking at prenatal clinics—as opposed to being diagnosed as gestational diabetes late in pregnancy—is increasingly prevalent, and in those regions of the United States with large minority populations is already the predominant form seen in pregnancy. With current trends in the incidence of type 2 diabetes in adolescents and young adults, it is safe to say we are just starting to grapple with the challenge of type 2 diabetes in pregnancy.

And a challenge it is, as this data from the United Kingdom shows. Table 1 summarizes the outcomes in comparison with regional and national population figures, with 2- to 3-fold increases in stillbirth, perinatal mortality and early neonatal death rates, and up to 6-fold increases in postnatal and neonatal mortality and late neonatal death rates. Just as in type 1 diabetes, it is clear that glycemic control at the time of conception is a major determinant of the successful outcome of pregnancy, and congenital cardiovascular abnormality is a major risk.[1,2] The authors are right to stress that "we need to dispel the myth that this form of diabetes is not serious."

It seems obvious that intensive prepregnancy counseling to achieve normal or near-normal glycemic control before conception would have the potential to improve outcomes. That is difficult enough to achieve in a system like the U.K. National Health Service, where, whatever doubts one may have about the system as a whole, there is unhindered access to primary care and prenatal services completely free at the point care. The problem in the United States is that those women with the greatest likelihood of having type 2 diabetes in their reproductive years are from sectors of the population that, for whatever reason, are least likely to have access to the appropriate services.

L. Kennedy, MD, FRCP

References

1. Schaefer-Graf UM, Buchanan TA, Xiong A: Patterns of congenital anomalies and relationship to initial maternal fasting glucose levels in pregnancies complicated by type 2 and gestational diabetes. *Am J Obstet Gynecol* 182:313-320, 2000.
2. Towner D, Kjos S, Leung B: Congenital malformations in pregnancies complicated by NIDDM. *Diabetes Care* 11:1446-1451, 1995.

Respiratory Failure Secondary to Diabetic Neuropathy Affecting the Phrenic Nerve

Tang EW, Jardine DL, Rodins K, et al (Christchurch Hosp, New Zealand)
Diabetic Med 20:599-601, 2003   65–3

Introduction.—The pathologic characteristics of diabetic mononeuropathy are not well known. The first known histologic report of a patient with type 2 diabetes mellitus complicated by neuropathy affecting the phrenic nerves was discussed.

Case Report.—Man, 74, was admitted to the hospital after being found unconscious in bed. He was stuporous and hypoxic with severe CO_2 retention. He was intubated and placed immediately on mechanical ventilation. He had a history of breathing that gradually worsened during a 6-week period, and a preference for sleeping upright. Diabetes mellitus and peripheral sensory neuropathy had been diagnosed 12 years previously. A year later, a truncal neuropathy developed, which produced bilateral pain and numbness in the T5-T11 dermatomes. Other diagnoses included hypertension (medically controlled), mild heart failure, and chronic obstructive pulmonary disease secondary to smoking. He regained consciousness and was extubated after 45 minutes of mechanical ventilation. His body mass index was 24, respiratory rate was 12-20 breaths/min, heart rate was 94 beats/min, and blood pressure was 100/54 mm Hg. His respiratory excursion was limited, despite use of accessory muscles. He had quadriceps wasting, associated with moderate weakness of hip flexion, and knee extension bilaterally. His ankle jerks were absent, plantar reflexes were downgoing, and he had reduced proprioception, pain, and light touch sensation in the feet. He required mechanical ventilation twice during the next 2 weeks for further episodes of respiratory failure. His chest radiograph was clear. Spirometry forced expiratory volume in 1 second was 34% of normal, forced vital capacity was 24% of normal, maximum inspiratory pressure was 10-cm water (normal, 103 cm), maximum expiratory pressure was 13-cm water (normal, 183 cm), and maximum minute ventilation was reduced. Phrenic nerve conduction studies revealed low-amplitude action potential on the right and absent conduction on the left, consistent with severe axonal neuropathy. The peripheral nerve amplitudes were also severely reduced; conduction velocity was preserved. Single-fiber electromyography showed changes consistent with denervation. Histologic analysis of the right pectoralis and intercostal muscles revealed denervation changes only. A diagnosis of diaphragmatic paralysis secondary to bilateral phrenic neuropathy was made; diabetes was the most likely cause. He died 2 weeks after hospital discharge from a lower respiratory tract infection, despite tracheostomy and bilateral positive airway pressure ventilatory assistance. Histologic findings of the phrenic nerve were consistent with severe diabetic neuropathy.

Conclusion.—Diabetic mononeuropathies are usually reversible, but the outcome in this patient would suggest that when both phrenic nerves are severely affected, the outcome is dismal.

▶ This is an interesting case report, which I have included because diabetic neuropathy is common, and, as the authors speculate, this particular manifestation may be underdiagnosed. One study has shown phrenic nerve latencies to be prolonged in 23% of patients with diabetes and breathlessness.[1] On a practical level, the authors also point out that nursing the patient in a supine position may be particularly inappropriate when there is any risk of impairment of diaphragmatic function.

L. Kennedy, MD, FRCP

Reference

1. Wolf E, Shochina M, Fidel Y, et al: Phrenic neuropathy in patients with diabetes mellitus. *Electromyogr Clin Neurophysiol* 23:523-530, 1983.

Estrogen Therapy and Risk of Cardiovascular Events Among Women With Type 2 Diabetes

Newton KM, LaCroix AZ, Heckbert SR, et al (Group Health Cooperative, Seattle; Univ of Wash, Seattle; Fred Hutchinson Cancer Research Ctr, Seattle)
Diabetes Care 26:2810-2816, 2003   65–4

Introduction.—Observational trials have reported that estrogen therapy alone or with progestin is linked with decreased risk of coronary events. Yet randomized controlled trials have reported that estrogen therapy with progestin is linked with increased coronary events and strokes and is not correlated with a decrease in cardiovascular events in females with pre-existing coronary disease. The risks and benefits of estrogen plus progestin therapy in females with diabetes mellitus remain uncertain. The relationship between estrogen therapy and risk of cardiovascular disease among women with type 2 diabetes was assessed in a retrospective, case-cohort study.

Methods.—The study included 6017 women (ages 45-80 years) with type 2 diabetes mellitus who were assessed between January 1, 1986, and December 31, 1992. Cardiovascular outcomes (nonfatal myocardial infarction in 215 patients, coronary revascularization in 253 patients, and cardiovascular deaths in 229 patients) were documented through December 31, 1998. The use of estrogen and progestin was determined through automated pharmacy records and modeled as a time-dependent variable. The median follow-up was 6.8 years. Multivariable-adjusted relative risk (RR) and 95% confidence intervals (CI) were determined.

Results.—The current use of estrogen alone (RR, 0.48; 95% CI, 0.30-0.78) or with progestin (RR, 0.43; 95% CI, 0.22-0.85) was linked with a reduced risk of cardiovascular events, compared to never having taken estrogen. The risk of cardiovascular events linked with a first episode of estrogen use (with or without progestin) of less than 25-months' duration (RR, 1.12; 95% CI, 0.49-2.54), a first episode of use of 25 months or more duration (RR, 0.32; 95% CI, 0.06-1.70), and a current use that was not the first episode (RR, 0.42; 95% CI, 0.42-0.67) suggested that recent initiation was not associated with an increase or reduction in risk.

Conclusion.—An association between estrogen therapy (with or without progestin), and a reduced risk of cardiovascular events among women with type 2 diabetes was observed. This relationship should be further investigated in large, randomized, controlled trials.

▶ So here is yet another observational study reporting a cardiovascular protective effect of estrogen therapy, this time solely in women with type 2 diabetes. There can be very few people, either in medicine and related professions or among postmenopausal women interested in the maintenance of their health, who are now unaware of the 2 major clinical trials (HERS and WHI) that fairly comprehensively torpedoed the results of previous observational studies that had led to the (almost) conventional wisdom that estrogen therapy helped to prevent cardiovascular disease in older women.[1,2]

In support of their findings, the authors of this article draw attention to 2 other studies—a case-control analysis,[3] and a cohort study[4]—that also suggest a cardiovascular benefit of hormone replacement therapy (HRT) in diabetic women; they also acknowledge that another, relatively small, observational study suggested increased risk of cardiovascular disease in diabetic women with estrogen with or without progestin.[5]

Confusing, isn't it? Well, in an excellent accompanying editorial, Elizabeth Barrett-Connor, one of the most experienced epidemiologists in the field of diabetes, points out the potential deficiencies of observational studies compared to clinical trials.[6] These include (1) preferential selection of "healthy/wealthy" women to receive HRT, with lower rates of smoking and higher rates of regular exercise; (2) higher rates of blood glucose monitoring in diabetic women taking estrogen; and (3) differential study entry or loss to follow-up by health status. She also points out that the package insert for conjugated equine estrogen therapy "cautioned against its use by women with diabetes, hypertension, or heart disease" so that in case-cohort studies, the bias would be toward heart disease diabetic cases being much less likely to have been prescribed estrogen than diabetic control subjects without heart disease.

It is hard to disagree with Barrett-Connor's contention that the favorable results in observational studies like that of Newton et al "likely ...are spurious consequences of biases related to the health advantage characteristics of women who use presumably preventive medications."

L. Kennedy, MD, FRCP

References

1. Hulley S, Grady D, Bush T, et al: Randomized trial of estrogen plus progestin for secondary prevention of coronary heart disease in postmenopausal women: Heart and Estrogen/progestin Replacement Study (HERS) Research Group. *JAMA* 280:605-613, 1998.
2. Rossouw JE, Anderson GL, Prentice RL, et al: Risks and benefits of estrogen plus progestin in healthy postmenopausal women: Principal results from the Women's Health Initiative randomized controlled trial. *JAMA* 288:321-333, 2002.
3. Kaplan RC, Heckbert SR, Weiss NS, et al: Postmenopausal estrogens and risk of myocardial infarction in diabetic women. *Diabetes Care* 21: 1117-1121, 1998.
4. Ferrara A, Quesenberry CP, Karter AJ, et al: Current use of unopposed estrogen and estrogen plus progestin and the risk of acute myocardial infarction among women with diabetes: The Northern California Kaiser Permanente Diabetes Registry, 1995-1998. *Circulation* 107:43-48, 2003.
5. Lokkegaard E, Pederson AT, Heitmann BL, et al: Relation between hormone replacement therapy and ischaemic heart disease in women: Prospective observational study. *BMJ* 326:426, 2003.
6. Barrett-Connor E: Diabetes and heart disease. *Diabetes Care* 26: 2947-2948, 2003.

Diabetes and Idiopathic Cardiomyopathy: A Nationwide Case-Control Study

Bertoni AG, Tsai A, Kasper EK, et al (Wake Forest Univ, Winston-Salem, North Carolina; Johns Hopkins Univ, Baltimore, Md)
Diabetes Care 26:2791-2795, 2003   65–5

Introduction.—Controversy exists concerning the link between diabetes and nonischemic idiopathic cardiomyopathy (ICM). Data are limited on the incidence of ICM in adults with diabetes. Data from the 1995 National Inpatient Sample were used to ascertain discharge rates and investigate whether diabetes is independently linked with ICM.

Methods.—The 1995 NIS includes demographic and diagnostic data regarding all discharges from more than 900 representative hospitals in 19 states. The ICD-9 codes were used to identify ICM, defined as discharges with a diagnosis of primary cardiomyopathy, yet without established risk factors for cardiomyopathy. Control subjects were chosen by stratified random sampling by age to yield 10/ICU case. Analyzed covariates included age, sex, median income, and diagnoses of diabetes and hypertension. Multivariate logistic regression was used to perform case-control analyses.

Results.—By the use of sampling weights, it was estimated that in 1995, the incidence of hospital discharge for ICM among persons diagnosed with diabetes was 7.6 per 1000 patients. The incidence of diabetes was markedly higher in the 44,837 ICM patients versus the 450,254 control subjects (26.6% vs 17.2%). This increased incidence corresponded to a relative odds ratio (OR) of 1.75 (95% confidence index [CI], 1.71-1.79). After adjusting for age, sex, hypertension, and median income, diabetes remained significantly correlated with ICM (OR, 1.58; 95% CI, 1.55-1.62).

Conclusion.—Hospitalization for ICM occurred at a much higher rate in persons with diabetes versus the general population. Diabetes was linked with ICM independently of age, sex, income, or hypertension. A relationship was seen between diabetes and ICM in males and females and African Americans and whites. The link between diabetes and ICM was strongest among patients discharged with microvascular complications of diabetes, indicating a possible link to hyperglycemia in relation to duration, severity, and/or susceptibility to myocardial injury.

▶ While it is widely recognized that diabetes is associated with a 2- to 4-fold increase in ischemic heart disease, I suspect that the entity of ICM as a diabetic complication is less well known among primary care physicians and internists without a particular interest in diabetes. Fig 1 from the original article gives a clue to the possible etiology of the condition, showing the greater association with microvascular than with macrovascular complications.

Once again, I will take the opportunity of drawing attention to an excellent accompanying editorial on the condition.[1] David Bell points out that it is more than 30 years since the existence of this condition was first proposed by Rubler et al.[2] He goes on to discuss the central role of diastolic dysfunction, attributable in large measure to the accumulation of advanced glycation end-products (AGEs), causing increased collagen crosslinks and myocardial fibrosis. Recent animal studies show that lysis of the increased collagen crosslinks decreases the fibrosis and improves diastolic function.[3] Other potential mechanisms associated with prolonged hyperglycemia include activation of protein kinase C β (PKC-β) activity and increases in myocardial free radicals and oxidants. Equally, the increase of free fatty acids seen with hyperglycemia may play a role—lipotoxicity—and in this regard, insulin resistance seems likely to be a co-culprit along with hyperglycemia. It turns out also that microalbuminuria is a good prescreening test, shown to correlate well with the degree of diastolic dysfunction.[4] The diagnosis can then be confirmed with echocardiography.

So, as Bell points out, there is plenty of scope with existing medications as follows: (1) β-blockers and thiazolidinediones shift the metabolism of the myocardium from the use of free fatty acids to glucose; (2) angiotensin-converting enzyme (ACE) inhibitors decrease left ventricular hypertrophy and myocardial fibrosis, prevent myocardial remodeling, and improve endothelial function; and (3) both thiazolidinediones and ACE inhibitors (and possibly also metformin) decrease insulin resistance—all can be used for the early treatment of this condition to reduce progression to heart failure. Drugs that prevent or reverse glycation would be an obvious useful development.

L. Kennedy, MD, FRCP

References

1. Bell DSH: Diabetic cardiomyopathy. *Diabetes Care* 26:2949-2950, 2003.
2. Rubler S, Dlugash J, Yuceoglu YZ, et al: New type of cardiomyopathy associated with diabetic glomerulosclerosis. *Am J Cardiol* 30:595-602, 1972.
3. Candido R, Forbes JM, Thomas MC, et al: A breaker of advanced glycation end products attenuates diabetes-induced myocardial structural changes. *Circ Res* 92:785-792, 2003.

4. Liu JE, Robbins DC, Palmieri V, et al: Association of albuminuria with systolic and diastolic left ventricular dysfunction in type 2 diabetes: The Strong Heart Study. *J Am Coll Cardiol* 42:2022-2028, 2003.

Glucose Control and Mortality in Critically Ill Patients

Finney SJ, Zekveld C, Elia A, et al (Royal Brompton Hosp, London)
JAMA 290:2041-2047, 2003   65–6

Introduction.—Hyperglycemia is common in patients who are critically ill, even with those who do not have diabetes mellitus. Aggressive glycemic control may decrease the mortality rate in these patients. The link between mortality rate, hyperglycemia control, and administration of exogenous insulin is not well defined. A single-center, prospective, observational trial was performed to determine whether blood glucose level is associated with a decreased mortality rate for patients who are critically ill.

Methods.—Data regarding all patients admitted to the adult ICU during the first 6 months of 2002 were obtained. The major end point was ICU mortality rate. The secondary end points were hospital mortality rate, ICU and hospital length of stay (LOS), and the predicted threshold glucose level linked with risk of death.

Results.—Of 531 patients admitted to ICU, 523 were evaluated for glycemic control. The 24-hour control of blood glucose levels varied. ICU and hospital mortality rates were 5.2% and 5.7%, respectively; the median LOS was 1.8 days (interquartile range, 0.9-3.7) for ICU and 6 days (interquartile range, 4.5-8.3) for hospital stay. Multivariable logistic regression showed that increased administration of insulin was positively and significantly linked with ICU mortality rate (odds ratio [OR], 1.02; 95% confidence interval [CI], 1.01-1.04) at a prevailing glucose level of 111 to 144 mg/dL (6.1-8.0 mmol/L for a 1-IU/day increase), indicating that mortality rate reductions may be attributed to glycemic control rather than with increased administration of insulin. The regression model indicates that a mortality rate benefit amasses below a predicted threshold glucose level of 144 to 200 mg/dL (8.0-11.1 mmol/L), with a speculative upper limit of 145 mg/dL (8.0 mmol/L) for the target glucose level.

Conclusion.—Increased insulin administration is positively correlated with death in the ICU, regardless of the prevailing blood glucose level. Control of glucose levels as opposed to absolute levels of exogenous insulin apparently is responsible for the mortality rate reduction associated with intensive insulin therapy reported by earlier studies.

▶ The publication by van den Berghe et al in 2001 of their study of intensive insulin therapy in a surgical ICU, which was featured as the first editor's choice in the 2002 YEAR BOOK OF ENDOCRINOLOGY, undoubtedly led to a major rethinking of the importance of controlling glucose in critically ill patients, whether or not they have diabetes. A valid criticism of the van den Berghe study, which would apply to any study of randomized intensive insulin therapy in critically ill patients, is that the necessarily unblinded design may have been associated with (unintentional) better overall care being given to the treatment group, and that that fact, rather than the improved glycemia, could conceivably account for the more favorable outcome.

The observational study of Finney et al presented here was undertaken as a direct result of the van den Berghe study, and the question I have to ask is whether it really sheds any new light on the subject. The study confirms that there is an association between lower blood glucose levels and improved outcome, but increased insulin administration was positively associated with death in the ICU. How should we interpret this? The authors suggest that "control of glucose levels rather than of absolute levels of exogenous insulin appear to account for the mortality benefit associated with intensive insulin therapy." What they seem to overlook entirely is that since their study is observational, and the protocol allowed for infusion rates is to be set "at the discretion of the attending/senior nurse unconstrained by a fixed regimen, with the goal of achieving rapid and tight control of blood glucose levels," it is inevitable that the patients with higher glucose levels would have had the highest insulin infusion rates, and those with near-normal glucose at the outset would have received much less insulin. It also strikes me as somewhat disingenuous to imply that in the ICU, lower blood glucose is good but it had better be achieved without increased use of insulin. How, pray, are we to accomplish that?

So, in my opinion, this study does not throw any more light on whether making a positive effort to achieve near-normal glucose levels in critically ill patients is truly a critical determinant of outcome. Instead, this study surely confirms that hyperglycemia, perhaps as a reflection of increased stress hormones or insulin resistance (neither of which were measured), is a risk factor for poor outcome in severely ill patients.

L. Kennedy, MD, FRCP

Reference

1. van den Berghe G, Woulters P, Weekers F, et al: Intensive insulin therapy in the surgical intensive care unit. *N Engl J Med* 345:1359-1367, 2001.

The Role of Hyperbaric Oxygen Therapy in Ischaemic Diabetic Lower Extremity Ulcers: A Double-blind Randomised-controlled Trial
Abidia A, Laden G, Kuhan G, et al (Univ of Hull, England; BUPA Hosp, Hull, England)
Eur J Vasc Endovasc Surg 25:513-518, 2003   65–7

Introduction.—Lower-extremity ulcers in patients with diabetes are a source of major concern because bacterial infection can lead to limb-threatening complications. Hyperbaric oxygen therapy is of potential benefit in cases of diabetic lower-extremity ulcers, but a lack of supporting research and relatively high costs have limited its use as an adjunctive treatment. The role of hyperbaric oxygen therapy in patients with peripheral arterial disease

(PAD) and diabetic lower-extremity ulcers was examined in a double-blind trial.

Methods.—The 18 patients recruited to the study were randomly assigned to receive 100% oxygen (treatment group) or air (control group), administered at 2.4 atmospheres of absolute pressure for 90 minutes daily, 5 days per week, for a total of 30 sessions. Wound care and use of antibiotics were standardized. The primary outcome was reduction in ulcer size at 6 weeks after the end of treatment.

Results.—Five of 8 ulcers in the treatment group, but only 1 of 8 ulcers in the control group, were healed with complete epithelialization at 6-week follow-up. The median decrease in wound areas was 100% in the treatment group and 52% in the control group at 6 weeks. At 6 months, the 2 groups had similar reduction in ulcer size (100% and 95%, respectively). Visits for dressing of the study ulcers were far more frequent in the control group; thus, the mean total cost per patient per year for ulcer dressing was £1972 in the treatment group versus £7946 in the control group. It was costly, but adjunctive hyperbaric oxygen reduced the average cost to £2960 per patient.

Discussion.—Among patients with PAD and nonhealing lower-extremity ulcers, hyperbaric oxygen treatment enhanced healing. The therapy may be a cost-effective, valuable adjunct when patients are unable to undergo reconstructive therapy.

▶ This is an encouraging pilot study—according to the authors, the first double-blinded, randomized controlled study of hyperbaric oxygen in the treatment of ischemic lower limb ulcers in diabetes—and should be the stimulus for a much larger study, which by necessity would need to be multicentered.

The authors' concerns that the length of time—realistically, the better part of half of every day, Monday through Friday for 6 weeks—the treatment requires could cause problems with, for example, full employment may be unfounded, since it is probably unfortunately true that few such patients will be in full employment. The economics used in working out the cost effectiveness of the treatment, based purely on a charge for time using the hyperbaric chamber and for the cost of dressings, which the authors say make the treatment cost-effective, would certainly be much more complex in the United States but would also give a truer reflection of total costs involved because these authors omit any consideration of medical and other salaries.

L. Kennedy, MD, FRCP

Effect of Metabolic Control on Homocysteine Levels in Type 2 Diabetic Patients: A 3-Year Follow-up

Passaro A, Calzoni F, Volpato S, et al (Univ of Ferrara, Italy; Univ of Pisa, Italy)
J Intern Med 254:264-271, 2003   65–8

Introduction.—A direct relationship between glycosylated hemoglobin A_{1c} (HbA_{1c}) and total homocysteine (tHcy) in type 2 diabetic patients (D2p) has been reported recently. To determine whether a real link exists between tHcy and metabolic control, a prospective study was performed in 3 groups of D2p with preserved kidney function and various grades of metabolic control. The impact of glucose and lipids on homocysteine levels was assessed in these patients.

Methods.—The study included 95 D2p who underwent baseline and 36-month determinations of values of clinical parameters, fasting plasma glucose, HbA_{1c}, serum lipids, blood urea nitrogen (BUN) and creatinine, vitamin B_{12}, folate, and tHcy. The methylenetetrahydrofolate reductase (MTHFR) C677T polymorphism was also examined. Participants were categorized according to their level of δHbA_{1c} into group A (±1 point), B (>1 point) increase), or C (>1 point decrease).

Results.—tHcy was decreased in participants whose HbA_{1c} decreased with time. Patients with worsened metabolic controls had increased tHcy levels, compared with those at baseline. A greater response to the improved metabolic control with tHcy reduction was seen in patients with the wild-type gene, compared with the response seen in those homozygous for the gene mutation. Multivariate analysis demonstrated MTHFR polymorphism and HbA_{1c} as strong determinants of changes in tHcy with time.

Conclusion.—tHcy is reduced in D2p, even with modest improvement of glycemic control. Patients homozygous for the MTHFR C677T mutation demonstrated the greatest changes in tHcy levels with concomitant changing of HbA_{1c}. These findings define a further mechanism through which hyperglycemia may promote cardiovascular damage in D2p.

▶ It is accepted that elevated tHcy is an independent risk factor for cardiovascular disease,[1,2] though whether this is specifically true in diabetic patients has been subject to debate.[3,4] The present study represents the strongest evidence to date that glycemic control in type 2 diabetes does have an influence on Hcy levels. Those patients whose HbA_{1c} worsened by more than 1% over a 3-year period had a significant rise in serum Hcy (group B), while those whose HbA_{1c} decreased by more than 1% had a significant fall in homocysteine. An interesting finding is that homozygosity for a mutation in the MTHFR gene, which reduces the enzymatic activity and leads to hyperhomocysteinemia, seems to be associated with a greater effect of glycemic control on Hcy levels, though the number of subjects in each of the groups in this analysis was quite small.

Just why improved glycemic control should lead to lower Hcy levels is not at all clear, and no further light is thrown on possible mechanisms by this study. It is disappointing that no details are given of the treatment regimens for diabetes.

L. Kennedy, MD, FRCP

References

1. Stampfer MJ, Malinow MR, Willett WC, et al: A prospective study of plasma homocysteine and risk of myocardial infarction in US physicians. *JAMA* 268:877-881, 1992.

2. Perry IJ, Refsum H, Morris RW, et al: Prospective study of serum homocysteine concentration and risk of stroke in middle-aged British men. *Lancet* 346:1395-1398, 1995.
3. Drzewoski J, Czupryniak L, Chwatko G, et al: Total plasma homocysteine and insulin levels in type 2 diabetic patients with secondary failure to oral agents. *Diabetes Care* 22:2097-2099, 1999.
4. Hoogeveen EK, Kostense PJ, Beks PJ, et al: Hyperhomocysteinemia is associated with an increased risk of cardiovascular disease, particularly in non-insulin-dependent diabetes mellitus: A population-based study. *Arterioscl Thromb Vasc Biol* 18:133-138, 1998.

66 Bone and Mineral Metabolism

Fractures in Patients With Primary Hyperparathyroidism: Nationwide Follow-up Study of 1201 Patients
Vestergaard P, Mosekilde L (Aarhus Univ Hosp, Denmark)
World J Surg 27:343-349, 2003   66–1

Introduction.—An increased fracture risk has been observed in patients with primary hyperparathyroidism (PHPT). Fracture rates have not been compared between patients who have and have not undergone parathyroid surgery. Increased spinal and femoral neck bone mineral densities have been reported in patients who have undergone surgery compared with those who have not. A large population-based cohort investigation of 1201 patients with PHPT and 3601 matched controls was performed to evaluate the fracture risk before and after the diagnosis of PHPT. The fracture risk was compared in patients who did and did not undergo surgery.

Methods.—All patients with a new case of PHPT diagnosed between January 1, 1982, and December 31, 1996, in Denmark (population 5 million) were evaluated. Every patient was compared with 3 age-, gender-, and status-matched controls. It was possible to match 299 nonsurgically treated patients with 299 surgically treated patients for age and gender.

Results.—Surgically treated patients were younger and had fewer fractures before diagnosis, compared with nonsurgically treated patients. Before diagnosis, the fracture risk was increased for both groups and remained similar after diagnosis. Differences in fracture risk were observed during the first year and more than 10 years after diagnosis in the surgical group. In the nonsurgical group, an increase in fracture risk was present at any time after diagnosis. Fracture-free survival was similar in both groups and persisted after adjusting for age, gender, and fracture before diagnosis. The fracture risk was significantly increased if a fracture occurred before diagnosis. Females had a higher fracture risk than males, and the fracture risk rose with increasing age at diagnosis. A trend toward lower bone mineral density in the spine was seen in the nonsurgical versus the surgical group; the difference remained after adjusting for age and gender. No difference was seen in the femoral neck. Serum calcium levels at the time of diagnosis were higher in the surgical group than in the nonsurgical group. A significantly higher risk of death after diagnosis was seen in the nonsurgical group compared with the surgical group. The mean survival time in the surgical group was longer than in the nonsurgical group; this could not be explained by the time interval between diagnosis and surgery, even after adjusting for age and gender. In the surgical group, 27 patients had fractures before and 31 had fractures after surgery; corresponding numbers for the nonsurgical group were 27 and 23, respectively (odds ratio, 1.39; 95% confidence interval, 0.19-9.94). Seventy-four patients in the surgical group and 126 in the nonsurgical groups died during follow-up (odds ratio, 0.45; 95% confidence interval, 0.36-0.56).

Conclusion.—There is an increased risk of fractures in untreated patients with PHPT. The risk is increased up to 10 years before diagnosis, is reduced immediately after surgery, and is increased again more than 10 years after surgery.

▶ This article from Denmark attempts to answer several very important questions regarding PHPT. First, do patients with PHPT have more fractures than normal subjects? Second, does surgical cure of hyperparathyroidism result in fewer fractures? And finally, do patients with untreated PHPT have higher death rates?

To answer these questions, the researchers analyzed all new cases of PHPT in Denmark between 1982 and 1996. Each patient with PHPT (n = 1201) was compared with 3 age-, gender-, and status-matched (death or emigration) controls (n = 3601). Patients with PHPT who received surgery (n = 299) were age- and gender-matched to 299 patients with PHPT who were managed nonsurgically. The results from this large historical cohort showed that before diagnosis of PHPT, both surgically and nonsurgically treated patients had an increased risk of fracture (especially of the upper extremities) compared with controls. Fracture risk was significantly increased by history of prior fracture, female gender, and advancing age. Patients who were referred for surgery tended to be younger, with higher calcium levels and lower bone density measurements than those treated nonsurgically. However, those who received nonsurgical treatment had significantly higher mortality rates than those treated surgically, even when adjusting for age and gender. After the diagnosis of PHPT, nonsurgically treated patients did not have higher fracture rates than the surgically treated patients, perhaps because those who were sent to surgery had more advanced disease (higher calcium levels and lower bone mineral densities). Patients treated surgically continued to have higher fracture rates up to 10 years after diagnosis of PHPT compared with controls, whereas fracture rates among nonsurgically treated patients were similar to those of controls.

Overall, these data strongly indicate that patients with PHPT have an increased fracture risk compared with controls and that this risk is not completely eliminated by parathyroid surgery. Among the surgically treated group, rates of total fractures, arm fractures, and "osteoporotic" fractures were significantly increased above normal controls. Among the nonsurgically treated group, rates of spine, femur, arm, Colles', and total fractures were significantly elevated.

This study also found that nonsurgical management of PHPT is associated with a much higher risk of death relative to surgically treated patients. Although this may be due to referral bias (physicians are less likely to refer older, sicker, elderly patients with PHPT for surgery than younger patients), it is also possible that cure of PHPT offers a distinct survival advantage. As surgery for PHPT becomes safer with use of local anesthesia and "minimally invasive parathyroidectomy," it may be appropriate to refer more elderly patients for surgical cure of PHPT. Prospective clinical trials randomizing elderly patients with PHPT to surgical versus nonsurgical treatments are needed to address this issue definitively.

C. Becker, MD

Effects of Estrogen Plus Progestin on Risk of Fracture and Bone Mineral Density: The Women's Health Initiative Randomized Trial
Cauley JA, for the Women's Health Initiative Investigators (Univ of Pittsburgh, Pa; et al)
JAMA 290:1729-1738, 2003   66–2

Introduction.—In the Women's Health Initiative trial of estrogen plus progestin therapy, the women assigned to active treatment had fewer fractures. It was hypothesized that the relative risk reduction of estrogen plus progestin on fractures differs according to risk factors for fractures.

Methods.—A randomized controlled trial was conducted between September 1993 and July 2002, in which 16,608 postmenopausal women aged 50 to 79 years with an intact uterus at baseline were recruited at 40 US centers. Follow-up was an average of 5.6 years. Participants were randomly assigned to receive either conjugated equine estrogen, 0.625 mg/d, plus medroxyprogesterone acetate, 2.5 mg/d, in 1 tablet or placebo. The primary outcome measures were all verified osteoporotic fracture events that occurred from enrollment to trial discontinuation (July 7, 2002); bone mineral density, measured in a subset of 1024 women at baseline and years 1 and 3; and a global index, created to summarize the balance of risks and benefits to test whether the risk-benefit profile varied across tertiles of fracture risk.

Results.—Fractures occurred in 833 women (8.6%) in the estrogen plus progestin group and 896 women (11.1%) in the placebo group (hazard ratio, [HR], 0.76; 95% confidence interval [CI], 0.69-0.83). In subgroup analyses, active treatment reduced the risk of hip fracture by 60% in women with baseline calcium intake of more than 1200 mg/d and not among women with lower calcium intake (P for interaction = .02). There was no evidence that the efficacy of active treatment differed according to any risk factors for fractures, including age, body mass index, smoking, history of falls, calcium intake, personal and family history of fractures, and past use of hormones. Estrogen plus progestin decreased the rate of fractures to a similar extent in women at low, medium, and high risk of fracture.

Conclusion.—Estrogen plus progestin increases bone mineral density and decreases the risk of fractures in healthy postmenopausal women. The reduced risk of fracture attributed to estrogen plus progestin appeared to be present in all subgroups. When considering the effects of hormone therapy on other important disease outcomes in a global model, there was no net benefit, even in women considered to be at high risk of fracture.

▶ One of the few positive findings to come out of the Women's Health Initiative[1] (WHI) was a significant reduction in fractures among women randomized to estrogen plus progestin (E+P), compared with placebo. Indeed, the WHI was the first randomized clinical trial to prove that E+P reduces the risk of fractures at all skeletal sites, including the hip, vertebrae, and wrist. And despite the increase in "global risk" and the negative risk-benefit profile of E+P that led to early cessation of the trial, it was hoped that a subgroup of women might be found for whom E+P was truly beneficial. This detailed analysis of the fracture data from the WHI by Cauley et al hammers a final nail into the coffin of E+P use for anything other than relief of vasomotor symptoms.

Of the 16,600 postmenopausal women enrolled in the WHI, over 1600 sustained a fracture during the trial. Baseline risk factors for fracture did not vary between the 2 treatment groups. A subgroup of 1024 women had bone density (BMD) measurements at the lumbar spine, total hip, or femoral neck. Of these, only 4% of the E+P and 6% of the placebo group had osteoporosis, defined as a T-score of less than −2.5. During an average follow-up of 5.6 years, 8.6% of women receiving E+P and 11.1% of those receiving placebo had fractures, representing a significant 24% fracture risk reduction for women receiving E+P. Hormone therapy reduced hip fractures by 33%, irrespective of age, smoking, history of falls, prior fractures, past use of hormone therapy, maternal fracture history, years since menopause, or overall "fracture risk score." With the use of Kaplan-Meier time plots, the differences in hip, wrist, vertebral, and total fractures between the 2 groups were evident by the second year and only increased with time.

Not surprisingly, BMD at both the spine and hip increased significantly in the E+P group compared with placebo. Somewhat surprisingly, however, the benefits of hormone therapy on fractures did not vary according to risk factors for fracture (such as age, body mass index, smoking, etc). Thus, the authors were unable to define a group of women at such high risk for fractures that the benefits of E+P outweighed the risks.

The women who participated in the WHI were not chosen according to risk for osteoporosis, and indeed, they may have been at much lower risk than the general population. Seventy percent of the participants had BMIs of 25 or above, and hip fracture rates were only 50% of expected for a similar age-matched cohort. BMD results revealed a very low prevalence of osteoporosis in the participants (approximately 5%). Nevertheless, the authors conclude that "treatment with estrogen plus progestin should not be recommended for prevention or for treatment of osteoporosis in women without vasomotor symptoms." How ironic that the first major clinical trial to prove that hormone therapy truly reduces fractures is also the one that argues against its use!

C. Becker, MD

Reference

1. Writing Group for the Women's Health Initiative Investigators: Risks and benefits of estrogen plus progestin in healthy postmenopausal women: Principal results from the Women's Health Initiative randomized controlled trial. *JAMA* 288:321-333, 2002.

Oral Alendronate Increases Bone Mineral Density in Postmenopausal Women With Primary Hyperparathyroidism

Chow CC, Chan WB, Li JKY, et al (Chinese Univ of Hong Kong; Yan Chai Hosp, Hong Kong; Alice Ho Miu Ling Nethersole Hosp, Hong Kong; et al)
J Clin Endocrinol Metab 88:581-587, 2003   66–3

Introduction.—About 80% of patients with primary hyperparathyroidism (PHP) are asymptomatic. Many are elderly and have multiple medical problems associated with an increased surgical risk. The management of these patients is controversial. Adherence to the National Institutes of Health guidelines is poor. The efficacy of oral alendronate, a potent second-generation bisphosphonate, was assessed in the management of postmenopausal women with PHP during a 48-week evaluation period, with further follow-up at 24 weeks after discontinuation of therapy.

Methods.—Forty postmenopausal women with PHP with a mean age of 70 years and a known mean duration of disease of 1.8 years were randomly assigned to receive either alendronate, 10 mg/d, or placebo for 48 weeks in a double-blind placebo-controlled trial. The primary end point was bone mineral density (BMD) at the femoral neck. Secondary end points were BMD at the lumbar spine and distal radius and serum albumin–adjusted calcium concentration. Patients were instructed to eat a normal diet and avoid extra vitamin D supplementation. The BMD was measured via dual-density x-ray absorptiometry at the femoral neck, lumbar spine, and distal third of the nondominant radius. The test drug was discontinued at 48 weeks; patients were reassessed at weeks 60 and 72.

Results.—Thirty-six women completed the trial. The patients were generally osteoporotic at baseline. At 48 weeks' evaluation, the change in BMD at the femoral neck was significantly different between the alendronate and placebo groups (+4.17% for alendronate vs −0.25% for placebo; $P = .011$). The BMD in the alendronate group decreased to +3.42% at 24 weeks after treatment withdrawal ($P = .012$ for trend of change over time). For the lumbar spine, the BMD at 48 weeks was +3.49% change for alendronate versus +0.19% for placebo ($P = .016$). At 24 weeks after treatment cessation, the BMD at the lumbar spine decreased to +2.41% ($P = .004$ for trend of change over time); no BMD change occurred for the placebo group. There were no between-group differences in change of BMD at the distal third of the radius at 48 weeks. For the alendronate group, the serum calcium concentration decreased significantly, from a mean of 2.82 mmol/L at baseline to 2.74 mmol/L at the end of 48 weeks; the concentration increased to 2.78 mmol/L at 24 weeks after drug withdrawal ($P = .003$ for trend of change over time). At 48 weeks, the change in serum PTH was not significant ($P = .110$), and the trend in change was not significant between groups. Eight patients had a 25-hydroxyvitamin D concentration below 10 ng/L, indicating underlying vitamin D deficiency. In the alendronate group, serum bone-specific alkaline phosphatase activity followed a trend of change that was opposite of BMD, with a progressive decrease from 21.1 to 7.3 IU/L ($P < .001$) at completion of 48 weeks of treatment; this increased to 15.0 IU/L at 24 weeks after withdrawal of treatment ($P = .088$; $P = .002$ for trend of change over time). Controls had no significant change in serum bone-specific alkaline phosphatase activity or in trend over time. A similar trend in change was observed in serum osteocalcin concentration and urinary N-telopeptide/creatinine ratio in the alendronate group; no changes were observed for controls. There were 2 serious adverse events in the alendronate group: dizziness that resulted in a fall severe enough to require hospitalization and methyldopa-induced hemolytic anemia in another patient.

Conclusion.—Alendronate therapy was safe and effective, and improved BMD at the femoral neck and lumbar spine. It had favorable effects on serum calcium concentration and markers of bone turnover in elderly postmenopausal women with PHP.

▶ In the 2003 YEAR BOOK OF ENDOCRINOLOGY, I reviewed a study by Parker et al[1] in which 32 patients with PHP were randomized to alendronate (ALN) 10 mg/d or placebo for 2 years. The ALN-treated group showed improvement in lumbar spine BMD but had higher PTH levels at 18 months. The current study by Chow et al is another look at the issue of medical therapy for PHP. In this double-blind, randomized, placebo-controlled trial, 40 postmenopausal women with PHP were randomized to either ALN 10 mg/d or placebo and followed up for 48 weeks. Although of shorter duration, this trial had more rigorous inclusion and exclusion criteria than the study by Parker et al (eg, the Parker trial included men and women and did not exclude patients receiving thiazide diuretics or glucocorticoids). Patients in the current study were instructed to get adequate calcium and vitamin D in the diet, but 20% had significant vitamin D deficiency (25-hydroxyvitamin D < 10 ng/L).

The mean age of the women was 70 years, and most had osteoporosis. Average baseline T scores on dual-energy x-ray absorptiometry were −2.07, −2.54, and −3.58 at the femoral neck, lumbar spine, and distal radius, respectively. At 48 weeks, the ALN-treated group showed statistically significant gains in BMD at the lumbar spine and femoral neck but not at the distal radius. Six months after withdrawal of ALN, there were significant losses of BMD from the spine and femoral neck, but overall, BMD remained higher than controls.

By 48 weeks, serum calcium concentrations had declined significantly in the ALN group without a compensatory increase in PTH. Calcium levels tended to increase 6 months after cessation of ALN but not back to pretreatment levels. All biochemical markers of bone turnover (bone-specific alkaline phosphatase, osteocalcin, and urinary N-telopeptide levels) showed the expected significant declines from bisphosphonate therapy, and partial reversal after ALN was stopped.

The authors do not indicate whether patients with vitamin D deficiency showed the same responses as those who were vitamin D replete. One would expect the vitamin D–deficient group to have higher average PTH levels and a blunted response to ALN, but these data are not reported.

The current study demonstrates that at least over the short-term, ALN increases BMD at both the spine and femoral neck, reduces bone turnover, and lowers serum calcium without a compensatory increase in PTH. Cessation of ALN after 48 weeks results in some reversal of these improvements and suggests that a longer duration of therapy may be desirable. We still do not know whether bisphosphonate therapy reduces fractures in patients with PHP, but there is cause for some optimism. It appears from this study and others[1,2] that ALN is an effective and well-tolerated medical therapy for treatment of PHP in older postmenopausal women.

C. Becker, MD

References

1. Parker CR, Blackwell PJ, Fairbairn KJ, et al: Alendronate in the treatment of primary hyperparathyroid-related osteoporosis: A 2-year study. *J Clin Endocrinol Metab* 87:4482-4489, 2002. (2003 YEAR BOOK OF ENDOCRINOLOGY, pp 262-263.)
2. Rossini M, Gatti D, Isaia G, et al: Effects of oral alendronate in elderly patients with osteoporosis and mild primary hyperparathyroidism. *J Bone Miner Res* 16:113-119, 2001.

Effects of Vitamin D and Calcium Supplementation on Falls: A Randomized Controlled Trial
Bischoff HA, Stähelin HB, Dick W, et al (Univ of Basel, Switzerland; Brigham and Women's Hosp, Boston; Inst for Clinical Osteology, Bad Pyrmont, Germany; et al)
J Bone Miner Res 18:343-351, 2003   66–4

Introduction.—Nearly 90% of hip fractures involve falls. Fractures caused by falls occur in approximately 5% of elderly persons every year. Of these, 1% to 2% involve the hip. Epidemiologic, clinical, and laboratory findings indicate a direct effect of vitamin D on muscle strength. A link between low vitamin D levels and reversible myopathy has been observed in patients with osteomalacia and uremia. It may be that vitamin D and calcium supplementation would improve musculoskeletal function and decrease falls. The effect of vitamin D and calcium supplementation on musculoskeletal function and on the mean number of falls and recurrent falls per person was examined in a randomized double blind investigation.

Methods.—One hundred twenty-two elderly women (mean age, 85.3 years; range, 63-99 years) in a long-stay geriatric care center were randomly assigned to receive either 1200 mg calcium plus 800 IU cholecalciferol (Cal+D-group) or 1200 mg calcium (Cal-group) daily during a 12-week period. The number of falls per person (0, 1, 2-5, 6-7, >7 falls) was compared between the Cal+D-group and the Cal-group. Falls were compared between treatment groups, after controlling for age, number of falls in a 6-week pretreatment period, and baseline 25-hydroxyvitamin D and 1,25-dihydroxyvitamin D serum concentrations. Among fallers during the treatment period, the crude excess fall rate (treatment − pretreatment falls) was compared between the 2 groups. The secondary outcome was change in musculoskeletal functions (summed score of knee flexor and extensor strength, grip strength, and the times up&go test).

Results.—There were significant increases in the median serum 25-hydroxyvitamin D (+71%) and 1,25-dihydroxyvitamin D (+8%) levels in the Cal+D-group. Before treatment initiation, the mean observed number of falls per person per week was 0.059 in the Cal+D-group and 0.056 in the Cal-group. During the 12-week treatment period, the mean number of falls per person per week was 0.034 in the Cal+D-group and 0.076 in the Cal-group. After adjustment, Cal+D-treatment accounted for a 49% decrease in falls (95% confidence interval, 14%-71%; $P < .01$). Among fallers during the treatment period, the crude average number of excessive falls was significantly higher in the Cal-group versus the Cal+D-group ($P = .045$). Musculoskeletal function improved significantly in the Cal+D-group versus the Cal-group ($P = .0094$).

Conclusion.—Vitamin D plus calcium supplementation during a 3-month period decreased the risk of falling by 49%, compared with supplementation with calcium alone in elderly postmenopausal women. Recurrent fallers appeared to benefit the most by this treatment. The impact of vitamin D on falls may be explained by the improvement in musculoskeletal function.

▶ Although only 5% of elderly people fall each year, falls account for over 90% of hip fractures. Any intervention that can reduce the risk of falling should have a major impact on the risk of hip fractures. In this excellent study from Switzerland, we have the first randomized controlled trial to look at the effect of calcium and vitamin D supplementation on falls among the elderly. One hundred twenty-two elderly women in long-stay geriatric care units, awaiting nursing home placement, were randomized to either calcium alone (600 mg twice daily) or calcium plus cholecalciferol (600 mg calcium plus 400 IU vitamin D twice daily) and followed up for 12 weeks. The 2 groups were well matched for average age (85 years), height, weight, body mass index, comorbidities, duration of stay, concomitant medications, walking aids, vitamin D therapy before study, and number of falls in the 6 weeks before treatment. Fifty percent of all the women had severe vitamin D deficiency (25-hydroxyvitamin D < 12 ng/mL), and 17% had secondary hyperparathyroidism. There were no differences between the treatment groups in baseline laboratory values.

By the end of 12 weeks of therapy, the women receiving calcium plus vitamin D had a significant 49% reduction in falls compared with the women receiving calcium alone ($P = .01$). There were 25 falls in the Cal+D-group and 55 falls in the Cal-group. Fig 1 (see original article) shows the distribution of fall probabilities according to treatment groups. To lend biologic plausibility to these impressive findings, the authors tested a variety of musculoskeletal functions both before and 3 months after starting therapy. All the musculoskeletal parameters improved significantly in the Cal+D-group relative to the Cal-group alone (*P* = .0094). Other studies have shown that vitamin D supplementation increases the number and cross-sectional area of fast-twitch muscle fibers, muscle strength, balance, and muscle function, while reducing body sway. We now have strong clinical evidence that an inexpensive, easily available, and safe intervention (calcium plus vitamin D) can dramatically reduce the risk of falling among very elderly women within 3 months of treatment. Calcium and vitamin D supplementation should be given to all elderly individuals and particularly to those with a history of falls.

C. Becker, MD

67 Thyroid Disorders

Combined Thyroxine/Liothyronine Treatment Does Not Improve Well-Being, Quality of Life, or Cognitive Function Compared to Thyroxine Alone: A Randomized Controlled Trial in Patients With Primary Hypothyroidism
Walsh JP, Shiels L, Lim EM, et al (Sir Charles Gairdner Hosp, Nedlands, Australia; Western Australian Ctr for Pathology and Med Research, Nedlands)
J Clin Endocrinol Metab 88:4543-4550, 2003   67–1

Background.—The standard replacement therapy for hypothyroidism is T_4. However, in some patients, the symptoms of poor health persist despite T_4 treatment. It is unclear whether this occurs because of comorbidity or because standard T_4 replacement is somehow inadequate for some patients. T_4 has little intrinsic biologic activity. Its metabolic effects are achieved by peripheral conversion to liothyronine (T_3). About 20% of the body's total T_3 production is attributable to the thyroid; thus, a true physiologic thyroid replacement regimen would include both T_4 and T_3. A recent study has reported that a combined T_4/T_3 treatment improved well-being and cognitive function compared with T_4 alone. The effects of combined T_4/T_3 treatment and T_4 treatment alone on symptoms of hypothyroidism, quality of life, cognitive function, and subjective satisfaction with T_4 therapy were compared.

Methods.—This randomized, double-blind, controlled, crossover trial enrolled 110 patients with primary hypothyroidism in which T_3 (10 µg) was substituted for 50 µg of the patient's usual T_4 dose.

Results.—No significant differences were noted between T_4 and combined T_4/T_3 treatment on tests of cognitive function, quality of life scores, Thyroid Symptom Questionnaire scores, patients' subjective assessments of satisfaction with treatment, or 8 of 10 visual analogue scales assessing symptoms. On the General Health Questionnaire-28 and visual analogue scales assessing anxiety and nausea, scores were significantly worse for combined treatment than for T_4 alone. Serum TSH levels were lower during T_4 treatment than during combined T_4/T_3 treatment, which was a potential confounding factor. However, subgroup analysis of patients with comparable serum TSH concentrations failed to demonstrate a benefit from combined treatment compared with T_4 alone.

Conclusions.—The use of combined T_4/T_3 treatment does not provide improved well-being, cognitive function, or quality of life in comparison with T_4 alone.

▶ This study was prompted by the study by Bunevicius et al[1] of 33 hypothyroid patients from Kaunas, Lithuania, which reported that substituting 12.5 μg of liothyronine (T_3) for 50 μg of the patient's usual dose of levothyroxine (T_4) resulted in improved mood, well-being, and cognitive function compared with T_4 alone, according to scores on standardized tests, and that the combination of T_4/T_3 was preferred by most patients. Walsh et al opined that if the Bunevicius study could be confirmed, then combined T_4/T_3 treatment might become the standard thyroid replacement therapy.

In the double-blind crossover Walsh study, 56 patients were randomized to T_4 followed by combined T_4/T_3 treatment, and 54 patients were randomized to combined treatment first followed by T_4. At study entry, patients reduced their daily T_4 dose by 50 μg and took the study medication, which was either 50 μg T_4 or 10 μg T_3. Their subjective satisfaction or dissatisfaction with their baseline treatment before commencement of the study was rated on a 4-point scale, ranging from "very satisfied: my thyroid treatment seems very effective" to "very dissatisfied: my thyroid treatment doesn't seem to work at all." Only about 45% were satisfied with their treatment. At the final visit, patients were again asked which treatment they preferred.

No benefit of T_4/T_3 treatment over standard T_4 treatment could be demonstrated on the quality of life, hypothyroid symptoms, cognitive function, subjective satisfaction with thyroid hormone replacement therapy, or treatment preference, and no subgroup could be identified that benefited symptomatically from T_4/T_3 treatment. Of most importance, there was no improvement in the clinical subgroup of patients complaining of persistent symptoms of hypothyroidism despite seemingly adequate T_4 replacement.

During combined T_4/T_3 treatment, the mean serum free T_4 concentration *decreased*, free T_3 was unchanged, and serum TSH *increased* compared with the values obtained during treatment with T_4 alone. Why this occurred was not entirely clear, but the authors were concerned that it may have masked a beneficial effect of T_4/T_3 therapy. A *post hoc* subgroup analysis, however, of patients who did not develop a high TSH with T_4/T_3 treatment identified no trend for an improved quality of life in this group.

These results differ substantially from those of Bunevicius et al.[1] There are several possible explanations for this: (1) the Bunevicius study was smaller (33 patients), (2) the majority of patients had thyroid cancer presumably being treated with T_4 suppressive therapy rather than standard therapy, and (3) the treatment periods were shorter (5 weeks) than those in the Walsh study (10 weeks). The treatments in the 2 studies differed slightly: Bunevicius et al added 12.5 μg T_3, whereas Walsh et al substituted 10 μg T_3 for 50 μg of the patients' usual T_4 dosage, which is unlikely to have confounded the results enough to account for the markedly different results in the 2 studies. The Walsh study was (1) larger than the Bunevicius study and (2) the number of subjects was determined by power calculations for the principal outcome analyses, which was not done in the Bunevicius study, and (3) avoided the problem of including patients being treated for thyroid cancer with supraphysiologic doses of thyroid hormone. In a post hoc analysis, Bunevicius and Prange[2] found that 11 patients with autoimmune thyroiditis had less mental improvement than did 15 thyroid cancer patients, suggesting that their observations might not be applicable to patients with primary hypothyroidism.

There is no doubt that a sizable number of patients undergoing thyroid hormone replacement therapy are dissatisfied with the way they feel, despite having normal thyroid function tests. In the Walsh study, 65% of the patients were dissatisfied with their treatment at baseline. A survey that was conducted in general practices in Bristol, United Kingdom,[3] attempted to determine the degree of dissatisfaction with T_4 therapy by using 2 survey instruments, one related to feelings of general well-being and the other containing questions related to the symptoms of hypothyroidism. Patients on T_4 scored worse on both surveys, but for the thyroid-specific survey, nearly half of the 583 responding patients with a recent normal TSH and about one third of the 551 responding controls had scores indicating dissatisfaction with their health status.

It simply is not known why so many hypothyroid patients experience persistent symptoms of ill health despite apparently adequate T_4 replacement, but adding T_3 to the regimen does not seem to solve this problem. Another large study[4] published in the same issue of the *Journal of Endocrinology and Metabolism* reached a similar negative conclusion regarding combination T_4/T_3 therapy.

One reason that patients do not feel well during levothyroxine replacement therapy may be that their TSH levels during treatment are not optimal. Recent studies[5,6] show that the serum TSH levels for healthy individuals are generally at the low end of the normal range for TSH established by the laboratory, especially in young and middle-aged persons,[6] and over time remain in a narrow range with minimal fluctuation.[5] For these reasons, I normally attempt to maintain the serum TSH around 1 to 2 µU/L in patients with primary hypothyroidism unless there is some compelling reason to do otherwise. The current evidence does not support the use of T_4/T_3 to achieve this goal.

E. L. Mazzaferri, MD

References

1. Bunevicius R, Kazanavicius G, Zalinkevicius R, et al: Effects of thyroxine as compared with thyroxine plus triiodothyronine in patients with hypothyroidism. *N Engl J Med* 340:424-429, 1999.
2. Bunevicius R, Prange AJ: Mental improvement after replacement therapy with thyroxine plus triiodothyronine: Relationship to cause of hypothyroidism. *Int J Neuropsychopharmacol* 3:167-174, 2000.
3. Saravanan P, Chau WF, Roberts N, et al: Psychological well-being in patients on 'adequate' doses of L-thyroxine: Results of a large, controlled community-based questionnaire study. *Clin Endocrinol (Oxf)* 57:577-585, 2002.
4. Sawka AM, Gerstein HC, Marriott MJ, et al: Does a combination regimen of thyroxine (T4) and 3,5,3'-triiodothyronine improve depressive symptoms better than T4 alone in patients with hypothyroidism? Results of a double-blind, randomized, controlled trial. *J Clin Endocrinol Metab* 88:4551-4555, 2003.

5. Andersen S, Pedersen KM, Bruun NH, et al: Narrow individual variations in serum t(4) and t(3) in normal subjects: A clue to the understanding of subclinical thyroid disease. *J Clin Endocrinol Metab* 87:1068-1072, 2002.
6. Hollowell JG, Staehling NW, Hannon WH, et al: Iodine nutrition in the United States. Trends and public health implications: Iodine excretion data from National Health and Nutrition Examination Surveys I and III (1971-1974 and 1988-1994). *J Clin Endocrinol Metab* 83:3401-3408, 1998.

Does a Combination Regimen of Thyroxine (T₄) and 3,5,3'-Triiodothyronine Improve Depressive Symptoms Better Than T₄Alone in Patients With Hypothyroidism? Results of a Double-blind, Randomized, Controlled Trial

Sawka AM, Gerstein HC, Marriott MJ, et al (McMaster Univ, Hamilton, Ont, Canada; St Joseph's Healthcare, Hamilton, Ont, Canada; Hamilton Health Sciences, Ont, Canada; et al)

J Clin Endocrinol Metab 88:4551-4555, 2003   67–2

Background.—Psychiatric symptoms may develop in patients with overt hypothyroidism. These symptoms may include depressed mood and cognitive dysfunction, which are generally reversible with levothyroxine replacement therapy. However, some patients who received levothyroxine replacement therapy have complained of depressive symptoms despite normal TSH measurements. At present, it is not known whether the addition of T_3 in these patients can reverse these psychiatric symptoms. Whether nonthyroidectomized primary hypothyroid patients with depressive symptoms experience an improved mood and sense of well-being when euthyroidism is maintained with a combination of T_3 and T_4 compared with T_4 therapy alone was determined.

Methods.—A group of 40 patients with depressive symptoms despite taking a stable dose of levothyroxine for treatment of hypothyroidism were randomly assigned to receive T_4 plus placebo or the combination of T_4 plus T_3 in a double-blind manner for 15 weeks. Study participants who were receiving combination therapy had their prestudy dose of T_4 reduced by 50%, and T_3 was initiated at a dosage of 12.5 µg twice daily. T_4 and T_3 doses were adjusted to maintain goal TSH concentrations within the normal range.

Results.—Compared with the group taking T_4 alone, the group receiving both T_4 plus T_3 did not report any improvement in self-rated mood and well-being scores, including subscales of the Symptom Check-List-90, the Comprehensive Epidemiological Screen for Depression, and the Multiple Outcome Study.

Conclusions.—These findings are not supportive of the routine use of combined T_3 and T_4 therapy in hypothyroid patients with depressive symptoms.

▶ About half of the patients taking levothyroxine (T_4) replacement are dissatisfied with how they feel, despite having serum TSH levels within the normal range established by the laboratory.[1,2] Depressive symptoms, which are especially common in hypothyroid patients as well as the general population, have been reported by Bunevicius et al[3,4] to respond to the addition of liothyronine (T_3) to T_4 replacement therapy. However, many of the Bunevicius patients who reported improvement in their mood had thyroid cancer and were likely taking supraphysiologic doses of thyroid hormone[3]; moreover, a post hoc analysis found that thyroid cancer patients had more improvement in mood than did a group with primary hypothyroidism.

The study from Ontario, Canada, by Sawka et al addresses whether there is an amelioration of depression in nonthyroidectomized primary hypothyroid patients treated with combined T_4 plus T_3 therapy. The selection criteria included the use of a stable, unchanged dose of T_4 for 6 months before randomization, a normal baseline serum TSH concentration, and evidence of depressive symptoms as defined by scores on a well-established general health questionnaire, and the Symptom Check-List-90, a self-report questionnaire, and on the Comprehensive Epidemiological Screen for Depression (CES-D).

All 20 participants randomized to receive T_3 had their prestudy dose of T_4 dropped by 50%, and T_3 was started at a dose 12.5 µg, twice daily, whereas the 20 participants randomized to receive T_4 therapy alone continued their usual dose of T_4 and received a placebo substitute for T_3. The study design did not have a crossover. Seven patients did not complete the full 15 weeks of the study after baseline assessment. Throughout the study, the serum TSH remained within the normal range, and the serum free T_4 and T_3 levels underwent the expected changes.

Combined T_4 plus T_3 therapy did not significantly affect the self-assessed scores of mood compared with T_4 plus placebo. Furthermore, the combination of T4 plus T_3 did not lead to a greater change in personal sense of well-being and social functioning.

This study is different than both the Bunevicius and Walsh studies in the type of patients that were enrolled and in the way patients were treated with a combination of T_4 plus T_3. To name a few, it included a uniform group of persons with a history of primary hypothyroidism and depressive symptoms, and avoided overreplacement with thyroid hormone. However, only 40 patients were studied (Walsh et al studied 110 patients and Bunevicius et al studied 33 persons) and there was a high dropout rate, and there was no objective assessment of mood and cognitive status by a psychiatrist. Nonetheless, the study fails to show a significant improvement in mood in an important subset of hypothyroid patients with depressive symptoms. Walsh et al[1] reported similar findings in a larger number of hypothyroid patients.

There is thus little evidence to support the routine use of the combination of T_4 plus T_3 in the treatment of patients with primary hypothyroidism. Why so many patients taking T_4 replacement are dissatisfied with how they feel, despite having serum TSH levels within the normal range established by the laboratory, remains an enigma.[1,2] However, there is strong evidence that even small elevations in serum TSH levels, in the range of 6.0 µU/L, cause a number of important adverse physiologic effects,[5] indicating that TSH levels during thyroid hormone replacement therapy must be carefully monitored and maintained around 1 to 2 µU/L in most patients. There seems to be no compelling reason to routinely add T_3 to standard T_4 therapy.

E. L. Mazzaferri, MD

References

1. Walsh JP, Shiels L, Lim EM, et al: Combined thyroxine/liothyronine treatment does not improve well-being, quality of life, or cognitive function compared to thyroxine alone: A randomized controlled trial in patients with primary hypothyroidism. *J Clin Endocrinol Metab* 88:4543-4550, 2003.
2. Saravanan P, Chau WF, Roberts N, et al: Psychological well-being in patients on 'adequate' doses of l-thyroxine: Results of a large, controlled community-based questionnaire study. *Clin Endocrinol (Oxf)* 57:577-585, 2002.
3. Bunevicius R, Kazanavicius G, Zalinkevicius R, et al: Effects of thyroxine as compared with thyroxine plus triiodothyronine in patients with hypothyroidism. *N Engl J Med* 340:424-429, 1999.
4. Bunevicius R, Prange AJ: Mental improvement after replacement therapy with thyroxine plus triiodothyronine: Relationship to cause of hypothyroidism. *Int J Neuropsychopharmacol* 3:167-174, 2000.
5. Cooper DS: Clinical practice. Subclinical hypothyroidism. *N Engl J Med* 345:260-265, 2001.

Maternal Hypothyroxinaemia During Early Pregnancy and Subsequent Child Development: A 3-year Follow-up Study
Pop VJ, Brouwers EP, Vader HL, et al (Univ of Tilburg, The Netherlands; Technical Univ of Eindhoven, The Netherlands; Univ of Amsterdam)
Clin Endocrinol (Oxf) 59:282-288, 2003   67–3

Background.—There has been a resurgence of interest in the relationship between maternal plasma thyroid hormone concentration during pregnancy and subsequent infant neurodevelopment. It is well known that both maternal thyroid dysfunction during pregnancy (especially hypothyroidism) and severe iodine deficiency adversely affect the outcome of neurodevelopment in children. Even in regions in which sufficient iodine intake is present in the general population, pregnant women often have lower free T_4(FT_4) plasma levels without elevated TSH levels. This condition is referred to as hypothyroxinemia and is generally regarded as normal. However, there is increasing concern that hypothyroxinemia during early gestation could be harmful to the offspring. The effects of maternal hypothyroxinemia during early gestation (FT_4 below the lowest 10th percentile and TSH within the reference range of 0.15 to 2.0 mIU/L) on infant development were assessed, together with any subsequent changes in FT_4 during gestation.

Methods.—Child development was evaluated with the Bayley Scales of Infant Development in children of women with hypothyroxinemia at 12 weeks' gestation and in children of women with FT_4 levels between the 50th and 90th percentiles at 12 weeks' gestation, matched for parity and gravidity (controls). Maternal thyroid function was assessed at 12, 24, and 32 weeks' gestation. The mental and motor functions of 63 patients and 63 controls were compared at 1 year of age, and those of 57 patients and 58 controls were compared at 2 years of age.

Results.—Children of women with hypothyroxinemia at 12 weeks' gestation demonstrated delayed mental and motor function in comparison with controls: 10 index points on the mental scale and 8 points on the motor scale at the age of 1 year, and 8 index points on the mental scale and 10 on the motor scale at 2 years of age. Children of hypothyroxinemic women in whom the FT_4 level was increased at 24 and 32 weeks' gestation had scores similar to those of controls, whereas in the controls, the developmental scores were not influenced by further declines in maternal FT_4 levels at 24 and 32 weeks' gestation.

Conclusions.—During early gestation, maternal hypothyroxinemia is an independent determinant of a delay in infant neurodevelopment. However, there appears to be no adverse effect on infant development when FT_4 concentrations increase during pregnancy in women who are hypothyroxinemic during early gestation.

▶ Because the fetal thyroid is unable to produce any T_4 before 12 to 14 weeks' gestation, maternal thyroid function during early pregnancy is an important determinant of early fetal brain development. It has been known for some time that both overt maternal hypothyroidism and severe iodine deficiency adversely affect neurologic development of the offspring. However, even in areas in which there is sufficient iodine uptake in the population, pregnant women often have serum FT_4 levels in the lower ranges of normal that are not accompanied by an elevation of TSH, which is defined as hypothyroxinemia and is generally regarded as a normal condition. In the past decade, a relationship has been established between mild maternal hypothyroidism during pregnancy and fetal neurodevelopment. Although adverse neurologic development of the fetus has been described in the setting of mild (subclinical) hypothyroidism with an elevated serum TSH level,[1,2] little is known about the relationship to child development of low-normal FT_4 levels that do not alter TSH during normal pregnancy.

Pop et al performed a longitudinal prospective study of maternal thyroid hormone levels and child development in women without subclinical thyroid dysfunction and an elevated serum TSH. After excluding 44 patients with subclinical thyroid dysfunction (TSH outside the reference range with normal FT_4) and others with various confounding factors such as a history of major depression or abortion, 125 children and their mothers were deemed eligible and stratified as follows: 63 cases of hypothyroxinemia at 12 weeks' gestation with an FT_4 below the 10th percentile and TSH within the reference range, and 62 controls with FT_4 levels at 12 weeks' gestation between the 50th and 90th percentiles and serum TSH within the reference range. All the children had normal Apgar scores at birth and normal screening results for congenital hypothyroidism, and came from families of similar socioeconomic status, parental education, income, and marital status, and were similar in breast-feeding status, mothers' lifestyle habits during pregnancy, and birth weight, sex, and gestational age.

The differences in mental and motor development in the cases and controls at 1 and 2 years' follow-up are shown in Table 2 of the original article. At 1 year of age, the group differences were statistically significant, with a mean difference of 10 index points on the mental scale and 8 on the motor scale. Among 19 children who had a delay in mental function (scores <84), 15 (79%) had hypothyroxinemic mothers. Similarly, among 21 children with a delay in motor function, 16 (76%) had hypothyroxinemic mothers. At age 2 years, 57 children of hypothyrox-inemic mothers had a significantly lower mean mental score (8 points) and motor score (10 points) than controls. Of 11 children with a delay on the mental scale, 8 (73%) had hypothyroxinemic mothers. Similarly, of 22 children with delayed motor function, 17 (77%) had hypothyroxinemic mothers. There was a significant correlation between maternal T_4 and mental scores ($R^2 = 0.13$, $P = .006$) and psychomotor scores ($R^2 = 0.23$, $P = .001$). Development was not affected in children of mothers who were hypothyroxinemic during early gestation but subsequent FT_4 concentrations increased during pregnancy.

The authors point out that the study had several limitations, perhaps the most important of which is that the subgroups defined according to maternal FT_4 patterns during pregnancy became rather small after cases with potentially confounding data had been excluded.

This study suggests that screening for FT_4 at 12 weeks' gestation could identify a subgroup of hypothyroxinemic women whose infants would likely benefit from an increase of maternal FT_4; however, the authors point out that it is not clear whether these women would benefit more from iodine treatment or thyroxine supplementation, and that more prospective studies are needed to answer this important question. In addition to the known risks of subclinical hypothyroidism on child neurologic development, this study adds concern about the even more subtle finding of maternal hypothyroxinemia.

E. L. Mazzaferri, MD

References

1. Pop VJ, Kuijpens JL, Van Baar AL, et al: Low maternal free thyroxine concentrations during early pregnancy are associated with impaired psychomotor development in infancy. *Clin Endocrinol (Oxf)* 50:149-155, 1999.
2. Haddow JE, Palomaki GE, Allan WC, et al: Maternal thyroid deficiency during pregnancy and subsequent neuropsychological development of the child. *N Engl J Med* 341:549-555, 1999.

Early Maternal Hypothyroxinemia Alters Histogenesis and Cerebral Cortex Cytoarchitecture of the Progeny
Lavado-Autric R, Ausó E, García-Velasco JV, et al (Universidad Autónoma de Madrid; Universidad Miguel Hernández, San Juan, Spain)
J Clin Invest 111:1073-1082, 2003   67–4

Introduction.—The importance of thyroid hormone transfer from the mother to the fetus during the second half of pregnancy has received increasing acceptance, along with increasing awarenesss of the significance of maternal thyroxine for the development of the brain early in pregnancy. Epidemiologic trials from both iodine-sufficient and iodine-deficient human populations strongly indicate that early maternal hypothyroxinemia increases the risk of neurodevelopmental deficits of the fetus, whether or not the mother is clinically hypothyroid. Neocortical cell migration is defective in the progeny of severely hypothyroid rat dams treated with methimazole. Early maternal thyroid hormone deficiency deranges the migratory patterns of cells into the cortex, either directly by reducing availability of the hormones to the developing brain or indirectly through poor placental function caused by maternal hypothyroidism. Rats were examined to determine whether such early migratory defects also occur in the progeny of hypothyroxinemic dams that, in contrast to those receiving methimazole, are not "clinically" hypothyroid.

Findings.—Young adult female rats were fed a low-iodine diet (LID) and 1% $KClO_4$ as drinking water to lower the initial content of iodine-containing compounds in the thyroid gland. Animals were divided into 3 groups: the LID-plus–potassium iodide (KI) group, the LID-1 group (fed LID alone), and the LID-2 group (fed LID containing 0.005% $KClO_4$). Blood was obtained 3 months later to determine T_4 and T_3. The T_4 values in LID-1 dams were below normal and the T_3 values were normal. In LID-2 dams, the T_3 values dropped, though considerably less than the T_4 values. Normal and LID-plus-KI pups demonstrated the normal "inside-out" gradient model of radial migration. Cell migration and cytoarchitecture in the sensory cortex and hippocampus of 40-day-old progeny of iodine-deficient dams were assessed. A significant proportion of cells at locations were aberrant or inappropriate with respect to their birth date. Most cells were neurons, as evaluated by single- and double-label immunostaining. The cytoarchitecture of the somatosensory cortex and hippocampus was also impacted. Layering was blurred; in the cortex, normal barrels were not formed.

Conclusion.—It is likely that this is the first direct evidence of an alteration in fetal brain histogenesis and cytoarchitecture that could only be associated with early maternal hypothyroxinemia. This condition may be 150 to 200 times more frequent than congenital hypothyroidism and should be prevented by mass screening of free thyroxine in early pregnancy and by early iodine supplementation to prevent iodine deficiency, however mild.

▶ There now is evidence that maternal thyroxine is important for the development of the fetal brain early in pregnancy before mid gestation, when there is no significant thyroxine secretion by the fetal thyroid gland and the mother is the only source of thyroid hormone. Experimental and epidemiologic studies show that maternal hypothyroxinemia early in the course of pregnancy results in neurodevelopmental impairment. Here the term "hypothyroxinemia" alone is synonymous with hypothyroidism, whether or not there is clinical or subclinical maternal hypothyroidism with TSH levels above normal values. Although much of the evidence to support this concept comes from studies of hypothyroxinemia caused by iodine deficiency (ID), maternal hypothyroxinemia and its attendant problems for the fetus have been described in The Netherlands[1] and the United States,[2] where ID is not present, and may be 150 to

200 times more common than the neurodevelopmental impairment associated with overt congenital hypothyroidism.[3]

The most marked CNS damage occurs in children with cretinism who are born in areas of severe ID, where both mother and child have hypothyroxinemia.[3] Here the neurologic deficits are profound and include severe mental deficiency and motor defects. More recently, it has become apparent that children of mothers with less severe hypothyroxinemia have mildly decreased mental and psychomotor development compared with the rest of the population, and that all degrees of ID affect thyroid function of the mother and the neonate, which in turn affects the mental development of the child. The damage increases with the degree of the ID, with overt endemic cretinism being the severest consequence. The key factor in the development of neurologic damage in the neonate is maternal hypothyroxinemia during early pregnancy.[4] Indeed, according to Delange,[4] ID results in a global loss of 10 to 15 IQ points at a population level and constitutes the world's single greatest cause of preventable brain damage and mental retardation.

Lavado-Autric et al investigated brain development in the progeny of hypothyroxinemic Wistar rats, some of which were prepared with LID and 1% $KClO_4$ as drinking water to lower the initial content of iodide-containing compounds in the thyroid gland. The rats were divided into 3 groups: the LID-plus-KI group, an LID-1 group fed an LID alone, and an LID-2 group fed LID containing $KClO_4$ to further decrease thyroid uptake of the small amounts of iodine contained in the LID. The effects of the different diets on T_4 and T_3 just before mating are summarized in Table 1 (see original article). The study provides histochemical evidence of aberrant or inappropriate cell migration and cytoarchitecture in the somatosensory cortex and hippocampus of the 40-day-old progeny of iodine-deficient dams. These and other abnormalities provide the first direct evidence of an alteration of fetal brain histogenesis and cytoarchitecture that might be related to early maternal hypothyroxinemia. The authors emphasize that because of obvious ethical constraints, direct evidence of a causal relationship between early maternal hypothyroxinemia and mental development can only be obtained in animal models.

The authors suggest that mass screening programs should be done on pregnant women early in gestation, with the tacit understanding that hypothyroxinemia will be treated. This can only be done after appropriate controlled randomized studies are performed.

E. L. Mazzaferri, MD

References

1. Pop VJ, Kuijpens JL, Van Baar AL, et al: Low maternal free thyroxine concentrations during early pregnancy are associated with impaired psychomotor development in infancy. *Clin Endocrinol (Oxf)* 50:149-155, 1999.
2. Haddow JE, Palomaki GE, Allan WC, et al: Maternal thyroid deficiency during pregnancy and subsequent neuropsychological development of the child. *N Engl J Med* 341:549-555, 1999.
3. Glinoer D, Delange F: The potential repercussions of maternal, fetal, and neonatal hypothyroxinemia on the progeny. *Thyroid* 10:871-887, 2000.
4. Delange F: Iodine deficiency as a cause of brain damage. *Postgrad Med J* 77:217-220, 2001.

Maternal Hypothyroidism May Affect Fetal Growth and Neonatal Thyroid Function

Blazer S, Moreh-Waterman Y, Miller-Lotan R, et al (Meyer Children's Hosp, Haifa, Israel; Technion–Israel Inst of Technology, Haifa, Israel)
Obstet Gynecol 102:232-241, 2003   67–5

Introduction.—It is possible that some pregnant women who are hypothyroid may be inadequately treated and may inadvertently undergo periods of hypothyroxinemia during gestation. These maternal events may affect fetal pituitary–thyroid axis function and manifest in the immediate postnatal days. Pituitary–thyroid axis function was examined in the early neonatal period of infants born to hypothyroid mothers who were considered to be adequately treated.

Methods.—Of 27,386 full-term newborn infants delivered during a 6-year period, 259 were born to 250 treated hypothyroid mothers (0.9%). Two hundred forty-six infants were included. One hundred thirty-nine term healthy neonates from healthy group-matched mothers acted as controls. Both study infants and controls underwent thyroid function testing in a prospective design. A single blood sample was obtained from each infant at 25 to 120 hours of life.

Results.—Compared with controls, serum TSH and free T_4 (FT_4) levels were higher in study neonates, particularly at 49 hours of life ($P < .005$ and $P < .03$, respectively). At 49 to 120 hours, 44.7% of newborns in the study group had serum FT_4 levels higher than the 95th percentile of controls ($P < .001$); 16.8% had significantly higher TSH levels ($P < .001$). Serum FT_4 correlated positively with TSH in controls ($r = 0.316$) and not study newborns ($r = 0.062$; $P = .36$). Neonatal TSH at 49 hours or older correlated positively with maternal TSH in the 18 cases in which maternal TSH values during pregnancy were available ($r = 0.751$; $P < .001$). Birth weight and head circumference were significantly less in study versus control neonates ($P < .001$).

Conclusion.—The impaired intrauterine growth and the unduly elevated serum levels of TSH and FT_4 detected in a substantial portion of study newborns may reflect an inadequate level of hormone replacement therapy of their hypothyroid mothers during pregnancy, despite an assumed adequate management. Close monitoring is recommended for maternal hypothyroidism.

▶ The fetal thyroid gland concentrates iodine and synthesizes thyroid hormone after 10 to 12 weeks' gestation. Before this time, fetal thyroid hormone requirement is supplied by the mother via the placenta. Beyond the first trimester, however, the fetal hypothalamic-pituitary-thyroid axis develops and functions independently, but the fetus continues to rely to some extent on maternal T_4.[1]

The prospective study by Blazer et al indicates that the pituitary-thyroid axis of newborn infants born to hypothyroid mothers is often adversely affected, even when the mother is apparently taking adequate thyroid hormone supplementation. Neonatal serum TSH and FT_4 levels were both significantly higher in a large subgroup of infants of hypothyroid mothers than in controls (normal neonates from healthy mothers). High postnatal FT_4 levels declined after birth more rapidly in the control infants than the study infants of hypothyroid mothers, who were smaller at birth and had smaller head circumferences than controls. Small head circumference and low birth weight are known to increase the risk of subsequent subnormal intellectual and psychologic performance, but this was not tested.[2]

There is one important limitation to this study: the frequency of thyroid function testing and the results of these tests during the pregnancy were unknown in the hypothyroid mothers. The replacement thyroid hormone dosage requirements increase about 50% in most pregnant women during the first trimester and return to the pregestational dosage shortly after delivery.[3] Why this occurs is usually not known but is sometimes caused by diminished absorption resulting from the effects of iron in prenatal vitamins.[4]

This study provides another piece of important information about the complexity of problems in the fetus of hypothyroid mothers, especially those taking thyroid hormone replacement therapy. It is not clear from this study whether the findings in the fetal pituitary–thyroid axis are caused by inadequate maternal thyroid hormone replacement, but this certainly is a possibility.

E. L. Mazzaferri, MD

References

1. Morreale de Escobar G, Obregon MJ, Escobar del Rey F: Is neuropsychological development related to maternal hypothyroidism or to maternal hypothyroxinemia? *J Clin Endocrinol Metab* 85:3975-3987, 2000.
2. Lundgren EM, Cnattingius S, Jonsson B, et al: Intellectual and psychological performance in males born small for gestational age with and without catch-up growth. *Pediatr Res* 50:91-96, 2001.
3. Mandel SJ, Larsen PR, Seely EW, et al: Increased need for thyroxine during pregnancy in women with primary hypothyrodism. *N Engl J Med* 323:91-96, 1990.
4. Chopra IJ, Baber K: Treatment of primary hypothyroidism during pregnancy: Is there an increase in thyroxine dose requirement in pregnancy? *Metabolism* 52:122-128, 2003.

Raloxifene Causing Malabsorption of Levothyroxine

Siraj ES, Gupta MK, Reddy SSK (Cleveland Clinic Foundation, Ohio)
Arch Intern Med 163:1367-1370, 2003   67–6

Background.—Many patients receiving thyroid hormone therapy are also taking other medications. It is important therefore that clinicians treating these patients be aware of the potential interactions between various drugs and thyroid hormone replacement. There appear to have been no previous reports of raloxifene hydrochloride, a selective estrogen receptor modulator, interfering with the absorption of levothyroxine. An elderly woman with chronic, treated primary hypothyroidism who had increasing levothyroxine requirements while taking raloxifene at the same time as levothyroxine was described.

> *Case Report.*—Woman, 79, receiving treatment for chronic hypothyroidism, was referred for increasing levothyroxine requirements. She underwent a subtotal thyroidectomy in 1970 and was prescribed levothyroxine sodium, after which she maintained normal TSH levels for several years with a daily levothyroxine sodium dose of 0.15 mg taken early in the morning. She was prescribed raloxifene for treatment of osteopenia several months before presentation. The raloxifene was also to be taken early in the morning. Within 2 to 3 months, an elevated TSH level of 14.5 µU/mL and symptoms of hypothyroidism resulted in an increase in levothyroxine sodium dosage to 0.2 mg/d. At presentation, after 9 months of raloxifene therapy, she had a TSH level of 9.36 µU/mL while taking 0.3 mg of levothyroxine sodium daily. For two 6- to 8-week periods, the ingestion of raloxifene and levothyroxine was separated by about 12 hours. The absorption of 1 mg of levothyroxine was tested with and without the coadministration of 60 mg of raloxifene on 2 separate occasions by collecting serial blood samples for 6 hours. Hypothyroidism was reproducible whenever levothyroxine and raloxifene were administered together and improved when they were administered separately.

Conclusions.—The combined administration of levothyroxine and raloxifene provided lower levels of serum thyroxine compared with the administration of levothyroxine alone. The mechanism by which the coadministration of raloxifene and levothyroxine caused malabsorption of levothyroxine has not been elucidated.

▶ Iron sulfate,[1] aluminum antacids,[2] calcium carbonate,[3] cholestyramine resin,[4,5] colestipol,[6] sucralfate,[7] and herbal remedies[8] have been reported to inhibit the absorption of levothyroxine in man. In addition, women with hypothyroidism that is being treated with levothyroxine often need higher doses when they are pregnant.[9] In older women, estrogens may induce lower free T_4 and higher TSH levels, leading to an increased requirement of thyroxine.[10] However, neither estrogens nor selective estrogen receptor modulators until now seem to have caused malabsorption of levothyroxine. The article by Siraj et al demonstrates that raloxifene (Evista) also interferes with levothyroxine absorption when the 2 drugs are administered simultaneously. Why this occurs is unknown.

It is prudent to advise patients to take levothyroxine in the morning shortly after arising and before breakfast, to avoid the malabsorption that may occur from high-fiber diets and other drugs the patient is taking. Each year or so for the past 3 decades, we discover another new cause of thyroxine malabsorption or another new instance in which the drug dose has to be modified.

It is common for patients taking thyroxine to have sudden changes in thyroid function tests while using the same dose of the drug. This is usually caused by concurrent use of another drug. For example, even though it is common knowledge that iron sulfate interferes with the absorption of thyroxine, this continues to be a frequent problem seen in practice, especially in pregnant women.[11] An occasional patient seems to malabsorb thyroxine,[12] but this is rare. When this diagnosis is entertained, a 6-hour absorption test can be done using 1.0 mg of levothyroxine, with blood specimens drawn at 0, 60, 90, 120, 180, 240, 300, and 360 minutes as was previously described[13] and as performed in this study.

E. L. Mazzaferri, MD

References

1. Campbell NR, Hasinoff BB, Stalts H, et al: Ferrous sulfate reduces thyroxine efficacy in patients with hypothyroidism. *Ann Intern Med* 117:1010-1013, 1992.
2. Sperber AD, Liel Y: Evidence for interference with the intestinal absorption of levothyroxine sodium by aluminum hydroxide. *Arch Intern Med* 152:183-184, 1992.
3. Singh N, Weisler SL, Hershman JM: The acute effect of calcium carbonate on the intestinal absorption of levothyroxine. *Thyroid* 11:967-971, 2001.
4. Northcutt RC, Stiel JN, Hollifield JW, et al: The influence of cholestyramine on thyroxine absorption. *JAMA* 208:1857-1861, 1969.
5. Rosenberg R: Malabsorption of thyroid hormone with cholestyramine administration. *Conn Med* 58:109, 1994.
6. Phillips WA, Schultz JR, Stafford WW: Effects of colestipol hydrochloride on drug absorption in the rat: I. Aspirin, L-thyroxine, phenobarbital, cortisone, and sulfadiazine. *J Pharm Sci* 63:1097-1103, 1974.
7. Sherman SI, Tielens ET, Ladenson PW: Sucralfate causes malabsorption of L-thyroxine. *Am J Med* 96:531-535, 1994.
8. Geatti O, Barkan A, Turrin D, et al: L-thyroxine malabsorption due to the injection of herbal remedies. *Thyroidology* 5:97-102, 1993.
9. Mandel SJ, Larsen PR, Seely EW, et al: Increased need for thyroxine during pregnancy in women with primary hypothyroidism. *N Engl J Med* 323:91-96, 1990.
10. Arafah BM: Increased need for thyroxine in women with hypothyroidism during estrogen therapy. *N Engl J Med* 344:1743-1749, 2001.
11. Chopra IJ, Baber K: Treatment of primary hypothyroidism during pregnancy: Is there an increase in thyroxine dose requirement in pregnancy? *Metabolism* 52:122-128, 2003.
12. Jauk B, Mikosch P, Gallowitsch HJ, et al: Unusual malabsorption of levothyroxine. *Thyroid* 10:93-95, 2000.
13. Ain KB, Refetoff S, Fein HG, et al: Pseudomalabsorption of levothyroxine. *JAMA* 266:2118-2120, 1991.

Treatment of Type II Amiodarone-Induced Thyrotoxicosis by Either Iopanoic Acid or Glucocorticoids: A Prospective, Randomized Study

Bogazzi F, Bartalena L, Cosci C, et al (Univ of Pisa, Italy; Univ of Insubria, Varese, Italy; National Research Council, Pisa, Italy; et al)

J Clin Endocrinol Metab 88:1999-2002, 2003　　　　　　　　　　　　67–7

Introduction.—Amiodarone-induced thyrotoxicosis (AIT) may occur either in persons with underlying thyroid disease (type I AIT) or in persons with apparently normal thyroid glands (type II AIT). Type II AIT, which is a destructive thyroiditis, frequently responds favorably to glucocorticoids. Iopanoic acid (IopAc) is an iodinated cholecystographic agent that inhibits deiodinase activity and diminishes the conversion of T_4 to T_3. Cholecystographic agents have recently been shown to restore euthyroidism in patients with type II AIT. Twelve patients with type II AIT treated with either IopAc or prednisone were compared in a prospective randomized trial.

Methods.—Patients were randomly assigned to treatment with either IopAc (500 mg twice daily) or prednisone (starting dosage, 30 mg/d for 2 weeks, gradually tapered and withdrawn after 3 months). Amiodarone was discontinued in all patients before randomization. Cure of the destructive thyroiditis was examined with the use of survival curves at 12 months.

Results.—Serum free T_3 levels normalized quickly in both groups after 7 days (from 0.75 to 0.46 ng/dL [$P < .01$], and from 0.58 ng/dL to 0.34 ng/dL [$P < .003$] in the IopAc and prednisone groups, respectively [P = not significant]). Serum free T_4 levels dropped at 6 months in the prednisone group (from 2.70 to 1.0 ng/dL [$P < .0001$]) but not in the IopAc group (from 2.90 to 2.30 ng/dL; $P = .39$) ($P = .005$, prednisone group vs IopAc group). All participants in both groups became euthyroid, and their amiodarone-induced destructive thyroiditis was cured, as demonstrated by normalization of both serum free T_4 and free T_3 levels during both drug therapies. Patients in the prednisone group were cured more rapidly than those in the IopAc group (43 vs 221 days; $P < .002$).

Conclusion.—Both prednisone and IopAc are effective in the treatment of type II AIT, but prednisone (glucocorticoids) is probably the drug of choice because of its more rapid curing action.

▶ Amiodarone is an effective antiarrhythmic drug that contains 75 mg of iodine per 200-mg tablet, which daily releases about 10% of it as free iodide, resulting in complex changes in thyroid function. Up to 20% of patients treated with amiodarone subsequently develop some thyroid dysfunction, and about 6% develop thyrotoxicosis.[1] There are 2 forms of AIT. Type I is a form of iodine-induced thyrotoxicosis that occurs in patients with Graves' disease or nodular goiter. It is characterized by goiter, the presence of thyroid autoantibodies, high thyroidal ^{131}I uptake, low interleukin-6 (IL-6) levels, and persistent thyrotoxicosis that responds to methimazole and perchlorate therapy. Type II AIT, which occurs in patients with a normal thyroid gland, is a form of destructive thyroiditis that causes the release of stored thyroid hormone and is characterized by a nontender thyroid gland associated with a low thyroidal ^{131}I uptake, high IL-6 levels, and transient thyrotoxicosis lasting for about 1 to 3 months, which promptly resolves when thyroid hormone stores are depleted. It is usually treated with glucocorticoids and is usually followed by transient, or more rarely, permanent hypothyroidism. However, it may not be possible to distinguish the 2 forms of AIT on the bases of these clinical features. A high thyroidal radioiodine uptake rules out type II AIT, but a low uptake may occur in patients with type II AIT because of the large iodine load. When there are mixed forms of AIT or the diagnosis is uncertain, thionamides, perchlorate ($KClO_4$), and glucocorticoids are usually given.[1]

Oral cholecystographic agents (OCAs), which inhibit the peripheral conversion of T_4 to T_3, have been used to treat spontaneous hyperthyroidism by lowering serum T_3 concentrations without lowering levels of T_4. These agents rapidly control thyrotoxicosis, but there is a high recurrence rate of hyperthyroidism caused by the escape phenomenon. Recently, Chopra and Baber[2] described 5 cardiac patients with type II AIT who were treated with a combination of an OCA (sodium ipodate [Oragrafin] or sodium iopanoate [Telepaque]) and propylthiouracil or methimazole. Amiodarone was discontinued in all patients, although this is not absolutely necessary,[3] and all 5 patients improved within a few days of treatment and either became euthyroid or hypothyroid in 15 to 31 weeks. They suggested that the combination of an OCA and a thionamide is a safe and effective form of therapy for type II AIT. Admittedly, this might be taking the hair of the dog that bit you, since both OCA agents and amiodarone inhibit peripheral conversion of T_4 to T_3.

In the Bogazzi study, glucocorticoids and iopanoic acid were compared head-to-head. Although both drugs resulted in rapid normalization of serum T_3 levels after 7 days' therapy, glucocorticoid therapy resulted in a rapid return of serum free T_4 (FT_4) to normal levels (about 14 days), while FT_4 remained elevated for 240 days with OCA therapy ($P < .005$). This resulted in a significantly shorter time for a cure (defined as cessation of hyperthyroidism) with glucocorticoid than with OCA therapy. For the short haul OCAs can be used, but glucocorticoid therapy is probably the treatment of choice.

E. L. Mazzaferri, MD

References

1. Daniels GH: Amiodarone-induced thyrotoxicosis. *J Clin Endocrinol Metab* 86:3-8, 2001.
2. Chopra IJ, Baber K: Use of oral cholecystographic agents in the treatment of amiodarone-induced hyperthyroidism. *J Clin Endocrinol Metab* 86:4707-4710, 2001.
3. Osman F, Franklyn JA, Sheppard MC, et al: Successful treatment of amiodarone-induced thyrotoxicosis. *Circulation* 105:1275-1277, 2002.

Antithyroid Drugs in the Management of Patients With Graves' Disease: An Evidence-Based Approach to Therapeutic Controversies
Cooper DS (Johns Hopkins Univ, Baltimore, Md)
J Clin Endocrinol Metab 88:3474-3481, 2003   67–8

Introduction.—Published guidelines have addressed the general subject of hyperthyroidism therapy. Yet, they have not been evidence-based and do not confront questions concerning choice of antithyroid agent, duration of use, proper dosage, patient selection, or pretreatment before radioiodine administration. A MEDLINE search was performed to address these questions.

Which Drug Is More Effective?—One retrospective trial suggested that methimazole led to a more rapid normalization of thyroid function than propylthiouracil (PTU). The retrospective design made it hard to determine whether patients were equivalent at baseline. Three prospective, randomized controlled trials (RCTs) compared methimazole and PTU head-to-head. Data suggested methimazole was somewhat more effective.

Which Drug Is Less Toxic?—Both PTU and methimazole are linked to minor reactions. Data suggest that the rate of side effects are dose related with methimazole. Data for PTU are not as clear. Some rare, yet major side effects are linked with PTU. Methimazole appears to be a safer drug, particularly when administered in dosages below 10 mg/d.

Which Drug Is Associated With Greater Patient Compliance?—One RCT that compared patients receiving methimazole, 30 mg/d as a single dose, and PTU, 100 mg every 6 hours, showed a compliance rate (>80% of medication being taken) of 83% for methimazole and 53% for PTU ($P < .01$). The major advantage of methimazole was probably that it was a single daily dose.

Which Drug Costs Less?—At lower doses, the cost of methimazole and PTU is similar; at higher doses, Tapazole and methimazole are more expensive.

What Are the Effects of PTU and Methimazole on the Efficacy of Subsequent Radioactive Iodine Therapy?—Several retrospective trials have reported PTU to significantly lower the efficacy of subsequent radioiodine treatment. Two retrospective and 2 prospective RCTs reported no alteration in the effectiveness of radioactive iodine therapy after methimazole, making it preferable for pretreatment.

How Long Should the Patient Be Treated to Maximize the Chances of Remission?—Retrospective trials have suggested that the chance of remission increases the longer antithyroid drugs are taken. Prospective randomized trials have not concurred. It appears that treating in excess of 12 to 18 months is not likely to yield a higher remission rate, compared with longer treatment periods.

Does the Antithyroid Drug Dose Influence the Chances of Remission?—One prospective RCT comparing traditional drug doses to high-dose treatment revealed a higher remission rate in patients receiving high-dose methimazole or PTU; follow-up was less than 2 years after drug discontinuation. Four recent RCTs showed no difference in remission rates in patients receiving high-dose antithyroid drugs supplemented with either T_4 or T_3, compared with a lower dose regimen titrated to maintain normal thyroid function. Recent evidence suggests that there is no advantage and potential harm with high-dose therapy.

What Antithyroid Drug Dose Should Be Used Initially?—The underlying disease activity and starting dose are both important factors. In patients with mild to moderate disease, an initial methimazole dose of 10 to 20 mg would be appropriate in most patients.

Would Administration of T_4 During or After Antithyroid Drug Therapy Enhance the Chances of Remission?—It appears that there is currently no rationale for using T_4 in combination with antithyroid drugs to enhance remission rates.

Is the Patient a Good Candidate for Primary Antithyroid Drug Therapy, or Is She Unlikely to Achieve a Remission, Making Radioiodine a Better Choice?—Most retrospective trials have reported the highest remission rates in patients with relatively small goiters in whom thyroid function tests are only slightly deranged. It appears that severe disease and large goiter are poor prognostic features for achieving a remission. This has not been observed in prospective trials.

Conclusion.—In general, methimazole is the preferred drug for management of hyperthyroidism due to Graves' disease. There is no advantage to larger doses, longer treatment regimens, or concomitant use of T_4. Few data show that antithyroid drug treatment prevents clinical or biochemical exacerbations after radioiodine.

▶ It is difficult to reconcile differences in the literature when there are conflicting data about the efficacy of treatments, which is true for antithyroid drugs. The review by Dr Cooper, an expert in the field, is a unique evidence-based summary of the clinical issues and controversies surrounding the antithyroid drugs in the management of thyrotoxic Graves' disease. His main findings are shown in Tables 1 and 2 (see original article).

He cites strong evidence that methimazole (MMI) is the preferred drug in the management of hyperthyroidism due to Graves' disease. However, this conclusion is not based on major differences in therapeutic efficacy between MMI and PTU. Cooper cites 3 prospective RCTs that performed head-to-head comparisons of the 2 drugs and concludes that although the data suggest MMI is somewhat more effective than PTU, only one small prospective randomized trial compared the drugs at therapeutically equivalent doses.

The conclusion that MMI is the preferred drug rests more on its safety profile and other features of the drug. Its rates of side effects are dose related, whereas this is less clear with PTU. For example, the reported rates of agranulocytosis for both drugs range from 0.2% to 0.5%, but the number of cases is very small in patients receiving MMI in dosages of less than 10 mg/d. In one large study,[1] there was an 8.6-fold increased risk of agranulocytosis with dosages of MMI greater than 40 mg/d ($P < .01$), and no cases of agranulocytosis were seen with MMI given in dosages of less than 30 mg/d, whereas the mean dosages of PTU did not differ among those who did or did not have this complication. Cooper concludes that MMI is a safer drug, especially when given in dosages below 10 mg/d, which is adequate in most patients with mild to moderate thyrotoxicosis.

Cooper found few data showing that antithyroid drug pretreatment prevents clinical or biochemical exacerbations after ^{131}I therapy for Graves' disease, but when an exacerbation of symptoms does occur, it is less severe in those who have been pretreated with the drugs. Yet there is good evidence that discontinuing antithyroid drugs before treatment with ^{131}I results in a mild deterioration of thyroid function, the clinical significance of which is uncertain. Endocrinologists often pretreat with antithyroid drugs when patients are elderly or have underlying conditions that might be exacerbated by the release of thyroid hormone that occurs shortly after ^{131}I therapy. There is now evidence[2] that lithium given after discontinuing antithyroid drugs prevents this rise in thyroid hormone levels and also leads to more rapid control of thyroid function after ^{131}I therapy.

There are many other advantages to using MMI. Cooper concludes that, in all likelihood, MMI has a major advantage over PTU in terms of compliance because it is effective when given in a single daily dose. At lower doses, the cost of MMI and PTU is similar, but at higher doses, MMI is more expensive. Moreover, MMI is preferable if one chooses to pretreat a patient with antithyroid drugs, because none of the studies of MMI demonstrate an alteration in the effectiveness of ^{131}I therapy, whereas the dose of ^{131}I could be increased by as much as 25% because of the putative radioresistant effects of PTU.

Cooper concludes that treatment for longer than 12 to 18 months is not likely to yield a higher remission rate as compared with longer periods. Also, he concludes that there is currently no rationale for using T_4 in combination with antithyroid drugs to enhance remission rates. He notes that the underlying disease activity and the starting dose of MMI are both important considerations, but an initial dose of 10 to 20 mg is appropriate in most cases. He cites a large body of retrospective data that support the notion that severe disease and large goiter are poor prognostic features for achieving a remission, although this has been difficult to demonstrate in prospective studies.

Endocrinologists will find this article very helpful and should read it in its entirety.

E. L. Mazzaferri, MD

References

1. Cooper DS, Goldminz D, Levin A, et al: Agranulocytosis associated with antithyroid drugs: Effects of patient age and drug dose. *Ann Intern Med* 98:26-29, 1983.
2. Bogazzi F, Bartalena L, Pinchera A, et al: Adjuvant effect of lithium on radioiodine treatment of hyperthyroidism. *Thyroid* 12:1153-1154, 2002.

Natural History of Benign Solid and Cystic Thyroid Nodules

Alexander EK, Hurwitz S, Heering JP, et al (Harvard Med School, Boston)

Ann Intern Med 138:315-318, 2003   67–9

Introduction.—Thyroid tumors are common and are frequently benign. The natural history of benign thyroid nodules has yet to be defined. The medical records of all patients from a single institution who were referred to a thyroid nodule clinic with benign cytologic findings on US-guided fine-needle aspiration (FNA) of a thyroid nodule between 1995 and 2000 and returned for a requested follow-up examination 1 month to 5 years later were reviewed retrospectively.

Methods.—Nodule dimensions were determined at initial and follow-up visits. Growth was defined as an increase in calculated volume of 15% or more. These findings were correlated with the time between examinations, age, gender, baseline serum TSH concentration, and cystic content of each nodule.

Results.—Nodule volume increased over time (*P* < .001). The estimated proportion of nodules with an increase in volume of 15% or more after 5 years was 89%. Nodules with higher cystic content were less likely to grow, compared with solid nodules (*P* = .01). Seventy-four of 330 nodules were reaspirated during the second visit. There was an average increase in volume of 69%, but only 1 of 74 reaspirated nodules was malignant.

Conclusion.—Because most solid, benign thyroid nodules grow, it is important to understand that increased nodule volume alone is not a reliable predictor of malignancy.

▶ Although most authorities suggest that FNA should be repeated when a thyroid nodule enlarges in the course of follow-up, relatively few studies have measured nodule growth by thyroid US during follow-up. Moreover, the definition of what comprises significant enlargement of a thyroid nodule is inconsistent and usually couched in terms of nodule diameter increasing more than 50%[1] or by 3 mm,[2] or nodule volume increasing by 15%[3] or more.

The study by Alexander et al provides important information about the natural history of benign thyroid nodules. Most nodules increased 15% or more in volume over 3 to 5 years, which was calculated by using the formula for a rotational ellipsoid (length × width × depth × π/6). Solid nodules grew more than cystic nodules, and only 1 malignant nodule was found among 74 nodules (64 patients) that underwent repeat FNA. It should be noted that a 15% change in the volume of a 4.7 × 2.3 × 2.3-mm nodule is only about a 1-mm increase in each of the 3 dimensions, which would be difficult to replicate. However, a 50% increase in the volume of the same nodule would be about a 5-mm increase in its largest diameter or a 4-mm change in each dimension, which is easy to replicate. Although only 24% of the patients seen in follow-up underwent repeat FNA, their nodules were larger on initial examination (2.7 cm vs 2.3 cm, *P* = .001) and increased more in volume (69% vs 14%) and diameter (2.9 mm vs 0.1 mm) during follow-up compared with the nodules that did not undergo repeat biopsy. The only nodule that was found to be malignant on repeat FNA, a poorly differentiated papillary thyroid carcinoma, had an 80% increase in volume, enlarging from 10.1 to 18.1 cm³ over 36 months.

These authors acknowledge a few limitations of this study, namely, follow-up evaluations were not chosen randomly, the time when growth occurred cannot be known precisely and may have been overestimated, and only a minority of benign nodules (22%) were rebiopsied. Although most were probably colloid nodules, the clinical diagnosis of the benign nodules is not mentioned.

Kung et al[4] recently reported that in pregnant women, the volume of a single colloid nodule or of a dominant benign nodule in a multinodular goiter increased from 60 (14-344) mm³ during the first trimester to 65 (26-472) mm³ by the third trimester ($P < .02$) and remained enlarged at 6 weeks ($P < .005$) and 3 months postpartum (P < .05). This is consistent with the Alexander study.

It is important to know that benign nodules grow during follow-up, although where we draw the line to repeat the FNA is still not clear but probably is close to a 50% change in volume (most newer US units calculate volume automatically), which for an average-sized 2- or 3-cm nodule is about a 3- or 4-mm increase in its largest dimension. Certain other characteristics of a nodule (blurred margins, microcalcifications, heterogeneous echogenicity, and intranodular Doppler flow) in addition to its size provide strong clues of malignancy.[5] This study also underscores the importance of performing US at baseline and during follow-up of thyroid nodules. Palpation of a thyroid nodule is simply not an accurate way of assessing size.

E. L. Mazzaferri, MD

References

1. Reverter JL, Lucas A, Salinas I, et al: Suppressive therapy with levothyroxine for solitary thyroid nodules. *Clin Endocrinol (Oxf)* 36:25-28, 1992.
2. Singer PA, Cooper DS, Daniels GH, et al: Treatment guidelines for patients with thyroid nodules and well-differentiated thyroid cancer. *Arch Intern Med* 156:2165-2172, 1996.
3. Berghout A, Wiersinga WM, Drexhage HA, et al: Comparison of placebo with L-thyroxine alone or with carbimazole for treatment of sporadic non-toxic goitre. *Lancet* 336:193-197, 1990.
4. Kung AWC, Chau MT, Lao TT, et al: The effect of pregnancy on thyroid nodule formation. *J Clin Endocrinol Metab* 87:1010-1014, 2002.
5. Papini E, Guglielmi R, Bianchini A, et al: Risk of malignancy in nonpalpable thyroid nodules: Predictive value of ultrasound and color-Doppler features. *J Clin Endocrinol Metab* 87:1941-1946, 2002.

68 Adrenal Disorders

Ten Years On: Safety of Short Synacthen Tests in Assessing Adrenocorticotropin Deficiency in Clinical Practice
Gleeson HK, Walker BR, Seckl JR, et al (Western Gen Hosp, Edinburgh, Scotland)
J Clin Endocrinol Metab 88:2106-2111, 2003   68–1

Background.—In screening patients for adrenocorticotropic hormone (ACTH) deficiency, the short synacthen test (SST) and the insulin tolerance test (ITT) have both been proposed. The SST offers the advantages of being cheaper, safer, and less taxing on the patient than the ITT. However, concern has arisen regarding whether the SST accurately detects adequate responses in stressful situations, with normal cortisol responses to the SST sometimes found in patients whose response to the ITT is subnormal. The predictive value for clinical outcome of a postoperative SST in patients with and without ACTH deficiency who were having pituitary surgery was evaluated.

Methods.—The biochemical results and clinical outcome of 63 patients who had not been diagnosed with ACTH deficiency (had passed the SST) were assessed.

Results.—New ACTH deficiency was found in 18.5% of the patients, and borderline SST results were obtained in 9 operations. Four of the latter group passed on retest, while 5 were not retested and continued to take hydrocortisone. Twelve of the 63 patients who had initially passed the SST developed ACTH deficiency. The postoperative SST had a false negative return in 2 cases, for a predictive value of 97%.

Conclusion.—The predictive value of the SST in excluding ACTH deficiency was similar to values found in other studies, but these patients should be closely monitored to ensure that any false-negative cases are detected promptly.

▶ In clinical practice, the "short ACTH stimulation test" has become a safe, inexpensive, and reasonably sensitive test to assess the adequacy of the entire hypothalamic-pituitary-adrenal axis. This premise is based on 3 requirements: first, a viable adrenal gland with an adequate supply of a preformed pool of hormone ready to be released; second, an adrenal that has been sufficiently primed by endogenous ACTH; and third, viable corticotrophs that have been stimulated by hypothalamic corticotropin-releasing hormone. Hence, a perfectly normal response to 250 µg of Cotrosyn validates healthy status of the entire axis. The unfortunate wrinkle here is that priming of the zona fasciculata is not an entirely all-or-none issue. Thus, a small but significant percentage of patients with ACTH deficiency may show preservation of a normal response to the standard high-dose ACTH stimulation test.

In various studies, the false-negative or "miss rate" for ACTH deficiency remains from 2% to as high as 10%. The introduction of the low-dose ACTH stimulation test was aimed to get around this issue. But unfortunately this has not found wide application since the sensitivity of this test has not been established with certainty. This study deals with patients who underwent pituitary surgery.

The authors have focused on the 63 patients who "passed the test," implying an adequate postoperative ACTH reserve. It is impressive that 12 of the 63 patients who passed the test eventually developed bona fide ACTH deficiency on subsequent testing. Undoubtedly, in some this may have been a reflection of radiation-induced delayed hypopituitarism. But in a few, ACTH deficiency occurred in the absence of radiotherapy. The authors note that the predictive value of the SST in excluding ACTH deficiency was 97%, with a "miss rate" of only 3%. With the combination of a high clinical suspicion and the benefits of annual repetition of the test, it appears that one can do well with this test without having to resort to the ITT or the low-dose Cortrosyn stimulation test.

Another spinoff from this study is the value of the 0900-hour plasma cortisol level as a predictor for the need for further assessment with dynamic testing of the hypothalamic-pituitary-adrenal axis. The authors found that a 0900-hour plasma cortisol level less than 400 nmol/L was 91% sensitive and 85% specific for the diagnosis of ACTH deficiency. Despite this perceived usefulness of a single plasma cortisol level, dynamic tests are often required to decide the need for lifelong glucocorticoid replacement therapy.

C. R. Kannan, MD

Randomized Placebo-controlled Trial of Androgen Effects on Muscle and Bone in Men Requiring Long-term Systemic Glucocorticoid Treatment
Crawford BAL, Liu PY, Kean MT, et al (Royal Prince Alfred Hosp, Sydney, Australia; Concord Hosp, Sydney, Australia; Univ of Sydney, Australia)
J Clin Endocrinol Metab 88:3167-3176, 2003   68–2

Background.—Significant adverse effects attend the long-term use of systemic glucocorticoid therapy, including muscle and bone loss together with decreased serum testosterone levels, and these effects may impair the quality of life. Androgen replacement therapy is known to increase muscle mass and strength and to restore deficits in bone mineral density (BMD) in androgen-deficient men, although minimal effects on muscle strength and bone mass have been seen in older men who have minimal androgen deficiency. The tissue-specific effects of dihydrotestosterone and estradiol, the 2 bioactive metabolites of testosterone, and their influence on the actions of androgen is unclear. The effect of testosterone and its minimally aromatizable analogue nandrolone on muscle mass, muscle strength, BMD, and quality of life was assessed.

Methods.—Fifty-one men (mean age, 60.3 years) whose mean daily prednisone dose was 12.6 mg were assessed for the effect of testosterone and nandrolone. Tests included dual x-ray absorptiometry, knee flexion and extension by isokinetic dynamometry, BMD, and the Qualeffo-41 questionnaire. The participants were randomly assigned to receive either testosterone (200 mg mixed esters), nandrolone decanoate (200 mg), or placebo every 2 weeks by IM injection over the course of 12 months. Evaluations of fasting blood and urine samples were carried out every 3 months, along with the administration of the questionnaires; every 6 months, measurements of BMD, body composition, and muscle strength were obtained.

Results.—Forty-three men completed 6 months of the study and 37 completed 12 months. Nandrolone treatment produced marked suppression of plasma total and free testosterone concentrations. After 6 and 12 months, lean muscle mass was increased with both treatments but not in the placebo group. The total body fat declined with testosterone and nandrolone but increased with placebo. Both nandrolone and testosterone treatment increased muscle strength. Only men receiving testosterone had significantly increased lumbar spine BMD. Hip and total body BMD showed no alterations. The overall quality of life was rated as better among the men receiving testosterone but not by those receiving nandrolone or placebo.

Conclusion.—High-dose glucocorticoids make valuable contributions with their anti-inflammatory and immunosuppressive effects, but there are complications. Androgen therapy to ameliorate these adverse effects was tested. Testosterone given at a standard androgen replacement dose increased muscle mass and strength, as well as lumbar BMD, and improved quality of life. Nandrolone increased muscle mass and strength but did not improve BMD or quality of life. Thus, it appears that aromatization is needed for the androgen action to influence bone, but not muscle.

▶ What we have here is a 3 for 1, folks! The triple threat of long-term glucocorticoid therapy involves loss of bone, loss of muscle, and loss of sexual function. Steroid-induced osteoporosis is finally receiving the attention it deserves, and the concomitant use of bisphosphonates has become the standard of care. While bisphosphonates cause significant increase in the lumbar spine BMD and reduce the incidence of fractures by 50%, these drugs do not have any beneficial effects on improving sexual function or in improving the sarcopenia of glucocorticoid use.

In this study, testosterone injections not only increased the lumbar spine BMD by an average of 4.7% but also increased skeletal muscle mass and improved quality of life (which I suppose is a euphemism for one who is not "dead in bed"!). Should we treat patients on glucocorticoid therapy as if they were hypotestosteronemic? While the total and free testosterone levels in the 3 groups of patients were not particularly low, the response to testosterone therapy showed dramatic improvement by both objective and subjective parameters. While the BMD data appear good, fracture data are not available for the use of testosterone therapy. The fact that testosterone needs to be aromatized to be effective on the bone is illustrated by the fact that nandrolone had no effect on the bone.

Of course, hormone therapy being what it is, long-term safety with this approach needs to be established. The effects on the prostate, on the cardiovascular and hemopoietic systems, and sleep apnea need to be carefully studied. Until such time, the short-term use of testosterone for 6 to 12 months in such patients should be a case-by-case decision.

C. R. Kannan, MD

Management of Occult Adrenocorticotropin-Secreting Bronchial Carcinoids: Limits of Endocrine Testing and Imaging Techniques

Loli P, Vignati F, Grossrubatscher E, et al (Niguarda Hosp, Milan, Italy; Busto Arsizio Hosp, Italy)

J Clin Endocrinol Metab 88:1029-1035, 2003   68–3

Background.—From 5% to 10% of all cases of adrenocorticotropin (ACTH)-dependent hypercortisolism result from the ectopic ACTH syndrome, with bronchial carcinoids usually the source of the ectopic ACTH. The clinical course of patients who have these small nonaggressive tumors may mimic that of patients with Cushing disease. Differential diagnosis is achieved with ACTH sampling from the inferior petrosal sinuses, but this method does not locate the source of the ectopic ACTH secretion. That requires imaging methods such as CT or MRI. Experience involving 6 patients who had truly occult bronchial carcinoids and underwent hormonal and conventional imaging and scintigraphic evaluations was documented.

Methods.—The patients all had hypercortisolism plus high plasma ACTH values.

Results.—The corticotropin-releasing hormone and high-dose dexamethasone tests indicated an ectopic source for the ACTH in half of the patients. All patients had negative markers for neuroendocrine neoplasia. Four patients had negative MRI results, with an equivocal hypointense area that could have been microadenoma in 2 cases. No CT or MRI evidence of an ectopic source of ACTH was initially found, all patients eventually had a chest lesion detected on CT scans.

The use of ^{111}In-pentetreotide scintigraphy (PS) identified 4 of the 6 ACTH-secreting tumors; in none of the cases were false-negative results obtained for PS. Two patients underwent pituitary microsurgery that proved unsuccessful; it was followed in 1 case by pituitary radiotherapy and adrenal steroidogenesis inhibitors and in the other by bilateral adrenalectomy. Two patients had anticipatory bilateral adrenalectomy. The bronchial carcinoid of each patient was eventually identified and removed, with ACTH immunoreactivity found in all but one case. Five of the 6 patients had lymph node metastases at surgery. Between 8 and 96 months after diagnosis, all patients achieved cure with removal of the primary lesion and metastases.

Conclusion.—Single diagnostic procedures were inadequate to definitively diagnose the presence of bronchial carcinoids in these patients. Dy-

namic endocrine testing was found to be misleading, and the imaging procedures were not accurate enough to localize these small, occult ectopic
sources of ACTH secretion. Plasma ACTH has been found to be a good
marker for the presence or persistence of disease, and the use of an intraoperative γ counter to identify PS-positive tissue was helpful.

▶ How do you find a needle in a haystack? One way is to use a "guiding light."
The guide here is radiolabelled pentetreotide, and the light here is a hand-held
γ probe during surgery. In this article, the authors have elucidated many of the
difficulties inherent to the elusive occult ectopic ACTH secreting tumors. The
difficulties were not related to the diagnosis. In fact, all of the 6 patients with
this disorder were diagnosed by means of standard endocrine testing, with
confirmation by bilateral selective inferior petrosal sinus sampling. The problem in all 6 patients was related to localization. Eventually CT of the chest revealed the presence of a bronchial carcinoid in all 6 patients after variable time
intervals since the original diagnosis.

Of more interest is the fact that PS identified the chest lesion in 2 patients at
the time of diagnosis of hypercortisolism, even with negative CT imaging. The
hand-held γ probe was effective for picking up foci that signaled the presence
of residual as well as metastatic disease. The intraoperative use of γ probes
following the preoperative IV administration of pentetreotide holds promise
for detection of these occult tumors.

In addition to the innovative imaging technique, this article is of interest to
the clinician at several levels. First, these 6 patients with Cushing syndrome
caused by ectopic secretion of ACTH had severe manifestations and expres-
sions of hypercortisolism. This blows the myth that the carcinoid-related
Cushing syndrome is of a mild nature. Second, some of these patients demonstrated preservation of corticotropin-releasing hormone responsiveness as
well as suppressibilty to high-dose dexamethasone administration. This confirms the old adage that the mimicry of carcinoid-related ectopic ACTH secreting syndrome to pituitary-dependent Cushing disease can be carried to the extreme where the lines blur. Third, the authors demonstrate the desmopresin
test was unreliable.

For many years now, desmopressin has been regarded as the less glamor-
ous sister of corticotropin-releasing hormone. In recent years, this test staged
a comeback as a confirmatory test for the distinction between pituitary-depen-
dant disease from ectopic ACTH secreting tumors. Obviously this is not so,
based on this report, and the desmopressin test is not quite ready for its close
up! Finally, the only reliable test for establishing the ectopic source of ACTH
secretion is the bilateral inferior petrosal sinus sampling study. And even with
that, there are gray zones in the ratio between the peripheral and the central
gradients. All in all, the ectopic ACTH secretion associated with occult bronchial carcinoid tumors brings real meaning to the term "conundrum" of
Cushing syndrome.

C. R. Kannan, MD

69 Pediatric Endocrinology

Obesity and Risk of Type 2 Diabetes and Cardiovascular Disease in Children and Adolescents
Goran MI, Ball GDC, Cruz ML (Univ of Southern California, Los Angeles)
J Clin Endocrinol Metab 88:1417-1427, 2003   69–1

Introduction.—The incidence of overweight and obesity continues to rise in children and adolescents. The annual obesity-associated hospital costs in children and adolescents aged 6 to 17 years have reached $127 million per year. The pathophysiology of type 2 diabetes and cardiovascular risk in obese children and adolescents was reviewed.

Scope of Problem.—Impaired glucose tolerance and type 2 diabetes are being diagnosed in overweight children and adolescents. These children demonstrate early signs of the insulin resistance syndrome and cardiovascular risk.

Risk Factors.—Several risk factors have been recognized as contributors to the development of type 2 diabetes and cardiovascular risk in young persons, including increased body fat and abdominal fat, insulin resistance, ethnicity (with greater risk in African American, Hispanic, and Native American children), and onset of puberty. There is no clear explanation concerning how these factors increase risk. They appear to manifest in an additive fashion. The constellation of the risk factors may be particularly problematic during the critical period of adolescent development in persons who may have compromised β-cell function and an inability to compensate for severe insulin resistance.

Pathophysiology.—The following 2 theories are being examined to explain why increased body fat causes or contributes to insulin resistance and the risk for diabetes and cardiovascular disease: (1) fat accumulation only becomes metabolically harmful when accumulated in specific depots, and (2) fat per se is not harmful, yet fat-derived metabolic products may contribute to insulin resistance. The development of type 2 diabetes may differ in children and adolescents from that in adults.

Conclusion.—It is possible that the development of type 2 diabetes in children and adolescents is different from that of adults. Since physical activity has the potential to have profound effects on decreasing the risk for obesity, type 2 diabetes, and cardiovascular disease and offers a natural and drug-free intervention approach, greater emphasis and research are required to determine optimal approaches.

▶ This particular subject—obesity and the risk of type 2 diabetes mellitus (T2DM) and cardiovascular disease in children and adolescents—is an ever expanding one. Goran et al have gathered a large number of studies, both acute, but especially over time, to define the problem and to note its prevalence.[1] Those of us who evaluate patients in pediatric endocrine clinics are inundated with obese, insulin-resistant children and with adolescents who meet the criteria for polycystic ovary disease (PCOS).[2] We are all frustrated with our inability to materially help these children, especially those of us who do not have the proper team approach—nutritionists, exercise physiologists, and social workers (at a minimum)—to this seemingly intractable problem.

The data presented put the public health and individual lifetime morbidity and mortality into sharp focus. Abnormalities in glucose tolerance are very common as in the transition from impaired fasting glucose (IFG) to impaired glucose tolerance (IGT) to T2DM and their attendant list of cardiovascular morbidities. The data are compelling. The pathophysiology involves insulin resistance, including the "natural" insulin resistance at puberty, and increased body fat with a likely redistribution toward the central ("apple") variety of regional distribution. In addition, there are abnormalities in blood pressure and its regulation and circulating lipid concentration, all of which are encompassed as the metabolic syndrome (syndrome X).

In addition, a number of the underlying factors that may contribute to the metabolic syndrome are reviewed: ethnicity (African Americans and Hispanic children and adolescents seem at increased risk); puberty (as noted above); and low birth weight along with marked catch-up (the thrifty gene and Barker hypotheses, see McChance et al[3]). A central role for the lack of physical activity is highlighted. A number of studies indicate that this particular factor—increasing the metabolic equivalents (mets) and decreasing sedentary activities has a very large role to reduce body weight and insulin resistance with proper dietary habits and psychological strategies to both treat the children with obesity, but more importantly, to prevent or delay its onset.

As proper pediatricians, it is incumbent upon us to give our patients anticipatory guidance. The lessening of the morbidity, especially as it relates to the cardiovascular system, bone (osteoporosis), fertility (PCOS), and carbohydrate metabolism (IFG, IGT, T2DM), must become a priority for the health of children. Not only will their lives be more enjoyable and productive, but the economic burden on the health care system will be markedly decreased.

A. D. Rogol, MD, PhD

References

1. American Diabetes Association: Type 2 diabetes in children and adolescents. *Pediatrics* 105:671-680, 2000.
2. Sinha R, Fisch G, Teague B, et al: Prevalence of impaired glucose tolerance among children and adolescents with marked obesity. *N Engl J Med* 346:802-810, 2002.

3. McChance DR, Pettitt DJ, Hanson RL, et al: Birth weight and non-insulin dependent diabetes: Thrifty genotype, thrifty phenotype, or surviving small baby genotype. *BMJ* 308:942-945, 1994.

Health-Related Quality of Life of Severely Obese Children and Adolescents

Schwimmer JB, Burwinkle TM, Varni JW (Univ of California, San Diego; Children's Hosp, San Diego, Calif; Texas A&M Univ, College Station)
JAMA 289:1813-1819, 2003   69–2

Introduction.—There is growing awareness of the long-term health complications of obesity in children and adolescents. Yet many pediatricians do not offer treatment to obese children and adolescents when no comorbid conditions are present. One of the most widespread consequences of childhood obesity may be the risk of psychological and social adjustment problems, including lower perceived competencies than normative samples on social, athletic, and appearance domains, as well as overall self-worth. The health-related quality of life (HR-QOL) of obese children and adolescents was compared with the HR-QOL of children and adolescents who are healthy and those diagnosed with cancer.

Methods.—One hundred six children and adolescents aged 5 to 18 years (mean, 12.1 years) referred to an academic children's hospital for assessment of obesity between January and June 2002 were assessed in a cross-sectional investigation. The mean body mass index (BMI) was 34.7, and the mean BMI z score was 2.6. The primary outcome measures were child self-report and parent proxy report via a pediatric QOL inventory generic scale (range, 0-100). For children aged 5 through 7 years, the inventory was administered by an interviewer. Scores were compared with previously published scores for healthy children and adolescents and children and adolescents with cancer.

Results.—Compared with healthy children and adolescents, obese children and adolescents reported significantly ($P < .001$) lower HR-QOL in all domains (mean total score, 67 and 83 for obese and healthy children, respectively). Obese children and adolescents were more likely to have impaired HR-QOL compared with healthy children and adolescents (odds ratio [OR], 5.5; 95% confidence interval [CI], 3.4-8.7) and were similar to children and adolescents with cancer (OR, 1.3; 95% CI, 0.8-2.3). Children and adolescents who had obstructive sleep apnea reported a significantly lower HR-QOL total score (mean, 53.8) than did obese children and adolescents without obstructive sleep apnea (mean, 67.9). The parent proxy report showed that BMI z score was significantly inversely correlated with total score ($r = -0.246$; $P = .01$), physical functioning ($r = -0.263$; $P < .01$), social functioning ($r = -0.347$; $P < .001$), and psychosocial functioning ($r = -0.209$; $P = .03$).

Conclusion.—Severely obese children and adolescents have lower HR-QOL than children who are healthy. They have similar HR-QOL as those with cancer. Physicians, parents, and teachers need to become aware of the risk of impaired HR-QOL among obese children and adolescents and focus on interventions that can imrove health outcomes.

▶ This is scary stuff! Obesity is one of the most stigmatizing and least socially acceptable conditions in childhood. Most of us who evaluate obese children and adolescents realize that they are unhappy; however, I, for one, had no idea of the depth of their disaffection. The likelihood of an obese child or adolescent having impaired HR-QOL was 5.5 times greater than that of a healthy child or adolescent.

The data were obtained from a well-validated inventory. The subject number is large, and a proper control group was analyzed. The other comparator group, those children with neoplastic diseases receiving chemotherapy, was chosen because they were subjectively and objectively "known" to have a much diminished QOL.

Valid data corroborated both comparator groups—the normal children scored as predicted, and those receiving chemotherapy had a significantly diminished QOL. The surprising data are not that the obese group had a lower-than-normal QOL, but that their objectively measured QOL was as low as children with neoplastic disease.

This should be a wake-up call, especially for those involved in school administration. There is a cadre of very unhappy students in their charge. The results of this study should have them revisit school menus and the decreasing amounts of physical activity during the school day and, perhaps, before and after the school day. Physical activity is important to the physical health and (now) the emotional health of the student body.

Parents, physicians, and other caregivers are also on notice to tend to the physical and emotional concomitants of obesity. Syndrome X and type 2 diabetes mellitus lurk not far behind childhood and adolescent obesity.

A. D. Rogol, MD, PhD

Final Height Outcome and Value of Height Prediction in Boys With Constitutional Delay in Growth and Adolescence Treated With Intramuscular Testosterone 125 mg per Month for 3 Months
Kelly BP, Paterson WF, Donaldson MDC (Royal Hosp for Sick Children, Yorkhill, Glasgow, Scotland)
Clin Endocrinol (Oxf) 58:267-272, 2003   69–3

Introduction.—Constitutional delay in growth and adolescence (CDGA) is a relatively frequent cause of short stature in boys. The clinical characteristics of CDGA are short stature, lack of pubertal progress, and delayed epiphyseal maturation in an otherwise healthy child. Basic treatment strategies include simple counseling with a prediction of final height based on skeletal age. When accelerated growth, accelerated development, or both are desired, an anabolic steroid or a short course of either oral or IM testosterone may be administered. Boys with CDGA were treated with a 3-month course of testosterone enanthate to verify that this approach does not impede final height prediction and to determine the accuracy of height prediction in these patients.

Methods.—Boys with CDGA who had attended the growth clinic, who were now at or close to final height, and who had received either testosterone or declined treatment were identified via retrospective case-note analysis. Bone age assessment was performed by a single observer with the RUS (TW2) method of Tanner and Whitehouse. Medical records were reviewed for age, bone age, height, pubertal stage, parental heights, and predicted final height. All participants were measured at 19 years of age or older. The primary outcome measures were comparison of final height in treated and untreated boys; and final height comparisons with midparental height and with height prediction (RUS [TW2] method) at the initial evaluation and at subsequent review.

Results.—Of 64 boys who met inclusion criteria, 41 had received testosterone and 23 were not treated. There were no significant between-group differences in age, height, midparental heights, or bone age. The mean final heights in both groups (treated, 168.9 cm; untreated, 168.2 cm) were closely associated with predicted final heights (170.0 cm vs 168.1 cm); these were only slightly less than midparental heights. Three participants had final heights below the initial height prediction range.

Conclusion.—A short-term course of testosterone enanthate administered IM in a moderate dose of 125 mg is efficacious in boys with CDGA. The treatment resulted in a rapid increase in height velocity, along with satisfaction with the treatment outcome. Bone age assessment via RUS (TW2) was accurate and clinically helpful.

▶ These data are important, although they represent a nonrandomized retrospective review. These experienced clinicians have followed up a large number of adolescent boys with CDGA. They rightly point out the expected result, to avoid the major side effect of any type of growth-promoting therapy— unmet expectations. Thus, they predicted adult height, told the boys that they would reach within the target range, and likely counseled them that they might do that quicker if they were treated. A surprising number (to me at least) chose not to receive therapy. All who were treated received the same therapy, testosterone enanthate, 125 mg/mo for 3 months. Thus, there is no mixing and matching of dose and duration as is common in previously performed studies.

Virtually all boys reached their target range, although it was below the population mean and in the lower portion of the target range. This is not unusual in previous studies of boys with CDGA. There were essentially no differences in the *measured* adult height (not final height, which has a quite different meaning) among the boys who were treated and those who were not.

My own experience is quite similar, although I have not had the follow-up of this group. Still, they were only able to follow-up approximately 60% of the boys treated. Many of the boys that I follow seem more concerned about the lack of sexual development than their height, but usually both are concerning. I cannot emphasize enough the necessity of reviewing the predicted height with the adolescent and his parents. At first, most boys think that the medications (either testosterone or GH) are magic and will put them into the (well) above-average category. My message is that the medication will permit one to reach his *genetically determined height percentile* perhaps earlier than without treatment.

A. D. Rogol, MD, PhD

Influence of Iodine-131 Dose on the Outcome of Hyperthyroidism in Children

Rivkees SA, Cornelius EA (Yale Univ, New Haven, Conn)
Pediatrics 111:745-749, 2003   69–4

Introduction.—There is increasing evidence that hypothyroidism should be a goal of therapy when using iodine-131 for the treatment of Graves' disease in children. The doses of iodine-131 for treating children with Graves' disease vary widely among institutions. The association between the dose of iodine-131 in children with hyperthyroidism and thyroid status at 1 year after treatment was examined retrospectively.

Methods.—The medical records of all pediatric patients younger than 18 years who received a single treatment of radioactive iodine for treatment of Graves' disease between 1991 and 2001 were reviewed.

Methods.—The outcome of iodine-131 treatment in children and adolescents with Graves' disease was assessed, as related to dose. A comparison was made of 3 iodine-131 doses: 72 to 108 Gy (80-120 µCi/g), 180-225 Gy (200-250 µCI/g), and 270 to 364 Gy (300-405 µCi/g) in 31 patients. Their age range was 7 to 18 years. Thyroid status was assessed more than 1 year after therapy by thyroid function tests.

Results.—Doses of 100 Gy (110 µCi/g), 200 Gy (220 µCi/g), and 300 Gy (330 µCi/g) produced hypothyroidism in 50%, 70%, and 95% of treated participants, respectively.

Conclusion.—To ensure ablation of thyroid tissue, doses of more than 270 Gy (300 µCi/g) are required, particularly when the thyroid is large.

▶ These are important data because they reassure us of the proper use of radioactive iodine (RAI) for Graves' disease and speak to the issue of dose. Many of our colleagues use exclusively antithyroid medication and send the most recalcitrant to surgery. I believe that to be "old-fashioned." The message here is that RAI therapy is effective and safe if given in a great enough dose. Virtually all children and adolescents who received at least 270 to 364 Gy (300-405 µCi/g estimated tissue) became hypothyroid quickly. This is the desired outcome, for it is relatively easy to treat hypothyroidism, and it avoids the multiple visits and tests for those children receiving antithyroid medication long term.

It is theoretically possible that lower doses, especially in the 72- to 108-Gy range, stun the thyroid for a while but do not destroy the follicles. This permits both the recurrence of Graves' disease and the possibility of adenoma formation. Data from children and adults confirm this hypothesis.[1]

My general practice is to use antithyroid medication for 6 weeks, double the dose if the underlying disease is not under control, and make plans for RAI after 12 weeks unless the child, or especially the parent, is adamantly against radioactivity. So far, I have followed (currently) only 1 patient who may need a second dose of RAI. It is imperative to work with our colleagues in nuclear medicine to be sure that our optimally prepared patients—off antithyroid medications for 5 to 7 days and on a relatively low-iodine diet, if the intake is quite high—are administered *ablative* doses of RAI.

A. D. Rogol, MD, PhD

Reference

1. Dobyns BM, Sheline GE, Workman JB, et al: Malignant and benign neoplasms of the thyroid in patients treated for hyperthyroidism: A report of the Cooperative Thyrotoxicosis Therapy Follow-up Study Group. *J Clin Endocrinol Metab* 38:976-998, 1974.

Diurnal Rhythms of Serum Total, Free and Bioavailable Testosterone and of SHBG in Middle-Aged Men Compared With Those in Young Men

Diver MJ, Imtiaz KE, Ahmad AM, et al (Royal Liverpool Univ Hosp, England)
Clin Endocrinol (Oxf) 58:710-717, 2003   69–5

Background.—Opinions differ in the literature regarding the association between advancing age and gradually diminishing concentrations of serum total testosterone in men. The apparent loss of diurnal rhythm in serum total testosterone in older men is reported to be caused partly by low concentrations of testosterone in the morning compared with the higher concentrations found in young men. The diurnal patterns of total, free, and bioavailable testosterone as well as sex hormone binding globulin (SHBG) in young men were compared with those measured in a group of middle-age men.

Methods.—The study groups included 10 fit, healthy graduate students, 23 to 33 years old and 8 healthy middle-age men, 55 to 64 years old, who engage in regular exercise. None of the subjects smoked or consumed more than 21 u of alcohol per week. None of the patients complained of or were diagnosed as having any endocrinopathy. Total, free, and bioavailable testosterone and SHBG were measured in blood samples obtained every 30 minutes throughout a 24-hour period in both groups.

Results.—Both the middle-age and the young groups showed a significant diurnal rhythm in all variables, with a minimum decline of 43% in total testosterone from peak to nadir in all subjects. A time series analysis of the data by least squares estimation showed no significant difference in mesor, amplitude, or acrophase for total testosterone between the 2 groups. A comparison of bioavailable testosterone in the 2 groups showed no significant difference in mesor or acrophase, but a significant difference was seen in amplitude. Both the young and middle-age groups demonstrated a significant circadian rhythm. A highly significant rhythm in free testosterone was evident in both the young and middle-age groups, with no significant difference between the groups in mesor or acrophase. Analysis of the SHBG data revealed a significant rhythm in the young group and the middle age group, but the acrophase occurred in mid-afternoon in both groups. The men in the middle-age group had a significantly greater amplitude, but no significant difference was observed in mesor or acrophase between the 2 groups. Acrophase for total, bioavailable, and free testosterone occurred between 7 and 7:30 hours. The acrophase for SHBG occurred at 3:12 PM in the young men and at 3:40 PM in the middle-age men.

Conclusions.—The diurnal rhythms for total, bioavailable, and free testosterone and SHBG are maintained in fit, healthy men well into middle age.

▶ This study shows that both younger and older men have a diurnal variation of serum total, free, and bioavailable testosterone, findings that contrast with previous observations.

A. W. Meikle, MD

What Happens to Testosterone After Prostate Radiation Monotherapy and Does It Matter?
Pickles T, Graham P, and Members of the British Columbia Cancer Agency Prostate Cohort Outcomes Initiative (British Columbia Cancer Agency, Vancouver, Canada; Univ of British Columbia, Vancouver, Canada; St George Hosp, Kogarah, New South Wales, Australia)
J Urol 167:2448-2452, 2002   69–6

Background.—Several small studies have reported temporary decreases, permanent decreases, or no change in testosterone levels after radiation monotherapy or radical prostatectomy. However, controversy is present as to the potential importance of this phenomenon in outcome; some studies have stated that decreases in testosterone levels after prostate radiation monotherapy are unlikely to have an effect on tumor progression, and others have argued that worse outcomes will result in some patient groups. Some studies have postulated that these decreased levels of testosterone will augment the success of radiation in some patient groups. The effects of decreased testosterone on biochemical and clinical outcomes were investigated, and prostate specific antigen (PSA) doubling time in men with relapse after primary treatment was determined.

Methods.—The study included 666 British men who were followed up after external beam radiation therapy without neoadjuvant or adjuvant androgen ablation. Serial testosterone and PSA were measured before and at 3- to 6-month intervals after therapy.

Results.—At a median nadir of 6 months, testosterone levels decreased to an average of 83% of baseline, with 7.5% of patients experiencing a decrease greater than 50%. All but 3% of patients with normal initial testosterone levels experienced recovery to at least normal levels, but only 60% of patients recovered to their individual pretreatment levels of testosterone. Multivariate analysis showed that patients with a low preintervention testosterone level, and patients treated with larger radiation volumes, had a low testosterone nadir. Univariate and multivariate analyses showed no effect of initial testosterone level, degree of decrease, and absolute testosterone nadir. PSA doubling times in patients with relapse were no different than times in patients with a small or large decrease in testosterone.

Conclusions.—A temporary decrease in testosterone occurs after radiation therapy to the prostate, but this temporary decrease has no effect on subsequent tumor outcome.

▶ External radiation therapy for treatment of prostate cancer transiently lowers serum testosterone concentrations.

A. W. Meikle, MD

70 Obesity

Relationship of Changes in Physical Activity and Mortality Among Older Women
Gregg EW, for the Study of Osteoporotic Fractures Research Group (Ctrs for Disease Control and Prevention, Atlanta, Ga; et al)
JAMA 289:2379-2386, 2003   70–1

Background.—Physical activity has been associated with a decreased mortality rate. However, whether changes in physical activity affect mortality rate among older women is unclear.

Methods.—Four U.S. research centers enrolled 9518 community-dwelling white women aged 65 years or older in this prospective cohort study. The women were assessed at baseline between 1986 and 1988. A median 5.7 years later, 7553 were available for reassessment.

Findings.—Compared with women who remained sedentary during follow-up, women who increased their levels of physical activity had a lower mortality rate from all causes, with a hazard ratio (HR) of 0.52. This finding was independent of age, smoking, body mass index, comorbid conditions, and baseline physical activity level. Among women increasing their levels of physical activity, the HR for death from cardiovascular disease was 0.64 and 0.49 from cancer. The relation between changes in physical activity and decreased mortality rate were comparable in women with and without chronic diseases but tended to be weaker in women at least 75 years old and in women with a poor health status. Women who were physically active at both assessments also had a reduced all-cause and cardiovascular mortality rate when compared with sedentary women.

Conclusions.—Among elderly women, increasing and maintaining physical activity levels may prolong life. However, this appears less beneficial among women aged 75 years and older and in those with poor health status.

▶ This study was chosen because few studies have examined the association between late-life physical activity changes and mortality rate. This interesting study supports the notion that being physically active and becoming physically active will lower mortality rates in older white women. How much physical activity is needed to achieve this benefit? The investigators noted that sedentary white women who increased their physical activity levels to approximately 1 mile per day of walking achieved a 40% to 57% lower all-cause cardiovascular disease and cancer mortality rates than sedentary white women.

E. T. Poehlman, PhD

Effects of the Amount and Intensity of Exercise on Plasma Lipoproteins
Kraus WE, Houmard JA, Duscha BD, et al (Duke Univ, Durham, NC; Durham Veterans Affairs Med Ctr, NC; East Carolina Univ, Greenville, NC; et al)
N Engl J Med 347:1483-1492, 2002   70–2

Introduction.—The association between increased physical activity and decreased risk of cardiovascular disease may be because of improvement in the lipoprotein profile. The amount of exercise training needed for optimal benefit is not known. The effects of the amount and intensity of exercise on lipoproteins were examined in a prospective, randomized trial.

Methods.—One hundred eleven sedentary, overweight males and females with mild-to-moderate dyslipidemia were randomly assigned to participate for 6 months in a control group or to participate for 8 months in 1 of 3 exercise groups: high-amount–high-intensity exercise, the caloric equivalent of jogging 20 miles (32.0 km) a week at 65% to 80% of peak oxygen consumption; low-amount–high-intensity exercise, the equivalent of jogging 12 miles (19.2 km) a week at 65% to 80% of peak oxygen consumption; or low-amount–moderate-intensity exercise, the equivalent of walking 12 miles a week at 40% to 55% of peak oxygen consumption. Research subjects were encouraged to maintain their baseline body weight. Eighty-four participants who complied with these guidelines were the basis for the main analysis. Detailed lipoprotein profiling was performed by means of nuclear MR spectroscopy with confirmation by measurement of cholesterol in lipoprotein subfractions.

Results.—A beneficial effect of exercise was observed on a variety of lipid and lipoprotein variables, particularly in the high-amount–high-intensity exercise group. The high amount of exercise produced greater improvements than lower amounts of exercise in 10 of 11 lipoprotein variables, and was always superior to the control condition in 11 of 11 variables. Both of the lower-amount exercise groups always had better responses than control subjects (22 of 22 comparisons).

Conclusion.—The highest amount of weekly exercise, with minimal weight change, resulted in the most widespread beneficial effects on the lipoprotein profile. Improvements were associated with the amount of activity and not with the intensity of exercise or improvement in fitness.

▶ This study was chosen because it compared the effects of 2 different amounts and intensities of exercise training on lipoproteins in a randomized controlled trial. The major finding in this study is that a higher amount of exercise (17-18 miles of jogging per week at a moderate pace) has a much greater benefit on lipids than a lower amount of exercise (approximately 11 miles/wk).

The other interesting finding is that the benefits achieved with the higher level of exercise appeared to be related to the volume of exercise achieved, whereas the intensity of exercise appeared to play a less important role in the improvements in the lipid profile.

E. T. Poehlman, PhD

What Level of Physical Activity Protects Against Premature Cardiovascular Death? The Caerphilly Study

Yu S, Yarnell JWG, Sweetnam PM, et al (Queen's Univ, Belfast, Northern Ireland)

Heart 89:502-506, 2003   70–3

Background.—There can be no doubt that leisure-time physical activity is associated with a decrease in all-cause mortality and may extend life by 1 to 2 years. It has been shown in many studies that leisure-time physical activity is associated with a reduction in premature death from cardiovascular disease and more specifically from coronary heart disease. However, the optimal intensity of physical activity has not been clearly determined. In addition, studies of leisure-time physical activity and cancer death have yielded inconsistent findings. The association of leisure-time physical activity with all-cause mortality and cause-specific mortality was examined, and the required level of intensity of activity important in the prevention of premature death was determined. Work-related physical activity was also examined.

Methods.—This prospective study used a whole population sample of men from South Wales, United Kingdom, and enrolled men ages 49 to 64 years without historical or clinical evidence of coronary heart disease at baseline examination. The main outcome measures were all-cause mortality and mortality from cardiovascular disease and coronary heart disease. The subjects were monitored for 11 years.

Results.—A graded, significant association was observed between total (cumulative) leisure-time physical activity and all-cause, coronary heart disease, and cardiovascular disease mortality. However, no association was observed with cancer deaths. Light- and moderate-intensity leisure-time physical activity was inconsistently and nonsignificantly related to all-cause mortality, coronary heart disease mortality, and cardiovascular disease mortality when adjusted for age or for other cardiovascular risk factors. In contrast, a significant dose-response relationship was noted for heavy-intensity leisure-time physical activity for all-cause, cardiovascular disease, and coronary heart disease mortality after adjustment for other risk factors.

Conclusions.—Among men with no evidence of coronary heart disease at baseline, only heavy or vigorous leisure exercise was independently associated with a reduced risk of premature death from cardiovascular disease.

▶ The optimal or ideal intensity of exercise needed to protect against premature cardiovascular death is still unclear. The principal message from this study is that only "heavy" or vigorous leisure time physical activity is associated with a lower risk of premature death from cardiovascular disease risk. The strengths of this study included its prospective design, length of follow-up, and a validated assessment of physical activity.

E. T. Poehlman, PhD

71 Pituitary

Withdrawal of Long-term Cabergoline Therapy for Tumoral and Nontumoral Hyperprolactinemia
Colao A, Di Sarno A, Cappabianca P, et al (Federico II Univ of Naples, Italy)
N Engl J Med 349:2023-2033, 2003   71–1

Background.—Prolactinoma is usually treated with a dopamine agonist, such as cabergoline. This observational prospective study analyzed the possibility of cabergoline withdrawal in patients whose hyperprolactinemia was controlled.

Study Design.—The study group consisted of 200 patients with hyperprolactinemia who had received cabergoline as first-line therapy, had serum PRL levels in the normal range, and whose tumors had decreased by at least 50%. The outer tumor border had to be at least 5 mm from the optic chiasm, without evidence of invasion. Patients were followed up for at least 24 months. If PRL levels were above the normal range at any point during follow-up, recurrence was diagnosed and cabergoline immediately restarted.

Findings.—Recurrence rates were 24% in patients with nontumoral hyperprolactinemia, 31% in patients with microprolactinomas, and 36% in patients with macroprolactinomas over 2 to 5 years of follow-up. No patients had tumor growth. PRL levels remained significantly lower than at diagnosis. The Kaplan-Meier estimate of 5-year recurrence was significantly higher among those with macroprolactinomas or microprolactinomas with visible tumor on MRI.

Conclusion.—These data support the concept of withdrawal of cabergoline therapy from patients with hyperprolactinemia after PRL levels normalize. Patients must be closely monitored for return of hyperprolactinemia, especially if tumor is still visible on MRI.

▶ This is an important article that shows that many patients treated long term with cabergoline can eventually be withdrawn from the drug. I found it hard to tease out what we want to know (or at least what I wanted to know) from this article and so I have rewritten the pertinent results here.

For patients with microadenomas (*n* = 105), 32 (30%) had recurrence of hyperprolactinemia after drug withdrawal, but none had MRI evidence of recurrent tumor. Of these, 17 of 42 (40%) had recurrence if residual tumor was visible on MRI and 15 of 63 (24%) had recurrence if no tumor was visible on MRI. For patients with macroadenomas (n = 70), 25 (36%) had recurrence of hyperprolactinemia after drug withdrawal, but none had MRI evidence of tumor growth. Of these, 14 of 24 (58%) had recurrence if residual tumor was visible on MRI, but only 12 of 46 (26%) had recurrence if no tumor was visible on MRI.

Why was there no tumor regrowth in those with persistent tumor on MRI? I don't know, but it may take a while for the tumor to grow or what is present has fibrosed down and cannot grow. My own practice is to withdraw patients by tapering them down to the lowest dose at which PRL levels do not rise. I have been hesitant to take people off entirely if there is tumor still visible on MRI, but I guess if it is not a particularly big remnant (How big is big?), it may be worth a trial off cabergoline, with careful observation such as was done here.

I also do not take people off if their PRL level remains slightly elevated and not normal, thinking that there is still persistent tumor activity. Certainly, in those with normal PRL levels on 0.5 mg once a week and no visible tumor on MRI, taking them off is relatively simple to do and in them I just follow PRL levels and do not repeat MRI scans.

Last year, I cited an article that showed the benefits of medical therapy for giant prolactinomas in contrast to what can be achieved by surgery in such patients.[1] In another 10 patients with giant prolactinomas, Corsello et al reported that significant tumor shrinkage was achieved in 9, with greater than 95% volume reduction in 3, greater than 50% reduction in 4, and 25% reduction in 2 by 12 months.[2] An improvement in visual field defects was shown in 6 of the 7 with visual impairment. Only 3 of their patients were followed past 1 year and these 3 had no further changes, but I have seen continued tumor size reduction occurring past 1 year, so we should keep going in these patients. No need for surgery and, in fact, surgery may be dangerous.

Why is there such a high recurrence rate for prolactinoma patients after what appears to be surgical cure compared to those with acromegaly or Cushing's disease? Amar et al[3] reported a recurrence rate of hyperprolactinemia in 18% of patients with normal (less than 20 µg/L) PRL levels 1 day postoperatively. However, when they subdivided their patients into those below and above 10 µg/L, they found that the 5-year recurrence rate was only 2% (2/132) of those with PRL levels less than 10 µg/L, but the rate was 84% (27/32) of those with PRL levels between 10 and 20 µg/L.

I think this just shows us that we have not had good criteria for cure. We require a normal IGF-I and suppressibility of GH by glucose in acromegaly and the development of actual ACTH/cortisol deficiency for Cushing's disease but have simply accepted a "normal" PRL for patients with prolactinomas without knowing what their premorbid PRL levels were. The actual reason for the authors publishing their article was different but was also important and that was to show that a PRL done on postoperative day 1 had poor predictive value for what the PRL was, even at 6 weeks, with 1 of their 133 patients with PRL levels less than 10 µg/L having a PRL more than 20 µg/L by 6 weeks and 14 of 46 patients with PRL levels between 10 and 20 µg/L having PRL values greater than 20 µg/L by 6 weeks. Another interesting finding from this article is that all of the recurrences occurred in patients with macroadenomas and none in those with microadenomas.

M. E. Molitch, MD

References

1. Shrivastava RK, Anginteanu MS, King WA, et al: Giant prolactinomas: Clinical management and long-term follow up. *J Neurosurg* 97:299-306, 2002. (2003 YEAR BOOK OF ENDOCRINOLOGY, p 359.)
2. Corsello SM, Ubertini G, Altomare M, et al: Giant prolactinomas in men: Efficacy of cabergoline treatment. *Clin Endocrinol* 58:662-670, 2003.
3. Amar AP, Couldwell WT, Chen JCT, et al: Predictive value of serum prolactin levels measured immediately after transsphenoidal surgery. *J Neurosurg* 97:307-314, 2002.

Diagnostic Reliability of a Single IGF-I Measurement in 237 Adults With Total Anterior Hypopituitarism and Severe GH Deficiency
Aimaretti G, Corneli G, Baldelli R, et al (Univ of Turin, Italy; Endocrinology Istituto Regina Elena IRCCS; La Sapienza Univ of Rome)
Clin Endocrinol (Oxf) 59:56-61, 2003   71–2

Background.—Within the appropriate clinical context, it is desirable to diagnose GH deficiency (GHD) in adults by a single test, usually either insulin-induced hypoglycemia or GH-releasing hormone (GHRH) plus arginine (ARG), although neither is considered completely reliable. The diagnostic sensitivity of a single IGF-I measurement in hypopituitary patients when compared to age-related persons with normative values was evaluated.

Study Design.—The study group consisted of 237 well-nourished adult patients, aged 20 to 80 years, with total anterior pituitary deficiency. Of these 237 patients, 225 had only the GHRH plus ARG test, 57 had the insulin-induced hypoglycemia test only, and 54 had both tests. IGF-I levels were compared to age-related normative values.

Findings.—Both average and individual IGF-I levels were significantly lower in patients with GHD than in age-matched healthy patients for each decade of life, except for those 70 to 80 years of age.

Conclusion.—Very low total IGF-I levels can be considered diagnostic of severe GHD in hypopituitary patients, who can thereby avoid provocative testing of GH secretion.

▶ Now we are getting somewhere. These were all patients who were panhypopituitary and had GH peaks less than the first percentile (3 μg for the insulin tolerance test and 9 μg by GHRH plus ARG). Of course, according to Hartman et al, they probably didn't even have to do a stimulation test with 3 or more pituitary hormone axes being deficient.[1] In any case, IGF-I levels were below the 10th percentile in 89.4% of patients up to 40 years of age and 53.0% of older patients, and below the 25th percentile in 97.6% of patients up to 40 years of age and 77.8% of the remaining patients.

My guess—I don't really remember anyone else ever saying this—is that the reason why the IGF-I level is less good an indicator of GHD is the very wide range seen in normal, especially as we get older. The lower limit of normal in "normal" older individuals actually is quite low, generally due to decreased GH levels themselves. When you look at this figure, those third percentile figures are very low. Based on this article, it would seem that a level of below the 25th percentile for age would qualify as being petty low. We still don't have a set of objective improvements with GH that we could use to define what cutoffs to use to indicate those who would respond best to therapy.

A little more on these 2 tests. Darzy et al compared the insulin-induced hypoglycemia test with the GHRH plus ARG stimulation test in patients who had undergone irradiation for nonpituitary brain tumors or leukemia.[2] They found that there was always a greater GH response to GHRH plus ARG than to insulin-induced hypoglycemia but that this increment was greatest within the first 5 years following irradiation, suggesting hypothalamic damage with a subsequent somatotroph atrophy due to either prolonged GHRH deficiency or delayed direct damage to the pituitary. They also opined that this makes the GHRH plus ARG test an unreliable test in the early years following irradiation in diagnosing GH deficiency, if the goal is to treat diagnosed GH deficiency.

M. E. Molitch, MD

References

1. Hartman ML, for the HypoCCS Advisory Board and the US HypoCCS Study Group: Which patients do not require a GH stimulation test for the diagnosis of adult GH deficiency? *J Clin Endocrinol Metab* 87:477-485, 2002. (2003 Year Book of Endocrinology, p 336.)
2. Darzy KH, Aimeretti G, Wieringa G, et al: The usefulness of the combined growth hormone (GH)–releasing hormone and arginine stimulation test in the diagnosis of radiation-induced GH deficiency is dependent on the post-irradiation time interval. *J Clin Endocrinol Metab* 88:95-102, 2003.

Men With Acquired Hypogonadotropic Hypogonadism Treated With Testosterone May be Fertile

Drincic A, Arseven OK, Sosa E, et al (Northwestern Univ, Chicago; Hospital de Especialidades, Centro Medico Nacional, Mexico City)
Pituitary 6:5-10, 2003   71–3

Background.—It has generally been assumed that men with acquired hypogonadotropic hypogonadism treated with testosterone are infertile. Spermatogenesis can be restored or initiated by treatment with pulsatile GnRH when the pituitary is intact, or with FSH in the form of human menopausal gonadotropin or recombinant FSH, and with LH, in the form of human chorionic gonadotropin (hCG). Once restored, spermatogenesis can usually be maintained by hCG treatment alone. In men with previously normal sperm production before the development of hypogonadotropic hypogonadism, spermatogenesis can usually be reinitiated with hCG treatment alone. Exogenous testosterone supplementation can be used to correct androgen deficiency when fertility is not desired. The finding of 2 patients with unexpected fertility and normal sperm counts after treatment with testosterone for acquired hypogonadotropic hypogonadism prompted an evaluation of spermatogenesis in additional men with this condition.

Methods.—A search of case records identified one similar case of unexpected fertility and normal sperm counts after testosterone therapy for acquired hypogonadotropic hypogonadism. Twelve consecutive patients with acquired hypogonadotropic hypogonadism were then evaluated for gonadal function and spermatogenesis while receiving testosterone. In 5 patients with proved spermatogenesis, exon 10 of the FSH receptor was sequenced to search for activating mutations.

Results.—The original 3 patients and 4 of the subsequent 12 patients had sperm concentrations of 15 million/mL or more. Two additional men had concentrations of 1 million/mL, and 6 patients were azoospermic. Residual LH and FSH levels were slightly higher in men who had maintained spermatogenesis before testosterone replacement. In the 5 cases studied for activating mutations, no such mutations were found in exon 10 of the FSH receptor.

Conclusions.—Sterility should not be assumed in men with acquired hypogonadotropic hypogonadism who are treated with testosterone. Semen analysis should be performed in such men as a routine procedure so that appropriate counseling can be provided regarding the potential for fertility.

▶ These findings really were a surprise. These were men who were panhypopituitary for a variety of reasons—usually surgery for pituitary adenomas—who were being treated generally with full hormone replacement, including exogenous testosterone. When the first 2 of these patients reported that their partners were pregnant, I kind of wondered what was going on at home, but then we did sperm counts, and they were positive! This prompted us to look at additional men, and 7 of 15 overall had sperm counts of at least 15 million. Why should patients who are clearly panhypopituitary be fertile? We postulated that perhaps only a minimal amount of FSH plus testosterone is needed to maintain spermatogenesis.

Men have been reported with FSHβ gene mutations who are azoospermic,[1,2] and with FSH receptor mutations who have sperm counts ranging from 0 to low normal.[3] Layman et al[4] have recently reported a woman and her brother with FSHβ gene mutations who had no FSH levels, but they had some evidence of puberty, the woman having Tanner stage II-III breast development with low estradiol levels but primary amenorrhea, and her brother having small testes but normal testosterone levels, erections, and ejaculation. He was azoospermic, and a testicular biopsy revealed sparse, small seminiferous tubules with germinal cell aplasia. Thus, complete absence of FSH from birth prevents initial spermatogenesis.

Haywood et al[5] created an interesting mouse model in which mice with a germline mutation in the GnRH gene are functionally deficient in LH and FSH but then have an FSH transgene inserted. By dissecting out the different roles of testosterone and FSH in this model, they determined that FSH has the dominant role in Sertoli cell development, although androgens could also independently stimulate Sertoli cell maturation and proliferation. FSH has a predominant effect on early mitotic germ cell (spermatogonia) proliferation, and FSH combines synergistically with androgens to have a marked effect on both meiotic and postmeiotic germ cell maturation. The fact that androgens could independently stimulate Sertoli cell maturation and proliferation may explain the results seen in our patients.

M. E. Molitch, MD

References

1. Phillip M, Arbelle JE, Segev Y, et al: Male hypogonadism due to a mutation in the gene for the β subunit of follicle-stimulating hormone. *N Engl J Med* 338:1729-1732, 1998.
2. Linstedt G, Nystrom E, Matthews C, et al: Follitropin (FSH) deficiency in an infertile male due to FSHβ gene mutation. A syndrome of normal puberty and virilization but underdeveloped testicles with azoospermia, low FSH but high lutropin and normal serum testosterone. *Clin Chem Lab Med* 36:663-665, 1998.
3. Tapanainen JS, Aittomaki K, Min J, et al: Men homozygous for an inactivating mutation of the FSH receptor gene present with variable suppression of spermatogenesis and fertility. *Nat Genet* 15:205-206, 1997.
4. Layman LC, Porto ALA, Xie J, et al: FSHβ gene mutations in a female with partial breast development and a male sibling with normal puberty and azoospermia. *J Clin Endocrinol Metab* 87:3702-3707, 2002.
5. Haywood M, Spaliviero J, Jimemez M, et al: Sertoli and germ cell development in hypogonadal (*hpg*) mice expressing transgenic follicle-stimulating hormone alone or in combination with testosterone. *Endocrinology* 144:509-517, 2003.

Subject Index

A

Abdominal
pain in adult celiac disease, 493
Absenteeism
infection-related, effects of multivitamin
and mineral supplement on, 163
ABVD
vs. MOPP/ABVD hybrid for advanced
Hodgkin's disease, 211
ACE (*see* Angiotensin, -converting
enzyme)
Acetaminophen
-induced acute liver failure, infection
and progression of hepatic
encephalopathy in, 525
ACTH
deficiency, safety of short synacthen
tests in assessing, 593
-secreting bronchial carcinoids, occult,
management of, 596
Activity
physical (*see* Physical, activity)
Acupuncture
vs. massage therapy and spinal
manipulation for low back pain, 55
Adenocarcinoma
esophagus or gastric cardia, in GERD
patients, endoscopy and mortality
from, 474
Adenoma
colorectal, and aspirin, 197
Adenosine
deaminase 1 activity, enzymatic,
increase in rheumatoid synovial
fibroblasts, 15
Adiposity
aminotransferase levels and, elevated,
517
Adolescents
constitutional delay in growth and
adolescence treated with IM
testosterone for 3 months, final
height outcome and value of height
prediction in boys with, 602
obesity in
risk of type 2 diabetes and
cardiovascular disease and, 599
severe, and health-related quality of
life, 601
Adrenal
disorders, 593
Adrenocorticotropin
deficiency, safety of short synacthen
tests in assessing, 593

-secreting bronchial carcinoids, occult,
management of, 596
African American(s)
hepatitis C and diabetes in, 524
HIV patients receiving dialysis, clinical
characteristics and antiretroviral
patterns of, 299
vs. caucasians, bone turnover and intact
PTH levels in patients with
end-stage renal disease in, 314
Aging
humans, determinants of glomerular
hypofiltration in, 230
Airway
hyperresponsiveness, methacholine,
body mass index associated with
development of, 334
pressure, continuous positive (*see* CPAP)
Albumin
synthesis rate increase in chronic renal
failure, 271
Alcohol
consumption and C-reactive protein
levels, 386
Aldosterone
-to-renin ratio increase in hypertensives,
prediction by CYP11B2
polymorphisms, 275
Alendronate
oral, bone mineral density in
postmenopausal women with
primary hyperparathyroidism
increased by, 565
/parathyroid hormone in osteoporosis
male, 47
postmenopausal, 45
Allograft
nephropathy, chronic, natural history
of, 294
Alteplase
/heparin in submassive pulmonary
embolism, 346
Amantadine
for influenza in older adults,
cost-effectiveness of, 139
Aminotransferase
levels, elevated, prevalence and etiology
of, 516
Amiodarone
-induced thyrotoxicosis, type II,
iopanoic acid or glucocorticoids
for, 585
ANCA
-associated vasculitis (*see* Vasculitis,
ANCA-associated)

O

Author Index

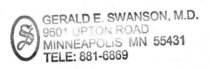

The year's best literature in one convenient volume!

YES! Please start my subscription to the *Year Book(s)* checked below with the current volume according to the terms described below.* I understand that I will have 30 days to examine each annual edition.

Please Print:

Name _____

Address _____

City _____ State _____ ZIP _____

Method of Payment

❏ Check (payable to **Elsevier**; add the applicable sales tax for your area)

❏ VISA ❏ MasterCard ❏ AmEx ❏ Bill me

Card number _____ Exp. date _____

Signature _____

❏ **Year Book of Allergy, Asthma and Clinical Immunology (YALI)**
$103.00 (Avail. November)

❏ **Year Book of Anesthesiology and Pain Management (YANE)**
$109.00 (Avail. August)

❏ **Year Book of Cardiology® (YCAR)**
$109.00 (Avail. August)

❏ **Year Book of Critical Care Medicine® (YCCM)**
$107.00 (Avail. June)

❏ **Year Book of Dentistry® (YDEN)**
$101.00 (Avail. August)

❏ **Year Book of Dermatology and Dermatologic Surgery™ (YDER)**
$111.00 (Avail. October)

❏ **Year Book of Diagnostic Radiology® (YRAD)**
$111.00 (Avail. November)

❏ **Year Book of Emergency Medicine® (YEMD)**
$111.00 (Avail. May)

❏ **Year Book of Endocrinology® (YEND)**
$108.00 (Avail. July)

❏ **Year Book of Family Practice™ (YFAM)**
$95.00 (Avail. June)

❏ **Year Book of Gastroenterology™ (YGAS)**
$104.00 (Avail. December)

❏ **Year Book of Hand Surgery® (YHND)**
$112.00 (Avail. April)

❏ **Year Book of Medicine® (YMED)**
$103.00 (Avail. July)

❏ **Year Book of Neonatal and Perinatal Medicine® (YNPM)**
$112.00 (Avail. September)

❏ **Year Book of Neurology and Neurosurgery® (YNEU)**
$107.00 (Avail. January)

❏ **Year Book of Nuclear Medicine® (YNUM)**
$106.00 (Avail. June)

❏ **Year Book of Obstetrics, Gynecology, and Women's Health® (YOBG)**
$111.00 (Avail. February)

❏ **Year Book of Oncology® (YONC)**
$112.00 (Avail. November)

❏ **Year Book of Ophthalmology® (YOPH)**
$112.00 (Avail. September)

❏ **Year Book of Orthopedics® (YORT)**
$112.00 (Avail. October)

❏ **Year Book of Otolaryngology— Head and Neck Surgery® (YOTO)**
$103.00 (Avail. July)

❏ **Year Book of Pathology and Laboratory Medicine® (YPAT)**
$112.00 (Avail. March)

❏ **Year Book of Pediatrics® (YPED)**
$98.00 (Avail. January)

❏ **Year Book of Plastic and Aesthetic Surgery® (YPRS)**
$111.00 (Avail. March)

❏ **Year Book of Psychiatry and Applied Mental Health® (YPSY)**
$101.00 (Avail. March)

❏ **Year Book of Pulmonary Disease® (YPDI)**
$105.00 (Avail. April)

❏ **Year Book of Rheumatology, Arthritis, and Musculoskeletal Disease™ (YRHE)**
$112.00 (Avail. January)

❏ **Year Book of Sports Medicine® (YSPM)**
$106.00 (Avail. December)

❏ **Year Book of Surgery® (YSUR)**
$105.00 (Avail. September)

❏ **Year Book of Urology® (YURO)**
$112.00 (Avail. November)

❏ **Year Book of Vascular Surgery® (YVAS)**
$112.00 (Avail. April)

© Elsevier 2004. *Offer valid in U.S. only. Prices subject to change without notice.* MO 10614 DE 6572

Order your Year Book today! Simply complete and detach this card and drop it in the mail to receive the latest information in your field.

Your Year Book service guarantee:

When you subscribe to a *Year Book*, you will receive notice of future annual volumes about two months before publication. To receive the new edition, do nothing—we'll send you the new volume as soon as it is available. (Applicable sales tax is added to each shipment.) If you want to discontinue, the advance notice allows you time to notify us of your decision. If you are not completely satisfied, you have 30 days to return any *Year Book*.

VISIT OUR HOME PAGE!
www.us.elsevierhealth.com/periodicals

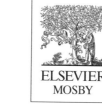

ELSEVIER
MOSBY